ADOLESCENT MEDICINE: STATE OF THE ART REVIEWS

Handbook of Adolescent Medicine
2nd Edition

GUEST EDITORS

Alain Joffe, MD, MPH
Margaret J. Blythe, MD

August 2009 • Volume 20 • Number 2

THE AMERICAN ACADEMY OF PEDIATRICS ®

ADOLESCENT MEDICINE CLINICS: STATE OF THE ART REVIEWS
August 2009
Editor: Diane E. Lundquist
Marketing Manager: Marirose Russo
Production Manager: Shannan Martin
Editorial Assistant: Carrie Peters

Volume 20, Number 2
ISBN 978-1-58110-334-2
ISSN 1934-4287
MA0479
SUB1006

Adolescent Medicine: State of the Art Reviews is published three times per year by the American Academy of Pediatrics, 141 Northwest Point Blvd, Elk Grove Village, IL 60007-1098. Periodicals postage paid at Arlington Heights, IL.

POSTMASTER: Send address changes to American Academy of Pediatrics, Department of Marketing and Publications, Attn: AM:STARs, 141 Northwest Point Blvd, Elk Grove Village, IL 60007-1098.

Subscriptions: Subscriptions to *Adolescent Medicine: State of the Art Reviews* (AM:STARs) are provided to members of the American Academy of Pediatrics Section on Adolescent Health as part of annual section membership dues. All others, please contact the AAP Customer Service Center at 866/843-2271 (7:00 am–5:30 pm Central Time, Monday–Friday) for pricing and information.

Adolescent Medicine: State of the Art Reviews

Official Journal of the American Academy of Pediatrics Section on Adolescent Health

EDITORS-IN-CHIEF

VICTOR C. STRASBURGER, MD, FAAP, Professor of Pediatrics, Division of Adolescent Medicine, University of New Mexico, School of Medicine, Albuquerque, New Mexico

DONALD E. GREYDANUS, MD, FAAP, Professor of Pediatrics, Michigan State University; and Pediatrics Program Director, Kalamazoo Center for Medical Studies, Kalamazoo, Michigan

GUEST EDITORS

ALAIN JOFFE, MD, MPH, FAAP, Director, Student Health and Wellness Center, Johns Hopkins University, Baltimore, Maryland

MARGARET J. BLYTHE, MD, FAAP, FSAM, Professor of Pediatrics and Adjunct Professor of Gynecology, Indiana University School of Medicine, Indianapolis, Indiana

HANDBOOK OF ADOLESCENT MEDICINE, 2ND EDITION

CONTENTS

Preface	**xiii**
1. Adolescent Health Statistics	**261**
2. Biological and Psychosocial Growth and Development	**350**
3. The Adolescent Office Visit	**386**
4. Endocrine/Metabolic	**416**
5. Gynecology	**457**
6. Contraception	**484**
7. Infectious Diseases	**566**
8. Cardiorespiratory	**637**
9. Genitourinary	**664**
10. Dermatology	**677**
11. Musculoskeletal and Sports Medicine	**695**
12. Mental Health, Psychotropic Medications, and Substance Abuse	**728**
13. Nutrition	**788**
14. Rheumatology and Miscellaneous Clinical Conditions	**794**
Adolescent Drug Formulary	**823**
Index	**857**

Preface
Handbook of Adolescent Medicine, 2nd Edition

This issue of *Adolescent Medicine: State of the Art Reviews* (AM:STARs) is a departure from what you are used to seeing in your mailbox. With the amount of information available to physicians growing exponentially and the pressure to see more patients each day also increasing, we have tried to develop this issue as a useful point-of-care tool for practicing physicians with a particular interest in adolescent medicine.

In assembling key reference materials that pertain specifically to adolescents, we tried to focus on problems clinicians who care for many teenagers are most likely to encounter on any given day. It includes material gathered from a variety of sources including past issues of AM:STARs, textbooks, classic review articles, insights of colleagues, and information from the Internet. In each instance, the material provided is succinct, usable, and, most importantly, timely.

We also tried to include evidence-based material that might not yet be easily available or identified, even in the library or from an Internet search. Because many of us are teachers as well as clinicians—whether that is with adolescents, their parents, community groups interested in adolescent health, medical students, or residents—we included information to support those efforts as well. Some of the teaching materials are intended to be photocopied and distributed to patients and their parents.

Because of the page limits of the AM:STARs format, we focused on including only the timeliest information to serve as an adjunct to traditional textbooks and reference materials. Our selections are highly personal, and we have chosen what we believe will be the most useful to you in your practice.

We would like to thank Diane Lundquist and Carrie Peters at the American Academy of Pediatrics for their efforts to bring this issue to fruition. Because much of the material was not submitted in Microsoft Word document form, they spent countless hours downloading materials, creating PDFs and resetting our materials.

Alain Joffe, MD, MPH
Margaret J. Blythe, MD
Guest Editors

 ISSN 1934-4287

Adolesc Med 20 (2009) 261–349

1. Adolescent Health Statistics

Alain Joffe, MD, MPH
E-mail address: ajoffe@jhu.edu.

 ISSN 1934-4287

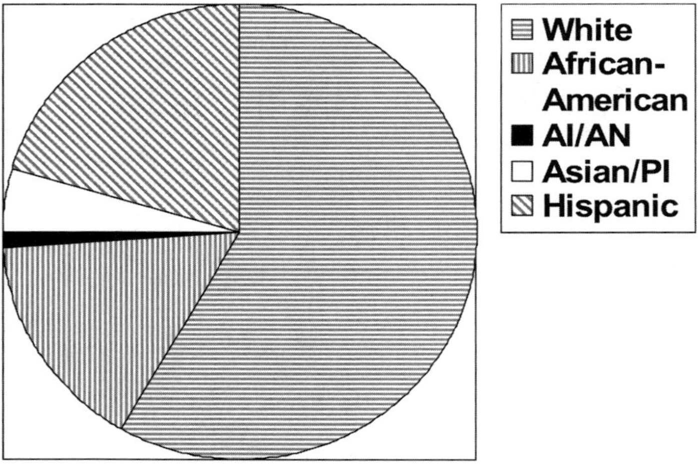

Fig 1.1. Projected racial/ethnic composition of US population aged 10 to 24 years, 2010. AI/AN indicates American Indian/Alaska Native; PI, Pacific Islander. Data source: US Census Bureau. National population projections: released 2008 (based on Census 2000) [release date: August 14, 2008]. Available at: www.census.gov/population/www/projections/summarytables.html. Accessed April 11, 2009.

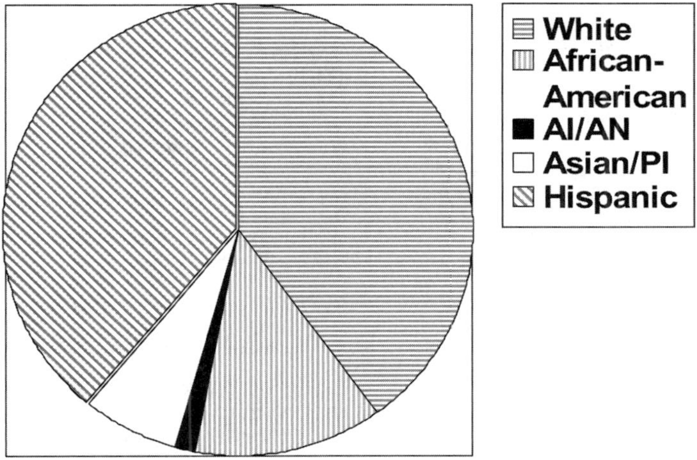

Fig 1.2. Projected racial/ethnic composition of US population aged 10 to 24 years, by 2050. AI/AN indicates American Indian/Alaska Native; PI, Pacific Islander. Data source: US Census Bureau. National population projections: released 2008 (based on Census 2000) [release date: August 14, 2008]. Available at: www.census.gov/population/www/projections/summarytables.html. Accessed April 11, 2009.

Table 1.1
Projections of the US population according to selected age groups and gender for the United States: 2010–2050

Age/Gender	2010	2020	2030	2040	2050
Total US population, *N*	310 233[a]	341 387	373 504	405 655	439 010
Both genders					
10–14, *n* (%)	20 395 (6.6)[b]	22 571	24 567 (6.6)	26 105	28 274 (6.4)
15–19	21 770 (7.0)	22 554	24 723 (6.6)	26 051	28 422 (6.5)
20–24	21 779 (7.0)	21 799	24 191 (6.5)	26 408	28 171 (6.4)
Males, *n* (%)					
10–14	10 421 (3.4)	11 514	12 527 (3.4)	13 304	14 403 (3.3)
15–19	11 159 (3.6)	11 513	12 612 (3.4)	13 506	14 472 (3.3)
20–24	11 100 (3.6)	11 072	12 266 (3.3)	13 379	14 259 (3.2)
Females, *n* (%)					
10–14	9975 (3.2)	11 057	12 040 (3.2)	12 802	13 872 (3.2)
15–19	10 611 (3.4)	11 041	12 112 (3.2)	12 995	13 950 (3.2)
20–24	10 680 (3.4)	10 728	11 926 (3.2)	13 029	13 913 (3.2)

[a] Numbers are in thousands.

[b] Percent of total US population for the specified age and gender group; percentages are rounded to the nearest tenth percent.

Data source: US Census Bureau. National population projections: released 2008 (based on Census 2000) [release date: August 14, 2008]. Available at: www.census.gov/population/www/projections/summarytables.html. Accessed April 5, 2009.

Table 1.2
Projections of population according to age and race/ethnicity for the United States: 2010–2050

Race/Ethnicity	2010, *n* (%)	2020, *n* (%)	2030, *n* (%)	2040, *n* (%)	2050, *n* (%)
Total US population	310 323[a]	341 387	373 504	405 655	439 010
10–14 y					
Non-Hispanic white	11 440 (3.7)[b]	11 564 (3.4)	11 640 (3.1)	11 039 (2.7)	10 862 (2.5)
Black	3021 (<0.01)	3163 (<0.01)	3403 (<0.01)	3452 (<0.01)	3621 (<0.01)
AI/AN	244 (<0.001)	301 (<0.001)	342 (<0.001)	358 (<0.001)	404 (<0.001)
Asian/PI	894 (0.003)	1131 (0.003)	1276 (0.003)	1519 (0.004)	1786 (0.004)
Hispanic	4513 (1.5)	6036 (1.8)	7436 (2.0)	9182 (2.3)	10 926 (2.5)
15–19 y					
Non-Hispanic white	12 472 (4.0)	11 632 (3.4)	11 794 (3.2)	11 479 (2.8)	11 014 (2.5)
Black	3410 (0.01)	3166 (<0.01)	3439 (<0.01)	3549 (<0.01)	3658 (<0.01)
AI/AN	268 (<0.001)	279 (<0.001)	337 (<0.001)	360 (<0.001)	390 (<0.001)
Asian/PI	932 (<0.01)	1182 (<0.001)	1368 (<0.001)	1580 (<0.001)	1873 (<0.001)
Hispanic	4473 (1.4)	5983 (1.8)	7382 (2.0)	9047 (2.2)	10 901 (2.5)
20–24 y					
Non-Hispanic white	13 049 (4.2)	11 561 (3.4)	11 714 (3.1)	11 818 (2.9)	11 247 (2.6)
Black	3330 (0.01)	3142 (<0.01)	3314 (<0.01)	3585 (<0.01)	3664 (<0.01)
AI/AN	275 (<0.001)	256 (<0.001)	315 (<0.001)	357 (<0.001)	376 (<0.001)
Asian/PI	938 (<0.01)	1147 (<0.01)	1419 (<0.01)	1604 (<0.01)	1889 (<0.01)
Hispanic	4010 (1.3)	5441 (1.6)	7089 (1.9)	8164 (2.0)	10 483 (2.4)

AI/AN indicates American Indian/Alaska Native; PI, Pacific Islander.

[a] Numbers in thousands.

[b] Percentage of total population accounted for by the indicated age and racial/ethnic group. For example, in 2050, 10- to 14-year-old Hispanics will account for 2.5% of the total US population.

Data source: US Census Bureau. National population projections: released 2008 (based on Census 2000) [release date: August 14, 2008]. Available at: www.census.gov/population/www/projections/summarytables.html. Accessed April 5, 2009.

Table 1.3
Healthy People 2010 national health objectives and leading health indicators pertinent to adolescents and young adults

Objective	Baseline Data (Year)	2000	Most Recent Data (Year)	2010 Goal
Overall mortality				
16-03: Reduce adolescent and young adult deaths				
10–14 y (16-03a)	21.5 (1998)[a,b]	20.3	18.1 (2005)	16.5[c]
15–19 y (16-03b)	69.5 (1998)[b]	67.1	65.1 (2005)	38.0[c]
20–24 y (16-03c)	92.7 (1998)[b]	93.6	97.6 (2004)	41.5[c]
15-15a: Unintentional injuries				
Reduce deaths from motor vehicle crashes (per 100 000 population), ages 15–24 y	25.6 (1999)[b]	26.3	25.3 (2005)	NA
26-01a: Alcohol-related motor vehicle crash deaths (per 100 000 population), ages 15–24 y	11.8[b]	—	12.2 (2000)	NA
26-06: Adolescents riding with a driver who has been drinking alcohol, grades 9–12	33% (1999)	—	29.1% (2007 YRBS)	30%
15-19: Seat belt use, 9th–12th grade	84% (1999)	—	88.9% (2007 YRBS)	92%
15-32: Homicides per 100 000 population				
Ages 10–14 y (not age-adjusted)	1.2 (1999)[b]	1.1	1.1 (2005)	NA
Ages 15–19 y (not age-adjusted)	10.4 (1999)[b]	9.5	9.9 (2005)	NA
18-01: Suicides per 100 000 standard population				
Ages 10–14 y (not age-adjusted)	1.2 (1999)[b]	1.5	1.3 (2005)	NA
Ages 15–19 y (not age-adjusted)	8.0 (1999)[b]	8.0	7.7 (2005)	NA
Ages 20–24 y (not age-adjusted)	12.3 (1999)[b]	12.5	12.4 (2005)	
18-02: Suicide attempts requiring medical attention, grades 9–12	2.6% (1999)	—	2.0% (2007 YRBS)	1.0%
15-38: Physical fighting among adolescents, grades 9–12	36% (1999)	—	35.5% (2007 YRBS)	32%
15-39: Weapon carrying by adolescents on school property, grades 9–12	6.9% (1999)	—	5.9% (2007 YRBS)	4.9%
19: Nutrition and overweight				
19-03b: Overweight or obesity in children and adolescents, 12–19 y	11% (1988–1994)	—	18% (2003–2006)	5%

(*Continued*)

Table 1.3
(Continued)

Objective	Baseline Data (Year)	2000	Most Recent Data (Year)	2010 Goal
22: Physical activity and fitness				
22-06: Moderate physical activity, grades 9–12	27% (1999)	—	27% (2005)	35%
22-07: Vigorous physical activity, grades 9–12	65% (1999)	—	64% (2007 YRBS)	85%
Males	72% (1999)	—	72% (2005)	
Females	57% (1999)	—	56% (2005)	
22-09: Participation in daily physical education in schools, grades 9–12	29% (1999)	—	30% (2007)	50%
15: Sexually transmitted diseases				
Reduce the proportion of adolescents and young adults (15–24 y) with *Chlamydia trachomatis* infection				
25-01a: Females in family planning clinics	5% (1997)	5.9%	7.1% (2006)	3%
25-01b: Females in STD clinics	12.2% (1997)	13.5%	14.8% (2006)	3%
25-10c: Males in STD clinics	15.7% (1997)	16.4%	20.8% (2006)	3%
25-01 d: Females in National Job Training Program, ≤24 y	10.1% (2002)	—	13.3% (2006)	6.8%
25: Responsible sexual behavior				
25-11: Never had sex or, if sexually active, use condoms	—	—	86.7% (2007 YRBS)	95%
25-11a: Never had sexual intercourse, grades 9–12	50% (1999)	—	52% (2007)	56%
25-11b: Had sex but not in last 3 mo, grades 9–12	27% (1999)	—	27% (2007)	30%
25-11c: Used condom at last sex, grades 9–12	58% (1999)	—	62% (2007)	65%
09: Family planning				
09-07: Adolescent pregnancy, aged 15–17 y (per 1000 population)	63 (1996)[b]	51	—	39[c]
26: Substance abuse				
26-10a: Adolescents not using alcohol or illicit drugs in past 30 d, 12–17 y	78% (2002)[b]	—	80% (2007)	91%[c]
26-10b: Adolescents using marijuana in past 30 d, 12–17 y	8.2% (2002)[b]	—	6.7% (2006)	0.7%

(Continued)

Table 1.3
(Continued)

Objective	Baseline Data (Year)	2000	Most Recent Data (Year)	2010 Goal
Binge drinking in the past 2 wk				
26-11a: High school seniors	32% (1998)	30%	25% (20006)	11%
26-11b: College students	39% (1998)	39%	40% (2006)	20%
26-11 d: 12- to 17-y-olds	10.7% (2002)[b]	—	10.3% (2006)	3.1%[c]
27: Tobacco use				
Adolescents (grades 9–12) past month use of				
27-02a: Tobacco products	40% (1999)	—	25.7% (2007 YRBS)	21%
27-02b: Cigarettes	35% (1999)	—	20% (2007 YRBS)	16%
27-02c: Spit tobacco	8% (1999)	—	7.9% (2007 YRBS)	1%
27-02d: Cigars	18% (1999)	—	13.6% (2007 YRBS)	8%
27-02e: Bidis	4% (2000)	—	3% (2006)	2%

NA indicates not applicable; YRBS, Youth Risk Behavior Surveillance System; STD, sexually transmitted disease; —, data not available.

[a] Age-adjusted per 100 000 population.

[b] Baseline revised.

[c] Target revised.

Data sources: Centers for Disease Control and Prevention. Wide-ranging Online Data for Epidemiologic Research (WONDER). Available at: http://wonder.cdc.gov/scripts/broker.exe. Accessed April 11, 2009; and Eaton DK, Kann L, Kinchen S, et al; Centers for Disease Control and Prevention. Youth Risk Behavior Surveillance: United States, 2007. *MMWR CDC Surveill Summ.* 2008;57(4):1–131. Available at: www.cdc.gov/mmwr/PDF/ss/ss5704.pdf. Accessed April 11, 2009.

Table 1.4
Other health indicators for adolescents (aged 12–17 years)

Indicator	
How would you describe your child's health?	82.8%, excellent/very good; 12.7%, good; 4.4%, fair/poor
No. of school days missed in past 12 mo due to illness or injury?	24.4%, no days; 56.8%, 1–5 d; 12.0%, 6–10 d; 6.7%, ≥11 d
Parent-rated severity of child's health condition	71.0%, no reported condition; 14.8%, minor/do not affect child; 14.2%, moderate or severe
How many children currently have ≥1 chronic health condition (from a list of 16 conditions)?	70.8%, no current conditions; 17.0%, 1 current chronic health condition (from list of 16); 12.2%, ≥2
How many children currently have ADD or ADHD?	88.0%, do not have; 3.2%, had ADD/ADHD but not now; 8.8%, currently have ADD/ADHD
How many children currently have anxiety problems?	93.4%, do not have; 2.5%, had anxiety but not now; 4.1%, currently have anxiety
How many children currently have asthma?	83.9%, do not have; 5.9%, had asthma but not now; 10.2%, currently have asthma
How many children currently have behavioral or conduct problems?	94.4%, do not have; 1.2%, had but not now; 4.2%, currently have behavioral or conduct problems
How many children currently have depression?	93.0%, do not have depression; 3.5%, had depression but not now; 3.5%, currently have depression
How many children currently have a learning disability?	86.4%, do not have a learning disability; 3.6%, had but do not have now; 10.0%, currently have a learning disability
How many children consistently exhibit problematic social behaviors?	90.7%, do not consistently exhibit problematic social behaviors; 9.3%, consistently exhibit problematic social behaviors
Percentage of children with ADD/ADHD taking medication	91.2%, do not currently have ADD/ADHD; 3.2%, currently have ADD/ADHD but not taking medication now; 5.2%, currently taking medication
Parent describes ADD/ADHD as mild, moderate, or severe?	91.3%, do not have ADD/ADHD; 4.5%, mild; 4.3%, ADD/ADHD is moderate or severe
How many children are taking medication for ADHD, emotions, concentration, or behavioral issues?	90.9%, not taking medication; 9.1%, taking medications for ADHD, emotions, concentration, or behavior
How many children exhibit ≥1 specific depressive behavior from a list of 3 (felt worthless/inferior; unhappy, sad, or depressed; withdrawn and does not get involved with others)?	93.8%, seldom or never exhibit behaviors; 4.5%, exhibit 1 behavior from list; 1.7%, exhibit 2 or 3 behaviors
Does child have health insurance coverage?	90.1%, insured at time of survey; 9.9%, uninsured
Consistent coverage during past 12 mo	85.2%, insured all year; 14.8%, currently uninsured or periods of no coverage
Type of health insurance at time of survey	24.1%, public insurance; 65.8%, private insurance; 10.0%, uninsured
How many children/youth had ≥1 preventive medical care visit during the past 12 mo?	84.2%, ≥1 preventive medical care visit; 15.8%, no preventive medical care visits;

(*Continued*)

Table 1.4
(Continued)

Indicator	
Of youth with current emotional, developmental, or behavioral problems requiring treatment or counseling, percentage receiving some type of mental health care in past year	66.3%, received needed mental health services; 33.7%,%, needed but did not get mental health services
During past 12 mo, was there any time when child needed health care but it was delayed or not received?	92.7%, no unmet needs; 7.3%, ≥1 unmet need
How many children/youth receive health care that meets AAP definition of medical home?	53.4%, have a medical home; 46.6%, do not have a medical home
Do you have ≥1 person you think of as your child's personal doctor or nurse?	90.9%, have a personal doctor or nurse; 9.1%, do not have a personal doctor or nurse
During the past month, how many children were engaged in school?	45.1%, always engaged; 30.3%, usually engaged; 24.6%, never, rarely, or sometimes engaged in school
How many children live in "working-poor" households?	90.4%, do not live in working-poor household; 9.6%, live in working-poor household;
During the past week, on how many days did all family members living in the household eat a meal together?	32.9%, every day; 36.4%, 4–6 d; 25.5%, 1–3 d; 5.2%, no days
During the past week, on how many nights did child get enough sleep for someone his or her age?	56.6%, every night; 31.7%, 4–6 nights; 11.7%, 0–3 nights
On average weekday, how much time does child usually watch television, watch videos, or play video games?	6.3%, none, do not watch television 41.9%, ≤1 h; 39.4%, 1–4 h; 12.5%, ≥4 h
How many children live in supportive neighborhoods?	85.3%, do; 14.7%, do not
How often do you feel your child is safe in your community or neighborhood?	86.6%, usually or always safe; 11.1%, sometimes safe; 2.3%, never safe
How often do you feel your child is safe at school?	86.4%, usually or always safe; 12.2%, sometimes safe; 1.4%, never safe

ADD indicates attention-deficit disorder; ADHD, attention-deficit/hyperactivity disorder; AAP, American Academy of Pediatrics.
Data source: National Survey of Children's Health, 2007. Available at: www.nschdata.org/Dataquery/SurveyAreas.aspx?yid=2. Accessed May 21, 2009.

Table 1.5

Percentage of high school students who rode in a car or other vehicle driven by someone who had been drinking alcohol[a] and who drove a car or other vehicle when they had been drinking alcohol,[a] according to gender: selected US sites, Youth Risk Behavior Survey, 2007

Category	Rode With a Driver Who Had Been Drinking Alcohol			Drove When Drinking Alcohol		
	Female	Male	Total	Female	Male	Total
State surveys, median (range), %[b]	27.7 (14.1–35.6)	26.7 (14.8–35.5)	27.4 (14.8–35.6)	8.6 (3.5–18.4)	12.3 (5.8–18.9)	10.4 (4.7–18.7)
Local surveys, median (range), %[c]	27.5 (18.4–40.2)	26.6 (17.6–36.5)	27.0 (18.0–38.4)	4.5 (1.7–11.1)	8.5 (3.4–14.8)	6.6 (2.8–12.9)

[a] One or more times during the 30 days before the survey.

[b] Data from 39 states.

[c] Data from 22 cities.

Data source: Eaton DK, Kann L, Kinchen S, et al; Centers for Disease Control and Prevention. Youth Risk Behavior Surveillance: United States, 2007. *MMWR CDC Surveill Summ.* 2008;57(4):1–131. Available at: www.cdc.gov/HealthyYouth/yrbs/pdf/yrbss07_mmwr.pdf. Accessed March 22, 2009.

Table 1.6

Percentage of high school students who experienced dating violence[a] and who were ever physically forced to have sexual intercourse,[b] according to gender, race/ethnicity, and grade: United States, Youth Risk Behavior Survey, 2007

Category	Dating Violence						Forced to Have Sexual Intercourse					
	Female		Male		Total		Female		Male		Total	
	%	95% CI	%	95% CI	%	95% CI	%	95% CI	%	95% CI	%	95% CI
Race/ethnicity												
White[c]	7.4	6.1–9.1	9.3	7.6–11.4	8.4	7.2–9.9	11.0	9.4–12.7	3.2	2.3–4.3	7.0	6.1–8.2
Black[c]	13.2	11.5–15.2	15.2	12.5–18.2	14.2	12.6–15.9	13.3	10.3–17.1	7.8	6.3–9.6	10.5	8.8–12.5
Hispanic	10.1	8.2–12.5	12.0	9.8–14.6	11.1	9.5–12.9	11.4	9.3–13.8	6.2	4.8–7.9	8.8	7.3–10.4
Grade												
9th	6.3	4.8–8.2	10.5	8.6–12.7	8.5	7.3–9.8	9.2	7.3–11.5	4.1	3.1–5.4	6.6	5.4–7.9
10th	8.8	6.6–11.5	9.1	7.5–10.9	8.9	7.4–10.7	13.1	10.6–16.0	3.4	2.5–4.7	8.2	6.6–10.0
11th	10.2	8.7–12.0	10.8	8.5–13.5	10.6	9.2–12.2	12.0	9.8–14.5	5.0	3.9–6.5	8.5	7.2–10.0
12th	10.1	8.3–12.2	14.1	11.8–16.7	12.1	10.6–13.8	10.9	9.2–12.8	5.7	4.3–7.5	8.3	7.3–9.5
Total	8.8	7.6–10.3	11.0	9.7–12.4	9.9	8.9–11.1	11.3	9.9–12.8	4.5	3.8–5.3	7.8	7.0–8.8

CI indicates confidence interval.

[a] Hit, slapped, or physically hurt on purpose by their boyfriend or girlfriend during the 12 months before the survey.

[b] When they did not want to.

[c] Non-Hispanic.

Data source: Centers for Disease Control and Prevention. Youth Risk Behavior Surveillance: United States, 2007. Surveillance Summaries. *MMWR CDC Surveill Summ.* 2008;57(SS-4):1–136. Available at: www.cdc.gov/mmwr/PDF/ss/ss5704.pdf. Accessed April 11, 2009.

Table 1.7
Percentage of high school students who felt sad or hopeless,[a,b] according to gender, race/ethnicity, and grade: United States, Youth Risk Behavior Survey, 2007

Category	Female		Male		Total	
	%	95% CI	%	95% CI	%	95% CI
Race/ethnicity						
White[c]	34.6	31.9–37.5	17.8	16.2–19.6	26.2	24.5–28.0
Black[c]	34.5	31.5–37.6	24.0	21.2–27.1	29.2	27.4–31.1
Hispanic	42.3	39.7–45.0	30.4	26.6–34.4	36.3	33.8–38.8
Grade						
9th	34.8	31.0–38.8	22.1	19.3–25.2	28.2	25.7–30.9
10th	37.7	34.2–41.5	20.3	18.3–22.5	28.9	26.9–31.1
11th	34.5	30.8–38.4	19.5	17.1–22.1	27.1	24.9–29.3
12th	35.9	32.8–39.1	22.6	19.7–25.9	29.4	27.1–31.8
Total	35.8	33.8–37.9	21.2	19.9–22.7	28.5	27.1–29.8

CI indicates confidence interval.

[a] Almost every day for ≥2 weeks in a row so that they stopped doing some usual activities.

[b] During the 12 months before the survey.

[c] Non-Hispanic.

Data source: Centers for Disease Control and Prevention. Youth Risk Behavior Surveillance: United States, 2007. Surveillance Summaries. *MMWR CDC Surveill Summ.* 2008;57(SS-4): 1–136. Available at: www.cdc.gov/mmwr/PDF/ss/ss5704.pdf. Accessed April 11, 2009.

Table 1.8

Percentage of high school students who seriously considered attempting suicide[a] and who made a plan about how they would attempt suicide,[a] according to gender, race/ethnicity, and grade: United States, Youth Risk Behavior Survey, 2007

Category	Seriously Considered Attempting Suicide						Made a Suicide Plan					
	Female		Male		Total		Female		Male		Total	
	%	95% CI	%	95% CI	%	95% CI	%	95% CI	%	95% CI	%	95% CI
Race/ethnicity												
White[b]	17.8	15.9–19.9	10.2	8.6–12.1	14.0	12.8–15.3	12.8	11.3–14.5	8.8	7.5–10.1	10.8	9.8–11.9
Black[b]	18.0	15.5–20.8	8.5	6.3–11.5	13.2	11.1–15.6	12.0	9.7–14.6	7.1	5.2–9.6	9.5	7.8–11.6
Hispanic	21.1	18.5–23.9	10.7	8.7–13.1	15.9	14.0–17.9	15.2	13.2–17.5	10.4	8.7–12.5	12.8	11.3–14.4
Grade												
9th	19.0	16.5–21.7	10.8	9.0–12.8	14.8	13.4–16.3	13.4	11.1–16.2	9.2	7.7–10.9	11.2	9.8–12.8
10th	22.0	19.4–24.9	9.3	7.6–11.3	15.6	13.9–17.4	16.1	13.7–18.9	8.9	7.2–11.0	12.5	10.7–14.4
11th	16.3	14.2–18.6	10.7	8.6–13.2	13.5	12.1–15.1	11.6	9.4–14.3	9.2	7.5–11.2	10.4	9.1–11.8
12th	16.7	13.8–20.0	10.2	8.5–12.2	13.5	11.7–15.5	11.7	9.8–13.8	9.5	7.9–11.4	10.6	9.4–12.0
Total	18.7	17.1–20.4	10.3	9.1–11.6	14.5	13.4–15.6	13.4	12.0–14.8	9.2	8.3–10.3	11.3	10.4–12.3

CI indicates confidence interval.

[a] During the 12 months before the survey.

[b] Non-Hispanic.

Data source: Centers for Disease Control and Prevention. Youth Risk Behavior Surveillance: United States, 2007. Surveillance Summaries. *MMWR CDC Surveill Summ.* 2008;57(SS-4):1–136. Available at: www.cdc.gov/mmwr/PDF/ss/ss5704.pdf. Accessed April 11, 2009.

Table 1.9
Percentage of high school students who attempted suicide[a,b] and whose suicide attempt resulted in an injury, poisoning, or an overdose that had to be treated by a doctor or nurse,[a] according to gender, race/ethnicity, and grade: United States, Youth Risk Behavior Survey, 2007

Category	Attempted Suicide						Suicide Attempt Treated by a Doctor or Nurse					
	Female		Male		Total		Female		Male		Total	
	%	95% CI	%	95% CI	%	95% CI	%	95% CI	%	95% CI	%	95% CI
Race/ethnicity												
White[c]	7.7	6.7–8.9	3.4	2.7–4.3	5.6	5.0–6.3	2.1	1.6–2.8	0.9	0.6–1.3	1.5	1.2–1.9
Black[c]	9.9	7.4–13.2	5.5	4.1–7.4	7.7	6.1–9.7	2.1	1.3–3.3	2.5	1.4–4.5	2.3	1.5–3.4
Hispanic	14.0	12.1–16.2	6.3	5.2–7.7	10.2	9.0–11.6	3.9	2.9–5.1	1.8	1.3–2.6	2.9	2.3–3.5
Grade												
9th	10.5	8.7–12.5	5.3	4.1–6.8	7.9	6.8–9.1	2.6	1.8–3.9	1.9	1.2–2.9	2.3	1.7–3.0
10th	11.2	9.1–13.7	4.9	4.0–5.9	8.0	6.9–9.4	3.1	2.3–4.0	1.0	0.6–1.8	2.0	1.6–2.6
11th	7.8	6.2–9.9	3.7	2.8–4.9	5.8	4.8–6.9	1.7	1.1–2.7	1.4	0.9–2.1	1.6	1.1–2.2
12th	6.5	5.2–8.1	4.2	3.2–5.6	5.4	4.4–6.5	1.8	1.2–2.8	1.5	0.9–2.4	1.7	1.1–2.4
Total	9.3	8.2–10.4	4.6	4.0–5.2	6.9	6.3–7.6	2.4	2.0–2.9	1.5	1.2–1.8	2.0	1.7–2.3

CI indicates confidence interval.

[a] During the 12 months before the survey.

[b] One or more times.

[c] Non-Hispanic.

Data source: Centers for Disease Control and Prevention. Youth Risk Behavior Surveillance: United States, 2007. Surveillance Summaries. *MMWR CDC Surveill Summ.* 2008;57(SS-4):1–136. Available at: www.cdc.gov/mmwr/PDF/ss/ss5704.pdf. Accessed April 11, 2009.

Table 1.10
Trends in the prevalence of selected risk behaviors for black students: national Youth Risk Behavior Survey, 1991–2007

1991	1993	1995	1997	1999	2001	2003	2005	2007	Changes from 1991–2007[1]	Change from 2005–2007[2]
Rarely or never wore a seat belt (When riding in a car driven by someone else.)										
34.5 (27.5–42.2)[3]	30.3 (26.0–34.9)	31.5 (27.0–36.4)	31.3 (26.1–37.0)	22.5 (18.1–27.6)	16.1 (12.5–20.6)	20.6 (17.0–24.7)	13.4 (10.3–17.3)	12.4 (10.0–15.4)	Decreased, 1991–2007	No change
Rode with a driver who had been drinking alcohol (In a car or other vehicle one or more times during the 30 days before the survey.)										
35.5 (31.8–39.3)	39.3 (36.7–42.0)	37.1 (33.6–40.7)	33.5 (29.2–38.0)	34.4 (28.4–40.9)	27.6 (24.3–31.1)	30.9 (27.7–34.2)	24.1 (22.0–26.4)	27.4 (23.7–31.5)	Decreased, 1991–2007	No change
Carried a weapon (For example, a gun, knife, or club on at least 1 day during the 30 days before the survey.)										
32.7 (29.5–36.2)	28.5 (26.2–30.9)	21.8 (17.9–26.3)	21.7 (18.0–26.0)	17.2 (12.4–23.3)	15.2 (12.9–17.8)	17.3 (14.0–21.2)	16.4 (14.8–18.1)	17.2 (15.2–19.4)	Decreased, 1991–2001 No change, 2001–2007	No change
Did not go to school because they felt unsafe at school or on their way to or from school (On at least 1 day during the 30 days before the survey.)										
NA[4]	7.1 (5.9–8.7)	7.7 (6.1–9.7)	6.8 (5.4–8.5)	6.0 (4.9–7.3)	9.8 (8.3–11.4)	8.4 (7.3–9.7)	8.7 (6.9–10.8)	6.6 (5.4–8.0)	No change, 1993–2007	No change
Attempted suicide (One or more times during the 12 months before the survey.)										
6.6 (4.8–9.0)	8.4 (6.9–10.0)	9.5 (7.8–11.7)	7.3 (6.0–9.0)	7.3 (5.4–9.8)	8.8 (7.6–10.1)	8.4 (6.8–10.3)	7.6 (5.7–10.1)	7.7 (6.1–9.7)	No change, 1991–2007	No change

(*Continued*)

Table 1.10
(Continued)

1991	1993	1995	1997	1999	2001	2003	2005	2007	Changes from 1991–2007[1]	Change from 2005–2007[2]
Current cigarette use (Smoked cigarettes on at least 1 day during the 30 days before the survey.)										
12.6 (10.2–15.5)	15.4 (12.9–18.2)	19.1 (16.1–22.6)	22.7 (19.0–26.8)	19.7 (15.8–24.3)	14.7 (12.0–17.9)	15.1 (12.4–18.2)	12.9 (11.1–14.8)	11.6 (9.5–14.1)	Increased, 1991–1997 Decreased, 1997–2007	No change
Current alcohol use (Had at least one drink of alcohol on at least 1 day during the 30 days before the survey.)										
42.0 (37.3–46.9)	42.5 (38.9–46.1)	42.0 (37.3–46.9)	36.9 (34.1–39.9)	39.9 (32.0–48.3)	32.7 (28.2–37.6)	37.4 (34.1–40.9)	31.2 (29.1–33.3)	34.5 (31.2–37.9)	Decreased, 1991–2007	No change
Current marijuana use (Used marijuana one or more times during the 30 days before the survey.)										
13.5 (10.4–17.3)	18.6 (15.2–22.6)	28.6 (23.4–34.4)	28.2 (25.0–31.7)	26.4 (20.0–34.0)	21.8 (17.9–26.4)	23.9 (20.8–27.2)	20.4 (18.3–22.7)	21.5 (18.4–25.0)	Increased, 1991–1995 Decreased, 1995–2007	No change
Lifetime methamphetamine use (Used methamphetamines [also called speed, crystal, crank, or ice] one or more times during their life.)										
NA	NA	NA	NA	1.7 (1.1–2.9)	2.1 (1.6–2.8)	3.1 (2.3–4.3)	1.7 (1.0–3.0)	1.9 (1.3–2.9)	No change, 1999–2007	No change
Ever had sexual intercourse										
81.5 (78.0–84.5)	79.7 (76.2–82.7)	73.4 (68.4–77.8)	72.7 (69.7–75.4)	71.2 (62.2–78.8)	60.8 (53.9–67.4)	67.3 (63.7–70.6)	67.6 (64.4–70.7)	66.5 (63.0–69.9)	Decreased, 1991–2001 No change, 2001–2007	No change
Had sexual intercourse with four or more persons during their life										
43.1 (39.5–46.7)	42.7 (38.8–46.7)	35.6 (31.2–40.3)	38.5 (34.9–42.3)	34.4 (24.7–45.7)	26.6 (22.9–30.6)	28.8 (26.3–31.5)	28.2 (25.6–30.9)	27.6 (24.8–30.6)	Decreased, 1991–2007	No change

(Continued)

Table 1.10
(Continued)

1991	1993	1995	1997	1999	2001	2003	2005	2007	Changes from 1991–2007[1]	Change from 2005–2007[2]
Used a condom during last sexual intercourse (Among students who were currently sexually active.)										
48.0 (44.1–51.9)	56.5 (52.6–60.3)	66.1 (61.0–70.9)	64.0 (61.0–66.8)	70.0 (64.1–75.2)	67.1 (63.4–70.6)	72.8 (68.8–76.4)	68.9 (65.0–72.5)	67.3 (62.6–71.6)	Increased, 1991–1999 No change, 1999–2007	No change
Ever taught in school about AIDS or HIV infection										
84.1 (80.0–87.5)	83.5 (80.0–86.4)	83.9 (79.3–87.6)	89.7 (87.9–91.3)	86.7 (82.2–90.3)	86.1 (83.4–88.4)	85.1 (81.3–88.2)	86.3 (82.7–89.3)	90.3 (88.6–91.8)	Increased, 1991–2007	Increased
Attended physical education classes daily (5 days in an average week when they were in school.)										
51.9 (44.9–58.8)	43.0 (37.6–48.6)	33.8 (29.1–39.0)	32.5 (26.9–38.7)	29.2 (20.1–40.3)	40.8 (29.8–52.9)	33.0 (26.8–39.8)	34.4 (25.7–44.3)	31.9 (26.0–38.4)	Decreased, 1991–1999 No change, 1999–2007	No change
Were obese[5] (Students who were $\geq 95^{th}$ percentile for body mass index, by age and sex, based on reference data.)										
NA	NA	NA	NA	12.4 (9.2–16.6)	16.0 (13.7–18.6)	16.2 (14.8–17.7)	16.0 (14.4–17.8)	18.3 (16.2–20.7)	Increased, 1999–2007	No change

The national Youth Risk Behavior Survey monitors priority health risk behaviors that contribute to the leading causes of death, disability, and social problems among youth and adults in the United States. The national Youth Risk Behavior Survey is conducted every 2 years during the spring semester and provides data representative of 9th- through 12th-grade students in public and private schools throughout the United States. NA indicates not available.

[a] Based on trend analyses using a logistic regression model controlling for gender, race/ethnicity, and grade.

[b] Based on *t* test analyses, $P < .05$.

(*Continued*)

Table 1.10
(Continued)

[c] 95% confidence interval.

[d] Previous Youth Risk Behavior Survey fact sheets used the term "overweight" to describe those youth with a BMI at ≥95th percentile for age and gender. However, this fact sheet uses the term "obese" rather than "overweight" in accordance with the 2007 recommendations from the Expert Committee on the Assessment, Prevention, and Treatment of Child and Adolescent Overweight and Obesity convened by the American Medical Association (AMA) and cofunded by the AMA in collaboration with the Health Resources and Services Administration and Centers for Disease Control and Prevention.

Data source: Centers for Disease Control and Prevention. National trends in risk behaviors. Available at: www.cdc.gov/HealthyYouth/yrbs/trends.htm. Accessed April 11, 2009.

Table 1.11
Trends in the prevalence of selected risk behaviors for Hispanic Students: national Youth Risk Behavior Survey, 1991–2007

1991	1993	1995	1997	1999	2001	2003	2005	2007	Changes from 1991–2007[1]	Change from 2005–2007[2]
Rarely or never wore a seat belt (When riding in a car driven by someone else.)										
31.3 (24.8–38.6)[3]	19.5 (16.1–23.5)	18.4 (13.7–24.2)	20.3 (14.6 –27.4)	14.4 (10.7–19.2)	14.5 (11.9–17.5)	20.2 (13.8–28.5)	10.6 (8.6–13.0)	12.9 (9.7–17.0)	Decreased, 1991–2007	No change
Rode with a driver who had been drinking alcohol (In a car or other vehicle one or more times during the 30 days before the survey.)										
46.9 (40.9–53.0)	42.3 (39.8–45.0)	49.5 (41.9–57.1)	42.8 (38.8–46.8)	39.5 (35.4–43.8)	38.3 (34.0–42.9)	36.4 (32.2–40.8)	36.1 (32.8–39.6)	35.5 (32.3–38.8)	Decreased, 1991–2007	No change
Carried a weapon (For example, a gun, knife, or club on at least 1 day during the 30 days before the survey.)										
25.8 (21.5–30.6)	24.4 (21.9–27.1)	24.7 (20.7–29.2)	23.3 (20.6–26.3)	18.7 (16.1–21.5)	16.5 (15.0–18.1)	16.5 (14.0–19.3)	19.0 (16.9–21.3)	18.5 (16.2–21.1)	Decreased, 1991–2001 No change, 2001–2007	No change
Did not go to school because they felt unsafe at school or on their way to or from school (On at least 1 day during the 30 days before the survey.)										
NA[4]	10.1 (8.5–11.9)	8.5 (6.0–11.7)	7.2 (5.6–9.1)	11.2 (8.2–15.1)	10.2 (8.9–11.7)	9.4 (8.0–11.1)	10.2 (8.7–12.1)	9.6 (7.8–11.8)	No change, 1993–2007	No change
Attempted suicide (One or more times during the 12 months before the survey.)										
7.9 (6.2–9.9)	13.6 (12.1–15.1)	13.4 (10.4–17.3)	10.7 (8.6–13.3)	12.8 (10.9–15.1)	12.1 (10.5–13.9)	10.6 (9.3–12.1)	11.3 (9.8–12.9)	10.2 (9.0–11.6)	Increased, 1991–1993 Decreased, 1993–2007	No change

(*Continued*)

Table 1.11
(Continued)

1991	1993	1995	1997	1999	2001	2003	2005	2007	Changes from 1991–2007[1]	Change from 2005–2007[2]
Current cigarette use (Smoked cigarettes on at least 1 day during the 30 days before the survey.)										
25.3 (22.5–28.2)	28.7 (25.8–31.8)	34.0 (28.7–39.6)	34.0 (31.3–36.9)	32.7 (29.0–36.6)	26.6 (22.4–31.2)	18.4 (16.1–20.9)	22.0 (18.7–25.8)	16.7 (13.5–20.4)	Increased, 1991–1995 Decreased, 1995–2007	Decreased
Current alcohol use (Had at least one drink of alcohol on at least 1 day during the 30 days before the survey.)										
54.3 (48.3–60.1)	50.8 (45.3–56.4)	54.7 (49.3–59.9)	53.9 (50.0–57.8)	52.8 (47.9–57.6)	49.2 (46.2–52.3)	45.6 (42.8–48.4)	46.8 (44.0–49.7)	47.6 (44.0–51.3)	Decreased, 1991–2007	No change
Current marijuana use (Used marijuana one or more times during the 30 days before the survey.)										
14.4 (11.2–18.3)	19.4 (16.8–22.3)	27.8 (22.3–34.1)	28.6 (24.7–33.0)	28.2 (23.8–33.0	24.6 (23.0–26.3)	23.8 (21.5–26.2)	23.0 (20.7–25.6)	18.5 (15.8–21.5)	Increased, 1991–1997 Decreased, 1997–2007	Decreased
Lifetime methamphetamine use (Used methamphetamines [also called speed, crystal, crank, or ice] one or more times during their life.)										
NA	NA	NA	NA	11.3 (7.2–17.2)	9.1 (7.3–11.2)	8.3 (6.5–10.5)	8.8 (6.8–11.3)	5.7 (4.1–7.9)	Decreased, 1999–2007	Decreased
Ever had sexual intercourse										
53.1 (49.4–56.7)	56.0 (51.8–60.2)	57.6 (48.6–66.1)	52.2 (48.4–55.8)	54.1 (49.0–59.0)	48.4 (43.8–53.0)	51.4 (48.1–54.8)	51.0 (46.5–55.4)	52.0 (48.3–55.6)	No change, 1991–2007	No change
Had sexual intercourse with four or more persons during their life										
16.8 (14.3–19.7)	18.6 (15.7–22.0)	17.6 (14.1–21.7)	15.5 (13.2–18.1)	16.6 (13.2–20.7)	14.9 (13. 2–16.7)	15.7 (13.5–18.1)	15.9 (13.6–18.5)	17.3 (15.2–19.5)	No change, 1991–2007	No change

(Continued)

Table 1.11
(Continued)

1991	1993	1995	1997	1999	2001	2003	2005	2007	Changes from 1991–2007[1]	Change from 2005–2007[2]
Used a condom during last sexual intercourse (Among students who were currently sexually active.)										
37.4 (31.3–44.0)	46.1 (41.6–50.6)	44.4 (33.4–56.0)	48.3 (42.6–54.0)	55.2 (48.1–62.0)	53.5 (48.2–58.7)	57.4 (51.9–62.8)	57.7 (53.4–61.8)	61.4 (56.7–65.9)	Increased , 1991-2007	No change
Ever taught in school about AIDS or HIV infection										
82.2 (76.2–87.0)	82.4 (79.7–84.8)	84.2 (80.8–87.0)	85.9 (82.9–88.4)	84.1 (81.1–86.7)	80.5 (76.0–84.3)	83.4 (80.0–86.3)	84.7 (82.0–87.1)	85.0 (82.9–86.8)	No change, 1991–2007	No change
Attended physical education classes daily (5 days in an average week when they were in school.)										
46.6 (40.7–52.5)	39.7 (35.6–44.0)	33.1 (25.7–41.5)	38.4 (34.5–42.5)	40.4 (31.2–50.2)	38.7 (32.5–45.3)	36.7 (28.9–45.3)	38.3 (27.8–50.1)	36.0 (28.4–44.3)	Decreased, 1991–2007	No change
Were obese[5] (Students who were ≥ 95th percentile for body mass index, by age and sex, based on reference data.)										
NA	NA	NA	NA	13.6 (11.4–16.1)	15.1 (12.4–18.3)	16.4 (14.0–19.2)	16.8 (14.5–19.4)	16.6 (14.7–18.7)	Increased, 1999–2007	No change

The national Youth Risk Behavior Survey monitors priority health risk behaviors that contribute to the leading causes of death, disability, and social problems among youth and adults in the United States. The national Youth Risk Behavior Survey is conducted every 2 years during the spring semester and provides data representative of 9th- through 12th-grade students in public and private schools throughout the United States. NA indicates not available.

[a] Based on trend analyses using a logistic regression model controlling for gender, race/ethnicity, and grade.

[b] Based on t test analyses, $P < .05$.

(Continued)

Table 1.11
(Continued)

[c] 95% confidence interval.

[d] Previous Youth Risk Behavior Survey fact sheets used the term “overweight” to describe those youth with a BMI at ≥95th percentile for age and gender. However, this fact sheet uses the term “obese” rather than “overweight” in accordance with the 2007 recommendations from the Expert Committee on the Assessment, Prevention, and Treatment of Child and Adolescent Overweight and Obesity convened by the American Medical Association (AMA) and cofunded by the AMA in collaboration with the Health Resources and Services Administration and Centers for Disease Control and Prevention.

Data source: Centers for Disease Control and Prevention. National trends in risk behaviors. Available at: www.cdc.gov/HealthyYouth/yrbs/trends.htm. Accessed April 11, 2009.

Table 1.12
Trends in the prevalence of selected risk behaviors for white students: national Youth Risk Behavior Survey, 1991–2007

1991	1993	1995	1997	1999	2001	2003	2005	2007	Changes from 1991–2007[1]	Change from 2005–2007[2]
Rarely or never wore a seat belt (When riding in a car driven by someone else.)										
23.9 (18.1–30.9)[3]	17.2 (14.3–20.6)	20.5 (16.4–25.2)	17.1 (13.2–21.8	15.5 (12.0–19.9)	13.6 (11.6–15.9)	16.9 (12.2–22.8)	9.4 (7.4–11.9)	10.1 (7.4–13.8)	Decreased, 1991–2007	No change
Rode with a driver who had been drinking alcohol (In a car or other vehicle one or more times during the 30 days before the survey.)										
40.5 (37.9–43.1)	34.1 (30.6–37.7)	37.7 (32.4–43.3)	36.9 (34.1–39.8)	32.4 (29.9–35.0)	30.3 (28.1–32.6)	28.5 (25.9–31.2)	28.3 (25.7–31.0)	27.9 (25.4–30.6)	Decreased, 1991–2007	No change
Carried a weapon (For example, a gun, knife, or club on at least 1 day during the 30 days before the survey.)										
25.1 (22.5–27.8)	20.6 (17.9–23.6)	18.9 (17.1–20.8)	17.0 (14.5–19.7)	16.4 (13.8–19.3)	17.9 (15.4–20.7)	16.7 (14.8–18.7)	18.7 (16.5–21.1)	18.2 (15.8–21.0)	Decreased, 1991–1999 No change, 1999–2007	No change
Did not go to school because they felt unsafe at school or on their way to or from school (On at least 1 day during the 30 days before the survey.)										
NA[4]	3.0 (2.3–3.8)	2.8 (2.1–3.7)	2.4 (1.8–3.2)	3.9 (2.8–5.6)	5.0 (3.9–6.3)	3.1 (2.5–3.8)	4.4 (2.9–6.5)	4.0 (3.2–4.9)	Increased, 1993–2007	No change
Attempted suicide (One or more times during the 12 months before the survey.)										
6.7 (5.7–7.9)	7.7 (6.8–8.8)	7.6 (6.6–8.9)	6.3 (5.2–7.6)	6.7 (5.3–8.4)	7.9 (6.9–9.1)	6.9 (5.9–8.0)	7.3 (6.3–8.4)	5.6 (5.0–6.3)	Decreased, 1991–2007	Decreased

(Continued)

Table 1.12
(Continued)

1991	1993	1995	1997	1999	2001	2003	2005	2007	Changes from 1991–2007[1]	Change from 2005–2007[2]
Current cigarette use (Smoked cigarettes on at least 1 day during the 30 days before the survey.)										
30.9 (27.6–34.5)	33.7 (31.4–36.0)	38.3 (35.6–41.1)	39.7 (37.3–42.2)	38.6 (35.5–41.9)	31.9 (29.6–34.4)	24.9 (22.4–27.5)	25.9 (22.9–29.2)	23.2 (20.4–26.2)	Increased, 1991–1997 Decreased, 1997–2007	No change
Current alcohol use (Had at least one drink of alcohol on at least 1 day during the 30 days before the survey.)										
52.9 (49.7–56.1)	49.9 (47.4–52.5)	54.1 (50.5–57.6)	54.0 (51.0–57.0)	52.5 (49.2–55.7)	50.4 (48.1–52.7)	47.1 (44.1–50.2)	46.4 (42.8–50.2)	47.3 (43.9–50.7)	No change, 1991–1995 Decreased, 1995–2007	No change
Current marijuana use (Used marijuana one or more times during the 30 days before the survey.)										
15.2 (12.5–18.3)	17.3 (14.6–20.3)	24.5 (22.0–27.3)	25.0 (22.0–28.3)	26.4 (23.3–29.7)	24.4 (22.4–26.6)	21.7 (19.4–24.2)	20.3 (18.1–22.6)	19.9 (17.4–22.6)	Increased, 1991–1999 Decreased, 1999–2007	No change
Lifetime methamphetamine use (Used methamphetamines [also called speed, crystal, crank, or ice] one or more times during their life.)										
NA	NA	NA	NA	10.3 (8.9–11.8)	11.4 (9.4–13.7)	8.1 (7.0–9.3)	6.5 (5.4–7.7)	4.5 (3.5–5.6)	No change, 1999–2001 Decreased, 2001–2007	Decreased
Ever had sexual intercourse										
50.0 (46.7–53.4)	48.4 (45.6–51.3)	48.9 (43.8–54.1)	43.6 (39.4–48.0)	45.1 (41.1–49.2)	43.2 (40.7–45.8)	41.8 (39.0–44.5)	43.0 (38.8–47.3)	43.7 (40.5–47.0)	Decreased, 1991–2007	No change
Had sexual intercourse with four or more persons during their life										
14.7 (13.0–16.7)	14.3 (12.3–16.6)	14.2 (11.8–16.8)	11.6 (10.2–13.2)	12.4 (10.4–14.7)	12.0 (10.6–13.5)	10.8 (9.4–12.4)	11.4 (9.7–13.3)	11.5 (9.6–13.7)	Decreased, 1991–2007	No change

(Continued)

Table 1.12
(Continued)

1991	1993	1995	1997	1999	2001	2003	2005	2007	Changes from 1991–2007[1]	Change from 2005–2007[2]
Used a condom during last sexual intercourse (Among students who were currently sexually active.)										
46.5 (41.8–51.2)	52.3 (48.2–56.3)	52.5 (48.4–56.6)	55.8 (53.8–57.8)	55.0 (49.8–60.2)	56.8 (53.7–59.9)	62.5 (59.2–65.6)	62.6 (60.0–65.2)	59.7 (56.8–62.5)	Increased, 1991–2007	No change
Ever taught in school about AIDS or HIV infection										
83.4 (79.7–86.5)	87.3 (83.8–90.1)	87.3 (76.1–93.6)	93.3 (91.8–94.5)	92.2 (90.2–93.8)	91.1 (89.6–92.5)	90.3 (88.3–92.0)	89.4 (86.9–91.5)	91.1 (89.6–92.4)	Increased, 1991–1997 Decreased, 1997–2007	No change
Attended physical education classes daily (5 days in an average week when they were in school.)										
38.6 (31.9–45.7)	32.1 (26.7–38.0)	21.7 (11.9–36.1)	23.8 (17.6–31.4)	28.3 (17.1–43.2)	29.5 (24.5–35.2)	24.9 (18.4–32.8)	31.7 (26.3–37.6)	28.9 (23.0–35.5)	Decreased, 1991–1995 No change, 1995–2007	No change
Were obese[5] (Students who were $\geq 95^{th}$ percentile for body mass index, by age and sex, based on reference data.)										
NA	NA	NA	NA	10.1 (8.3–12.2)	8.8 (7.8–9.8)	10.4 (8.6–12.4)	11.8 (10.7–12.9)	10.8 (9.3–12.4)	No change, 1999–2007	No change

The national Youth Risk Behavior Survey monitors priority health risk behaviors that contribute to the leading causes of death, disability, and social problems among youth and adults in the United States. The national Youth Risk Behavior Survey is conducted every 2 years during the spring semester and provides data representative of 9th- through 12th-grade students in public and private schools throughout the United States. NA indicates not available.

[a] Based on trend analyses using a logistic regression model controlling for gender, race/ethnicity, and grade.

[b] Based on t test analyses, $P < .05$.

(Continued)

Table 1.12
(Continued)

[c] 95% confidence interval.

[d] Previous Youth Risk Behavior Survey fact sheets used the term "overweight" to describe those youth with a BMI at ≥95th percentile for age and gender. However, this fact sheet uses the term "obese" rather than "overweight" in accordance with the 2007 recommendations from the Expert Committee on the Assessment, Prevention, and Treatment of Child and Adolescent Overweight and Obesity convened by the American Medical Association (AMA) and cofunded by the AMA in collaboration with the Health Resources and Services Administration and Centers for Disease Control and Prevention.

Data source: Centers for Disease Control and Prevention. National trends in risk behaviors. Available at: www.cdc.gov/HealthyYouth/yrbs/trends.htm. Accessed April 11, 2009.

Table 1.13
Percentage of high school students who were obese[a,b] and who were overweight,[b,c] according to gender, race/ethnicity, and grade: United States, Youth Risk Behavior Survey, 2007

Category	Obese						Overweight					
	Female		Male		Total		Female		Male		Total	
	%	95% CI	%	95% CI	%	95% CI	%	95% CI	%	95% CI	%	95% CI
Race/ethnicity												
White[d]	6.8	5.2–8.9	14.6	13.0–16.4	10.8	9.3–12.4	12.8	10.9–15.0	15.7	14.4–17.1	14.3	12.9–15.7
Black[d]	17.8	15.0–20.9	18.9	16.1–22.1	18.3	16.2–20.7	21.4	18.5–24.7	16.6	14.1–19.3	19.0	17.2–20.9
Hispanic	12.7	10.6–15.1	20.3	17.8–23.0	16.6	14.7–18.7	17.9	15.3–21.0	18.3	16.0–20.8	18.1	16.1–20.3
Grade												
9th	10.7	8.8–13.0	16.6	14.5–18.9	13.8	12.5–15.2	18.3	15.4–21.6	17.0	14.7–19.6	17.6	15.5–20.1
10th	9.8	8.1–11.9	16.4	14.0–19.1	13.2	11.5–15.0	14.2	11.9–16.9	17.7	15.1–20.6	16.0	14.4–17.6
11th	8.1	6.5–10.1	17.3	15.2–19.6	12.7	11.3–14.4	14.2	11.9–16.8	15.9	13.6–18.6	15.1	13.3–17.1
12th	9.3	7.6–11.4	14.7	12.6–17.2	12.0	10.5–13.7	13.1	11.1–15.5	14.9	12.7–17.4	14.0	12.5–15.6
Total	9.6	8.3–11.0	16.3	15.1–17.5	13.0	11.9–14.1	15.1	13.8–16.5	16.4	15.4–17.5	15.8	14.8–16.8

CI indicates confidence interval.

[a] Students who were at ≥95th percentile for BMI, according to age and gender, based on reference data.

[b] Previous Youth Risk Behavior Survey reports used the term "overweight" to describe youth with a BMI at ≥95th percentile for age and gender and "at risk for overweight" for those with a BMI at ≥85th percentile and <95th percentile. However, this report uses the terms "obese" and "overweight" in accordance with the 2007 recommendations from the Expert Committee on the Assessment, Prevention, and Treatment of Child and Adolescent Overweight and Obesity convened by the American Medical Association (AMA) and cofunded by the AMA in collaboration with the Health Resources and Services Administration and Centers for Disease Control and Prevention.

[c] Students who were at ≥85th percentile but <95th percentile for BMI, according to age and gender, based on reference data.

[d] Non-Hispanic.

Data source: Centers for Disease Control and Prevention. Youth Risk Behavior Surveillance: United States, 2007. Surveillance Summaries. *MMWR CDC Surveill Summ.* 2008;57(SS-4):1–136. Available at: www.cdc.gov/mmwr/PDF/ss/ss5704.pdf. Accessed April 11, 2009.

Table 1.14

Percentage of high school students who described themselves as slightly or very overweight and who were trying to lose weight, according to gender, race/ethnicity, and grade: United States, Youth Risk Behavior Survey, 2007

Category	Described Themselves as Overweight						Were Trying to Lose Weight					
	Female		Male		Total		Female		Male		Total	
	%	95% CI	%	95% CI	%	95% CI	%	95% CI	%	95% CI	%	95% CI
Race/ethnicity												
White[a]	34.0	31.9–36.1	23.6	22.0–25.3	28.8	27.3–30.3	62.3	60.1–64.4	29.0	27.0–31.1	45.6	43.8–47.4
Black[a]	30.1	27.4–33.0	19.1	16.8–21.7	24.6	22.7–26.6	49.5	46.2–52.8	24.9	21.6–28.4	37.1	34.8–39.4
Hispanic	39.3	36.3–42.4	28.3	24.7–32.1	33.8	31.1–36.6	62.1	57.6–66.3	38.5	34.2–42.9	50.2	46.7–53.7
Grade												
9th	33.6	30.3–37.1	24.3	22.4–26.4	28.8	27.1–30.6	58.6	54.9–62.1	31.0	28.5–33.8	44.4	42.2–46.6
10th	33.8	31.1–36.6	24.8	22.6–27.2	29.2	27.3–31.2	60.2	56.9–63.4	31.6	28.8–34.6	45.8	43.5–48.1
11th	36.2	32.9–39.6	25.8	23.0–28.7	31.0	28.6–33.4	61.3	58.4–64.1	30.1	26.6–33.8	45.8	43.5–48.1
12th	34.9	30.9–39.1	21.6	19.1–24.2	28.3	25.9–30.8	61.6	59.0–64.1	28.7	25.6–32.1	45.3	43.5–47.2
Total	34.5	32.9–36.1	24.2	23.0–25.3	29.3	28.2–30.4	60.3	58.4–62.1	30.4	28.8–32.1	45.2	43.8–46.7

CI indicates confidence interval.

[a] Non-Hispanic.

Data source: Centers for Disease Control and Prevention. Youth Risk Behavior Surveillance: United States, 2007. Surveillance Summaries. *MMWR CDC Surveill Summ.* 2008;57(SS-4):1–136. Available at: www.cdc.gov/mmwr/PDF/ss/ss5704.pdf. Accessed April 11, 2009.

Table 1.15
Percentage of high school students who ate less food, fewer calories, or low-fat foods[a] and who exercised,[a] according to gender, race/ethnicity, and grade: United States, Youth Risk Behavior Survey, 2007

Category	Ate Less Food, Fewer Calories, or Low-Fat Foods to Lose Weight or to Keep From Gaining Weight						Exercised to Lose Weight or to Keep From Gaining Weight					
	Female		Male		Total		Female		Male		Total	
	%	95% CI	%	95% CI	%	95% CI	%	95% CI	%	95% CI	%	95% CI
Race/ethnicity												
White[b]	58.4	56.3–60.5	28.3	26.8–29.8	43.3	41.8–44.8	71.5	69.0–73.9	53.3	51.4–55.2	62.4	60.8–63.9
Black[b]	34.6	32.0–37.3	21.0	19.0–23.2	27.8	25.9–29.8	50.7	47.6–53.7	53.7	50.2–57.2	52.2	49.9–54.5
Hispanic	52.0	48.2–55.7	32.3	29.4–35.3	42.1	39.5–44.7	66.4	62.7–69.9	60.1	55.9–64.2	63.2	60.1–66.3
Grade												
9th	50.5	46.7–54.2	27.3	25.0–29.8	38.6	36.0–41.1	70.6	67.5–73.6	58.7	56.3–61.0	64.5	62.6–66.3
10th	53.0	50.0–55.9	29.1	26.2–32.1	40.9	38.7–43.2	67.7	64.6–70.8	54.2	51.5–56.8	60.9	59.1–62.6
11th	54.0	51.4–56.5	29.8	26.1–33.8	42.0	39.5–44.5	65.0	62.3–67.7	54.9	51.9–57.9	59.9	57.6–62.2
12th	56.4	53.5–59.3	27.4	24.2–30.8	42.0	39.8–44.3	63.7	60.7–66.5	51.1	48.0–54.3	57.5	55.1–59.8
Total	53.2	51.2–55.1	28.3	27.2–29.5	40.6	39.4–41.9	67.0	65.2–68.7	55.0	53.6–56.4	60.9	59.8–62.1

CI indicates confidence interval.

[a] To lose weight or to keep from gaining weight during the 30 days before the survey.

[b] Non-Hispanic.

Data source: Centers for Disease Control and Prevention. Youth Risk Behavior Surveillance: United States, 2007. Surveillance Summaries. *MMWR CDC Surveill Summ.* 2008;57(SS-4):1–136. Available at: www.cdc.gov/mmwr/PDF/ss/ss5704.pdf. Accessed April 11, 2009.

Table 1.16

Percentage of high school students who did not eat for ≥24 hours[a] and who took diet pills, powders, or liquids,[a,b] according to gender, race/ethnicity, and grade: United States, Youth Risk Behavior Survey, 2007

Category	Did Not Eat for ≥24 h to Lose Weight or to Keep From Gaining Weight						Took Diet Pills, Powders, or Liquids to Lose Weight or to Keep From Gaining Weight[b]					
	Female		Male		Total		Female		Male		Total	
	%	95% CI	%	95% CI	%	95% CI	%	95% CI	%	95% CI	%	95% CI
Race/ethnicity												
White[c]	16.7	15.5–18.1	5.7	4.3–7.3	11.2	10.3–12.1	8.3	7.1–9.6	3.7	3.0–4.7	6.0	5.3–6.8
Black[c]	13.2	11.0–15.8	7.4	5.9–9.3	10.3	9.0–11.9	3.9	2.8–5.5	3.6	2.5–5.1	3.7	2.9–4.8
Hispanic	17.4	15.3–19.8	10.7	8.1–14.0	14.1	12.4–15.9	7.8	5.9–10.1	5.1	3.8–6.9	6.4	5.1–8.0
Grade												
9	16.8	15.0–18.9	6.5	5.1–8.2	11.6	10.5–12.8	6.1	4.6–8.0	2.9	2.1–4.0	4.4	3.6–5.4
10	19.1	16.7–21.7	6.5	4.9–8.6	12.7	11.1–14.5	6.9	5.7–8.2	3.8	2.9–5.0	5.3	4.4–6.4
11	14.8	12.7–17.2	8.1	6.1–10.8	11.5	10.0–13.2	7.4	5.9–9.2	5.0	3.7–6.7	6.2	5.2–7.5
12	13.6	11.6–16.0	8.0	5.5–11.6	10.9	9.1–12.9	10.2	8.4–12.4	5.7	4.0–8.0	8.0	6.7–9.4
Total	16.3	15.2–17.3	7.3	6.1–8.6	11.8	11.0–12.6	7.5	6.6–8.4	4.2	3.5–5.1	5.9	5.2–6.5

CI indicates confidence interval.

[a] To lose weight or to keep from gaining weight during the 30 days before the survey.

[b] Without a doctor's advice.

[c] Non-Hispanic.

Data source: Centers for Disease Control and Prevention. Youth Risk Behavior Surveillance: United States, 2007. Surveillance Summaries. *MMWR CDC Surveill Summ.* 2008;57(SS-4):1–136. Available at: www.cdc.gov/mmwr/PDF/ss/ss5704.pdf. Accessed April 11, 2009.

Table 1.17
Percentage of high school students who vomited or took laxatives,[a] according to gender, race/ethnicity, and grade: United States, Youth Risk Behavior Survey, 2007

Category	Female		Male		Total	
	%	95% CI	%	95% CI	%	95% CI
Race/ethnicity						
White[b]	6.9	5.6–8.5	1.3	0.9–2.1	4.1	3.4–5.0
Black[b]	3.5	2.6–4.7	2.5	1.8–3.6	3.0	2.5–3.7
Hispanic	7.0	5.4–8.9	3.7	2.6–5.2	5.3	4.3–6.7
Grade						
9	5.5	4.4–7.0	2.1	1.5–3.0	3.8	3.1–4.7
10	7.6	5.6–10.3	1.8	1.2–2.5	4.7	3.6–6.1
11	5.7	4.2–7.6	2.1	1.3–3.4	4.0	3.0–5.2
12	6.6	5.2–8.3	2.6	1.6–4.2	4.6	3.7–5.7
Total	6.4	5.5–7.4	2.2	1.7–2.8	4.3	3.7–5.0

CI indicates confidence interval.
[a] To lose weight or to keep from gaining weight during the 30 days before the survey.
[b] Non-Hispanic.
Data source: Centers for Disease Control and Prevention. Youth Risk Behavior Surveillance: United States, 2007. Surveillance Summaries. *MMWR CDC Surveill Summ.* 2008;57(SS-4): 1–136. Available at: www.cdc.gov/mmwr/PDF/ss/ss5704.pdf. Accessed April 11, 2009.

Table 1.18
Deaths and death rates (per 100,000 population in specified group) according to age, gender, race, and Hispanic origin and age-adjusted death rates according to gender, race, and Hispanic origin: United States, 2005 (final) and 2006 (preliminary)

Race and Hispanic Origin, Gender, and Age	2006		2005	
	n	Rate	*n*	Rate
All races				
Total, both genders				
5–14 y	6153	15.3	6602	16.3
15–24 y	34 829	82.1	34 234	81.4
Males				
5–14 y	3617	17.5	3853	18.6
15–24 y	26015	119.1	25509	117.8
Females				
5–14 y	2536	12.9	2749	13.9
15–24 y	8814	42.8	8725	42.7
White				
Total, both genders				
5–14 y	4464	14.3	4710	15.0
15–24 y	25 843	77.9	25 410	77.1
Males				
5–14 y	2630	16.4	2749	17.1
15–24 y	19 146	111.7	18 792	110.4
Females				
5–14 y	1833	12.0	1961	12.8
15–24 y	6698	41.8	6618	41.5
Non–Hispanic white				
Total, both genders				
5–14 y	3370	14.1	3681	15.2
15–24 y	20127	76.3	19683	74.8
Males				
5–14 y	1989	16.2	2163	17.4
15–24 y	14596	107.9	14267	105.8
Females				
5–14 y	1381	11.9	1518	12.9
15–24 y	5530	43.1	5416	42.2
Black				
Total, both genders				
5–14 y	1394	21.2	1543	23.3
15–24 y	7470	111.9	7371	112.3
Males				
5–14 y	832	24.9	909	27.0
15–24 y	5786	171.1	5709	172.1

(*Continued*)

Table 1.18
(Continued)

Race and Hispanic Origin, Gender, and Age	2006		2005	
	n	Rate	*n*	Rate
Females				
5–14 y	562	17.3	634	19.4
15–24 y	1684	51.1	1662	51.2
Non-Hispanic black				
Total, both genders				
5–14 y	1363	21.9	1500	24.0
15–24 y	7335	115.4	7244	115.8
Males				
5–14 y	816	25.8	885	27.8
15–24 y	5685	176.7	5615	177.7
Females				
5–14 y	547	17.9	615	20.0
15–24 y	1650	52.6	1629	52.6
AI/AN				
Total, both genders				
5–14 y	90	16.7	110	19.8
15–24 y	654	109.2	635	107.4
Males				
5–14 y	46	16.8	64	22.7
15–24 y	469	153.2	439	145.1
Females				
5–14 y	45	17.0	46	16.8
15–24 y	185	63.2	196	67.9
API				
Total, both genders				
5–14 y	205	10.9	239	12.9
15–24 y	862	43.6	818	41.8
Males				
5–14 y	109	11.4	131	14.0
15–24 y	615	60.8	569	56.9
Females				
5–14 y	96	10.3	108	11.9
15–24 y	247	25.6	249	26.1
Hispanic				
Total, both genders				
5–14 y	1121	14.0	1068	13.7
15–24 y	5834	79.1	5837	81.2
Males				
5–14 y	658	16.0	612	15.3
15–24 y	4638	118.8	4604	120.4

(*Continued*)

Table 1.18
(Continued)

Race and Hispanic Origin, Gender, and Age	2006		2005	
	n	Rate	*n*	Rate
Females				
5–14 y	463	11.8	456	12.0
15–24 y	1196	34.5	1233	36.6

AI/AN indicates American Indian/Alaska Native (includes Elutes and Eskimos); API, Asian/Pacific Islander (includes Chinese, Filipino, Hawaiian, Japanese, and other Asian or Pacific Islander).

Data source: Heron MP, Hoyert DL, Xu J, et al. Deaths: preliminary data for 2006. *Natl Vital Stat Rep*. 2008;56(16). Available at: www.cdc.gov/nchs/data/nvsr/nvsr56/nvsr56_16.pdf. Accessed March 17, 2009.

Table 1.19
Deaths, percentage of total deaths, and death rates for the 5 leading causes of death in selected adolescent age groups according to race and gender: United States, 2004

Race, Gender, Age, and Cause of Death	No. of Deaths	Percent of Total	Rate[a]
All races, both genders, 10–14 y			
All causes	3946	100.00	18.7
1. Unintentional injuries	1540	39.0	7.3
2. Malignant neoplasms	493	12.5	2.3
3. Suicide	283	7.2	1.3
4. Homicide	207	5.2	1.0
5. Congenital malformations[b]	184	4.7	0.9
All races, both genders, 15–19 y			
All causes	13 706	100.0	66.1
1. Unintentional injuries	6825	49.8	32.9
2. Homicide	1932	14.1	9.3
3. Suicide	1700	12.4	8.2
4. Malignant neoplasms	731	5.3	3.5
5. Diseases of heart	366	2.7	1.8
All races, both genders, 20–24 y			
All causes	19 715	100.0	94.0
1. Unintentional injuries	8624	43.7	41.1
2. Homicide	3153	16.0	15.0
3. Suicide	2616	13.3	12.5
4. Malignant neoplasms	978	5.0	4.7
5. Diseases of heart	672	3.4	3.2
All races, males, 10–14 y			
All causes	2354	100.0	21.7
1. Unintentional injuries	979	41.6	9.0
2. Malignant neoplasms	269	11.4	2.5
3. Suicide	185	7.9	1.7
4. Homicide	138	5.9	1.3
5. Congenital malformations	100	4.2	0.9
All races, males, 15–19 y			
All causes	9678	100.0	91.0
1. Unintentional injuries	4744	49.0	44.6
2. Homicide	1631	16.9	15.3
3. Suicide	1345	13.9	12.6
4. Malignant neoplasms	435	4.5	4.1
5. Diseases of heart	240	2.5	2.3

(*Continued*)

Table 1.19
(Continued)

Race, Gender, Age, and Cause of Death	No. of Deaths	Percent of Total	Rate[a]
All races, males, 20–24 y			
All causes	14 909	100.00	138
1. Unintentional injuries	6679	44.8	61.8
2. Homicide	2749	18.4	25.4
3. Suicide	2251	15.1	20.8
4. Malignant neoplasms	592	4.0	5.5
5. Disease of heart	451	3.0	4.2
All races, females, 10–14 y			
All causes	1592	100.0	15.4
1. Unintentional injury	561	35.2	5.4
2. Malignant neoplasms	224	14.1	2.2
3. Suicide	98	6.2	1.0
4. Congenital malformations	84	5.3	0.8
5. Diseases of heart	73	4.6	0.7
All races, females, 15–19 y			
All causes	4028	100.0	39.9
1. Unintentional injuries	2081	51.7	20.6
2. Suicide	355	8.8	3.5
3. Homicide	301	7.5	3.0
4. Malignant neoplasms	296	7.3	2.9
5. Diseases of heart	126	3.1	1.2
All races, females, 20–24 y			
All causes	4806	100.0	47.3
1. Unintentional injuries	1945	40.5	19.1
2. Homicide	404	8.4	4.0
3. Malignant neoplasms	386	8.0	3.8
4. Suicide	365	7.6	3.6
5. Diseases of heart	221	4.6	2.2
White, both genders, 10–14 y			
All causes	2857	100.0	17.4
1. Unintentional injuries	1161	40.6	7.1
2. Malignant neoplasms	378	13.2	2.3
3. Suicide	217	7.6	1.3
4. Congenital malformations	140	4.9	0.9
5. Homicide	105	3.7	0.6
White, both genders, 15–19 y			
All causes	10 450	100	64.4
1. Unintentional injuries	5850	56.0	36.0
2. Suicide	1425	13.6	8.8
3. Homicide	822	7.9	5.1
4. Malignant neoplasms	581	5.6	3.6
5. Diseases of heart	233	2.2	1.4

(Continued)

Table 1.19
(Continued)

Race, Gender, Age, and Cause of Death	No. of Deaths	Percent of Total	Rate[a]
White, both genders, 20–24 y			
All causes	14, 563	100.0	88.3
1. Unintentional injuries	7324	50.3	44.4
2. Suicide	2185	15.0	13.2
3. Homicide	1304	9.0	7.9
4. Malignant neoplasms	742	5.1	4.5
5. Diseases of heart	445	3.1	2.7
White, males, 10–14 y			
All causes	1727	100.0	20.6
1. Unintentional injuries	749	43.4	8.9
2. Malignant neoplasms	211	12.2	2.5
3. Suicide	142	8.2	1.7
4. Congenital malformations	77	4.5	0.9
5. Homicide	73	4.2	0.9
White, males, 15–19 y			
All causes	7267	100.0	87.1
1. Unintentional injuries	4045	55.7	48.5
2. Suicide	1132	`5.6	13.6
3. Homicide	660	9.1	7.9
4. Malignant neoplasm	350	4.8	4.2
5. Diseases of heart	153	2.1	1.8
White, males, 20–24 y			
All causes	11 039	100.0	129.1
1. Unintentional injuries	5725	51.9	67.0
2. Suicide	1884	17.1	22.0
3. Homicide	1067	9.7	12.5
4. Malignant neoplasms	451	4.1	5.3
5. Diseases of heart	306	2.8	3.6
White, females, 10–14 y			
All causes	1130	100.0	14.2
1. Unintentional injuries	412	36.5	5.2
2. Malignant neoplasms	167	14.8	2.1
3. Suicide	75	6.6	0.9
4. Congenital malformations	63	5.6	0.8
5. Diseases of heart	45	4.0	0.6
White, females, 15–19 y			
All causes	3183	100.0	40.4
1. Unintentional injuries	1805	56.7	22.9
2. Suicide	293	9.2	3.7
3. Malignant neoplasms	231	7.3	2.9
4. Homicide	162	5.1	2.1
5. Congenital malformations	81	2.5	1.0

(Continued)

Table 1.19
(Continued)

Race, Gender, Age, and Cause of Death	No. of Deaths	Percent of Total	Rate[a]
White, females, 20–24 y			
All causes	3524	100.0	44.3
1. Unintentional injuries	1599	45.4	20.1
2. Suicide	301	8.5	3.8
3. Malignant neoplasms	291	8.3	2.7
4. Homicide	237	6.7	3.0
5. Diseases of heart	139	3.9	1.7
Black, both genders, 10–14 y			
All causes	899	100.0	25.3
1. Unintentional injuries	301	33.5	8.5
2. Malignant neoplasms	91	10.1	2.6
3. Homicide	87	9.7	2.4
4. Diseases of heart	53	5.9	1.5
5. Suicide	48	5.3	1.4
Black, both genders, 15–19 y			
All causes	2680	100.0	81.4
1. Homicide	1042	38.9	31.6
2. Unintentional injuries	712	26.6	21.6
3. Suicide	155	5.8	4.7
4. Malignant neoplasms	126	4.7	3.8
5. Diseases of heart	118	4.4	3.6
Black, both genders, 20–24 y			
All causes	4369	100.0	138.8
1. Homicide	1761	40.3	55.9
2. Unintentional injuries	949	21.7	30.1
3. Suicide	310	7.1	9.8
4. Diseases of heart	198	4.5	6.3
5. Malignant neoplasms	185	4.2	5.9
Black, males, 10–14 y			
All causes	516	100.0	28.6
1. Unintentional injuries	183	35.5	10.1
2. Homicide	60	11.6	3.3
3. Malignant neoplasms	44	8.5	2.4
4. Suicide	29	5.6	1.6
5. Diseases of heart	26	5.0	1.4
Black, males, 15–19 y			
All causes	2019	100.0	121.0
1. Homicide	915	45.3	54.8
2. Unintentional injuries	520	25.8	31.2
3. Suicide	124	6.1	7.4
4. Diseases of heart	80	4.0	4.8
5. Malignant neoplasms	69	3.4	4.1

(Continued)

Table 1.19
(Continued)

Race, Gender, Age, and Cause of Death	No. of Deaths	Percent of Total	Rate[a]
Black, males, 20–24 y			
All causes	3317	100.0	210.1
1. Homicide	1607	48.4	101.8
2. Unintentional injuries	708	21.3	44.8
3. Suicide	272	8.2	17.2
4. Diseases of heart	127	3.8	8.0
5. Malignant neoplasms	107	3.2	6.8
Black, females, 10–14 y			
All causes	383	100.0	21.9
1. Unintentional injuries	118	30.8	6.7
2. Malignant neoplasms	47	12.3	2.7
3. Diseases of heart	27	7.0	1.5
4. Homicide	27	7.0	1.5
5. Suicide	19	5.0	[c]
Black, females, 15–19 y			
All causes	661	100.0	40.7
1. Unintentional injuries	192	29.0	11.8
2. Homicide	127	19.2	7.8
3. Malignant neoplasms	57	8.6	3.5
4. Diseases of heart	38	5.7	2.3
5. Suicide	31	4.7	1.9
Black, females, 20–24 y			
All causes	1052	100.0	67.0
1. Unintentional injuries	241	22.9	15.4
2. Homicide	154	14.6	9.8
3. Malignant neoplasms	78	7.4	5.0
4. Diseases of heart	71	6.7	4.5
5. Pregnancy[d]	62	5.9	4.0
AI/AN, both genders, 10–14 y			
All causes	74	100.0	24.5
1. Unintentional injuries	39	52.7	12.9
2. Suicide	10	13.5	[c]
3. Homicide	4	5.4	[c]
4. Septicemia	2	2.7	[c]
5. Congenital malformations	2	2.7	[c]
AI/AN, both genders, 15–19 y			
All causes	260	100.0	87.0
1. Unintentional injuries	122	46.9	40.8
2. Suicide	69	26.5	23.1
3. Homicide	29	11.2	9.7
4. Diseases of heart	7	2.7	[c]
5. Malignant neoplasms	6	2.3	[c]

(Continued)

Table 1.19
(Continued)

Race, Gender, Age, and Cause of Death	No. of Deaths	Percent of Total	Rate[a]
AI/AN, both genders, 20–24 y			
All causes	333	100.0	116.6
1. Unintentional injuries	173	52.0	60.6
2. Suicide	53	15.9	18.6
3. Homicide	38	11.4	13.3
4. Malignant neoplasms	10	3.0	[c]
5. Diseases of heart	6	1.8	[c]
AI/AN, males, 10–14 y			
All causes	42	100.0	27.5
1. Unintentional injuries	22	52.4	14.4
2. Suicide	6	14.3	[c]
3. Homicide	2	4.8	[c]
4. Miscellaneous conditions (7) each associated with 1 death			
AI/AN, males 15–19 y			
All causes	171	100.0	112.5
1. Unintentional injuries	78	45.6	51.3
2. Suicide	49	28.7	32.2
3. Homicide	22	12.9	14.5
4. Malignant neoplasms	4	2.3	[c]
5. Congenital malformations	3	1.8	[c]
AI/AN, males, 20–24 y			
All causes	238	100.0	161.2
1. Unintentional injuries	125	52.5	84.7
2. Suicide	43	18.1	29.1
3. Homicide	31	13.0	21.0
4. Malignant neoplasms	5	2.1	[c]
5. Diseases of heart	3	1.3	[c]
AI/AN, females, 10–14 y			
All causes	32	100.0	21.5
1. Unintentional injuries	17	53.1	[c]
2. Suicide	4	12.5	[c]
3. Homicide	2	6.3	[c]
4. Septicemia	1	3.1	[c]
4. Congenital malformations	1	3.1	[c]
AI/AN, females, 15–19 y			
All causes	89	100.0	60.7
1. Unintentional injuries	44	49.4	30.0
2. Suicide	20	22.5	13.6
3. Homicide	7	7.9	[c]
4. Diseases of heart	5	5.6	[c]
5. Malignant neoplasms	2	2.2	[c]

(*Continued*)

Table 1.19
(Continued)

Race, Gender, Age, and Cause of Death	No. of Deaths	Percent of Total	Rate[a]
AI/AN, females, 20–24 y			
All causes	95	100.0	68.9
1. Unintentional injuries	48	50.5	34.8
2. Suicide	10	10.5	c
3. Homicide	7	7.4	c
4. Malignant neoplasms	5	5.3	c
5. Diseases of heart	3	3.2	c
API, both genders, 10–14 y			
All causes	116	100.0	12.7
1. Unintentional injuries	39	33.6	4.3
2. Malignant neoplasms	23	19.8	2.5
3. Suicide	8	6.9	c
4. Homicide	6	5.2	c
5. Congenital malformations	5	4.3	c
API, both genders, 15–19 y	316	100.0	34.7
1. Unintentional injuries	141	44.6	15.5
2. Suicide	51	16.1	5.6
3. Homicide	39	12.3	4.3
4. Malignant neoplasms	18	5.7	c
5. Congenital malformations	10	3.2	c
API, both genders, 20–24 y			
All causes	450	100.0	43.3
1. Unintentional injuries	178	39.6	17.1
2. Suicide	68	15.1	6.5
3. Homicide	50	11.1	4.8
4. Malignant neoplasms	41	9.1	3.9
5. Diseases of heart	23	5.1	2.2
API, males, 10–14 y			
All causes	69	100.0	14.7
1. Unintentional injuries	25	36.2	5.3
2. Malignant neoplasms	13	18.8	c
3. Suicide	8	11.6	c
4. Influenza/pneumonia	3	4.3	c
4. Congenital malformations	3	4.3	c
4. Homicide	3	4.3	c
API, males, 15–19 y			
All causes	221	100	47.2
1. Unintentional injuries	101	45.7	21.6
2. Suicide	40	18.1	8.5
3. Homicide	34	15.4	7.3
4. Malignant neoplasms	12	5.4	c
5. Diseases of heart	5	2.3	c

(Continued)

Table 1.19
(Continued)

Race, Gender, Age, and Cause of Death	No. of Deaths	Percent of Total	Rate[a]
API, males, 20–24 y			
All causes	315	100.0	59.9
1. Unintentional injuries	121	38.4	23.0
2. Suicide	52	16,5	9.9
3. Homicide	44	14.0	8.4
4. Malignant neoplasms	29	9.2	5.5
5. Diseases of heart	15	4.8	[c]
API, females, 10–14 y			
All causes	47	100.0	10.6
1. Unintentional injuries	14	29.8	[c]
2. Malignant neoplasms	10	21.3	[c]
3. Homicide	3	6.4	[c]
4. Pregnancy	2	4.3	[c]
4. Congenital malformations	2	4.3	[c]
API, females, 15–19 y			
All causes	95	100.0	21.5
1. Unintentional injuries	40	42.1	9.1
2. Suicide	11	11.6	[c]
3. Malignant neoplasms	6	6.3	[c]
4. Congenital malformations	5	5.3	[c]
4. Homicide	5	5.3	[c]
API, females, 20–24			
All causes	135	100.0	26.3
1. Unintentional injuries	57	42.2	11.1
2. Suicide	16	11.9	[c]
3. Malignant neoplasms	12	8.9	[c]
4. Diseases of heart	8	5.9	[c]
5. Cerebrovascular diseases/homicide	6/6	4.4/4.4	[c]
Hispanic, both genders, 10–14 y			
All causes	618	100.0	16.3
1. Unintentional injuries	213	34.5	5.6
2. Malignant neoplasms	112	18.1	3.0
3. Homicide	40	6.5	1.1
4. Suicide	39	6.3	1.0
5. Congenital malformations	34	5.5	0.9
Hispanic, both genders, 15–19 y			
All causes	2141	100.0	64.2
1. Unintentional injuries	956	44.7	28.7
2. Homicide	492	23.0	14.8
3. Suicide	214	10.0	6.4
4. Malignant neoplasms	137	6.4	4.1
5. Diseases of heart	43	2.0	1.3

(*Continued*)

Table 1.19
(Continued)

Race, Gender, Age, and Cause of Death	No. of Deaths	Percent of Total	Rate[a]
Hispanic, both genders, 20–24 y			
All causes	3287	100.0	87.3
1. Unintentional injuries	1416	43.1	37.6
2. Homicide	743	22.6	19.7
3. Suicide	357	10.9	9.5
4. Malignant neoplasms	168	5.1	4.5
5. Diseases of heart	86	2.6	2.3
Hispanic, males, 10–14 y			
All causes	383	100	19.8
1. Unintentional injuries	139	36.3	7.2
2. Malignant neoplasms	60	15.7	3.1
3. Homicide	28	7.3	1.4
4. Congenital malformations	25	6.5	1.3
5. Suicide	24	6.3	1.2
Hispanic, males, 15–19 y			
All causes	1662	100.0	96.5
1. Unintentional injuries	740	44.5	43.0
2. Homicide	445	26.8	25.8
3. Suicide	170	10.2	9.9
4. Malignant neoplasms	94	5.7	5.5
5. Diseases of heart	33	2.0	1.9
Hispanic, males, 20–24 y			
All causes	2714	100.0	130.9
1. Unintentional injuries	1186	43.7	57.2
2. Homicide	680	25.1	32.8
3. Suicide	317	11.7	15.3
4. Malignant neoplasms	113	4.2	5.5
5. Diseases of heart	68	2.5	3.3
Hispanic, females, 10–14 y			
All causes	235	100.0	12.7
1. Unintentional injuries	74	31.5	4.0
2. Malignant neoplasms	52	22.1	2.8
3. Suicide	15	6.4	[c]
4. Homicide	12	5.1	[c]
5. Congenital malformations	9	3.8	[c]
Hispanic, females, 15–19 y			
All causes	479	100.0	29.7
1. Unintentional injuries	216	45.1	13.4
2. Homicide	47	9.8	2.9
3. Suicide	44	9.2	2.7
4. Malignant neoplasms	43	9.0	2.7
5. Pregnancy	11	2.3	

(*Continued*)

Table 1.19
(Continued)

Race, Gender, Age, and Cause of Death	No. of Deaths	Percent of Total	Rate[a]
Hispanic, females, 20–24 y			
All causes	573	100.0	33.9
1. Unintentional injuries	230	40.1	13.6
2. Homicide	63	11.0	3.7
3. Malignant neoplasms	55	9.6	3.3
4. Suicide	40	7.0	2.4
5. Diseases of heart	18	3.1	[c]

AI/AN indicates American Indian/Alaska Native; API, Asian/Pacific Islander.

[a] Per 100 000 population in specified group.

[b] Congenital malformations, deformations, and chromosomal abnormalities.

[c] Figure does not meet standards of reliability or precision.

[d] Pregnancy, childbirth, and the puerperium.

Data source: Heron M. Deaths: leading causes for 2004. *Natl Vital Stat Rep*. 2007;56(5):1–95. Available at: www.cdc.gov/nchs/data/nvsr/nvsr56/nvsr56_05.pdf. Accessed March 19, 2009.

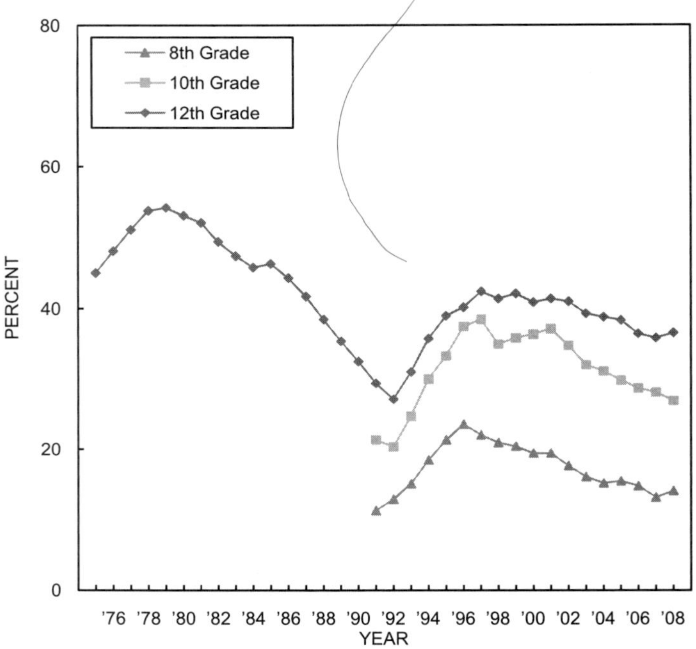

Fig 1.3. Trends in annual prevalence of an illicit drug-use index. Reproduced from: Johnston LD, O'Malley PM, Bachman JG, Schulenberg JE. Various stimulant drugs show continuing gradual declines among teens in 2008, most illicit drugs hold steady [press release]. Available at: www.monitoringthefuture.org/data/08data.html#2008data-drugs. Accessed April 11, 2009.

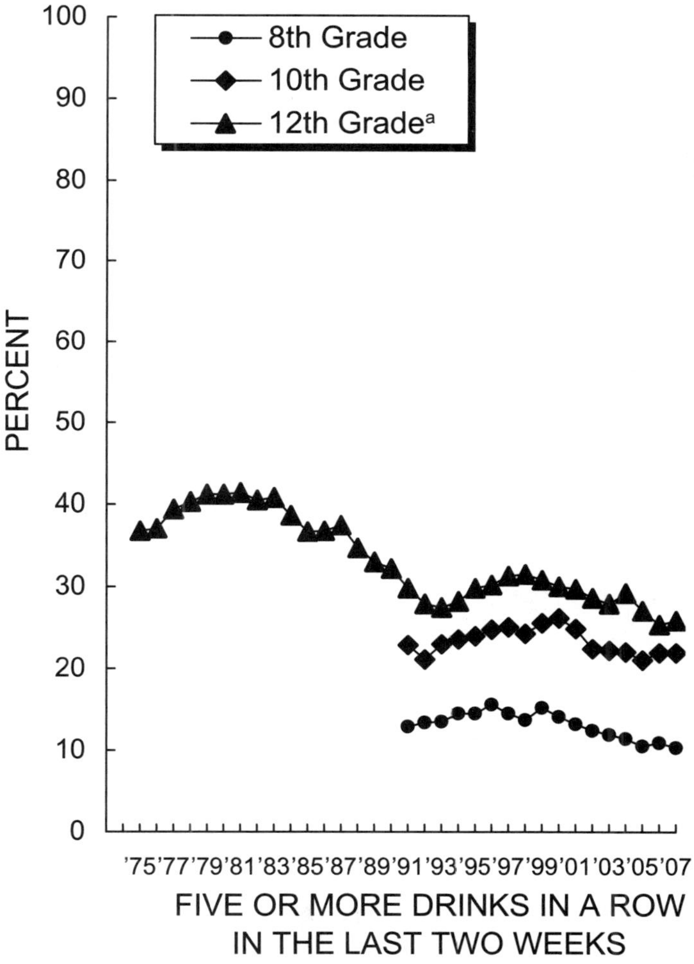

Fig 1.4. Alcohol: trends in 2-week prevalence of heavy drinking in grades 8, 10, and 12. [a]Due to a coding error, previously released versions of this figure contained values that were slightly off for the measure of ≥5 drinks in a row for 2005 and 2006. These values have been corrected here. Reproduced from: Johnston LD, O'Malley PM, Bachman JG, Schulenberg JE. *Monitoring the Future National Survey Results on Drug Use, 1975–2007: Volume I, Secondary School Students*. Bethesda, MD: National Institute on Drug Abuse; 2008:242. NIH publication No. 08-6418A. Available at: http://monitoringthefuture.org/pubs/monographs/vol1_2007.pdf. Accessed April 11, 2009.

Table 1.20

Trends in lifetime prevalence of use of various drugs in grades 8, 10, and 12

	Lifetime																		
	1991	1992	1993	1994	1995	1996	1997	1998	1999	2000	2001	2002	2003	2004	2005	2006	2007	2008	2007–2008 Change
Any illicit drug[a]																			
8th grade	18.7	20.6	22.5	25.7	28.5	31.2	29.4	29.0	28.3	26.8	26.8	24.5	22.8	21.5	21.4	20.9	19.0	19.6	0.6
10th grade	30.6	29.8	32.8	37.4	40.9	45.4	47.3	44.9	46.2	45.6	45.6	44.6	41.4	39.8	38.2	36.1	35.6	34.1	−1.6
12th grade	44.1	40.7	42.9	45.6	48.4	50.8	54.3	54.1	54.7	54.0	53.9	53.0	51.1	51.1	50.4	48.2	46.8	47.4	0.6
Any illicit drug other than marijuana[a,b]																			
8th grade	14.3	15.6	16.8	17.5	18.8	19.2	17.7	16.9	16.3	15.8[†]	17.0	13.7	13.6	12.2	12.1	12.2	11.1	11.2	0.1
10th grade	19.1	19.2	20.9	21.7	24.3	25.5	25.0	23.6	24.0	23.1[†]	23.6	22.1	19.7	18.8	18.0	17.5	18.2	15.9	−2.2s
12th grade	26.9	25.1	26.7	27.6	28.1	28.5	30.0	29.4	29.4	29.0[†]	30.7	29.5	27.7	28.7	27.4	26.9	25.5	24.9	−0.6
Any illicit drug including inhalants[a,c]																			
8th grade	28.5	29.6	32.3	35.1	38.1	39.4	38.1	37.8	37.2	35.1	34.5	31.6	30.3	30.2	30.0	29.2	27.7	28.3	0.6
10th grade	36.1	36.2	38.7	42.7	45.9	49.8	50.9	49.3	49.9	49.3	48.8	47.7	44.9	43.1	42.1	40.1	39.8	38.7	−1.2
12th grade	47.6	44.4	46.6	49.1	51.5	53.5	56.3	56.1	56.3	57.0	56.0	54.6	52.8	53.0	53.5	51.2	49.1	49.3	0.3
Marijuana/hashish																			
8th grade	10.2	11.2	12.6	16.7	19.9	23.1	22.6	22.2	22.0	20.3	20.4	19.2	17.5	16.3	16.5	15.7	14.2	14.6	0.4
10th grade	23.4	21.4	24.4	30.4	34.1	39.8	42.3	39.6	40.9	40.3	40.1	38.7	36.4	35.1	34.1	31.8	31.0	29.9	−1.1
12th grade	36.7	32.6	35.3	38.2	41.7	44.9	49.6	49.1	49.7	48.8	49.0	47.8	46.1	45.7	44.8	42.3	41.8	42.6	0.8
Inhalants[c,d]																			
8th grade	17.6	17.4	19.4	19.9	21.6	21.2	21.0	20.5	19.7	17.9	17.1	15.2	15.8	17.3	17.1	16.1	15.6	15.7	0.2
10th grade	15.7	16.6	17.5	18.0	19.0	19.3	18.3	18.3	17.0	16.6	15.2	13.5	12.7	12.4	13.1	13.3	13.6	12.8	−0.9
12th grade	17.6	16.6	17.4	17.7	17.4	16.6	16.1	15.2	15.4	14.2	13.0	11.7	11.2	10.9	11.4	11.1	10.5	9.9	−0.6

(Continued)

Table 1.20
(Continued)

	Lifetime																		
	1991	1992	1993	1994	1995	1996	1997	1998	1999	2000	2001	2002	2003	2004	2005	2006	2007	2008	2007–2008 Change
Nitrites[e]																			
8th grade	—	8	—	—	—	—	—	—	—	—	—	—	—	—	—	—	—	—	—
10th grade	—	1	—	—	—	—	—	—	—	—	—	—	—	—	—	—	—	—	—
12th grade	1.6	1.5	1.4	1.7	1.5	1.8	2.0	2.7	1.7	0.8	1.9	1.5	1.6	1.3	1.1	1.2	1.2	0.6	−0.7
Hallucinogens[b,f]																			
8th grade	3.2	3.8	3.9	4.3	5.2	5.9	5.4	4.9	4.8	4.6[†]	5.2	4.1	4.0	3.5	3.8	3.4	3.1	3.3	0.2
10th grade	6.1	6.4	6.8	8.1	9.3	10.5	10.5	9.8	9.7	8.9[†]	8.9	7.8	6.9	6.4	5.8	6.1	6.4	5.5	−0.9
12th grade	9.6	9.2	10.9	11.4	12.7	14.0	15.1	14.1	13.7	13.0[†]	14.7	12.0	10.6	9.7	8.8	8.3	8.4	8.7	0.4
LSD																			
8th grade	2.7	3.2	3.5	3.7	4.4	5.1	4.7	4.1	4.1	3.9	3.4	2.5	2.1	1.8	1.9	1.6	1.6	1.9	0.3
10th grade	5.6	5.8	6.2	7.2	8.4	9.4	9.5	8.5	8.5	7.6	6.3	5.0	3.5	2.8	2.5	2.7	3.0	2.6	−0.4
12th grade	8.8	8.6	10.3	10.5	11.7	12.6	13.6	12.6	12.2	11.1	10.9	8.4	5.9	4.6	3.5	3.3	3.4	4.0	0.5
Hallucinogens other than LSD[b]																			
8th grade	1.4	1.7	1.7	2.2	2.5	3.0	2.6	2.5	2.4	2.3[†]	3.9	3.3	3.2	3.0	3.3	2.8	2.6	2.5	−0.1
10th grade	2.2	2.5	2.8	3.8	3.9	4.7	4.8	5.0	4.7	4.8[†]	6.6	6.3	5.9	5.8	5.2	5.5	5.7	4.8	−0.9 s
12th grade	3.7	3.3	3.9	4.9	5.4	6.8	7.5	7.1	6.7	6.9[†]	10.4	9.2	9.0	8.7	8.1	7.8	7.7	7.8	0.1
PCP[e]																			
8th grade	—	8	—	—	—	—	—	—	—	—	—	—	—	—	—	—	—	—	—
10th grade	—	—	—	—	—	—	—	—	—	—	—	—	—	—	—	—	—	—	—
12th grade	2.9	2.4	2.9	2.8	2.7	4.0	3.9	3.9	3.4	3.4	3.5	3.1	2.5	1.6	2.4	2.2	2.1	1.8	−0.3
Ecstasy (MDMA)[g]																			
8th grade	—	8	—	—	—	3.4	3.2	2.7	2.7	4.3	5.2	4.3	3.2	2.8	2.8	2.5	2.3	2.4	0.1
10th grade	—	1	—	—	—	5.6	5.7	5.1	6.0	7.3	8.0	6.6	5.4	4.3	4.0	4.5	5.2	4.3	−1.0
12th grade	—	1	—	—	—	6.1	6.9	5.8	8.0	11.0	11.7	10.5	8.3	7.5	5.4	6.5	6.5	6.2	−0.3

(Continued)

Table 1.20
(Continued)

	Lifetime																		
	1991	1992	1993	1994	1995	1996	1997	1998	1999	2000	2001	2002	2003	2004	2005	2006	2007	2008	2007–2008 Change
Cocaine																			
8th grade	2.3	2.9	2.9	3.6	4.2	4.5	4.4	4.6	4.7	4.5	4.3	3.6	3.6	3.4	3.7	3.4	3.1	3.0	−0.1
10th grade	4.1	3.3	3.6	4.3	5.0	6.5	7.1	7.2	7.7	6.9	5.7	6.1	5.1	5.4	5.2	4.8	5.3	4.5	−0.8
12th grade	7.8	6.1	6.1	5.9	6.0	7.1	8.7	9.3	9.8	8.6	8.2	7.8	7.7	8.1	8.0	8.5	7.8	7.2	−0.6
Crack																			
8th grade	1.3	1.6	1.7	2.4	2.7	2.9	2.7	3.2	3.1	3.1	3.0	2.5	2.5	2.4	2.4	2.3	2.1	2.0	−0.1
10th grade	1.7	1.5	1.8	2.1	2.8	3.3	3.6	3.9	4.0	3.7	3.1	3.6	2.7	2.6	2.5	2.2	2.3	2.0	−0.3
12th grade	3.1	2.6	2.6	3.0	3.0	3.3	3.9	4.4	4.6	3.9	3.7	3.8	3.6	3.9	3.5	3.5	3.2	2.8	−0.5
Other cocaine[h]																			
8th grade	2.0	2.4	2.4	3.0	3.4	3.8	3.5	3.7	3.8	3.5	3.3	2.8	2.7	2.6	2.9	2.7	2.6	2.4	−0.2
10th grade	3.8	3.0	3.3	3.8	4.4	5.5	6.1	6.4	6.8	6.0	5.0	5.2	4.5	4.8	4.6	4.3	4.8	4.0	−0.8
12th grade	7.0	5.3	5.4	5.2	5.1	6.4	8.2	8.4	8.8	7.7	7.4	7.0	6.7	7.3	7.1	7.9	6.8	6.5	−0.4
Heroin[i]																			
8th grade	1.2	1.4	1.4	2.0	2.3	2.4	2.1	2.3	2.3	1.9	1.7	1.6	1.6	1.6	1.5	1.4	1.3	1.4	0.0
10th grade	1.2	1.2	1.3	1.5	1.7	2.1	2.1	2.3	2.3	2.2	1.7	1.8	1.5	1.5	1.5	1.4	1.5	1.2	−0.4 s
12th grade	0.9	1.2	1.1	1.2	1.6	1.8	2.1	2.0	2.0	2.4	1.8	1.7	1.5	1.5	1.5	1.4	1.5	1.3	−0.3
With a needle[j]																			
8th grade	—	—	—	—	1.5	1.6	1.3	1.4	1.6	1.1	1.2	1.0	1.0	1.1	1.0	1.0	0.9	0.9	0.0
10th grade	−1	—	—	—	1.0	1.1	1.1	1.2	1.3	1.0	0.8	1.0	0.9	0.8	0.8	0.9	0.9	0.7	−0.2
12th grade	−1	—	—	—	0.7	0.8	0.9	0.8	0.9	0.8	0.7	0.8	0.7	0.7	0.9	0.8	0.7	0.7	0.0
Without a needle[j]																			
8th grade	—	—	—	—	1.5	1.6	1.4	1.5	1.4	1.3	1.1	1.0	1.1	1.0	0.9	0.9	0.7	0.9	0.2
10th grade	−1	—	—	—	1.1	1.7	1.7	1.7	1.6	1.7	1.3	1.3	1.0	1.1	1.1	1.0	1.1	0.8	−0.2
12th grade	−1	—	—	—	1.4	1.7	2.1	1.6	1.8	2.4	1.5	1.6	1.8	1.4	1.3	1.1	1.4	1.1	−0.3

(Continued)

Table 1.20
(Continued)

	Lifetime																		
	1991	1992	1993	1994	1995	1996	1997	1998	1999	2000	2001	2002	2003	2004	2005	2006	2007	2008	2007–2008 Change
Narcotics other than heroin[k,l]																			
8th grade	−8	—	—	—	—	—	—	—	—	—	—	—	—	—	—	—	—	—	
10th grade	−1	—	—	—	—	—	—	—	—	—	—	—	—	—	—	—	—	—	—
12th grade	6.6	6.1	6.4	6.6	7.2	8.2	9.7	9.8	10.2	10.6	9.9[‡]	13.5	13.2	13.5	12.8	13.4	13.1	13.2	0.1
Amphetamines[k]																			
8th grade	10.5	10.8	11.8	12.3	13.1	13.5	12.3	11.3	10.7	9.9	10.2	8.7	8.4	7.5	7.4	7.3	6.5	6.8	0.3
10th grade	13.2	13.1	14.9	15.1	17.4	17.7	17.0	16.0	15.7	15.7	16.0	14.9	13.1	11.9	11.1	11.2	11.1	9.0	−2.1 ss
12th grade	15.4	13.9	15.1	15.7	15.3	15.3	16.5	16.4	16.3	15.6	16.2	16.8	14.4	15.0	13.1	12.4	11.4	10.5	−0.9
Methamphetamine[m,n]																			
8th grade	−8	—	—	—	—	—	—	—	4.5	4.2	4.4	3.5	3.9	2.5	3.1	2.7	1.8	2.3	0.5
10th grade	−1	—	—	—	—	—	—	—	7.3	6.9	6.4	6.1	5.2	5.3	4.1	3.2	2.8	2.4	−0.4
12th grade	−1	—	—	—	—	—	—	—	8.2	7.9	6.9	6.7	6.2	6.2	4.5	4.4	3.0	2.8	−0.3
Crystal meth (ice)[n]																			
8th grade	—	—	—	—	—	—	—	—	—	—	—	—	—	—	—	—	—	—	—
10th grade	−1	—	—	—	—	—	—	—	—	—		—	—	—	—	—	—	—	—
12th grade	3.3	2.9	3.1	3.4	3.9	4.4	4.4	5.3	4.8	4.0	4.1	4.7	3.9	4.0	4.0	3.4	3.4	2.8	−0.6
Sedatives (barbiturates)[k]																			
8th grade	−8	—	—	—	—	—	—	—	—	—	—	—	—	—	—	—	—	—	
10th grade	−1	—	—	—	—	—	—	—	—	—	—	—	—	—	—	—	—	—	—
12th grade	6.2	5.5	6.3	7.0	7.4	7.6	8.1	8.7	8.9	9.2	8.7	9.5	8.8	9.9	10.5	10.2	9.3	8.5	−0.9
Methaqualone[e,k]																			
8th grade	−8	—	—	—	—	—	—	—	—	—	—	—	—	—	—	—	—	—	
10th grade	−1	—	—	—	—	—	—	—	—	—	—	—	—	—	—	—	—	—	—
12th grade	1.3	1.6	0.8	1.4	1.2	2.0	1.7	1.6	1.8	0.8	1.1	1.5	1.0	1.3	1.3	1.2	1.0	0.8	−0.2

(Continued)

Table 1.20
(Continued)

	Lifetime																		
	1991	1992	1993	1994	1995	1996	1997	1998	1999	2000	2001	2002	2003	2004	2005	2006	2007	2008	2007–2008 Change
Tranquilizers[b,k]																			
8th grade	3.8	4.1	4.4	4.6	4.5	5.3	4.8	4.6	4.4	4.4‡	5.0	4.3	4.4	4.0	4.1	4.3	3.9	3.9	0.0
10th grade	5.8	5.9	5.7	5.4	6.0	7.1	7.3	7.8	7.9	8.0‡	9.2	8.8	7.8	7.3	7.1	7.2	7.4	6.8	−0.6
12th grade	7.2	6.0	6.4	6.6	7.1	7.2	7.8	8.5	9.3	8.9‡	10.3	11.4	10.2	10.6	9.9	10.3	9.5	8.9	−0.6
Rohypnol[o]																			
8th grade	−8	—	—	—	—	1.5	1.1	1.4	1.3	1.0	1.1	0.8	1.0	1.0	1.1	1.0	1.0	0.7	−0.3
10th grade	−1	—	—	—	—	1.5	1.7	2.0	1.8	1.3	1.5	1.3	1.0	1.2	1.0	0.8	1.3	0.9	−0.4
12th grade	−1	—	—	—	—	1.2	1.8	3.0	2.0	1.5	1.7	—	—	—	—	—	—	—	
Alcohol[p]																			
Any use																			
8th grade	70.1	69.3‡	55.7	55.8	54.5	55.3	53.8	52.5	52.1	51.7	50.5	47.0	45.6	43.9	41.0	40.5	38.9	38.9	0.1
10th grade	83.8	82.3‡	71.6	71.1	70.5	71.8	72.0	69.8	70.6	71.4	70.1	66.9	66.0	64.2	63.2	61.5	61.7	58.3	−3.4 ss
12th grade	88.0	87.5‡	80.0	80.4	80.7	79.2	81.7	81.4	80.0	80.3	79.7	78.4	76.6	76.8	75.1	72.7	72.2	71.9	−0.2
Been drunk[n]																			
8th grade	26.7	26.8	26.4	25.9	25.3	26.8	25.2	24.8	24.8	25.1	23.4	21.3	20.3	19.9	19.5	19.5	17.9	18.0	0.1
10th grade	50.0	47.7	47.9	47.2	46.9	48.5	49.4	46.7	48.9	49.3	48.2	44.0	42.4	42.3	42.1	41.4	41.2	37.2	−4.0 sss
12th grade	65.4	63.4	62.5	62.9	63.2	61.8	64.2	62.4	62.3	62.3	63.9	61.6	58.1	60.3	57.5	56.4	55.1	54.7	−0.4
Flavored alcoholic beverages[e,m]																			
8th grade	−8	—	—	—	—	—	—	—	—	—	—	—	—	37.9	35.5	35.5	34.0	32.8	−1.3
10th grade	−1	—	—	—	—	—	—	—	—	—	—	—	—	58.6	58.8	58.1	55.7	53.5	−2.3
12th grade	—	—	—	—	—	—	—	—	—	—	—	—	—	71.0	73.6	69.9	68.4	65.5	−2.9

(Continued)

Table 1.20
(Continued)

	Lifetime																		
	1991	1992	1993	1994	1995	1996	1997	1998	1999	2000	2001	2002	2003	2004	2005	2006	2007	2008	2007–2008 Change
Cigarettes																			
Any use																			
8th grade	44.0	45.2	45.3	46.1	46.4	49.2	47.3	45.7	44.1	40.5	36.6	31.4	28.4	27.9	25.9	24.6	22.1	20.5	−1.7
10th grade	55.1	53.5	56.3	56.9	57.6	61.2	60.2	57.7	57.6	55.1	52.8	47.4	43.0	40.7	38.9	36.1	34.6	31.7	−2.9 ss
12th grade	63.1	61.8	61.9	62.0	64.2	63.5	65.4	65.3	64.6	62.5	61.0	57.2	53.7	52.8	50.0	47.1	46.2	44.7	−1.5
Smokeless tobacco[q]																			
8th grade	22.2	20.7	18.7	19.9	20.0	20.4	16.8	15.0	14.4	12.8	11.7	11.2	11.3	11.0	10.1	10.2	9.1	9.8	0.8
10th grade	28.2	26.6	28.1	29.2	27.6	27.4	26.3	22.7	20.4	19.1	19.5	16.9	14.6	13.8	14.5	15.0	15.1	12.2	−2.9 ss
12th grade	—	32.4	31.0	30.7	30.9	29.8	25.3	26.2	23.4	23.1	19.7	18.3	17.0	16.7	17.5	15.2	15.1	15.6	0.5
Steroids[r]																			
8th grade	1.9	1.7	1.6	2.0	2.0	1.8	1.8	2.3	2.7	3.0	2.8	2.5	2.5	1.9	1.7	1.6	1.5	1.4	−0.2
10th grade	1.8	1.7	1.7	1.8	2.0	1.8	2.0	2.0	2.7	3.5	3.5	3.5	3.0	2.4	2.0	1.8	1.8	1.4	−0.4
12th grade	2.1	2.1	2.0	2.4	2.3	1.9	2.4	2.7	2.9	2.5	3.7	4.0	3.5	3.4	2.6	2.7	2.2	2.2	0.0

Level of significance of difference between the 2 most recent classes: s = .05; ss = .01; and sss = .001. — indicates data not available; ‡, some change in the question (see relevant footnote for that drug; any apparent inconsistency between the change estimate and the prevalence estimates for the 2 most recent years is a result of rounding).

Approximate Weighted *N*s	1991	1992	1993	1994	1995	1996	1997	1998	1999	2000	2001	2002	2003	2004	2005	2006	2007	2008
8th-graders	17 500	18 600	18 300	17 300	17 500	17 800	18 600	18 100	16 700	16 700	16 200	15 100	16 500	17 000	16 800	16 500	16 100	15 700
10th-graders	14 800	14 800	15 300	15 800	17 000	15 600	15 500	15 000	13 600	14 300	14 000	14 300	15 800	16 400	16 200	16 200	16 100	15 100
12th-graders	15 000	15 800	16 300	15 400	15 400	14 300	15 400	15 200	13 600	12 800	12 800	12 900	14 600	14 600	14 700	14 200	14 500	14 000

(Continued)

Table 1.20
(Continued)

[a] For 12th-graders only: use of “any illicit drug” includes any use of marijuana, LSD, other hallucinogens, crack, other cocaine, or heroin; or any use of narcotics other than heroin, amphetamines, sedatives (barbiturates), or tranquilizers not under a doctor’s orders. For 8th- and 10th-graders only: the use of narcotics other than heroin and sedatives (barbiturates) has been excluded because these younger respondents seem to overreport use (perhaps because they include the use of nonprescription drugs in their answers).

[b] In 2001 the question text was changed on half of the questionnaire forms for each age group. “Other psychedelics” was changed to “other hallucinogens,” and “shrooms” was added to the list of examples. For the tranquilizer list of examples, Miltown was replaced with Xanax. For 8th-, 10th-, and 12th-graders: the 2001 data presented here are based on the changed forms only; *N* is one half of *N* indicated. In 2002 the remaining forms were changed to the new wording. The data are based on all forms beginning in 2002. Data for any illicit drug other than marijuana and data for hallucinogens are also affected by these changes and have been handled in a parallel manner.

[c] For 12th-graders only: data are based on 5 of 6 forms in 1991–1998; *N* is five sixths of *N* indicated. Data are based on 3 of 6 forms beginning in 1999; *N* is three sixths of *N* indicated.

[d] Inhalants are unadjusted for underreporting of amyl and butyl nitrites.

[e] For 12th-graders only: data are based on 1 of 6 forms; *N* is one sixth of *N* indicated.

[f] Hallucinogens are unadjusted for underreporting of PCP.

[g] For 8th- and 10th-graders only: data are based on 1 of 2 forms in 1996; *N* is one half of *N* indicated. Data are based on one third of *N* indicated in 1997–2001 due to changes in the questionnaire forms. Data are based on 2 of 4 forms beginning in 2002; *N* is one half of *N* indicated. For 12th-graders only: data are based on 1 of 6 forms in 1996–2001; *N* is one sixth of *N* indicated. Data based on 2 of 6 forms beginning in 2002; *N* is two sixths of *N* indicated.

[h] For 12th-graders only: data are based on 4 of 6 forms; *N* is four sixths of *N* indicated.

[i] In 1995 the heroin question was changed in 1 of 2 forms for 8th- and 10th-graders and in 3 of 6 forms for 12th-graders. Separate questions were asked for use with and without injection. In 1996, the heroin question was changed in all remaining 8th- and 10th-grade forms. Data presented here represent the combined data from all forms.

[j] For 8th- and 10th-graders only: data are based on 1 of 2 forms in 1995; *N* is one half of *N* indicated. Data are based on all forms beginning in 1996. For 12th-graders only: data are based on 3 of 6 forms; *N* is three sixths of *N* indicated.

[k] Only drug use not under a doctor’s orders is included here.

(*Continued*)

Table 1.20
(Continued)

[l] In 2002 the question text was changed in half of the questionnaire forms. The list of examples of narcotics other than heroin was updated: Talwin, laudanum, and paregoric (all of which had negligible rates of use by 2001) were replaced with Vicodin, OxyContin, and Percocet. The 2002 data presented here are based on the changed forms only; *N* is one half of *N* indicated. In 2003, the remaining forms were changed to the new wording. The data are based on all forms beginning in 2003.
[m] For 8th- and 10th-graders only: data are based on 1 of 4 forms; *N* is one third of *N* indicated.
[n] For 12th-graders only: data are based on 2 of 6 forms; *N* is 2 sixths of *N* indicated.
[o] For 8th- and 10th-graders only: data are based on 1 of 2 forms in 1996; *N* is one half of *N* indicated. Data are based on 3 of 4 forms in 1997–1998; *N* is two thirds of *N* indicated. Data based on 2 of 4 forms in 1999–2001; *N* is one third of *N* indicated. Data are based on 1 of 4 forms beginning in 2002; *N* is one sixth of *N* indicated. For 12th-graders only: data are based on 1 of 6 forms in 1996–2001; *N* is one sixth of *N* indicated. Data are based on 2 of 6 forms beginning in 2002; *N* is two sixths of *N* indicated. Data for 2001 and 2002 are not comparable because of changes in the questionnaire forms.
[p] For 8th-, 10th-, and 12th-graders: in 1993, the question text was changed slightly in half of the forms to indicate that a "drink" meant "more than just a few sips." The 1993 data are based on the changed forms only; *N* is one half of *N* indicated for these groups. In 1994 the remaining forms were changed to the new wording. The data are based on all forms beginning in 1994. In 2004, the question text was changed slightly in half of the forms. An examination of the data did not show any effect from the wording change. The remaining forms were changed in 2005.
[q] For 8th- and 10th-graders only: data are based on 1 of 2 forms for 1991–1996 and on 2 of 4 forms beginning in 1997; *N* is one half of *N* indicated. For 12th-graders only: data are based on 1 of 6 forms; *N* is one sixth of *N* indicated.
[r] For 8th-, 10th-, and 12th-graders: in 2006, the question text was changed slightly in some of the forms. An examination of the data did not show any effect from the wording change. In 2007 the remaining forms were changed in a like manner. In 2008 the question text was changed slightly. An examination of the data did not show any effect from the wording change. For 12th-graders only: data are based on 2 of 6 forms in 1991–2005; *N* is two sixths of *N* indicated. Data are based on 3 of 6 forms beginning in 2006; *N* is three sixths of *N* indicated.
[s] For 12th-graders only: data are based on 2 of 6 forms in 2002–2005; *N* is two sixths of *N* indicated. Data are based on 3 of 6 forms beginning in 2006; *N* is three sixths of *N* indicated.
[t] For 12th-graders only: data based on 2 of 6 forms in 2000; *N* is two sixths of *N* indicated. Data based on 3 of 6 forms in 2001; *N* is three sixths of *N* indicated. Data are based on 1 of 6 forms beginning in 2002; *N* is one sixth of *N* indicated.
[u] Data are based on 2 of 6 forms in 2000; *N* is two sixths of *N* indicated. Data are based on 3 of 6 forms beginning in 2001; *N* is three sixths of *N* indicated.
[v] The 2003 flavored alcoholic beverage data were created by adjusting the 2004 data to reflect the change in the 2003 and 2004 "alcopops" data.

(*Continued*)

Table 1.20
(Continued)

[w] Daily use is defined as use on ≥20 occasions in the past 30 days except for cigarettes and smokeless tobacco, for which actual daily use is measured, and for ≥5 drinks, for which the prevalence of having ≥5 drinks in a row in the last 2 weeks is measured.

[x] For 12th-graders only: because of a coding error, previously released versions of this table contained values that were slightly off for the measure of ≥5 drinks in a row for 2005 and 2006; these have been corrected here. For 8th- and 10th-graders only: the 1991–2007 estimates for ≥5 drinks in a row differ slightly from some previous reports because of a consistent error in the data-editing process before 2008. The revised data, which have been entered into this table for those years (1991–2007) average ~2 percentage points lower than those previously reported.

Johnston LD, O'Malley PM, Bachman JG, Schulenberg JE. *Monitoring the Future National Results on Adolescent Drug Use: Overview of Key Findings, 2008*. Bethesda, MD: National Institute on Drug Abuse. 2009. NIH publication No. 09–7401 Available at: http://monitoringthefuture.org/pubs/monographs/overview2008.pdf. Accessed April 11, 2009.

Table 1.21
Trends in annual prevalence of use of various drugs in grades 8, 10, and 12

	Annual																		2007–2008 Change
	1991	1992	1993	1994	1995	1996	1997	1998	1999	2000	2001	2002	2003	2004	2005	2006	2007	2008	
Any illicit drug[a]																			
8th grade	11.3	12.9	15.1	18.5	21.4	23.6	22.1	21.0	20.5	19.5	19.5	17.7	16.1	15.2	15.5	14.8	13.2	14.1	0.8
10th grade	21.4	20.4	24.7	30.0	33.3	37.5	38.5	35.0	35.9	36.4	37.2	34.8	32.0	31.1	29.8	28.7	28.1	26.9	−1.2
12th grade	29.4	27.1	31.0	35.8	39.0	40.2	42.4	41.4	42.1	40.9	41.4	41.0	39.3	38.8	38.4	36.5	35.9	36.6	0.6
Any illicit drug other than marijuana[a,b]																			
8th grade	8.4	9.3	10.4	11.3	12.6	13.1	11.8	11.0	10.5	10.2‡	10.8	8.8	8.8	7.9	8.1	7.7	7.0	7.4	0.4
10th grade	12.2	12.3	13.9	15.2	17.5	18.4	18.2	16.6	16.7	16.7‡	17.9	15.7	13.8	13.5	12.9	12.7	13.1	11.3	−1.7 s
12th grade	16.2	14.9	17.1	18.0	19.4	19.8	20.7	20.2	20.7	20.4‡	21.6	20.9	19.8	20.5	19.7	19.2	18.5	18.3	−0.3
Any illicit drug including inhalants[a,c]																			
8th grade	16.7	18.2	21.1	24.2	27.1	28.7	27.2	26.2	25.3	24.0	23.9	21.4	20.4	20.2	20.4	19.7	18.0	19.0	1.0
10th grade	23.9	23.5	27.4	32.5	35.6	39.6	40.3	37.1	37.7	38.0	38.7	36.1	33.5	32.9	31.7	30.7	30.2	28.8	−1.3
12th grade	31.2	28.8	32.5	37.6	40.2	41.9	43.3	42.4	42.8	42.5	42.6	42.1	40.5	39.1	40.3	38.0	37.0	37.3	0.3
Marijuana/hashish																			
8th grade	6.2	7.2	9.2	13.0	15.8	18.3	17.7	16.9	16.5	15.6	15.4	14.6	12.8	11.8	12.2	11.7	10.3	10.9	0.6
10th grade	16.5	15.2	19.2	25.2	28.7	33.6	34.8	31.1	32.1	32.2	32.7	30.3	28.2	27.5	26.6	25.2	24.6	23.9	−0.6
12th grade	23.9	21.9	26.0	30.7	34.7	35.8	38.5	37.5	37.8	36.5	37.0	36.2	34.9	34.3	33.6	31.5	31.7	32.4	0.7
Inhalants[c,d]																			
8th grade	9.0	9.5	11.0	11.7	12.8	12.2	11.8	11.1	10.3	9.4	9.1	7.7	8.7	9.6	9.5	9.1	8.3	8.9	0.6
10th grade	7.1	7.5	8.4	9.1	9.6	9.5	8.7	8.0	7.2	7.3	6.6	5.8	5.4	5.9	6.0	6.5	6.6	5.9	−0.7
12th grade	6.6	6.2	7.0	7.7	8.0	7.6	6.7	6.2	5.6	5.9	4.5	4.5	3.9	4.2	5.0	4.5	3.7	3.8	0.1

(Continued)

Table 1.21
(Continued)

	Annual																		2007–2008 Change
	1991	1992	1993	1994	1995	1996	1997	1998	1999	2000	2001	2002	2003	2004	2005	2006	2007	2008	
Nitrites[e]																			
8th grade	—	8	—	—	—	—	—	—	—	—	—	—	—	—	—	—	—	—	—
10th grade	—	1	—	—	—	—	—	—	—	—	—	—	—	—	—	—	—	—	—
12th grade	0.9	0.5	0.9	1.1	1.1	1.6	1.2	1.4	0.9	0.6	0.6	1.1	0.9	0.8	0.6	0.5	0.8	0.6	−0.2
Hallucinogens[b,f]																			
8th grade	1.9	2.5	2.6	2.7	3.6	4.1	3.7	3.4	2.9	2.8‡	3.4	2.6	2.6	2.2	2.4	2.1	1.9	2.1	0.2
10th grade	4.0	4.3	4.7	5.8	7.2	7.8	7.6	6.9	6.9	6.1‡	6.2	4.7	4.1	4.1	4.0	4.1	4.4	3.9	−0.5
12th grade	5.8	5.9	7.4	7.6	9.3	10.1	9.8	9.0	9.4	8.1‡	9.1	6.6	5.9	6.2	5.5	4.9	5.4	5.9	0.5
LSD																			
8th grade	1.7	2.1	2.3	2.4	3.2	3.5	3.2	2.8	2.4	2.4	2.2	1.5	1.3	1.1	1.2	0.9	1.1	1.3	0.2
10th grade	3.7	4.0	4.2	5.2	6.5	6.9	6.7	5.9	6.0	5.1	4.1	2.6	1.7	1.6	1.5	1.7	1.9	1.8	−0.1
12th grade	5.2	5.6	6.8	6.9	8.4	8.8	8.4	7.6	8.1	6.6	6.6	3.5	1.9	2.2	1.8	1.7	2.1	2.7	0.6
Hallucinogens other than LSD[b]																			
8th grade	0.7	1.1	1.0	1.3	1.7	2.0	1.8	1.6	1.5	1.4‡	2.4	2.1	2.1	1.9	2.0	1.8	1.6	1.6	0.0
10th grade	1.3	1.4	1.9	2.4	2.8	3.3	3.3	3.4	3.2	3.1‡	4.3	4.0	3.6	3.7	3.5	3.7	3.8	3.3	−0.5
12th grade	2.0	1.7	2.2	3.1	3.8	4.4	4.6	4.6	4.3	4.4‡	5.9	5.4	5.4	5.6	5.0	4.6	4.8	5.0	0.2
PCP[e]																			
8th grade	−8	—	—	—	—	—	—	—	—	—	—	—	—	—	—	—	—	—	
10th grade	−1	—	—	—	—	—	—	—	—	—	—	—	—	—	—	—	—	—	
12th grade	1.4	1.4	1.4	1.6	1.8	2.6	2.3	2.1	1.8	2.3	1.8	1.1	1.3	0.7	1.3	0.7	0.9	1.1	0.2
Ecstasy (MDMA)[g]																			
8th grade	−8	—	—	—	—	2.3	2.3	1.8	1.7	3.1	3.5	2.9	2.1	1.7	1.7	1.4	1.5	1.7	0.2
10th grade	−1	—	—	—	—	4.6	3.9	3.3	4.4	5.4	6.2	4.9	3.0	2.4	2.6	2.8	3.5	2.9	−0.6
12th grade	−1	—	—	—	—	4.6	4.0	3.6	5.6	8.2	9.2	7.4	4.5	4.0	3.0	4.1	4.5	4.3	−0.2

(Continued)

Table 1.21
(Continued)

	Annual																		2007–2008 Change
	1991	1992	1993	1994	1995	1996	1997	1998	1999	2000	2001	2002	2003	2004	2005	2006	2007	2008	
Cocaine																			
8th grade	1.1	1.5	1.7	2.1	2.6	3.0	2.8	3.1	2.7	2.6	2.5	2.3	2.2	2.0	2.2	2.0	2.0	1.8	−0.2
10th grade	2.2	1.9	2.1	2.8	3.5	4.2	4.7	4.7	4.9	4.4	3.6	4.0	3.3	3.7	3.5	3.2	3.4	3.0	−0.5
12th grade	3.5	3.1	3.3	3.6	4.0	4.9	5.5	5.7	6.2	5.0	4.8	5.0	4.8	5.3	5.1	5.7	5.2	4.4	−0.8
Crack																			
8th grade	0.7	0.9	1.0	1.3	1.6	1.8	1.7	2.1	1.8	1.8	1.7	1.6	1.6	1.3	1.4	1.3	1.3	1.1	−0.2
10th grade	0.9	0.9	1.1	1.4	1.8	2.1	2.2	2.5	2.4	2.2	1.8	2.3	1.6	1.7	1.7	1.3	1.3	1.3	−0.1
12th grade	1.5	1.5	1.5	1.9	2.1	2.1	2.4	2.5	2.7	2.2	2.1	2.3	2.2	2.3	1.9	2.1	1.9	1.6	−0.4 s
Other cocaine[h]																			
8th grade	1.0	1.2	1.3	1.7	2.1	2.5	2.2	2.4	2.3	1.9	1.9	1.8	1.6	1.6	1.7	1.6	1.5	1.4	−0.1
10th grade	2.1	1.7	1.8	2.4	3.0	3.5	4.1	4.0	4.4	3.8	3.0	3.4	2.8	3.3	3.0	2.9	3.1	2.6	−0.5
12th grade	3.2	2.6	2.9	3.0	3.4	4.2	5.0	4.9	5.8	4.5	4.4	4.4	4.2	4.7	4.5	5.2	4.5	4.0	−0.5
Heroin[i]																			
8th grade	0.7	0.7	0.7	1.2	1.4	1.6	1.3	1.3	1.4	1.1	1.0	0.9	0.9	1.0	0.8	0.8	0.8	0.9	0.0
10th grade	0.5	0.6	0.7	0.9	1.1	1.2	1.4	1.4	1.4	1.4	0.9	1.1	0.7	0.9	0.9	0.9	0.8	0.8	0.0
12th grade	0.4	0.6	0.5	0.6	1.1	1.0	1.2	1.0	1.1	1.5	0.9	1.0	0.8	0.9	0.8	0.8	0.9	0.7	−0.2
With a needle[j]																			
8th grade	—	—	—	—	0.9	1.0	0.8	0.8	0.9	0.6	0.7	0.6	0.6	0.7	0.6	0.5	0.6	0.5	0.0
10th grade	−1	—	—	—	0.6	0.7	0.7	0.8	0.6	0.5	0.4	0.6	0.5	0.5	0.5	0.5	0.5	0.5	0.0
12th grade	−1	—	—	—	0.5	0.5	0.5	0.4	0.4	0.4	0.3	0.4	0.4	0.4	0.5	0.5	0.4	0.4	0.0
Without a needle[j]																			
8th grade	—	—	—	—	0.8	1.0	0.8	0.8	0.9	0.7	0.6	0.6	0.6	0.6	0.5	0.5	0.5	0.6	0.1
10th grade	−1	—	—	—	0.8	0.9	1.1	1.0	1.1	1.1	0.7	0.8	0.5	0.7	0.7	0.6	0.6	0.6	0.0
12th grade	−1	—	—	—	1.0	1.0	1.2	0.8	1.0	1.6	0.8	0.8	0.8	0.7	0.8	0.6	1.0	0.5	−0.5 ss

(Continued)

Table 1.21
(Continued)

	Annual																		2007–2008 Change
	1991	1992	1993	1994	1995	1996	1997	1998	1999	2000	2001	2002	2003	2004	2005	2006	2007	2008	
Narcotics other than heroin[k,l]																			
8th grade	−8		—	—	—	—	—	—	—	—	—	—	—	—	—	—	—	—	
10th grade	−1	—	—	—	—	—	—	—	—	—	—	—	—	—	—	—	—	—	—
12th grade	3.5	3.3	3.6	3.8	4.7	5.4	6.2	6.3	6.7	7.0	6.7‡	9.4	9.3	9.5	9.0	9.0	9.2	9.1	0.0
OxyContin[m,s]																			
8th grade	−8	—	—	—	—	—	—	—	—	—	—	1.3	1.7	1.7	1.8	2.6	1.8	2.1	0.3
10th grade	−1	—	—	—	—	—	—	—	—	—	3.0	3.6	3.5	3.2	3.8	3.9	3.6	−0.3	
12th grade	−1	—	—	—	—	—	—	—	—	—	—	4.0	4.5	5.0	5.5	4.3	5.2	4.7	−0.5
Vicodin[m,s]																			
8th grade	−8	—	—	—	—	—	—	—	—	—	—	2.5	2.8	2.5	2.6	3.0	2.7	2.9	0.2
10th grade	−1	—	—	—	—	—	—	—	—	—	6.9	7.2	6.2	5.9	7.0	7.2	6.7	−0.5	
12th grade	−1	—	—	—	—	—	—	—	—	—	—	9.6	10.5	9.3	9.5	9.7	9.6	9.7	0.1
Amphetamines[k]																			
8th grade	6.2	6.5	7.2	7.9	8.7	9.1	8.1	7.2	6.9	6.5	6.7	5.5	5.5	4.9	4.9	4.7	4.2	4.5	0.3
10th grade	8.2	8.2	9.6	10.2	11.9	12.4	12.1	10.7	10.4	11.1	11.7	10.7	9.0	8.5	7.8	7.9	8.0	6.4	−1.6 ss
12th grade	8.2	7.1	8.4	9.4	9.3	9.5	10.2	10.1	10.2	10.5	10.9	11.1	9.9	10.0	8.6	8.1	7.5	6.8	−0.7
Ritalin[m,n]																			
8th grade	−8	—	—	—	—	—	—	—	—	—	2.9	2.8	2.6	2.5	2.4	2.6	2.1	1.6	−0.4
10th grade	−1	—	—	—	—	—	—	—	—	—	4.8	4.8	4.1	3.4	3.4	3.6	2.8	2.9	0.2
12th grade	−1	—	—	—	—	—	—	—	—	—	5.1	4.0	4.0	5.1	4.4	4.4	3.8	3.4	−0.4
Methamphetamine[m,n]																			
8th grade	−8	—	—	—	—	—	—	—	3.2	2.5	2.8	2.2	2.5	1.5	1.8	1.8	1.1	1.2	0.1
10th grade	−1	—	—	—	—	—	—	—	4.6	4.0	3.7	3.9	3.3	3.0	2.9	1.8	1.6	1.5	−0.1
12th grade	−1	—	—	—	—	—	—	—	4.7	4.3	3.9	3.6	3.2	3.4	2.5	2.5	1.7	1.2	−0.5

(*Continued*)

Table 1.21
(Continued)

	Annual																		2007–2008 Change
	1991	1992	1993	1994	1995	1996	1997	1998	1999	2000	2001	2002	2003	2004	2005	2006	2007	2008	
Crystal meth (LCE)[n]																			
8th grade	—	—	—	—	—	—	—	—	—	—	—	—	—	—	—	—	—	—	
10th grade	−1	—	—	—	—	—	—	—	—	—	—	—	—	—	—	—	—	—	
12th grade	1.4	1.3	1.7	1.8	2.4	2.8	2.3	3.0	1.9	2.2	2.5	3.0	2.0	2.1	2.3	1.9	1.6	1.1	−0.6 s
Sedatives (barbiturates)[k]																			
8th grade	−8	—	—	—	—	—	—	—	—	—	—	—	—	—	—	—	—	—	
10th grade	−1	—	—	—	—	—	—	—	—	—	—	—	—	—	—	—	—	—	
12th grade	3.4	2.8	3.4	4.1	4.7	4.9	5.1	5.5	5.8	6.2	5.7	6.7	6.0	6.5	7.2	6.6	6.2	5.8	−0.4
Methaqualone[e,k]																			
8th grade	−8	—	—	—	—	—	—	—	—	—	—	—	—	—	—	—	—	—	
10th grade	−1	—	—	—	—	—	—	—	—	—	—	—	—	—	—	—	—	—	
12th grade	0.5	0.6	0.2	0.8	0.7	1.1	1.0	1.1	1.1	0.3	0.8	0.9	0.6	0.8	0.9	0.8	0.5	0.5	0.0
Tranquilizers[b,k]																			
8th grade	1.8	2.0	2.1	2.4	2.7	3.3	2.9	2.6	2.5	2.6‡	2.8	2.6	2.7	2.5	2.8	2.6	2.4	2.4	0.0
10th grade	3.2	3.5	3.3	3.3	4.0	4.6	4.9	5.1	5.4	5.6‡	7.3	6.3	5.3	5.1	4.8	5.2	5.3	4.6	−0.7
12th grade	3.6	2.8	3.5	3.7	4.4	4.6	4.7	5.5	5.8	5.7‡	6.9	7.7	6.7	7.3	6.8	6.6	6.2	6.2	0.0
OTC cough/cold medicines[m,n]																			
8th grade	−8	—	—	—	—	—	—	—	—	—	—	—	—	—	—	4.2	4.0	3.6	−0.5
10th grade	−1	—	—	—	—	—	—	—	—	—	—	—	—	—	5.3	5.4	5.3	−0.1	
12th grade	−1	—	—	—	—	—	—	—	—	—	—	—	—	—	6.9	5.8	5.5	−0.3	

(Continued)

Table 1.21
(Continued)

	Annual																		2007–2008 Change
	1991	1992	1993	1994	1995	1996	1997	1998	1999	2000	2001	2002	2003	2004	2005	2006	2007	2008	
Rohypnol[o]																			
8th grade	−8	—	—	—	—	1.0	0.8	0.8	0.5	0.5	0.7	0.3	0.5	0.6	0.7	0.5	0.7	0.5	−0.2
10th grade	−1	—	—	—	1.1	1.3	1.2	1.0	0.8	1.0	0.7	0.6	0.7	0.5	0.5	0.7	0.4	−0.3	
12th grade	−1	—	—	—	1.1	1.2	1.4	1.0	0.8	0.9‡	1.6	1.3	1.6	1.2	1.1	1.0	1.3	0.3	
GHB[m,t]																			
8th grade	−8	—	—	—	—	—	—	—	—	1.2	1.1	0.8	0.9	0.7	0.5	0.8	0.7	1.1	0.4 s
10th grade	−1	—	—	—	—	—	—	—	—	1.1	1.0	1.4	1.4	0.8	0.8	0.7	0.6	0.5	0.0
12th grade	−1	—	—	—	—	—	—	—	—	1.9	1.6	1.5	1.4	2.0	1.1	1.1	0.9	1.2	0.3
Ketamine[m,u]																			
8th grade	−8	—	—	—	—	—	—	—	—	1.6	1.3	1.3	1.1	0.9	0.6	0.9	1.0	1.2	0.2
10th grade	−1	—	—	—	—	—	—	—	—	2.1	2.1	2.2	1.9	1.3	1.0	1.0	0.8	1.0	0.2
12th grade	−1	—	—	—	—	—	—	—	—	2.5	2.5	2.6	2.1	1.9	1.6	1.4	1.3	1.5	0.2
Alcohol																			
Any use[p]																			
8th grade	54.0	53.7‡	45.4	46.8	45.3	46.5	45.5	43.7	43.5	43.1	41.9	38.7	37.2	36.7	33.9	33.6	31.8	32.1	0.3
10th grade	72.3	70.2‡	63.4	63.9	63.5	65.0	65.2	62.7	63.7	65.3	63.5	60.0	59.3	58.2	56.7	55.8	56.3	52.5	−3.8 sss
12th grade	77.7	76.8‡	72.7	73.0	73.7	72.5	74.8	74.3	73.8	73.2	73.3	71.5	70.1	70.6	68.6	66.5	66.4	65.5	−0.9
Been drunk[n]																			
8th grade	17.5	18.3	18.2	18.2	18.4	19.8	18.4	17.9	18.5	18.5	16.6	15.0	14.5	14.5	14.1	13.9	12.6	12.7	0.1
10th grade	40.1	37.0	37.8	38.0	38.5	40.1	40.7	38.3	40.9	41.6	39.9	35.4	34.7	35.1	34.2	34.5	34.4	30.0	−4.3 sss
12th grade	52.7	50.3	49.6	51.7	52.5	51.9	53.2	52.0	53.2	51.8	53.2	50.4	48.0	51.8	47.7	47.9	46.1	45.6	−0.5
Flavored alcoholic beverages[e,m,v]																			
8th grade	−8	—	—	—	—	—	—	—	—	—	—	—	—	30.4	27.9	26.8	26.0	25.0	−1.0
10th grade	−1	—	—	—	—	—	—	—	—	—	—	—	—	49.7	48.5	48.8	45.9	43.4	−2.4
12th grade	−1	—	—	—	—	—	—	—	—	—	—	—	55.2	55.8	58.4	54.7	53.6	51.8	−1.9

(Continued)

Table 1.21
(Continued)

	Annual																		2007–2008 Change
	1991	1992	1993	1994	1995	1996	1997	1998	1999	2000	2001	2002	2003	2004	2005	2006	2007	2008	
Bidis[m,n]																			
8th grade	—	—	—	—	—	—	—	—	—	3.9	2.7	2.7	2.0	1.7	1.6	—	—	—	
10th grade	−1	—	—	—	—	—	—	—	—	6.4	4.9	3.1	2.8	2.1	1.6	—	—	—	
12th grade	−1	—	—	—	—	—	—	—	—	9.2	7.0	5.9	4.0	3.6	3.3	2.3	1.7	1.9	0.2
Kreteks[m,n]																			
8th grade	−8	—	—	—	—	—	—	—	—	—	2.6	2.6	2.0	1.9	1.4	—	—	—	
10th grade	−1	—	—	—	—	—	—	—	—	6.0	4.9	3.8	3.7	2.8	—	—	—		
12th grade	−1	—	—	—	—	—	—	—	—	10.1	8.4	6.7	6.5	7.1	6.2	6.8	6.8	0.0	
Steroids[r]																			
8th grade	1.0	1.1	0.9	1.2	1.0	0.9	1.0	1.2	1.7	1.7	1.6	1.5	1.4	1.1	1.1	0.9	0.8	0.9	0.1
10th grade	1.1	1.1	1.0	1.1	1.2	1.2	1.2	1.2	1.7	2.2	2.1	2.2	1.7	1.5	1.3	1.2	1.1	0.9	−0.1
12th grade	1.4	1.1	1.2	1.3	1.5	1.4	1.4	1.7	1.8	1.7	2.4	2.5	2.1	2.5	1.5	1.8	1.4	1.5	0.1

See relevant footnotes in Table 1.20.

Johnston LD, O'Malley PM, Bachman JG, Schulenberg JE. *Monitoring the Future National Results on Adolescent Drug Use: Overview of Key Findings, 2008*. Bethesda, MD: National Institute on Drug Abuse. 2009. NIH publication No. 09–7401 Available at: http://monitoringthefuture.org/pubs/monographs/overview2008.pdf. Accessed April 11, 2009.

Table 1.22
Trends in 30-day prevalence of use of various drugs in grades 8, 10, and 12

	30-Day																		2007–2008 Change
	1991	1992	1993	1994	1995	1996	1997	1998	1999	2000	2001	2002	2003	2004	2005	2006	2007	2008	
Any illicit drug[a]																			
8th grade	5.7	6.8	8.4	10.9	12.4	14.6	12.9	12.1	12.2	11.9	11.7	10.4	9.7	8.4	8.5	8.1	7.4	7.6	0.2
10th grade	11.6	11.0	14.0	18.5	20.2	23.2	23.0	21.5	22.1	22.5	22.7	20.8	19.5	18.3	17.3	16.8	16.9	15.8	−1.1
12th grade	16.4	14.4	18.3	21.9	23.8	24.6	26.2	25.6	25.9	24.9	25.7	25.4	24.1	23.4	23.1	21.5	21.9	22.3	0.5
Any illicit drug other than marijuana[a,b]																			
8th grade	3.8	4.7	5.3	5.6	6.5	6.9	6.0	5.5	5.5	5.6‡	5.5	4.7	4.7	4.1	4.1	3.8	3.6	3.8	0.1
10th grade	5.5	5.7	6.5	7.1	8.9	8.9	8.8	8.6	8.6	8.5‡	8.7	8.1	6.9	6.9	6.4	6.3	6.9	5.3	−1.6 sss
12th grade	7.1	6.3	7.9	8.8	10.0	9.5	10.7	10.7	10.4	10.4‡	11.0	11.3	10.4	10.8	10.3	9.8	9.5	9.3	−0.2
Any illicit drug including inhalants[a,c]																			
8th grade	8.8	10.0	12.0	14.3	16.1	17.5	16.0	14.9	15.1	14.4	14.0	12.6	12.1	11.2	11.2	10.9	10.1	10.4	0.3
10th grade	13.1	12.6	15.5	20.0	21.6	24.5	24.1	22.5	23.1	23.6	23.6	21.7	20.5	19.3	18.4	17.7	18.1	16.8	−1.3
12th grade	17.8	15.5	19.3	23.0	24.8	25.5	26.9	26.6	26.4	26.4	26.5	25.9	24.6	23.3	24.2	22.1	22.8	22.8	0.0
Marijuana/hashish																			
8th grade	3.2	3.7	5.1	7.8	9.1	11.3	10.2	9.7	9.7	9.1	9.2	8.3	7.5	6.4	6.6	6.5	5.7	5.8	0.1
10th grade	8.7	8.1	10.9	15.8	17.2	20.4	20.5	18.7	19.4	19.7	19.8	17.8	17.0	15.9	15.2	14.2	14.2	13.8	−0.3
12th grade	13.8	11.9	15.5	19.0	21.2	21.9	23.7	22.8	23.1	21.6	22.4	21.5	21.2	19.9	19.8	18.3	18.8	19.4	0.7
Inhalants[c,d]																			
8th grade	4.4	4.7	5.4	5.6	6.1	5.8	5.6	4.8	5.0	4.5	4.0	3.8	4.1	4.5	4.2	4.1	3.9	4.1	0.2
10th grade	2.7	2.7	3.3	3.6	3.5	3.3	3.0	2.9	2.6	2.6	2.4	2.4	2.2	2.4	2.2	2.3	2.5	2.1	−0.4
12th grade	2.4	2.3	2.5	2.7	3.2	2.5	2.5	2.3	2.0	2.2	1.7	1.5	1.5	1.5	2.0	1.5	1.2	1.4	0.2

(Continued)

Table 1.22
(Continued)

	30-Day																		2007–2008 Change
	1991	1992	1993	1994	1995	1996	1997	1998	1999	2000	2001	2002	2003	2004	2005	2006	2007	2008	
Nitrites[e]																			
8th grade	—	—	—	—	—	—	—	—	—	—	—	—	—	—	—	—	—	—	
10th grade	—	—	—	—	—	—	—	—	—	—	—	—	—	—	—	—	—	—	
12th grade	0.4	0.3	0.6	0.4	0.4	0.7	0.7	1.0	0.4	0.3	0.5	0.6	0.7	0.7	0.5	0.3	0.5	0.3	−0.2
Hallucinogens[b,f]																			
8th grade	0.8	1.1	1.2	1.3	1.7	1.9	1.8	1.4	1.3	1.2‡	1.6	1.2	1.2	1.0	1.1	0.9	1.0	0.9	0.0
10th grade	1.6	1.8	1.9	2.4	3.3	2.8	3.3	3.2	2.9	2.3‡	2.1	1.6	1.5	1.6	1.5	1.5	1.7	1.3	−0.4
12th grade	2.2	2.1	2.7	3.1	4.4	3.5	3.9	3.8	3.5	2.6‡	3.3	2.3	1.8	1.9	1.9	1.5	1.7	2.2	0.5 s
LSD																			
8th grade	0.6	0.9	1.0	1.1	1.4	1.5	1.5	1.1	1.1	1.0	1.0	0.7	0.6	0.5	0.5	0.4	0.5	0.5	0.0
10th grade	1.5	1.6	1.6	2.0	3.0	2.4	2.8	2.7	2.3	1.6	1.5	0.7	0.6	0.6	0.6	0.7	0.7	0.7	0.0
12th grade	1.9	2.0	2.4	2.6	4.0	2.5	3.1	3.2	2.7	1.6	2.3	0.7	0.6	0.7	0.7	0.6	0.6	1.1	0.5 ss
Hallucinogens other than LSD[b]																			
8th grade	0.3	0.4	0.5	0.7	0.8	0.9	0.7	0.7	0.6	0.6‡	1.1	1.0	1.0	0.8	0.9	0.7	0.7	0.7	0.0
10th grade	0.4	0.5	0.7	1.0	1.0	1.0	1.2	1.4	1.2	1.2‡	1.4	1.4	1.2	1.4	1.3	1.3	1.4	1.0	−0.5 ss
12th grade	0.7	0.5	0.8	1.2	1.3	1.6	1.7	1.6	1.6	1.7‡	1.9	2.0	1.5	1.7	1.6	1.3	1.4	1.6	0.3
PCP[e]																			
8th grade	—	—	—	—	—	—	—	—	—	—	—	—	—	—	—	—	—		
10th grade	—	—	—	—	—	—	—	—	—	—	—	—	—	—	—	—	—	—	
12th grade	0.5	0.6	1.0	0.7	0.6	1.3	0.7	1.0	0.8	0.9	0.5	0.4	0.6	0.4	0.7	0.4	0.5	0.6	0.1
Ecstasy (MDMA)[g]																			
8th grade	—	—	—	—	—	1.0	1.0	0.9	0.8	1.4	1.8	1.4	0.7	0.8	0.6	0.7	0.6	0.8	0.2
10th grade	—	—	—	—	—	1.8	1.3	1.3	1.8	2.6	2.6	1.8	1.1	0.8	1.0	1.2	1.2	1.1	−0.1
12th grade	—	—	—	—	—	2.0	1.6	1.5	2.5	3.6	2.8	2.4	1.3	1.2	1.0	1.3	1.6	1.8	0.2

(Continued)

Table 1.22
(Continued)

	30-Day																		2007–2008 Change
	1991	1992	1993	1994	1995	1996	1997	1998	1999	2000	2001	2002	2003	2004	2005	2006	2007	2008	
Cocaine																			
8th grade	0.5	0.7	0.7	1.0	1.2	1.3	1.1	1.4	1.3	1.2	1.2	1.1	0.9	0.9	1.0	1.0	0.9	0.8	−0.1
10th grade	0.7	0.7	0.9	1.2	1.7	1.7	2.0	2.1	1.8	1.8	1.3	1.6	1.3	1.7	1.5	1.5	1.3	1.2	0.0
12th grade	1.4	1.3	1.3	1.5	1.8	2.0	2.3	2.4	2.6	2.1	2.1	2.3	2.1	2.3	2.3	2.5	2.0	1.9	−0.1
Crack																			
8th grade	0.3	0.5	0.4	0.7	0.7	0.8	0.7	0.9	0.8	0.8	0.8	0.8	0.7	0.6	0.6	0.6	0.6	0.5	−0.2
10th grade	0.3	0.4	0.5	0.6	0.9	0.8	0.9	1.1	0.8	0.9	0.7	1.0	0.7	0.8	0.7	0.7	0.5	0.5	0.0
12th grade	0.7	0.6	0.7	0.8	1.0	1.0	0.9	1.0	1.1	1.0	1.1	1.2	0.9	1.0	1.0	0.9	0.9	0.8	−0.1
Other cocaine[h]																			
8th grade	0.5	0.5	0.6	0.9	1.0	1.0	0.8	1.0	1.1	0.9	0.9	0.8	0.7	0.7	0.7	0.7	0.6	0.6	0.0
10th grade	0.6	0.6	0.7	1.0	1.4	1.3	1.6	1.8	1.6	1.6	1.2	1.3	1.1	1.5	1.3	1.3	1.1	1.0	−0.1
12th grade	1.2	1.0	1.2	1.3	1.3	1.6	2.0	2.0	2.5	1.7	1.8	1.9	1.8	2.2	2.0	2.4	1.7	1.7	0.0
Heroin[i]																			
8th grade	0.3	0.4	0.4	0.6	0.6	0.7	0.6	0.6	0.6	0.5	0.6	0.5	0.4	0.5	0.5	0.3	0.4	0.4	0.0
10th grade	0.2	0.2	0.3	0.4	0.6	0.5	0.6	0.7	0.7	0.5	0.3	0.5	0.3	0.5	0.5	0.5	0.4	0.4	−0.1
12th grade	0.2	0.3	0.2	0.3	0.6	0.5	0.5	0.5	0.5	0.7	0.4	0.5	0.4	0.5	0.5	0.4	0.4	0.4	0.0
With a needle[j]																			
8th grade	—	—	—	—	0.4	0.5	0.4	0.5	0.4	0.3	0.4	0.3	0.3	0.3	0.3	0.2	0.3	0.3	0.0
10th grade	—	—	—	—	0.3	0.3	0.3	0.4	0.3	0.3	0.2	0.3	0.2	0.3	0.3	0.3	0.3	0.2	−0.1
12th grade	—	—	—	—	0.3	0.4	0.3	0.2	0.2	0.2	0.2	0.3	0.3	0.2	0.3	0.3	0.2	0.2	0.0
Without a needle[j]																			
8th grade	—	—	—	—	0.3	0.4	0.4	0.3	0.4	0.3	0.4	0.3	0.3	0.3	0.2	0.2	0.2	0.2	0.0
10th grade	—	—	—	—	0.3	0.3	0.4	0.5	0.5	0.4	0.2	0.4	0.2	0.3	0.3	0.3	0.2	0.3	0.0
12th grade	—	—	—	—	0.6	0.4	0.6	0.4	0.4	0.7	0.3	0.5	0.4	0.3	0.5	0.3	0.4	0.2	−0.2

(*Continued*)

Table 1.22
(Continued)

	30-Day																		2007–2008 Change
	1991	1992	1993	1994	1995	1996	1997	1998	1999	2000	2001	2002	2003	2004	2005	2006	2007	2008	
Narcotics other than heroin[k,l]																			
8th grade	—	—	—	—	—	—	—	—	—	—	—	—	—	—	—	—	—	—	—
10th grade	—	—	—	—	—	—	—	—	—	—	—	—	—	—	—	—	—	—	—
12th grade	1.1	1.2	1.3	1.5	1.8	2.0	2.3	2.4	2.6	2.9	3.0‡	4.0	4.1	4.3	3.9	3.8	3.8	3.8	0.0
Amphetamines[k]																			
8th grade	2.6	3.3	3.6	3.6	4.2	4.6	3.8	3.3	3.4	3.4	3.2	2.8	2.7	2.3	2.3	2.1	2.0	2.2	0.2
10th grade	3.3	3.6	4.3	4.5	5.3	5.5	5.1	5.1	5.0	5.4	5.6	5.2	4.3	4.0	3.7	3.5	4.0	2.8	−1.2 sss
12th grade	3.2	2.8	3.7	4.0	4.0	4.1	4.8	4.6	4.5	5.0	5.6	5.5	5.0	4.6	3.9	3.7	3.7	2.9	−0.8 ss
Methamphetamine[m,n]																			
8th grade	—	—	—	—	—	—	—	—	1.1	0.8	1.3	1.1	1.2	0.6	0.7	0.6	0.6	0.7	0.1
10th grade	—	—	—	—	—	—	—	—	1.8	2.0	1.5	1.8	1.4	1.3	1.1	0.7	0.4	0.7	0.4 s
12th grade	—	—	—	—	—	—	—	—	1.7	1.9	1.5	1.7	1.7	1.4	0.9	0.9	0.6	0.6	−0.1
Crystal meth (ice)[n]																			
8th grade	—	—	—	—	—	—	—	—	—	—	—	—	—	—	—	—	—	—	—
10th grade	—	—	—	—	—	—	—	—	—	—	—	—	—	—	—	—	—	—	—
12th grade	0.6	0.5	0.6	0.7	1.1	1.1	0.8	1.2	0.8	1.0	1.1	1.2	0.8	0.8	0.9	0.7	0.6	0.6	0.0
Sedatives (barbiturates)[k]																			
8th grade	—	—	—	—	—	—	—	—	—	—	—	—	—	—	—	—	—	—	—
10th grade	—	—	—	—	—	—	—	—	—	—	—	—	—	—	—	—	—	—	—
12th grade	1.4	1.1	1.3	1.7	2.2	2.1	2.1	2.6	2.6	3.0	2.8	3.2	2.9	2.9	3.3	3.0	2.7	2.8	0.1
Methaqualone[e,k]																			
8th grade	—	—	—	—	—	—	—	—	—	—	—	—	—	—	—	—	—	—	—
10th grade	—	—	—	—	—	—	—	—	—	—	—	—	—	—	—	—	—	—	—
12th grade	0.2	0.4	0.1	0.4	0.4	0.6	0.3	0.6	0.4	0.2	0.5	0.3	0.4	0.5	0.5	0.4	0.4	0.2	−0.1

(Continued)

Table 1.22
(Continued)

	30-Day																		2007–2008 Change
	1991	1992	1993	1994	1995	1996	1997	1998	1999	2000	2001	2002	2003	2004	2005	2006	2007	2008	
Tranquilizers[b,k]																			
8th grade	0.8	0.8	0.9	1.1	1.2	1.5	1.2	1.2	1.1	1.4‡	1.2	1.2	1.4	1.2	1.3	1.3	1.1	1.2	0.1
10th grade	1.2	1.5	1.1	1.5	1.7	1.7	2.2	2.2	2.2	2.5‡	2.9	2.9	2.4	2.3	2.3	2.4	2.6	1.9	−0.7 sss
12th grade	1.4	1.0	1.2	1.4	1.8	2.0	1.8	2.4	2.5	2.6‡	2.9	3.3	2.8	3.1	2.9	2.7	2.6	2.6	0.0
Rohypnol[o]																			
8th grade	—	—	—	—	—	0.5	0.3	0.4	0.3	0.3	0.4	0.2	0.1	0.2	0.2	0.4	0.3	0.1	−0.3
10th grade	—	—	—	—	—	0.5	0.5	0.4	0.5	0.4	0.2	0.4	0.2	0.3	0.2	0.2	0.2	0.2	0.0
12th grade	—	—	—	—	—	0.5	0.3	0.3	0.3	0.4	0.3	—	—	—	—	—	—	—	—
Alcohol[p]																			
Any use																			
8th grade	25.1	26.1‡	24.3	25.5	24.6	26.2	24.5	23.0	24.0	22.4	21.5	19.6	19.7	18.6	17.1	17.2	15.9	15.9	0.1
10th grade	42.8	39.9‡	38.2	39.2	38.8	40.4	40.1	38.8	40.0	41.0	39.0	35.4	35.4	35.2	33.2	33.8	33.4	28.8	−4.7 sss
12th grade	54.0	51.3‡	48.6	50.1	51.3	50.8	52.7	52.0	51.0	50.0	49.8	48.6	47.5	48.0	47.0	45.3	44.4	43.1	−1.3
Been drunk[n]																			
8th grade	7.6	7.5	7.8	8.7	8.3	9.6	8.2	8.4	9.4	8.3	7.7	6.7	6.7	6.2	6.0	6.2	5.5	5.4	−0.1
10th grade	20.5	18.1	19.8	20.3	20.8	21.3	22.4	21.1	22.5	23.5	21.9	18.3	18.2	18.5	17.6	18.8	18.1	14.4	−3.7 sss
12th grade	31.6	29.9	28.9	30.8	33.2	31.3	34.2	32.9	32.9	32.3	32.7	30.3	30.9	32.5	30.2	30.0	28.7	27.6	−1.1
Flavored alcoholic beverages[e,m]																			
8th grade	—	—	—	—	—	—	—	—	—	—	—	—	—	14.6	12.9	13.1	12.2	10.2	−2.0 ss
10th grade	—	—	—	—	—	—	—	—	—	—	—	—	—	25.1	23.1	24.7	21.8	20.2	−1.6
12th grade	—	—	—	—	—	—	—	—	—	—	—	—	—	31.1	30.5	29.3	29.1	27.4	−1.8

(Continued)

Table 1.22
(Continued)

	30-Day																		2007–2008 Change
	1991	1992	1993	1994	1995	1996	1997	1998	1999	2000	2001	2002	2003	2004	2005	2006	2007	2008	
Cigarettes																			
Any use																			
8th grade	14.3	15.5	16.7	18.6	19.1	21.0	19.4	19.1	17.5	14.6	12.2	10.7	10.2	9.2	9.3	8.7	7.1	6.8	−0.2
10th grade	20.8	21.5	24.7	25.4	27.9	30.4	29.8	27.6	25.7	23.9	21.3	17.7	16.7	16.0	14.9	14.5	14.0	12.3	−1.7 s
12th grade	28.3	27.8	29.9	31.2	33.5	34.0	36.5	35.1	34.6	31.4	29.5	26.7	24.4	25.0	23.2	21.6	21.6	20.4	−1.2
Smokeless tobacco[q]																			
8th grade	6.9	7.0	6.6	7.7	7.1	7.1	5.5	4.8	4.5	4.2	4.0	3.3	4.1	4.1	3.3	3.7	3.2	3.5	0.3
10th grade	10.0	9.6	10.4	10.5	9.7	8.6	8.9	7.5	6.5	6.1	6.9	6.1	5.3	4.9	5.6	5.7	6.1	5.0	−1.1
12th grade	—	11.4	10.7	11.1	12.2	9.8	9.7	8.8	8.4	7.6	7.8	6.5	6.7	6.7	7.6	6.1	6.6	6.5	−0.1
Steroids[r]																			
8th grade	0.4	0.5	0.5	0.5	0.6	0.4	0.5	0.5	0.7	0.8	0.7	0.8	0.7	0.5	0.5	0.5	0.4	0.5	0.1
10th grade	0.6	0.6	0.5	0.6	0.6	0.5	0.7	0.6	0.9	1.0	0.9	1.0	0.8	0.8	0.6	0.6	0.5	0.5	0.0
12th grade	0.8	0.6	0.7	0.9	0.7	0.7	1.0	1.1	0.9	0.8	1.3	1.4	1.3	1.6	0.9	1.1	1.0	1.0	0.0
Marijuana/hashish																			
Daily[w]																			
8th grade	0.2	0.2	0.4	0.7	0.8	1.5	1.1	1.1	1.4	1.3	1.3	1.2	1.0	0.8	1.0	1.0	0.8	0.9	0.1
10th grade	0.8	0.8	1.0	2.2	2.8	3.5	3.7	3.6	3.8	3.8	4.5	3.9	3.6	3.2	3.1	2.8	2.8	2.7	−0.1
12th grade	2.0	1.9	2.4	3.6	4.6	4.9	5.8	5.6	6.0	6.0	5.8	6.0	6.0	5.6	5.0	5.0	5.1	5.4	0.4
Alcohol[p,w]																			
Any daily use																			
8th grade	0.5	0.6‡	1.0	1.0	0.7	1.0	0.8	0.9	1.0	0.8	0.9	0.7	0.8	0.6	0.5	0.5	0.6	0.7	0.2
10th grade	1.3	1.2‡	1.8	1.7	1.7	1.6	1.7	1.9	1.9	1.8	1.9	1.8	1.5	1.3	1.3	1.4	1.4	1.0	−0.4 ss
12th grade	3.6	3.4‡	3.4	2.9	3.5	3.7	3.9	3.9	3.4	2.9	3.6	3.5	3.2	2.8	3.1	3.0	3.1	2.8	−0.3

(Continued)

Table 1.22
(Continued)

	30-Day																		2007–2008 Change
	1991	1992	1993	1994	1995	1996	1997	1998	1999	2000	2001	2002	2003	2004	2005	2006	2007	2008	
Been drunk																			
Daily[n,w]																			
8th grade	0.1	0.1	0.2	0.3	0.2	0.2	0.2	0.3	0.4	0.3	0.2	0.3	0.2	0.2	0.2	0.2	0.2	0.2	0.0
10th grade	0.2	0.3	0.4	0.4	0.6	0.4	0.6	0.6	0.7	0.5	0.6	0.5	0.5	0.4	0.4	0.5	0.5	0.3	−0.2 ss
12th grade	0.9	0.8	0.9	1.2	1.3	1.6	2.0	1.5	1.9	1.7	1.4	1.2	1.6	1.8	1.5	1.6	1.3	1.4	0.1
≥5 drinks in a row in last 2 wk[x]																			
8th grade	10.9	11.3	11.3	12.1	12.3	13.3	12.3	11.5	13.1	11.7	11.0	10.3	9.8	9.4	8.4	8.7	8.3	8.1	−0.2
10th grade	21.0	19.1	21.0	21.9	22.0	22.8	23.1	22.4	23.5	24.1	22.8	20.3	20.0	19.9	19.0	19.9	19.6	16.0	−3.7 sss
12th grade	29.8	27.9	27.5	28.2	29.8	30.2	31.3	31.5	30.8	30.0	29.7	28.6	27.9	29.2	27.1	25.4	25.9	24.6	−1.3
Cigarettes																			
Any daily use																			
8th grade	7.2	7.0	8.3	8.8	9.3	10.4	9.0	8.8	8.1	7.4	5.5	5.1	4.5	4.4	4.0	4.0	3.0	3.1	0.0
10th grade	12.6	12.3	14.2	14.6	16.3	18.3	18.0	15.8	15.9	14.0	12.2	10.1	8.9	8.3	7.5	7.6	7.2	5.9	−1.3 s
12th grade	18.5	17.2	19.0	19.4	21.6	22.2	24.6	22.4	23.1	20.6	19.0	16.9	15.8	15.6	13.6	12.2	12.3	11.4	−0.9
≥ pack per day																			
8th grade	3.1	2.9	3.5	3.6	3.4	4.3	3.5	3.6	3.3	2.8	2.3	2.1	1.8	1.7	1.7	1.5	1.1	1.2	0.0
10th grade	6.5	6.0	7.0	7.6	8.3	9.4	8.6	7.9	7.6	6.2	5.5	4.4	4.1	3.3	3.1	3.3	2.7	2.0	−0.7 s
12th grade	10.7	10.0	10.9	11.2	12.4	13.0	14.3	12.6	13.2	11.3	10.3	9.1	8.4	8.0	6.9	5.9	5.7	5.4	−0.2

(Continued)

Table 1.22
(Continued)

	30-Day																		2007–2008 Change
	1991	1992	1993	1994	1995	1996	1997	1998	1999	2000	2001	2002	2003	2004	2005	2006	2007	2008	
Smokeless tobacco																			
Daily[q]																			
8th grade	1.6	1.8	1.5	1.9	1.2	1.5	1.0	1.0	0.9	0.9	1.2	0.8	0.8	1.0	0.7	0.7	0.8	0.8	−0.1
10th grade	3.3	3.0	3.3	3.0	2.7	2.2	2.2	2.2	1.5	1.9	2.2	1.7	1.8	1.6	1.9	1.7	1.6	1.4	−0.2
12th grade	—	4.3	3.3	3.9	3.6	3.3	4.4	3.2	2.9	3.2	2.8	2.0	2.2	2.8	2.5	2.2	2.8	2.7	−0.1

See relevant footnotes in Table 1.20.

Johnston LD, O'Malley PM, Bachman JG, Schulenberg JE. *Monitoring the Future National Results on Adolescent Drug Use: Overview of Key Findings, 2008*. Bethesda, MD: National Institute on Drug Abuse. 2009. NIH publication No. 09–7401 Available at: http://monitoringthefuture.org/pubs/monographs/overview2008.pdf. Accessed April 11, 2009.

Table 1.23
Percentage of high school students who currently smoked >10 cigarettes per day[a] and who tried to quit smoking cigarettes,[b] according to gender, race/ethnicity, and grade: United States, Youth Risk Behavior Survey, 2007

Category	Smoked >10 Cigarettes per Day						Tried to Quit Smoking Cigarettes					
	Female		Male		Total		Female		Male		Total	
	%	95% CI	%	95% CI	%	95% CI	%	95% CI	%	95% CI	%	95% CI
Race/ethnicity												
White[c]	8.0	5.8–10.8	15.7	12.7–19.2	11.9	9.8–14.3	55.6	50.3–60.7	43.8	40.2–47.4	49.4	46.2–52.6
Black[c]	1.7	0.4–6.6	8.6	4.4–15.9	6.1	3.2–11.4	67.5	58.6–75.3	53.6	43.0–64.0	58.4	50.0–66.4
Hispanic	4.8	2.1–10.6	8.4	4.6–14.8	6.8	4.1–11.0	47.2	39.4–55.2	49.2	43.9–54.5	48.3	43.5–53.2
Grade												
9th	6.7	3.2–13.7	12.6	7.9–19.5	10.1	6.8–14.8	53.2	42.9–63.2	45.3	39.2–51.6	48.6	42.4–54.9
10th	5.3	3.1–8.7	12.6	7.5–20.3	9.0	6.2–13.0	54.0	46.2–61.7	49.9	40.8–58.9	51.9	45.1–58.5
11th	8.1	4.7–13.6	9.9	5.7–16.5	9.0	5.6–14.3	56.1	48.9–63.2	44.9	37.8–52.2	49.9	44.9–55.0
12th	7.8	4.7–12.5	19.2	14.2–25.4	13.6	10.1–18.0	56.4	51.2–61.5	41.1	33.7–48.9	48.5	43.3–53.7
Total	7.1	5.4–9.3	13.8	11.4–16.7	10.7	9.0–12.6	55.1	50.9–59.3	45.1	42.1–48.1	49.7	47.2–52.2

CI indicates confidence interval.
[a] On the days they smoked during the 30 days before the survey, among the 20.0% of students nationwide who currently smoked cigarettes.
[b] During the 12 months before the survey, among the 20.0% of students nationwide who currently smoked cigarettes.
[c] Non-Hispanic.
Data source: Centers for Disease Control and Prevention. Youth Risk Behavior Surveillance: United States, 2007. *MMWR CDC Surveill Summ.* 2008;57(4):1–131. Available at: www.cdc.gov/mmwr/PDF/ss/ss5704.pdf. Accessed April 11, 2009.

Table 1.24
Percentage of high school students who tried marijuana for the first time before the age of 13 years, according to gender, race/ethnicity, and grade: United States, Youth Risk Behavior Survey, 2007

Category	Female		Male		Total	
	%	95% CI	%	95% CI	%	95% CI
Race/ethnicity						
White[a]	4.4	3.3–5.8	10.0	7.3–13.6	7.2	5.6–9.3
Black[a]	4.9	3.5–6.6	14.2	11.1–18.1	9.5	7.4–12.0
Hispanic	7.1	5.3–9.6	12.4	9.8–15.6	9.8	8.2–11.7
Grade						
9th	6.1	4.6–8.1	13.3	10.4–16.9	9.8	7.9–12.2
10th	5.7	4.1–7.8	11.7	9.1–14.8	8.7	7.0–10.7
11th	4.2	3.2–5.7	10.1	7.8–12.9	7.2	5.7–9.0
12th	4.2	3.0–5.8	9.1	6.8–12.0	6.6	5.2–8.4
Total	5.2	4.2–6.4	11.2	9.3–13.5	8.3	7.0–9.7

CI indicates confidence interval.
[a] Non-Hispanic.
Data source: Centers for Disease Control and Prevention. Youth Risk Behavior Surveillance: United States, 2007. *MMWR CDC Surveill Summ.* 2008;57(4):1–131. Available at: www.cdc.gov/mmwr/PDF/ss/ss5704.pdf. Accessed April 11, 2009.

Table 1.25
Percentage of high school students who smoked a whole cigarette and who drank alcohol[a] for the first time before the age of 13 years, according to gender, race/ethnicity, and grade: United States, Youth Risk Behavior Survey, 2007

Category	Smoked a Whole Cigarette Before Age 13 y						Drank Alcohol Before Age 13 y					
	Female		Male		Total		Female		Male		Total	
	%	95% CI	%	95% CI	%	95% CI	%	95% CI	%	95% CI	%	95% CI
Race/ethnicity												
White[b]	12.2	9.9–14.9	16.5	12.5–21.5	14.4	11.5–17.9	17.8	15.7–20.1	25.0	21.0–29.4	21.5	18.8–24.4
Black[b]	10.5	8.6–12.7	14.6	11.6–18.2	12.5	10.6–14.7	22.7	19.3–26.6	30.7	26.5–35.4	26.7	24.2–29.4
Hispanic	11.9	10.0–14.1	16.8	14.0–20.0	14.3	12.4–16.4	24.2	22.0–26.6	33.6	31.1–36.2	29.0	27.5–30.5
Grade												
9th	13.2	10.8–15.9	19.2	15.3–23.9	16.3	13.6–19.4	27.1	23.9–30.4	34.5	30.0–39.3	30.9	28.1–33.9
10th	12.9	9.9–16.7	15.7	12.2–19.9	14.3	11.7–17.4	22.2	19.2–25.4	26.6	23.5–30.0	24.4	22.1–26.9
11th	9.2	7.3–11.7	14.6	12.1–17.6	12.0	10.0–14.4	13.8	11.6–16.4	25.1	22.8–27.6	19.6	17.7–21.5
12th	11.5	9.0–14.5	15.2	11.8–19.2	13.3	10.7–16.4	14.8	12.3–17.7	21.2	17.2–25.8	18.0	15.2–21.1
Total	11.9	10.3–13.6	16.4	13.5–19.7	14.2	12.2–16.5	20.0	18.2–21.9	27.4	24.8–30.2	23.8	21.9–25.7

CI indicates confidence interval.
[a] Other than a few sips.
[b] Non-Hispanic.
Data source: Centers for Disease Control and Prevention. Youth Risk Behavior Surveillance: United States, 2007. *MMWR CDC Surveill Summ.* 2008;57(4):1–131. Available at: www.cdc.gov/mmwr/PDF/ss/ss5704.pdf. Accessed April 11, 2009.

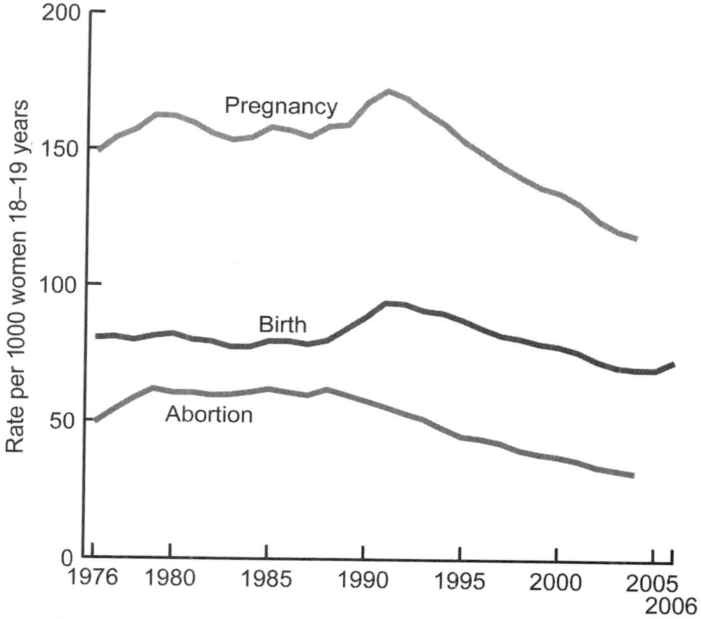

Fig 1.5. Pregnancy, birth, and abortion rates for teenagers aged 18 to 19 years: United States. Reproduced from: Ventura SJ, Abma JC, Mosher WD, Henshaw SK. Estimated pregnancy rates by outcome for the United States, 1990–2004. *Natl Vital Stat Rep*. 2008;56(15):5.

Table 1.26
Birth rates for women aged 15 to 19 years, according to age, race, and Hispanic origin of mother (United States, 1991, 2004, and 2005 [final] and 2006 [preliminary], and percent change in rates (1991–2005 and 2005–2006)

Age, Race, and Hispanic Origin of Mother	Year				Percent Change, 2005–2006	Percent Change, 1991–2005
	2006	2005	2004	1991		
10–14 y						
All races and origins[a]	0.6	0.7	0.7	1.4	−14	−50
Non-Hispanic white[b]	0.2	0.2	0.2	0.5	0[c]	−60
Non-Hispanic black[b]	1.6	1.7	1.6	4.9	−6	−65
American Indian or Alaska Native total[b,d]	0.9	0.9	0.9	1.6	0[c]	−44
Asian or Pacific Islander total[b,d]	0.2	0.2	0.2	0.8	0[c]	−75
Hispanic[e]	1.3	1.3	1.3	2.4	0[c]	−46
15–19 y						
All races and origins[a]	41.9	40.5	41.1	61.8	3	−34
Non-Hispanic white[b]	26.6	25.9	26.7	43.4	3	−40
Non-Hispanic black[b]	63.7	60.9	63.1	118.2	5	−48
American Indian or Alaska Native total[b,d]	54.7	52.7	52.5	84.1	4	−37
Asian or Pacific Islander total[b,d]	16.7	17.0	17.3	27.3	−2	−38
Hispanic[e]	83.0	81.7	82.6	104.6	2	−22
15–17 y						
All races and origins[a]	22.0	21.4	22.1	38.6	3	−45
Non-Hispanic white[b]	11.8	11.5	12.0	23.6	3	−51
Non-Hispanic black[b]	36.1	34.9	37.1	86.1	3	−59
American Indian or Alaska Native total[b,d]	30.5	30.5	30.0	51.9	0[c]	−41
Asian or Pacific Islander total[b,d]	8.7	8.2	8.9	16.3	6	−50
Hispanic[e]	47.9	48.5	49.7	69.2	−1	−30
18–19 y						
All races and origins[a]	73.0	69.9	70.0	94.0	4	−26
Non-Hispanic white[b]	49.3	48.0	48.7	70.6	3	−32
Non-Hispanic black[b]	108.4	103.0	103.9	162.2	5	−36
American Indian or Alaska Native total[b,d]	92.8	87.6	87.0	134.2	6	−35
Asian or Pacific Islander total[b,d]	28.9	30.1	29.6	42.2	−4	−29
Hispanic[e]	139.7	134.6	133.5	155.5	4	−13

Data for 2006 are based on a continuous file of records received from the states. Rates per 1000 women in the specified group are shown.

[a] Includes Hispanic origin not stated.

[b] Race and Hispanic origin are reported separately on birth certificates. Persons of Hispanic origin may be of any race. Race categories are consistent with the 1977 Office of Management and Budget (OMB) standards. Twenty-three states reported multiple-race data for 2006. The multiple-race data for these states were bridged to the single-race categories of the 1977 OMB standards for comparability with other states.

[c] Zero percent change.

[d] Data for persons of Hispanic origin are included in the data for each race group according to the person's reported race.

[e] Includes all persons of Hispanic origin of any race.

Data source: Hamilton BE, Martin JA, Ventura SJ. Births: Preliminary data for 2006. *Natl Vital Stat Rep*. 2007;56(7):1–18. Available at: www.cdc.gov/nchs/data/nvsr/nvsr56/nvsr56_07.pdf. Accessed April 11, 2009.

Table 1.27
Percentage of high school students who ever had sexual intercourse and who had sexual intercourse for the first time before the age of 13 years, according to gender, race/ethnicity, and grade: United States, Youth Risk Behavior Survey, 2007

Category	Ever Had Sexual Intercourse						Had First Sexual Intercourse Before Age 13 y					
	Female		Male		Total		Female		Male		Total	
	%	95% CI	%	95% CI	%	95% CI	%	95% CI	%	95% CI	%	95% CI
Race/ethnicity												
White[a]	43.7	40.8–46.7	43.6	39.7–47.6	43.7	40.5–47.0	3.1	2.6–3.7	5.7	3.9–8.3	4.4	3.4–5.7
Black[a]	60.9	56.2–65.4	72.6	68.5–76.3	66.5	63.0–69.9	6.9	5.6–8.5	26.2	23.0–29.6	16.3	14.7–18.0
Hispanic	45.8	41.0–50.7	58.2	54.0–62.4	52.0	48.3–55.6	4.5	3.3–6.1	11.9	10.1–13.9	8.2	7.1–9.3
Grade												
9th	27.4	24.2–30.9	38.1	33.8–42.6	32.8	29.7–36.1	4.9	3.8–6.1	13.5	11.1–16.3	9.2	7.6–11.1
10th	41.9	37.4–46.6	45.6	41.1–50.2	43.8	39.8–47.9	4.7	3.3–6.8	9.1	7.5–11.0	6.9	5.8–8.2
11th	53.6	47.7–59.4	57.3	53.2–61.3	55.5	51.3–59.6	3.4	2.5–4.7	9.9	7.4–13.1	6.6	5.1–8.6
12th	66.2	62.7–69.6	62.8	57.4–68.0	64.6	60.7–68.3	2.4	1.6–3.6	6.7	5.2–8.5	4.5	3.4–5.8
Total	45.9	43.1–48.6	49.8	46.7–52.9	47.8	45.1–50.6	4.0	3.5–4.5	10.1	8.6–12.0	7.1	6.2–8.1

CI indicates confidence interval.

[a] Non-Hispanic.

Data source: Centers for Disease Control and Prevention. Youth Risk Behavior Surveillance: United States, 2007. *MMWR CDC Surveill Summ.* 2008;57(4):1–131. Available at: www.cdc.gov/mmwr/PDF/ss/ss5704.pdf. Accessed April 11, 2009.

Table 1.28
Percentage of high school students who used a condom during last sexual intercourse[a] and who used birth control pills before last sexual intercourse,[a,b] according to gender, race/ethnicity, and grade: United States, Youth Risk Behavior Survey, 2007

Category	Condom Use						Birth Control Pill Use					
	Female		Male		Total		Female		Male		Total	
	%	95% CI	%	95% CI	%	95% CI	%	95% CI	%	95% CI	%	95% CI
Race/ethnicity												
White[c]	53.9	48.6–59.1	66.4	62.1–70.4	59.7	56.8–62.5	24.0	20.7–27.6	17.0	14.2–20.3	20.8	18.5–23.3
Black[c]	60.1	53.5–66.3	74.0	69.8–77.8	67.3	62.6–71.6	12.1	8.6–16.8	6.3	3.9–10.0	9.1	6.6–12.5
Hispanic	52.1	45.3–58.8	69.9	65.2–74.1	61.4	56.7–65.9	9.1	6.3–13.1	9.0	6.7–12.0	9.1	7.1–11.5
Grade												
9th	61.0	54.1–67.4	75.8	68.8–81.6	69.3	63.4–74.6	9.2	6.0–14.0	8.3	5.4–12.6	8.7	6.0–12.5
10th	59.5	52.6–66.1	73.2	67.6–78.2	66.1	62.5–69.5	13.7	9.5–19.4	9.5	6.2–14.1	11.6	8.9–15.1
11th	55.1	50.1–60.1	69.3	62.9–75.0	62.0	58.1–65.8	18.9	15.2–23.2	11.0	7.4–16.0	15.0	12.2–18.3
12th	49.9	44.9–54.9	59.6	55.2–63.9	54.2	50.7–57.7	25.6	21.4–30.3	20.8	16.7–25.7	23.5	20.5–26.8
Total	54.9	51.8–58.1	68.5	65.4–71.4	61.5	59.4–63.6	18.7	16.5–21.1	13.1	10.9–15.5	16.0	14.2–17.9

CI indicates confidence interval.
[a] Among the 35.0% of students nationwide who were currently sexually active.
[b] To prevent pregnancy.
[c] Non-Hispanic.
Data source: Centers for Disease Control and Prevention. Youth Risk Behavior Surveillance: United States, 2007. *MMWR CDC Surveill Summ.* 2008;57(4):1–131. Available at: www.cdc.gov/mmwr/PDF/ss/ss5704.pdf. Accessed April 11, 2009.

Table 1.29

Percentage of high school students who drank alcohol or used drugs before last sexual intercourse[a] and who were ever taught in school about AIDS or HIV infection, according to gender, race/ethnicity, and grade: United States, Youth Risk Behavior Survey, 2007

Category	Drank Alcohol or Used Drugs Before Last Sexual Intercourse						Were Taught in School About AIDS or HIV Infection					
	Female		Male		Total		Female		Male		Total	
	%	95% CI	%	95% CI	%	95% CI	%	95% CI	%	95% CI	%	95% CI
Race/ethnicity												
White[b]	19.8	16.3–23.9	30.5	26.1–35.2	24.8	22.3–27.5	91.7	89.8–93.3	90.5	88.8–92.0	91.1	89.6–92.4
Black[b]	12.9	9.7–16.8	19.8	15.5–24.9	16.4	13.4–20.0	91.8	89.8–93.5	88.8	85.8–91.2	90.3	88.6–91.8
Hispanic	16.5	12.7–21.2	25.9	22.0–30.2	21.4	18.2–25.1	84.8	81.8–87.3	85.1	82.9–87.1	85.0	82.9–86.8
Grade												
9th	20.4	14.4–28.1	22.9	18.1–28.6	21.8	17.2–27.2	87.7	84.9–90.1	86.4	83.9–88.5	87.1	84.9–89.0
10th	20.0	14.7–26.5	27.4	21.9–33.8	23.6	19.3–28.4	90.3	87.8–92.3	89.2	86.9–91.1	89.7	88.0–91.2
11th	14.8	11.1–19.5	28.3	23.5–33.7	21.6	18.7–24.8	92.6	90.1–94.6	91.0	88.5–93.0	91.8	89.6–93.6
12th	17.3	14.1–21.0	29.1	24.8–33.7	22.6	19.9–25.5	90.9	88.5–92.8	89.1	87.2–90.8	90.0	88.3–91.5
Total	17.7	15.1–20.7	27.5	24.6–30.6	22.5	20.7–24.5	90.2	88.5–91.7	88.7	87.4–89.9	89.5	88.1–90.7

CI indicates confidence interval.

[a] Among the 35.0% of students nationwide who were currently sexually active.

[b] Non-Hispanic.

Data source: Centers for Disease Control and Prevention. Youth Risk Behavior Surveillance: United States, 2007. *MMWR CDC Surveill Summ.* 2008;57(4):1–131. Available at: www.cdc.gov/mmwr/PDF/ss/ss5704.pdf. Accessed April 11, 2009.

Table 1.30
HIV/AIDS-related data for adolescents and young adults: United States: Estimated numbers of cases of HIV according to year of diagnosis and selected characteristics, 2004–2007, in 34 states and 5 US-dependent areas with confidential name-based HIV infection reporting

Age at Diagnosis, y	Year of Diagnosis			
	2004	2005	2006	2007
<13	212	189	169	159
13–14	41	40	45	40
15–19	1081	1216	1409	1703
20–24	3714	3875	4184	4907
Total cases all ages[a]	38 398	38 032	38 531	44 084

[a]Refers to all cases HIV/AIDS in the United States.
Data adapted from Centers for Disease Control and Prevention. Cases of HIV infection and AIDS in the United States and dependent areas, 2007: HIV/AIDS surveillance report—volume 19. Available at: www.cdc.gov/hiv/topics/surveillance/resources/reports/2007report/default.htm. Accessed March 22, 2009.

Table 1.31
HIV/AIDS-related data for adolescents and young adults: United States: Estimated number,[a] percentage, and rate[b] of persons with new HIV infections according to race/ethnicity and gender in the United States in 2006

	n (95% CI)	% of Total Cases[c]	Rate (95% CI)
White, non-Hispanic			
Males aged 13–29 y	4050 (3310–4790)	25	18.1 (14.8–21.4)
Females aged 13–29 y	1050 (730–1370)	32	4.9 (3.4–6.4)
Black, non-Hispanic			
Males aged 13–29 y	6760 (5970–7550)	42	128.4 (113.3–243.3)
Females aged 13–29 y	2810 (2350–3270)	32	53.6 (44.8–62.3)
Hispanic			
Males aged 13–29	3010 (2300–3720)	41	42.8 (32.7–53.0)
Females aged 13–29 y	820 (540–1110)	36	13.5 (8.9–18.3)
Totals			
Males aged 13–29 y	13 820 (12540–15100)	35	39.9 (36.2–43.6)
Females aged 13–29 y	4680 (4020–5350)	32	14.3 (12.3–16.3)

[a] Incidence estimates were adjusted for reporting delays and reclassification of cases reported without information regarding an HIV-transmission category but were not adjusted for underreporting. Estimates are rounded to the nearest 10.

[b] Per 100 000 population. CI indicates confidence interval.

[c] Percentage of total cases within a specified racial/ethnic category was accounted for by 13- to 29-year-old males or females.

Data source: Centers for Disease Control and Prevention. Subpopulation estimates from the HIV incidence surveillance system: United States, 2006. *MMWR Morb Mortal Wkly Rep*. 2008;57(36): 985–989. Available at: www.cdc.gov/mmwr/preview/mmwrhtml/mm5736a1.htm. Accessed March 22, 2009.

Table 1.32
HIV/AIDS-related data for adolescents and young adults: United States: Estimated[a] number and percentage of HIV/AIDS[b] diagnoses and estimated annual percentage change among 13- to 24-year-old men who have sex with men, according to selected characteristics: 2001–2006, 33 states

	Year of Diagnosis						Total 2001–2006, *n* (%)	EAPC 2001–2006 (95% CI)
	2001, *n* (%)[c]	2002, *n* (%)	2003, *n* (%)	2004, *n* (%)	2005, *n* (%)	2006, *n* (%)		
White, non-Hispanic	430 (6)	460 (7)	507 (8)	530 (8)	591 (8)	703 (10)	3221 (8)	9.4 (6.2 to 12.7)
Black, non-Hispanic	938 (16)	957 (17)	1113 (20)	1316 (23)	1523 (25)	1811 (27)	7658 (22)	14.9 (12.4 to 17.4)
Hispanic	330 (11)	371 (12)	360 (12)	431 (14)	449 (14)	481 (14)	2422 (13)	7.9 (3.8 to 12.0)
API	9 (7)	9 (7)	16 (9)	16 (9)	26 (12)	32 (15)	108 (10)	30.8 (11.8 to 53.0)
AI/AN	8 (11)	9 (12)	11 (15)	13 (17)	9 (11)	18 (20)	68 (14)	12.8 (−4.1 to 32.6)
Total	1725 (11)	1818 (11)	2028 (13)	2328 (15)	2624 (16)	3061 (18)	13 584 (14)	12.4 (10.6 to 14.2)

[a] Numbers were adjusted for reporting delays and missing risk factors. EAPC indicates estimated annual percentage change; CI, confidence interval; API, Asian/Pacific Islander; AI/AN, American Indian/Alaska Native.

[b] Diagnosis of HIV infection, regardless of whether AIDS was also diagnosed.

[c] Percentage of cases within specified racial/ethnic group and of total cases accounted for by 13- to 24-year-olds.

Data adapted from Centers for Disease Control and Prevention. Trends in HIV/AIDS diagnoses among men who have sex with men: 33 states, 2001–2006. *MMWR Morb Mortal Wkly Rep*. 2008;57(25):681–686. Available at: www.cdc.gov/mmwr/PDF/wk/mm5725.pdf. Accessed March 22, 2009.

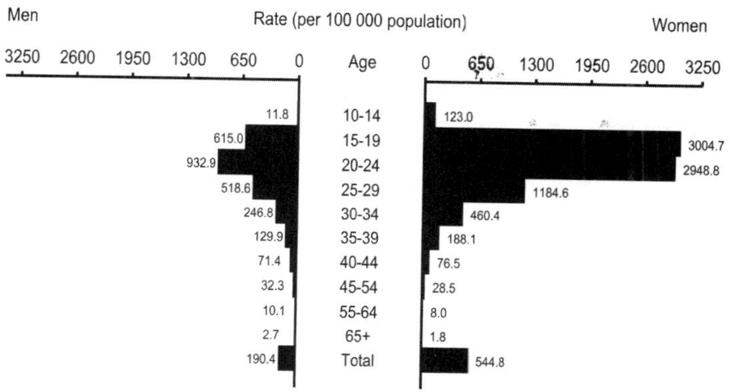

Fig 1.6. Chlamydia: age- and sex-specific rates, United States, 2007. Reproduced from Centers for Disease Control and Prevention. *Sexually Transmitted Diseases Surveillance, 2007*. Atlanta, GA: Department of Health and Human Services; 2008:13. Available at: www.cdc.gov/std/stats07/main.htm. Accessed April 11, 2009.

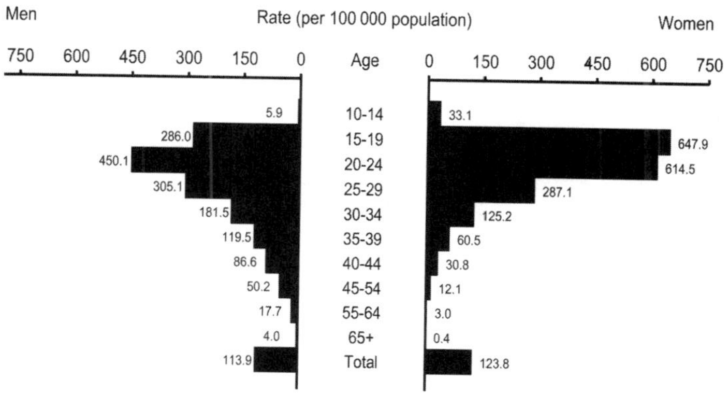

Fig 1.7. Gonorrhea: age- and sex-specific rates, United States, 2007. Reproduced from Centers for Disease Control and Prevention. *Sexually Transmitted Diseases Surveillance, 2007*. Atlanta, GA: Department of Health and Human Services; 2008:26. Available at: www.cdc.gov/std/stats07/main.htm. Accessed April 11, 2009.

Table 1.33
Chlamydia: rates per 100 000 population according to race/ethnicity, age group, and gender: United States, 2003–2007

Gender/Age Group	2003	2004	2005	2006	2007
White, non-Hispanic					
Males	1.8	1.9	2.1	1.4	1.5
10–14 y					
15–19 y	137.3	146.7	153.2	155.4	176.2
20–24 y	327.1	350.5	391.5	398.9	423.9
Females	53.1	51.5	50.5	44.9	42.2
10–14 y					
15–19 y	1393.3	1402.3	1412.8	1374.9	1432.7
20–24 y	1362.2	1425.4	1508.7	1508.7	1581.4
Black, non-Hispanic					
Males	43.8	46.3	48.7	54.7	54.9
10–14 y					
15–19 y	1711.0	1840.6	2073.2	2195.4	2550.8
20–24 y	2426.8	2673.0	2927.8	2980.0	3420.5
Females	477.2	487.3	460.9	462.2	469.4
10–14 y					
15–19 y	8399.4	8687.4	8716.3	8858.2	9646.7
20–24 y	7405.0	7762.9	7754.4	7942.6	8671.5
Hispanic					
Males	9.3	12.1	9.9	11.8	10.9
10–14 y					
15–19 y	463.0	474.9	511.2	519.5	562.8
20–24 y	640.1	686.3	782.9	838.3	857.9
Females	120.3	109.8	106.8	98.6	102.3
10–14 y					
15–19 y	2797.2	2725.0	2784.1	2845.8	2951.9
20–24 y	2928.8	2891.6	3134.6	3301.5	3348.4
API					
Males	1.6	1.2	3.6	0.7	1.5
10–14 y					
15–19 y	106.7	114.9	164.2	95.2	128.0
20–24 y	243.0	269.6	321.8	238.5	260.9
Females	35.6	32.9	26.7	23.2	28.9
10–14 y					
15–19 y	919.6	856.3	840.9	729.3	823.8
20–24 y	1046.1	1056.5	1144.8	1032.1	1072.8
AI/AN					
Males	16.1	27.2	22.1	17.6	16.4
10–14 y					
15–19 y	717.0	677.8	775.9	879.6	786.8
20–24 y	977.9	1113.2	1215.3	1187.9	1163.3

(Continued)

Table 1.33
(Continued)

Gender/Age Group	2003	2004	2005	2006	2007
Females 10–14 y	252.4	214.2	295.9	284.7	227.1
15–19 y	4295.6	4323.7	4617.5	4672.9	4360.4
20–24 y	4462.0	4512.3	4669.1	5008.6	4626.3

API indicates Asian/Pacific Islander; AI/AN, American Indian/Alaska Native.
Adapted from Centers for Disease Control and Prevention. *Sexually Transmitted Diseases Surveillance, 2007*. Atlanta, GA: Department of Health and Human Services; 2008. Available at: www.cdc.gov/std/stats07/main.htm. Accessed April 11, 2009.

Table 1.34
Gonorrhea: rates per 100 000 population according to race/ethnicity, age group, and gender: United States, 2003–2007

Gender/Age Group	2003	2004	2005	2006	2007
White, non-Hispanic					
Males	10.8	0.7	0.5	0.8	0.3
10–14 y					
15–19 y	37.7	37.7	39.5	38.4	39.7
20–24 y	93.5	89.3	97.6	99.4	94.4
Females	11.6	10.1	10.7	9.0	7.6
10–14 y					
15–19 y	204.7	200.4	203.6	208.3	200.6
20–24 y	206.3	207.1	225.1	233.2	226.6
Black, non-Hispanic					
Males	34.6	30.7	32.8	33.5	32.7
10–14 y					
15–19 y	1447.2	1360.8	1376.4	1467.6	1537.8
20–24 y	2558.2	2357.1	2333.5	2421.0	2451.3
Females	184.4	169.2	160.2	168.6	159.4
10–14 y					
15–19 y	2905.9	2723.6	2730.3	2829.6	2955.7
20–24 y	2670.3	2542.6	2542.0	2663.3	2789.2
Hispanic					
Males	3.8	2.5	2.6	3.5	3.2
10–14 y					
15–19 y	123.8	122.0	119.9	131.3	130.7
20–24 y	197.0	193.8	218.3	232.6	223.0
Females	17.9	17.2	16.1	15.4	15.6
10–14 y					
15–19 y	315.1	298.4	308.9	319.2	290.3
20–24 y	298.6	288.0	314.0	326.7	304.3
API					
Males	0.6	1.2	0.3	0.3	0.00
10–14 y					
15–19 y	26.3	25.8	41.2	27.0	26.4
20–24 y	54.0	65.4	88.0	66.8	59.3
Females	6.9	5.5	5.8	4.9	4.9
10–14 y					
15–19 y	100.1	85.3	107.1	98.7	86.1
20–24 y	116.2	109.4	117.4	97.9	97.2
AI/AN					
Males	5.7	5.8	7.4	1.4	2.6
10–14 y					
15–19 y	140.7	136,3	167.5	214.1	125.1
20–24 y	218.5	295.1	312.9	317.3	228.2

(Continued)

Table 1.34
(Continued)

Gender/Age Group	2003	2004	2005	2006	2007
Females					
10–14 y	42.7	27.7	34.7	33.2	26.1
15–19 y	481.1	556.1	575.2	548.9	455.7
20–24 y	532.1	590.4	625.0	634.8	578.7

API indicates Asian/Pacific Islander; AI/AN, American Indian/Alaska Native.
Adapted from Centers for Disease Control and Prevention. *Sexually Transmitted Diseases Surveillance, 2007*. Atlanta, GA: Department of Health and Human Services; 2008. Available at: www.cdc.gov/std/stats07/main.htm. Accessed April 11, 2009.

Table 1.35
Syphilis: rates per 100 000 population according to race/ethnicity, age group, and gender: United States, 2003–2007

Gender/Age group	2003	2004	2005	2006	2007
White, non-Hispanic					
Males	0.0	0.0	0.0	0.0	0.0
10–14 y					
15–19 y	0.4	0.5	0.5	0.6	0.7
20–24 y	2.4	2.8	3.4	3.7	4.1
Females	0.0	0.0	0.0	0.0	0.0
10–14 y					
15–19 y	0.4	0.4	0.5	0.5	0.7
20–24 y	0.6	0.9	0.8	0.7	1.1
Black, non-Hispanic					
Males	0.1	0.1	0.1	0.1	0.3
10–14 y					
15–19 y	5.9	7.1	10.6	14.7	17.8
20–24 y	21.1	25.0	30.2	41.0	57.5
Females	0.2	0.4	0.5	0.6	0.5
10–14 y					
15–19 y	7.4	6.3	8.2	10.6	10.4
20–24 y	10.9	13.2	13.5	14.8	16.0
Hispanic					
Males	0.0	0.0	0.1	0.0	0.0
10–14 y					
15–19 y	1.7	1.9	2.0	2.5	3.5
20–24 y	6.8	7.5	8.2	9.2	14.2
Females	0.3	0.1	0.0	0.0	0.0
10–14 y					
15–19 y	2.2	1.3	1.6	1.6	1.5
20–24 y	2.2	1.9	2.9	1.8	2.3
API					
Males	0.0	0.0	0.0	0.0	0.0
10–14 y					
15–19 y	1.2	1.9	0.9	0.2	0.0
20–24 y	2.3	3.1	2.3	2.3	2.5
Females	0.0	0.0	0.0	0.0	0.0
10–14 y					
15–19 y	0.2	0.5	0.2	0.0	0.0
20–24 y	0.4	0.6	0.8	0.2	0.4
AI/AN					
Males	0.0	0.0	0.0	0.0	0.0
10–14 y					
15–19 y	0.0	2.7	0.9	0.0	1.8
20–24 y	3.0	3.9	6.6	6.3	5.6

(Continued)

Table 1.35
(Continued)

Gender/Age group	2003	2004	2005	2006	2007
Females	0.9	0.0	0.0	1.0	0.0
10–14 y					
15–19 y	0.0	2.8	3.7	0.0	4.5
20–24 y	0.0	3.9	0.9	1.1	6.6

API indicates Asian/Pacific Islander; AI/AN, American Indian/Alaska Native.

Adapted from Centers for Disease Control and Prevention. *Sexually Transmitted Diseases Surveillance, 2007*. Atlanta, GA: Department of Health and Human Services; 2008. Available at: www.cdc.gov/std/stats07/main.htm. Accessed April 11, 2009.

Adolesc Med 20 (2009) 350–385

2. Biological and Psychosocial Growth and Development

PUBERTAL FAST FACTS

Endocrine

- Adrenal androgen production (dehydroepiandrosterone [DHEA], DHEA sulfate, and androstenedione) begins at ~6 to 8 years of age, before changes in gonadotropin secretion can be detected. Although adrenal androgens are not necessary for pubertal development to occur, they do stimulate the appearance of pubic and axillary hair in girls
- Early in puberty, the hypothalamus begins to secrete gonadotropin-releasing hormone (GnRH) in a pulsatile manner; initially, this occurs only during sleep. This phenomenon is seen even in agonadal children, which suggests the maturation of the pulse generator in the hypothalamus. GnRH secretion stimulates secretion of luteinizing hormone (LH) and, to a lesser extent, follicle-stimulating hormone (FSH) by the pituitary gland. The sensitivity of the hypothalamus and pituitary gland to negative feedback by estradiol (E_2) and testosterone lessens, further augmenting secretion of LH and FSH
- LH stimulates androgen production in ovarian thecal cells. In the testes, LH stimulates Leydig cells to produce testosterone
- In mid- to late puberty, FSH stimulates Sertoli cells to produce sperm. FSH stimulates ovarian follicle growth and the production of aromatase. Aromatase converts androgens to estrogens in the FSH-stimulated granulose cells
- At mid- to late puberty, governed by a separate mechanism from that described above, midcycle surges of estradiol trigger an LH surge that results in ovulation
- A variety of regulatory influences on the maturation of the hypothalamic-pituitary-gonadal (HPG) axis were recently identified. These influences include leptin (produced by fat cells) and the GPR54 G-protein-coupled receptor and its ligand (kisspeptins), derived from the *KiSS-1* gene. Leptin may provide a link between fat mass and the hypothalamus; there are leptin receptors throughout the HPG axis, and leptin accelerates

Alain Joffe, MD, MPH.
E-mail address: ajoffe@jhu.edu.

GnRH activity. Kisspeptins are thought to stimulate LH production through GnRH at the hypothalamic level

- Growth hormone is the key hormone that influences growth. Its secretion by the pituitary gland is stimulated by growth-hormone–releasing hormone and inhibited by somatostatin. Growth hormone stimulates production (in the liver) of insulin-like growth factors (IGFs) I and II, which in turn inhibit production of growth hormone. IGF-I stimulates bone and muscle growth. Peak IGF levels are demonstrated 1 to 2 years after achievement of peak height velocity

Body Composition/Nutrition

- Weight gained during puberty accounts for ~50% of adult ideal body weight
- Changes in body composition differ between boys and girls during puberty:
  - lean body mass decreases from 80% to 75% in girls while increasing from 80%/85% to 90% in boys;
  - percentage body fat increases from 16% to 27% in girls; and
  - lean body mass/fat mass ratio decreases from 5:1 at start of the female growth spurt to 3:1 at menarche
- At peak growth, girls attain a weight-gain velocity of 8 kg/year (95% range: 5.5–10.5). Boys attain a peak weight-gain velocity of 9 kg/year (95% range: 6–12.5)
- By the end of puberty, boys have 50% more lean body mass than girls; girls have twice the body fat of boys
- Growth demands during puberty require only an excess of 130 to 150 kcal/day over maintenance needs. Hence, the increased energy requirements during puberty result from increased maintenance and activity needs rather than growth. Adolescents who participate in sports may need 1000 kcal/day or more (even as much as 6000 kcal/day) depending on the type, duration, and intensity of the exercise/activity
- Eleven- to 14-year-old girls and boys require 1 g/kg per day of protein; this decreases to 0.9 and 0.8 g/kg per day of protein for 15- to 18-year-old boys and girls, respectively
- The prepubertal basal iron requirement for boys and girls is 10 mg/day. Girls require an additional 5 mg/day during the growth spurt and with menarche; boys require an additional 2 mg/day during growth
- The recommended daily allowance for calcium intake during adolescence is 1300 mg/day. The American Academy of Pediatrics recommends that adolescents consume 400 IU of vitamin D daily

Stature/Skeletal Changes

- Increases in foot-size velocity and height velocity precede the appearance of secondary sexual characteristics by ~4 to 6 months (data available for girls only)
- Growth during puberty accounts for 20% to 25% of adult height

- Growth in stature occurs first by increased leg length followed by increased growth of the trunk. Growth of the trunk contributes relatively more to pubertal growth than does increase in leg length
- Peak height velocity occurs sooner in girls than in boys. Boys average 28 cm of growth during puberty versus 25 cm for girls
- Ninety-five percent of girls complete growth by 16 years; the comparable figure for boys is 18 years
- Approximately 33% to 60% of adult bone mass accrues during adolescence/young adulthood
- By the end of puberty, boys have 50% more skeletal mass than girls
- Bone maturation is under the influence of multiple hormones: thyroxine, adrenal androgens, and gonadal sex steroids, especially estrogen
- Growth in hips and shoulders differs between girls and boys. Hips and shoulders grow equally in boys, resulting in a shoulder-to-hip ratio of 1.37 throughout puberty. In girls, hips widen more than shoulders; thus, the shoulder-to-hip ratio declines from 1.37 to 1.25 as puberty progresses

Sexual Maturation

See insert for figures 2.9–2.12, showing stages of pubertal development.

Boys

- The penis doubles in size, and the testes, prostate, and epididymis increase sevenfold
- Sperm are usually apparent in urine and semen by Tanner stage 3, and ejaculation usually occurs by Tanner stage 4

Girls

- Approximately 85% of girls will have breast development as the first secondary sexual characteristic to appear
- The uterus and ovaries increase in size approximately five- to sevenfold
- Ninety-five percent of girls will start to menstruate between 10.5 and 14.5 years of age; 98% of girls will have menstruated by the age of 15 years. Mean age of menarche is 12.43 years (black girls: 12.06 years; Hispanic girls: 12.25 years; white girls: 12.55 years)
- Menarche occurs when percentage body fat reaches 17%; regular cycles (or restoration of menses after amenorrhea) occur with a percentage body fat of 22%
- In young adolescents, the mean cycle interval is 32 days (90% range: 21–45). Menses typically lasts $\leq$7 days, and a girl will use between 3 and 6 pads/tampons per day
- Menarche typically occurs within 2 to 3 years of thelarche: Tanner stage 3 in 20% to 26% of girls and Tanner stage 4 in 47% to 62%
- Frequency of ovulation is related to age at menarche and time since menarche. If age of menarche is at <12 years, the time from menarche until 50% of cycles are ovulatory is approximately one year; that interval increases to 3 years if menarche occurs between 12 and 12.9 years and 4.5 years occurs after 13 years

REFERENCES

1. American Academy of Pediatrics, Committee on Adolescence; American College of Obstetricians and Gynecologists, Committee on Adolescent Health Care. Menstruation in girls and adolescents: using the menstrual cycle as a vital sign. *Pediatrics* 2006;118(5):2245–2250
2. Carswell JM, Stafford DEJ. Normal physical growth and development. In: Neinstein LS, Gordon CM, Katzman DK, Rosen DS, Woods ER, eds. *Adolescent Health Care: A Practical Guide*. 5th ed. Philadelphia, PA: Lippincott, Williams & Wilkins; 2009:3–26
3. DiVall SA, Radovick S. Endocrinology of female puberty. *Curr Opin Endocrinol Diabetes Obes*. 2009;16(1):1–4
4. Ford KR, Khoury JC, Biro FM. Early markers of pubertal onset: height and foot size. *J Adolesc Health*. 2009;44(5):500–501
5. Gordon CM, Laufer MR. The physiology of puberty. In: Emans SJ, Laufer MR, Goldstein DP, eds. *Pediatric and Adolescent Gynecology*. 5th ed. Philadelphia, PA: Lippincott, Williams & Wilkins; 2005:120–155
6. Kreipe RE. Normal somatic adolescent growth and development. In: McAnarney ER, Kreipe RE, Orr DP, Comerci GD, eds. *Textbook of Adolescent Medicine*. Philadelphia, PA: W. B. Saunders; 1992:44–67

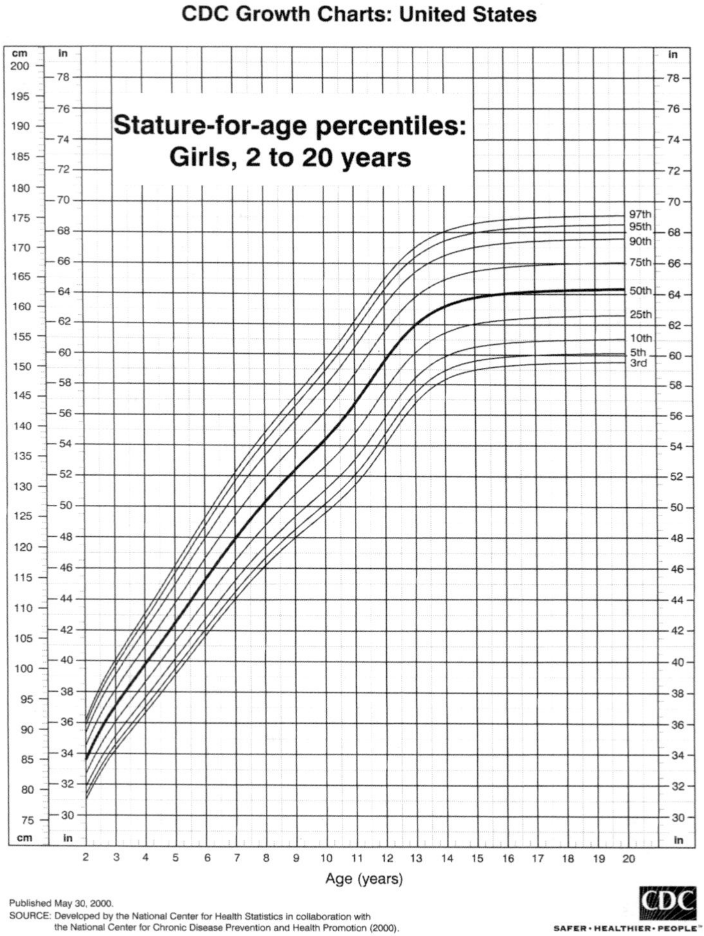

Fig 2.1. Stature-for-age percentiles: girls, 2 to 20 years. (Reproduced with permission from www.cdc.gov/growthcharts/clinical_charts.htm#Set1. Accessed August 5, 2009).

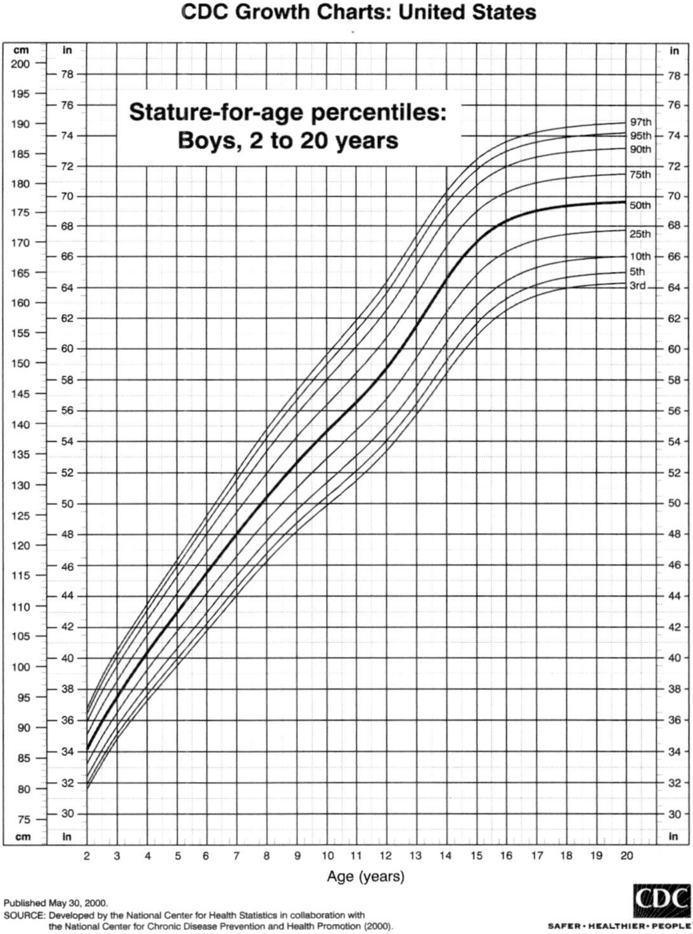

Fig 2.2. Stature-for-age percentiles: boys, 2 to 20 years. (Reproduced with permission from www.cdc.gov.growthcharts/clinical_charts.htm#Set1. Accessed August 5, 2009).

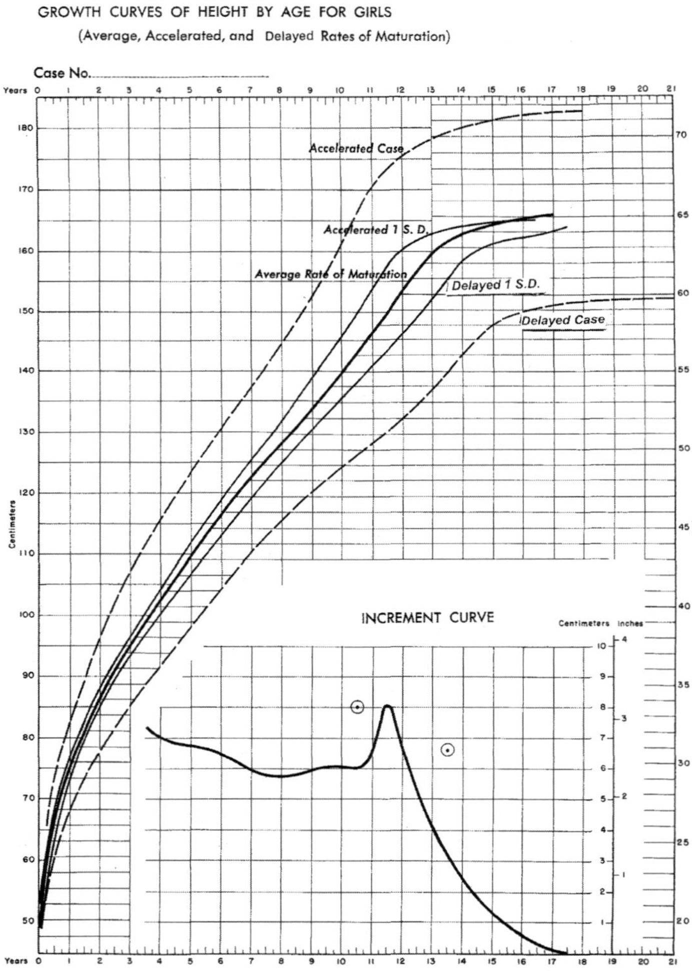

Fig 2.3. Growth curves of height by age for girls (Average, accelerated, and delayed rates of maturation) (Reprinted with permission from Bayer LM, Bayley N. *Growth Diagnosis*, 2nd ed. Chicago, Il; University of Chicago Press, 1976: 53.)

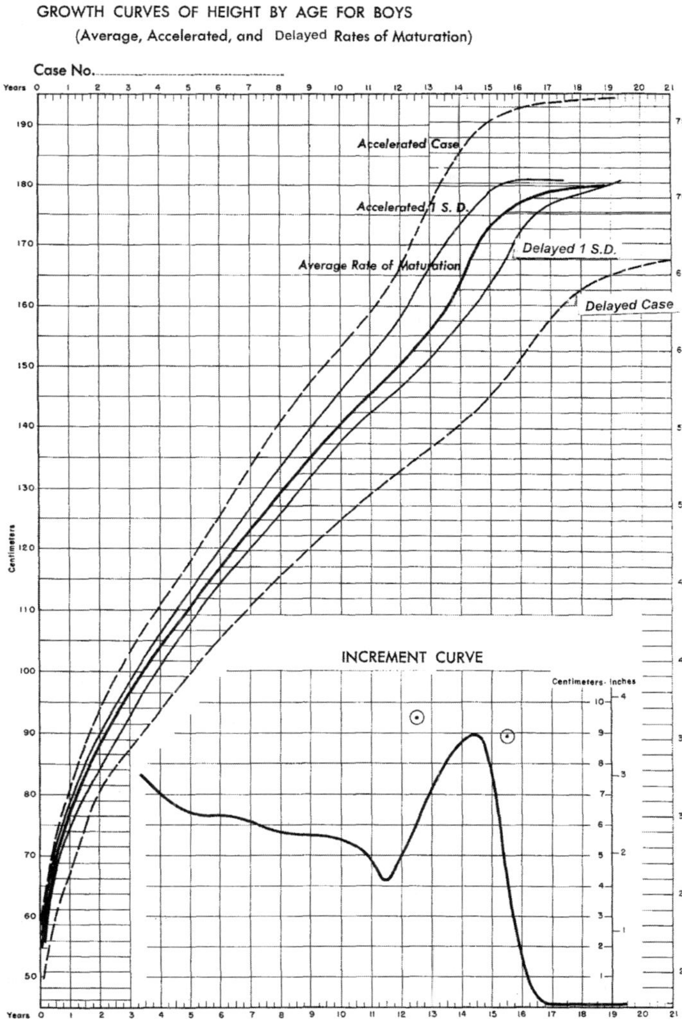

Fig 2.4. Growth curves of height by age for boys (average, accelerated, and delayed rates of maturation). (Reprinted with permission from Bayer LM, Bayley N. *Growth Diagnosis*, 2nd ed. Chicago, Il; University of Chicago Press, 1976: 51).

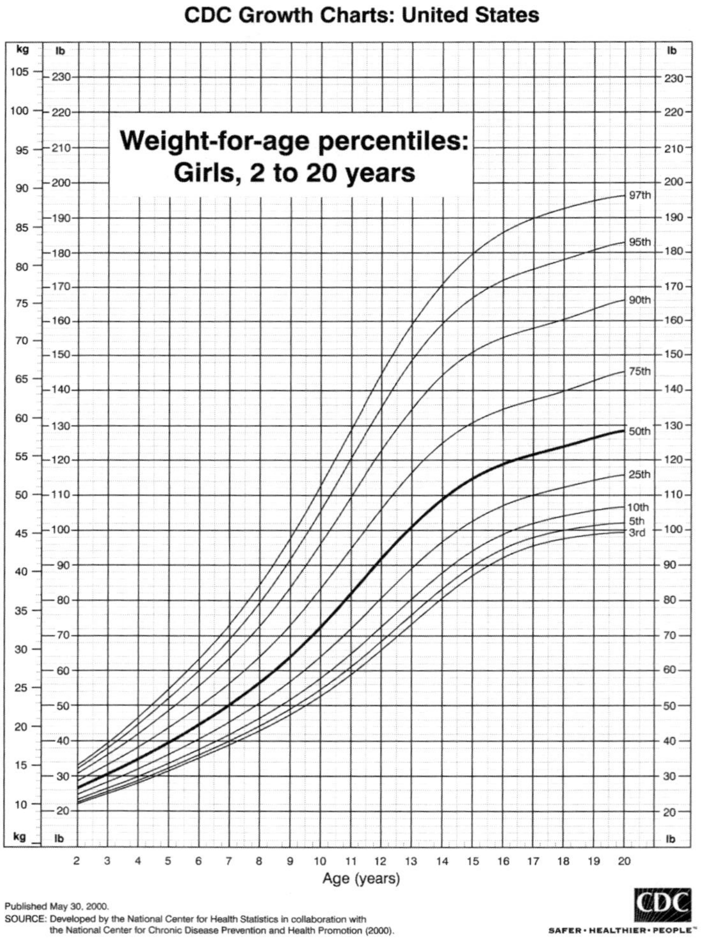

Fig 2.5. Weight-for-age percentiles: girls, 2 to 20 years. (Reproduced with permission from www.cdc.gov/growthcharts/clinical_charts.htm#Set1. Accessed August 5, 2009).

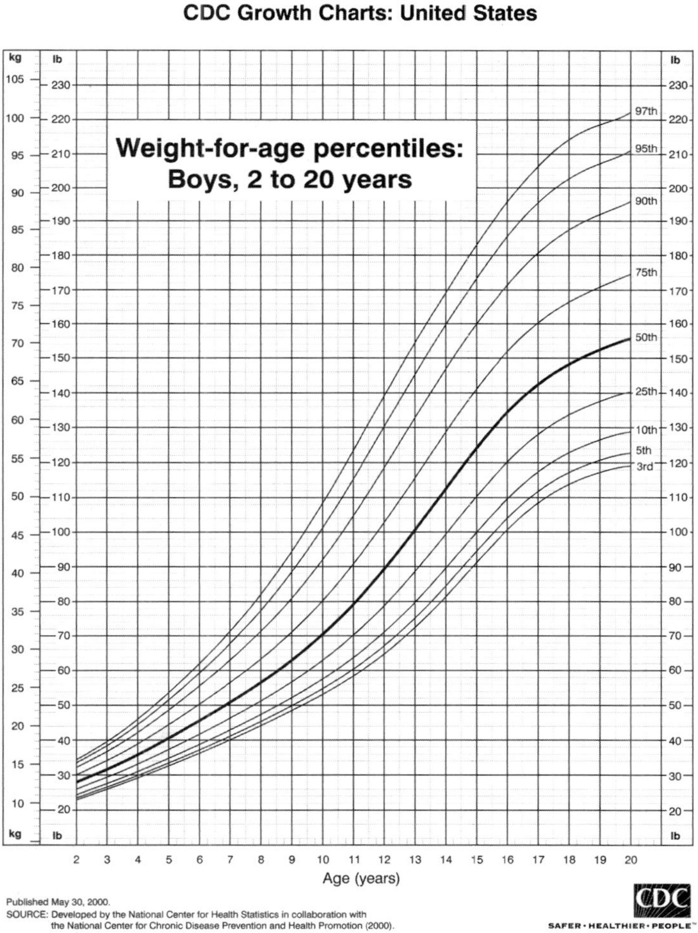

Fig 2.6. Weight-for-age percentiles: boys, 2 to 20 years. (Reproduced with permission from www.cdc.gov/growthcharts/clinical_charts.htm#Set1. Accessed August 5, 2009).

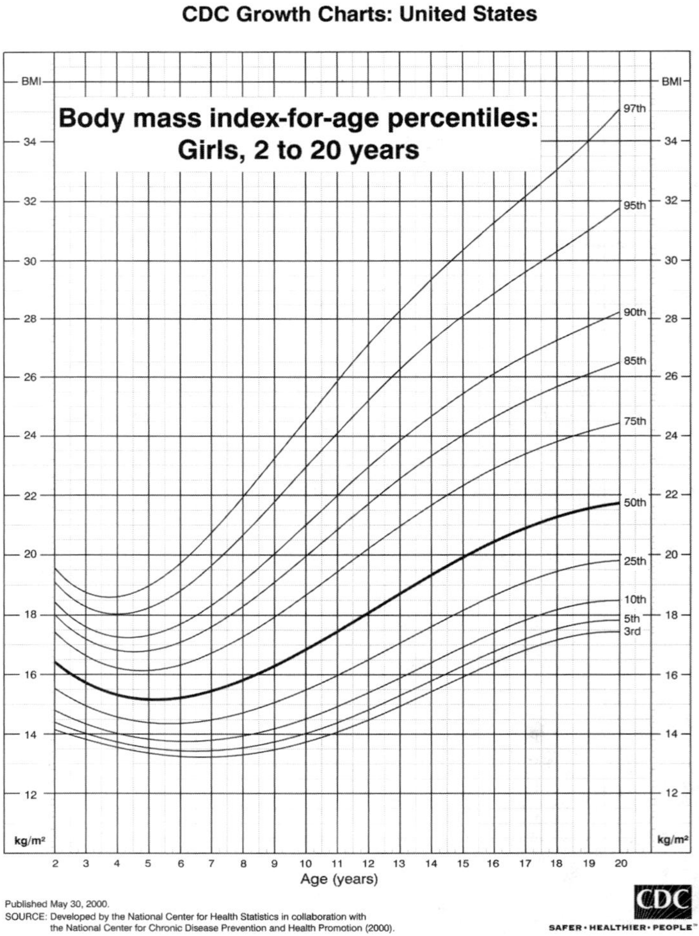

Fig 2.7. BMI-for-age percentiles, girls. (Reproduced with permission from www.cdc.gov/growthcharts/clinical_charts.htm#Set1. Accessed August 5, 2009).

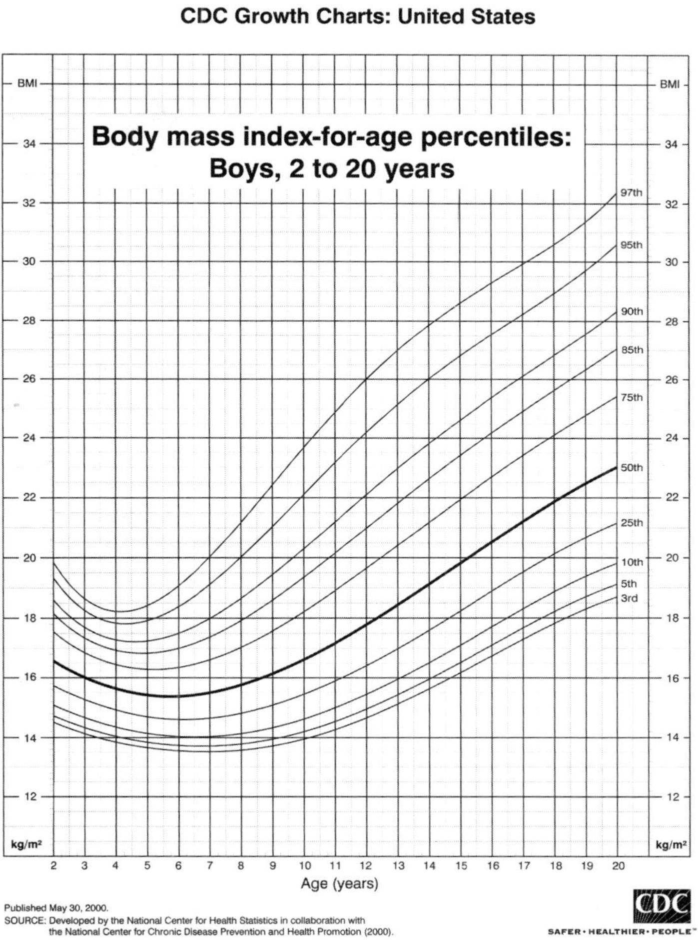

Fig 2.8. BMI-for-age percentiles, boys. (Reproduced with permission from www.cdc.gov/growthcharts/clinical_charts.htm#Set1. Accessed August 5, 2009).

See the color insert for figures 2.9–2.12, showing stages of pubertal development in boys and girls.

Table 2.1
BMI for Selected Weight and Stature

Guidelines for Adolescent Preventive Services

Body Mass Index for Selected Weight and Stature

Stature m (in)

Weight kg (lb)	1.24 (49)	1.27 (50)	1.30 (51)	1.32 (52)	1.35 (53)	1.37 (54)	1.40 (55)	1.42 (56)	1.45 (57)	1.47 (58)	1.50 (59)	1.52 (60)	1.55 (61)	1.57 (62)	1.60 (63)	1.63 (64)	1.65 (65)	1.68 (66)	1.70 (67)	1.73 (68)	1.75 (69)	1.78 (70)	1.80 (71)	1.83 (72)	1.85 (73)	1.88 (74)	1.90 (75)	1.93 (76)
20 (45)	13	13	12	12	11	11	10	10	10	9	9	9	8															
23 (50)	15	14	13	13	12	12	12	11	11	10	10	10	9	9	9	9	8											
25 (55)	16	15	15	14	14	13	13	12	12	12	11	11	10	10	10	9	9	9										
27 (60)	18	17	16	16	15	15	14	13	13	13	12	12	11	11	11	10	10	10	9	9								
29 (65)	19	18	17	17	16	16	15	15	14	14	13	13	12	12	12	11	11	10	10	10	10							
32 (70)	21	20	19	18	17	17	16	16	15	15	14	14	13	13	12	12	12	11	11	11	10	10						
34 (75)	22	21	20	20	19	18	17	17	16	16	15	15	14	14	13	13	12	12	12	11	11	11	10					
36 (80)	24	22	21	21	20	19	19	18	17	17	16	16	15	15	14	14	13	13	13	12	12	11	11	11				
39 (85)	25	24	23	22	21	21	20	19	18	18	17	17	16	16	15	15	14	14	13	13	13	12	12	12	11			
41 (90)	27	25	24	23	22	22	21	20	19	19	18	18	17	17	16	15	15	14	14	14	13	13	13	12	12	12		
43 (95)	28	27	25	25	24	23	22	21	20	20	19	19	18	17	17	16	16	15	15	14	14	13	13	13	12	12		
45 (100)	29	28	27	26	25	24	23	22	22	21	20	20	19	18	18	17	17	16	16	15	15	14	14	14	13	13	13	12
48 (105)	31	30	28	27	26	25	24	24	23	22	21	21	20	19	19	18	17	17	16	16	16	15	15	14	14	13	13	13
50 (110)	32	31	30	29	27	27	25	25	24	23	22	22	21	20	19	19	18	18	17	17	16	16	15	15	15	14	14	13
52 (115)	34	32	31	30	29	28	27	26	25	24	23	23	22	21	20	20	19	18	18	17	17	16	16	16	15	15	14	14
54 (120)	35	34	32	31	30	29	28	27	26	25	24	24	23	22	21	20	20	19	19	18	18	17	17	16	16	15	15	15
57 (125)	37	35	34	33	31	30	29	28	27	26	25	25	24	23	22	21	21	20	20	19	19	18	17	17	17	16	16	15
59 (130)	38	37	35	34	32	31	30	29	28	27	26	26	25	24	23	22	22	21	20	20	19	19	18	18	17	17	16	16
61 (135)	40	38	36	35	34	33	31	30	29	28	27	27	25	25	24	23	22	22	21	20	20	19	19	18	18	17	17	16
64 (140)	41	39	38	36	35	34	32	31	30	29	28	27	26	26	25	24	23	22	22	21	21	20	20	19	19	18	18	17
66 (145)	43	41	39	38	36	35	34	33	31	30	29	28	27	27	26	25	24	23	23	22	21	21	20	20	19	19	18	18
68 (150)	44	42	40	39	37	36	35	34	32	31	30	29	28	28	27	26	25	24	24	23	22	21	21	20	20	19	19	18
70 (155)	46	44	42	40	39	37	36	35	33	33	31	30	29	29	27	26	26	25	24	23	23	22	22	21	21	20	19	19
73 (160)	47	45	43	42	40	39	37	36	35	34	32	31	30	29	28	27	27	26	25	24	24	23	22	22	21	21	20	19
77 (170)	50	48	46	44	42	41	39	38	37	36	34	33	32	31	30	29	28	27	27	26	25	24	24	23	23	22	21	21
79 (175)		49	47	46	44	42	40	39	38	37	35	34	33	32	31	30	29	28	27	27	26	25	24	24	23	22	22	21
82 (180)		51	48	47	45	44	42	40	39	38	36	35	34	33	32	31	30	29	28	27	27	26	25	24	24	23	23	22
84 (185)			50	48	46	45	43	42	40	39	37	36	35	34	33	32	31	30	29	28	27	26	26	25	25	24	23	23
86 (190)				49	47	46	44	43	41	40	39	37	36	35	34	32	32	31	30	29	28	27	27	26	25	24	24	23
88 (195)				51	49	47	45	44	42	41	39	38	37	36	35	33	32	31	31	30	29	28	27	26	26	25	25	24
91 (200)					50	48	46	45	43	42	40	39	38	37	35	34	33	32	31	30	30	29	28	27	27	26	25	24
93 (205)						50	47	46	44	43	41	40	39	38	36	35	34	33	32	31	30	29	29	28	27	26	26	25
95 (210)							49	47	45	44	42	41	40	39	37	36	35	34	33	32	31	30	29	28	28	27	26	26
98 (215)							50	48	46	45	43	42	41	40	38	37	36	35	34	33	32	31	30	29	28	28	27	26
100 (220)								49	47	46	44	43	42	40	39	38	37	35	35	33	33	31	31	30	29	28	28	27
102 (225)								51	49	47	45	44	42	41	40	38	37	36	35	34	33	32	31	30	30	29	28	27
104 (230)									50	48	46	45	43	42	41	39	38	37	36	35	34	33	32	31	30	30	29	28
107 (235)										49	47	46	44	43	42	40	39	38	37	36	35	34	33	32	31	30	30	29
109 (240)										50	48	47	45	44	43	41	40	39	38	36	36	34	34	33	32	31	30	29
111 (245)											49	48	46	45	43	42	41	39	38	37	36	35	34	33	32	31	31	30
113 (250)											50	49	47	46	44	43	42	40	39	38	37	36	35	34	33	32	31	30
116 (255)												50	48	47	45	44	42	41	40	39	38	37	36	35	34	33	32	31
118 (260)													49	48	46	44	43	42	41	39	39	37	36	35	34	33	33	32
120 (265)													50	49	47	45	44	43	42	40	39	38	37	36	35	34	33	32
122 (270)														50	48	46	45	43	42	41	40	39	38	37	36	35	34	33
125 (275)															49	47	46	44	43	42	41	39	38	37	36	35	35	33
127 (280)															50	48	47	45	44	42	41	40	39	38	37	36	35	34
129 (285)															50	49	47	46	45	43	42	41	40	39	38	37	36	35
132 (290)																50	48	47	46	44	43	42	41	39	38	37	36	35
134 (295)																50	49	47	46	45	44	42	41	40	39	38	37	36
136 (300)																	50	48	47	45	44	43	42	41	40	39	38	37

Reprinted with permission from American Medical Association. *Guidelines for Adolescent Preventive Services*. Chicago, IL: American Medical Association; 1995.

Table 2.2
Descriptions of stages of pubertal development in boys and girls

Breast development

- B1: No palpable breast tissue; the areola is small and flat, and the nipple is elevated.
- B2: Breast tissue (bud) is palpable but only under the areola; the breast tissue and papilla elevate together as a small mound. The areola's diameter increases.
- B3: Both the areola and the breast tissue continue to enlarge, but there is no separation of the areola from the breast tissue (smooth contour).
- B4[a]: The areola and papilla form a secondary mound distinct from the breast tissue.
- B5: The areola and breast tissue form a smooth contour (no separation of areola); only the papilla projects above breast tissue.

Genital development

- G1: The testes, scrotum, and penis resemble those of a child.
- G2: Testes begin to increase in volume, and the scrotal skin thins and reddens. Slight penile enlargement may occur.
- G3: Penis enlarges, especially in length. Testicular volume increases, and scrotum continues to thin.
- G4: Penis enlarges, especially in diameter. The scrotal skin darkens, and the glans penis becomes more prominent.
- G5: Scrotum, penis, and testes are now all adult in size and appearance.

Pubic hair development

- Girls
  - PH1: No true pubic hair is present; fine vellus hairs cover the pubis.
  - PH2: Sparse growth of pubic hair confined in distribution to the medial labia. The hair is slightly pigmented, long, and "downy"; it tends to be straight to slightly curved.
  - PH3: The hair becomes darker, more curly, and coarser. It spreads to the mons pubis (sparsely).
  - PH4: Pubic hair is adult in nature, but the amount is less than that seen in adult women. The hair does not extend to the medial surface of the thighs.
  - PH5: Pubic hair is now adult-like in quantity, type, and distribution and has spread to the medial thighs. No hair extends up the linea alba or beyond the inverse triangle[b]
- Boys
  - PH1: Same as for girls.
  - PH2: Same as for girls. Distribution is limited to the base of the penis.
  - PH3: Same characteristics as for girls. Spreads out laterally from the base of the penis.
  - PH4: Same characteristics as for girls. No hair on the medial aspects of the thighs.
  - PH5: Same as for girls. Hair growth extends to the medial thighs.[b]

B*n* indicates stage of breast development; G*n*, stage of genital development in boys; PH*n*, stage of pubic hair (distribution and appearance).

[a] According to Tanner, ~25% of girls do not pass through stage 4 of breast development. In some women, the elevation of the areola to form a separate mound persists into adulthood.

[b] In ~10% of women and 80% of men, pubic hair may continue to spread beyond the inverse triangle (ie, up the linea alba) through the mid-20s; this is referred to as pubic hair stage 6 (PH6).

Adapted from Tanner JM. *Growth at Adolescence*. 2nd ed. Oxford, United Kingdom: Blackwell Scientific Publications; 1962:32–33; and Johnson RL, Tanner NM. Approaching the adolescent patient. In: Hofman A, Greydanus D, eds. *Adolescent Medicine*. 2nd ed. Norwalk, CT: Appleton and Lange; 1989:29–31.

Table 2.3
Comparison of the sequence of pubertal events in boys and girls

Girls		Boys	
B2	Appearance of breast buds (8–13 y)	G2	Testes enlarge (10–13.5 y)
PH2	Appearance of pubic hair (8–14 y)	G3	
		Penile enlargement begins	(11–14.5 y)
PHV	Peak height velocity	PH2	Pubic hair appears (10–15 y)
		Spermarche	Sperm detectable in urine
B3		G4	
PH3		PH3	
PH4		PHV	Peak height velocity
B4		PH4	
Menarche	(10–16.5 y)	G5	
PH5		PH5	
B5		Strength spurt	

The sequence of events occurs in order from top to bottom; the numbers in parentheses refer to the typical age range for the appearance of the indicated pubertal event. B*n* indicates stage of breast development; G*n*, stage of genital development in boys (as assessed by appearance of scrotum and enlargement of the penis and testicles); PH*n*, stage of pubic hair (distribution and appearance). For descriptions of each stage, see Table 2.2.
Adapted from Root AW. Endocrinology of puberty. I. Normal sexual maturation. *J Pediatr.* 1973;83(1):1–19; and Tanner JM. *Growth at Adolescence*. 2nd ed. Oxford, United Kingdom: Blackwell Scientific; 1962. Recent research data suggest that the age of onset of some pubertal events has shifted downward since these publications appeared.

Table 2.4
Duration of intervals between pubertal stages in girls and boys

Girls	Mean (95% range), y	Boys	Mean (97.5% range), y
B2–B3	0.86 (0.21–1.03)	G2–G3	1.12 (0.41–2.18)
B2–B4	1.80 (0.69–3.63)	G2–G5	3.05 (1.86–4.72)
B2–B5	4.00 (1.51–8.99)	G3–G4	0.81 (0.24–1.64)
B3–B4	0.89 (0.13–2.19)	G4–G5	1.01 (0.38–1.92)
B3–B5	3.08 (0.95–7.55)		
B4–B5	1.96 (0.12–6.82)		
PH2–PH3	0.62 (0.16–1.27)	PH2–PH3	0.44 (0.11–0.87)
PH2–PH4	1.13 (0.50–2.04)	PH2–PH5	1.59 (0.82–2.67)
PH2–PH5	2.49 (1.39–3.10)	PH3–PH4	0.42 (0.31–0.54)
PH3–PH4	0.51 (0.18–0.93)	PH4–PH5	0.72 (0.20–1.45)
PH3–PH5	1.85 (0.94–3.85)		
PH4–PH5	1.30 (0.57–2.37)		

For descriptions of pubertal stages, see Table 2.2. CI indicates confidence interval; B*n*, stage of breast development; G*n*, stage of genital development in boys; PH*n*, stage of pubic hair (distribution and appearance).

Adapted from Friedman IM, Goldberg E. Reference materials for the practice of adolescent medicine. *Pediatr Clin North Am.* 1980;27(1):193–209; Marshall WA, Tanner JM. Variations in patterns of pubertal changes in girls. *Arch Dis Child.* 1969;44(235):291–303; and Marshall WA, Tanner JM. Variations in patterns of pubertal changes in boys. *Arch Dis Child.* 1970;45(239):13–23.

Table 2.5
Testicular volumes in adolescent boys

	SMR1		SMR2		SMR3		SMR4		SMR5	
	Left	Right	Left	Right	Left	Right	Left	Right	Left	Right
Volume (SD), mL	4.8 (2.8)	5.2 (3.9)	6.4 (3.2)	7.1 (3.9)	14.6 (6.5)	14.8 (6.1)	19.8 (6.2)	20.4 (6.8)	28.3 (8.5)	30.2 (9.6)
Dimensions (cm) for a given volume, mL	5 ($1.8^a \times 2.7^b$) 6 (1.9 × 2.8)		8 (2.1 × 3.1) 10 (2.2 × 3.5)		12 (2.4 × 3.8) 15 cm^3 (2.6 × 4.1)		20 (3.9 × 4.3)		25 (4.1 × 4.8)	
According to pubic hair stage, mean (SD)	PH1: 6.0 mL (2.6)		PH2: 6.8 mL (3.6)							
				PH3: 9.3 mL (3.8)						
				PH4: 12.6 mL (4.2)						
					PH5: 16.3 mL (4.6)					
						PH6: 18.9 mL (4.0)				

SMR indicates sexual maturity rating (mean of genital and pubic hair ratings); PH*n*, stage of pubic hair (distribution and appearance).
[a] Shortest dimension of testis.
[b] Longest dimension of testis.
Adapted from Friedman IM, Goldberg E. Reference materials for the practice of adolescent medicine. *Pediatr Clin North Am*. 1980;27(1):193–209; and Neinstein L, Kaufman FR. Normal physical growth and development. In: Neinstein L. *Adolescent Health Care: A Practical Guide*. 4th ed. Philadelphia, PA: Lippincott, Williams & Wilkins; 2002:45.

Table 2.6
Median ages at entry into each maturity stage and fiducial limits[a] for pubic hair and breast development in girls according to race

Stage	Age at Entry for Girls, y					
	Non-Hispanic White		Non-Hispanic Black		Mexican American	
	Median	98.3% FLs	Median	98.3% FLs	Median	98.3% FLs
Pubic hair						
PH2	10.57[b]	10.29, 10.85	9.43[b]	9.05, 9.74	10.39	—
PH3	11.80[b]	11.54, 12.07	10.57[b]	10.30, 10.83	11.70[b]	11.14, 12.27
PH4	13.00[b]	12.71, 13.30	11.90[b]	11.38, 12.42	13.19[b]	12.88, 13.52
PH5	16.33[b]	15.86, 16.88	14.70[b]	14.32, 15.11	16.30[b]	15.90, 16.76
Breast development						
B2	10.38[b]	10.11, 10.65	9.48[b]	9.14, 9.76	9.80	0.00, 11.78
B3	11.75[b]	11.49, 12.02	10.79[b]	10.50, 11.08	11.43	8.64, 14.50
B4	13.29[b]	12.97, 13.61	12.24[b]	11.87, 12.61	13.07[b]	12.79, 13.36
B5	15.47[b]	15.04, 15.94	13.92[b]	13.57, 14.29	14.70[b]	14.37, 15.04

FL indicates fiducial limit; PH*n*, stage of pubic hair (distribution and appearance); B*n*, stage of breast development.

[a] Calculated 98.3% fiducial limits to adjust for multiple comparisons between races for an overall α value of .05.

[b] Significant pairwise racial difference: $P < .05$.

Adapted from Sun SS, Schubert CM, Chumlea WC, et al. National estimates of the timing of sexual maturation and racial differences among US children. *Pediatrics*. 2002;110(5):911–919.

Table 2.7
Mean ages and SEs for being in a stage for pubic hair and breast development in girls according to race

Stage	Age in Stage, y								
	Non-Hispanic White			Non-Hispanic Black			Mexican American		
	n	Mean	SE	*n*	Mean	SE	*n*	Mean	SE
Pubic hair									
PH2	67	10.96[a]	0.23	85	10.25[a]	0.15	105	11.17[a]	0.21
PH3	61	12.41[a]	0.19	98	11.37[a]	0.23	108	12.84[a]	0.18
PH4	154	15.11[a]	0.18	184	13.69[a]	0.31	177	14.61[a]	0.26
PH5	133	16.53[a]	0.17	282	16.05[a]	0.14	161	16.61[a]	0.12
Breast development									
B2	82	11.05[a]	0.18	99	10.25[a]	0.20	129	10.70	0.21
B3	80	12.80[a]	0.19	106	11.94[a]	0.22	131	12.61[a]	0.2
B4	110	15.16[a]	0.32	112	13.61[a]	0.34	97	14.03[a]	0.27
B5	173	16.25[a]	0.18	338	15.78[a]	0.14	254	16.21[a]	0.12

PH*n* indicates stage of pubic hair (distribution and appearance); B*n*, stage of breast development.

[a] Significant pair-wise racial difference, $P < .05$.

Adapted from Sun SS, Schubert CM, Chumlea WC, et al. National estimates of the timing of sexual maturation and racial differences among US children. *Pediatrics*. 2002;110(5):911–919.

Table 2.8
Median ages of entry into each stage and fiducial limits[a] for pubic hair and genitalia development in boys according to race

Stage	Age at Entry for Boys, y					
	Non-Hispanic White		Non-Hispanic Black		Mexican American	
	Median	98.3% FLs	Median	98.3% FLs	Median	98.3% FLs
Pubic hair						
PH2	11.98[b]	11.69, 12.29	11.16[b]	10.89, 11.43	12.30[b]	12.06, 12.56
PH3	12.65	12.37, 12.95	12.51[b]	12.26, 12.77	13.06[b]	12.79, 13.36
PH4	13.56	13.27, 13.86	13.73	13.49, 13.99	14.08	13.83, 14.32
PH5	15.67	15.30, 16.05	15.32	14.99, 15.67	15.75	15.46, 16.03
Genitalia development						
G2	10.03	9.61, 10.40	9.20[b]	8.62, 9.64	10.29[b]	9.94, 10.60
G3	12.32	12.00, 12.67	11.78[b]	11.50, 12.08	12.53[b]	12.29, 12.79
G4	13.52	13.22, 13.83	13.40	13.15, 13.66	13.77	13.51, 14.03
G5	16.01[b]	15.57, 16.50	15.00[b]	14.70, 15.32	15.76[b]	15.39, 16.14

FL indicates fiducial limit; PH*n*, stage of pubic hair (distribution and appearance); G*n*, stage of genital development.

[a] Calculated 98.3% fiducial limits to adjust for multiple comparisons between races for an overall α value of .05.

[b] Significant pairwise racial difference: $P < .05$.

Adapted from Sun SS, Schubert CM, Chumlea WC, et al. National estimates of the timing of sexual maturation and racial differences among US children. *Pediatrics*. 2002;110(5):911–919.

Table 2.9
Mean ages for being in a stage for pubic hair and genitalia development in boys according to race

Stage	Age in Stage, y								
	Non-Hispanic White			Non-Hispanic Black			Mexican American		
	n	Mean	SE	*n*	Mean	SE	*n*	Mean	SE
Pubic hair									
PH2	42	11.81	0.16	106	11.48[a]	0.13	50	12.20[a]	0.24
PH3	39	13.03	0.27	86	12.79[a]	0.19	55	13.44[a]	0.26
PH4	75	14.89	0.18	94	15.21	0.26	93	15.25	0.16
PH5	133	16.84	0.13	238	16.67[a]	0.08	211	17.14[a]	0.1
Genitalia development									
G2	136	11.08	0.18	181	10.79	0.13	183	11.09	0.17
G3	63	12.55	0.29	113	12.03[a]	0.28	80	12.97[a]	0.28
G4	91	15.29	0.19	98	15.07	0.33	104	15.38	0.19
G5	120	16.64	0.15	253	16.42[a]	0.09	219	16.85[a]	0.13

FL indicates fiducial limit; PH*n*, stage of pubic hair (distribution and appearance); G*n*, stage of genital development.

[a] Significant pairwise racial difference: $P < .05$.

Adapted from Sun SS, Schubert CM, Chumlea WC, et al. National estimates of the timing of sexual maturation and racial differences among US children. *Pediatrics*. 2002;110(5):911–919.

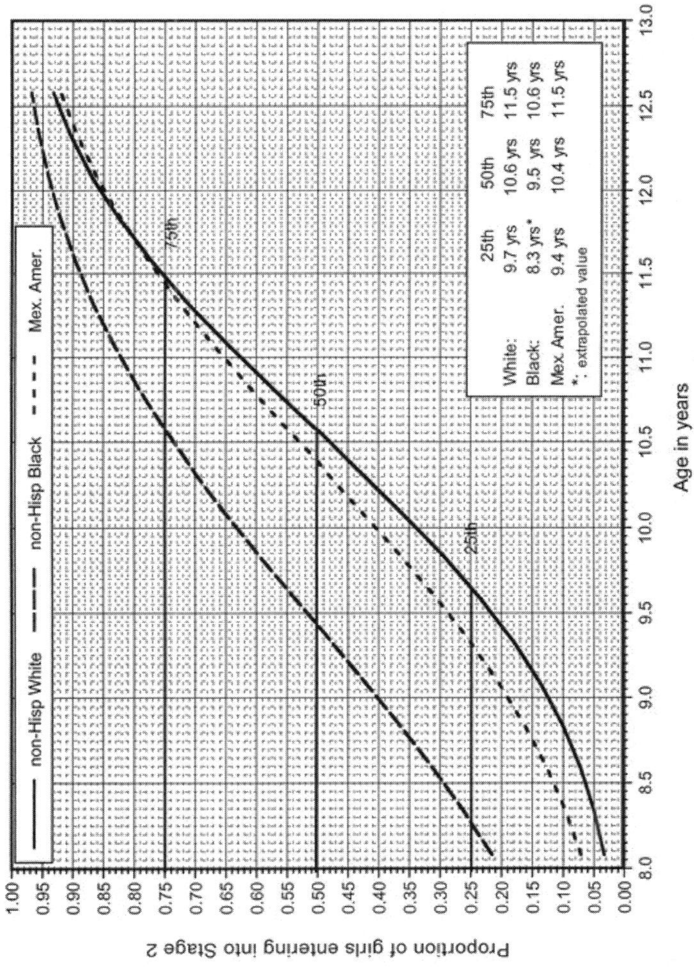

Fig 2.13. Reference data for age at onset of transition from stage 1 to stage 2 of pubic hair in girls. non-Hisp indicates non-Hispanic; Mex. Amer., Mexican American. [a]Extrapolated value. (Reproduced with permission from Sun SS, Schubert CM, Chumlea WC. National estimates of the timing of sexual maturation and racial differences among US children. *Pediatrics*. 2002;110[5]:911–919).

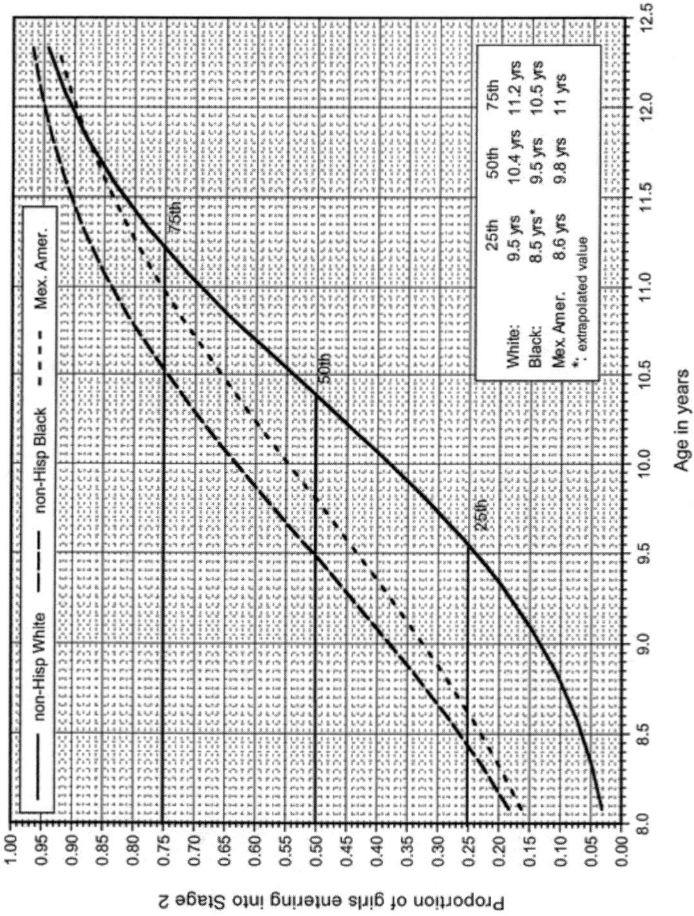

Fig 2.14. Reference data for age at onset of transition from stage 1 to stage 2 of breast development in girls. non-Hisp indicates non-Hispanic; Mex. Amer., Mexican American. [a]Extrapolated value. (Reproduced with permission from Sun SS, Schubert CM, Chumlea WC. National estimates of the timing of sexual maturation and racial differences among US children. *Pediatrics*. 2002;110[5]:911–919).

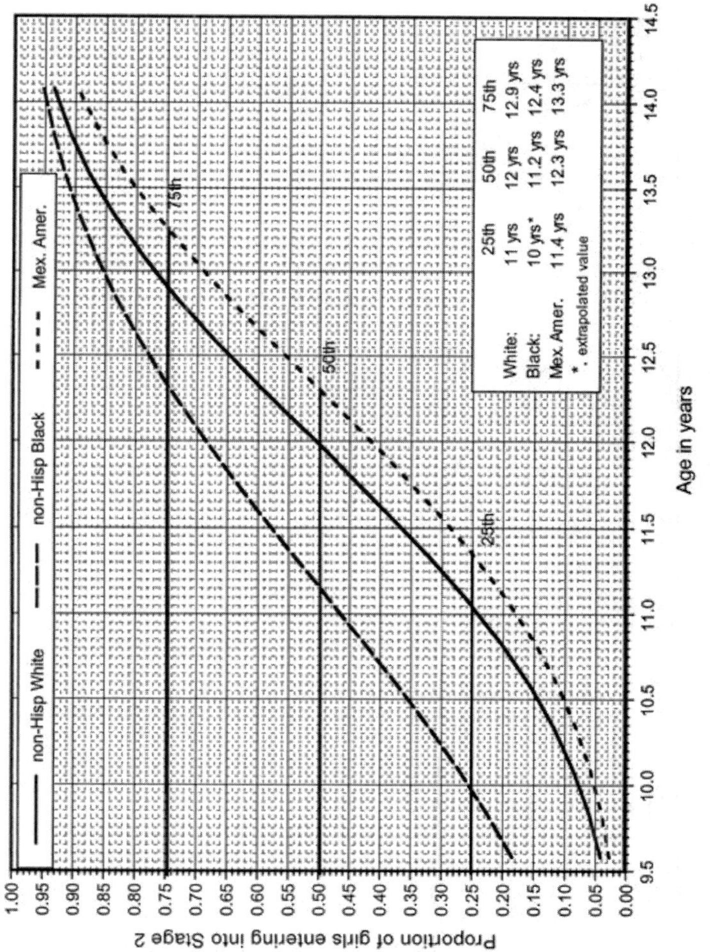

Fig 2.15. Reference data for age at onset of transition from stage 1 to stage 2 of pubic hair in boys. non-Hisp indicates non-Hispanic; Mex. Amer., Mexican American. [a]Extrapolated value. (Reproduced with permission from Sun SS, Schubert CM, Chumlea WC. National estimates of the timing of sexual maturation and racial differences among US children. *Pediatrics*. 2002;110[5]:911–919).

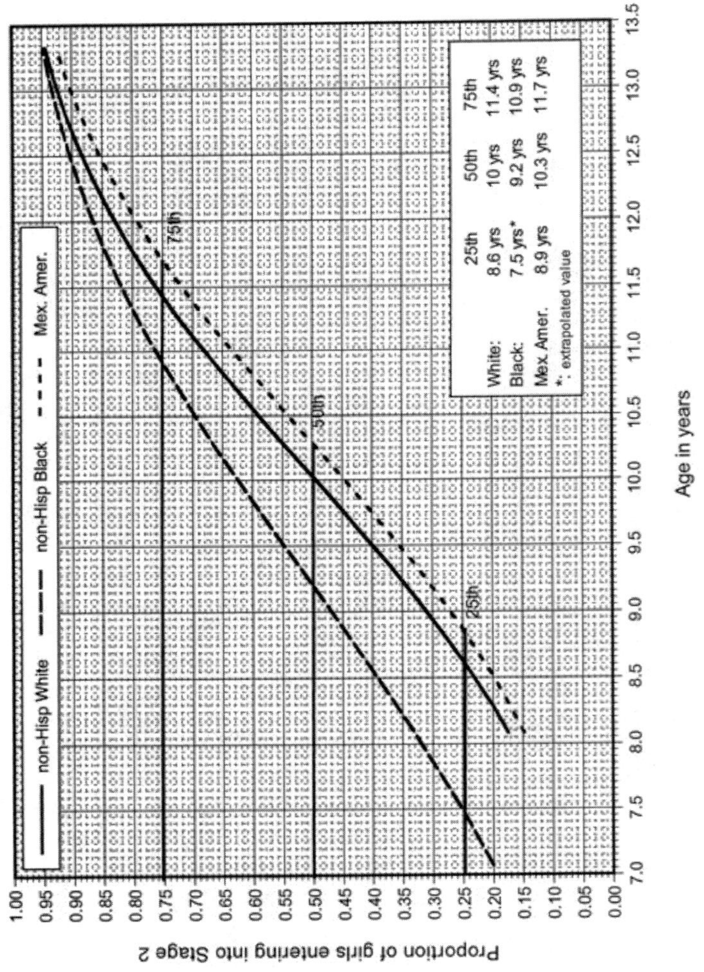

Fig 2.16. Reference data for age at onset of transition from stage 1 to stage 2 of genitalia development in boys. non-Hisp indicates non-Hispanic; Mex. Amer., Mexican American. [a]Extrapolated value. (Reproduced with permission from Sun SS, Schubert CM, Chumlea WC. National estimates of the timing of sexual maturation and racial differences among US children. *Pediatrics*. 2002;110[5]: 911–919).

Table 2.10
Strengths checklists oriented toward individual adolescents

Circle of Courage: Core Values for Nurturing Children	Basics of Parenting Adolescents	Desirable Youth Outcomes: The 5 Cs	READY for Life Checklist	Bright Futures Strengths During Adolescence	APA Factors Promoting Reliance and Positive Outcome	Criteria for the Assessment and Rating of Behavioral Adjustment
Spirit of generosity: the child can say, "I have a purpose for my life."	Teenagers need parent or an environment that will: love and connect; monitor and observe; guide and limit; model and consult: provide and advocate	Contribution	R: Relationships with friends, other students, co-workers, and family	Good physical health and nutrition	Stable, positive relationship with at least 1 caring adult	Relationships
Spirit of independence: the child can say, "I have power to make decisions."		Confidence	E: Energy to find things you enjoy	Appropriate weight	Religious and spiritual anchors	Satisfied internal status
Spirit of mastery: the child can say, "I can succeed."		Competence	A: Awareness of the world around you, your place in the world, and your contribution	Positive body image	Positive family environment	Coping patterns
Spirit of belonging: the child can say, "I am loved."		Connection	D: Independent decision-maker; knows how to get things done and can control behavior	Healthy habits and responsibility for health	Emotional intelligence and ability to cope with stress	

(Continued)

Table 2.10
(Continued)

Circle of Courage: Core Values for Nurturing Children	Basics of Parenting Adolescents	Desirable Youth Outcomes: The 5 Cs	READY for Life Checklist	Bright Futures Strengths During Adolescence	APA Factors Promoting Reliance and Positive Outcome	Criteria for the Assessment and Rating of Behavioral Adjustment
		Character	Y: Says "yes" to healthy behavior; eat well, play hard, work hard	Regular oral health care Physical activity Positive attitude Anger-management skills Safe experimentation Has confidants and capacity for intimacy Social competence Experiences hope, joy, success, love Self-esteem and expects success Learns stress management Demonstrates independence Individual identity Respects rights and need of others Establishes goals		

APA indicates American Psychological Association.
Adapted from Duncan PM, Garcia AC, Frankowski BL, et al. Inspiring healthy adolescent choices: a rationale for and guide to strength promotion in primary care. *J Adolesc Health*. 2007;41(6):525–535 with permission from Elsevier. More detailed information about the sources of each column heading can be found in the references on pages 533–535.

Table 2.11
Features of an office setting that supports adolescent strengths

Features of Positive Developmental Settings			Implications for the Medical Office
Feature	Descriptors	Opposite Poles	
Physical and psychological safety	Safe and health-promoting facilities and practices that increase safe peer group interaction and decrease unsafe or confrontational peer interactions	Physical and health dangers; fear; feeling of insecurity; sexual and physical harassment; and verbal abuse	Establish confidentiality policies and inform adolescent of what constitutes protected information; ensure privacy in changing areas and during specimen collection
Appropriate structure	Limit setting; clear and consistent rules and expectations; firm-enough control; continuity and predictability; clear boundaries; and age-appropriate monitoring	Chaotic; disorganized; laissez-faire; rigid; overcontrolled; and autocratic	Explain (verbally or in writing) to the adolescent what topics will be covered during the visit and options for follow-up; as patients mature, introduce the idea of an examination or confidential conversations without the parent present
Supportive relationships	Warmth; closeness; connectedness; good communication; caring; support; guidance; secure attachment; and responsiveness	Cold; distant; overcontrolling; ambiguous support; untrustworthy; focused on winning; inattentive; unresponsive; and rejecting	All staff should address adolescents directly and pause to allow adolescents enough time to respond; ask questions that show interest in or knowledge of the adolescent's stage of life
Opportunities to belong	Opportunities for meaningful inclusion, regardless of one's gender, ethnicity, sexual orientation, or disabilities; social inclusion, social engagement, and integration; opportunities for sociocultural identify formation; and support for cultural and bicultural competence	Exclusion; marginalization; and intergroup conflict	Offer appointment times for adolescents separate from times when smaller children or adults are seen; offer reading materials, furniture, and posters appropriate for adolescents

(Continued)

Table 2.11
(Continued)

Features of Positive Developmental Settings			Implications for the Medical Office
Feature	Descriptors	Opposite Poles	
Positive social norms	Rules of behavior; expectations; injunctions; ways of doing things; values and morals; and obligations for service	Normlessness; anomie, laissez-faire practices; antisocial and amoral norms that encourage violence; reckless behavior; consumerism; poor health practice; and conformity	Model respectful interactions with patients; discuss strengths and accomplishments and/or goals with the patient; express concern (without judgment) for the implications of risky behavior; share information to dispel myths about the prevalence of risky behaviors (eg, explain that ″most people your age are not sexually active″)
Support for efficacy and mattering	Youth-based; empowerment practices that support autonomy; making a real difference in one's community; and being taken seriously; practice that includes enabling, responsibility granting, and meaningful challenge; practices, that focus on improvement rather than on relative current performance levels	Unchallenging; overcontrolling; disempowering, and disabling; practices that undermine motivation and desire to learn, such as excessive focus on current relative performance level rather than improvement	Verbally, and with posters and other materials, acknowledge the adolescent's responsibility for his or her own health; direct recommendations regarding medications, diet, etc, primarily to the adolescent and secondarily to the parent; ask for adolescent feedback on the office experience and quality of service; encourage youth to consider making a difference in their community
Opportunities for skill building	Opportunities to learn physical, intellectual, psychological, emotional, and social skills; exposure to intentional learning experience; opportunities to learn cultural literacies, media literacy, communication skills, and good opportunities to develop social and cultural capital	Practices that promote bad physical habits and habits of mind; and practices that undermine school and learning	Have health information materials geared to adolescents; encourage problem solving and critical thinking about media messages; use motivational interviewing or reflective listening to help adolescents think through the consequences of their behaviors

(Continued)

Table 2.11
(Continued)

Features of Positive Developmental Settings			Implications for the Medical Office
Feature	Descriptors	Opposite Poles	
Integration of family, school, and community efforts	Concordance; coordination; and synergy among family, school, and community	Discordance; lack of communication; and conflict	Post or mention volunteer opportunities and community events that are appropriate for adolescents; contact area schools to find out if and how they are engaging positive youth-development concepts; try to the use the same materials and language they use to discuss strengths

Adapted from Duncan PM, Garcia AC, Frankowski BL, et al. Inspiring healthy adolescent choices: a rationale for and guide to strength promotion in primary care. *J Adolesc Health*. 2007;41(6):525–535, with permission from Elsevier. Features of positive developmental settings are drawn from: Eccles US, Gootman JA. Community programs to promote youth development. Washington, DC: National Academy Press, 2002. Available at: http://books.nap.edu/openbook.php?record_id=10022+page=86. Accessed August 5, 2009.

Table 2.12
Characteristics of adolescence

Characteristic	Early Adolescence	Midadolescence	Late Adolescence
Growth	Secondary sexual characteristics have begun to appear	Secondary sexual characteristics well advanced	Physically mature; statural and reproductive growth virtually complete
	Growth rapidly accelerating; reaches peak velocity	Growth decelerating; stature reaches 95% of adult height	
Cognition	Concrete thought dominant	Rapidly gaining competence in abstract thought	Established abstract thought processes
	Existential orientation	Capable of perceiving future implications of current acts and decisions but variably applied	Future oriented
	Cannot perceive long-range implications of current decisions and acts	Reverts to concrete operations under stress	Capable of perceiving and acting on long-range options
Psychosocial self	Preoccupation with rapid body change	Reestablishes body image as growth decelerates and stabilizes	Emancipation completed
		Preoccupation with fantasy and idealism in exploring expanded cognition and future options	Intellectual and functional identity established
		Development of a sense of omnipotence and invincibility	May experience "crisis of 21" when facing societal demands for autonomy
Family	Defining independence-dependence boundaries	Major conflicts over control	Transposition of child-parent dependency relationship to the adult-adult model
	No major conflicts over parental control	Struggle for emancipation	
Peer group	Seeks peer affiliation to counter instability generated by rapid change	Strong need for identification to affirm self-image	Recedes in importance in favor of individual friendships
	Compares own normality and acceptance with same-sex/age mates	Looks to peer group to define behavioral code during emancipation	

(Continued)

Table 2.12
(Continued)

Characteristic	Early Adolescence	Midadolescence	Late Adolescence
Sexuality	Self-exploration and evaluation	Multiple plural relationships Heightened sexual activity	Forms stable relationships Capable of mutuality and reciprocity in caring for another rather than former narcissistic orientation
	Limited dating	Testing ability to attract opposite sex and parameters of masculinity of femininity	Plans for future in thinking of marriage, family
	Limited intimacy	Preoccupation with romantic fantasy	Intimacy involves commitment rather than exploration and romanticism
Age range	Initiates between ages 11 and 13 y and merges with midadolescence at 14–15 y	Begins around 14–15 y and blends into late adolescence about age 17 y	~17–21 y upper end particularly variable; dependent on cultural, economic, and educational factors

Editor's note: Not all adolescents are heterosexual, although the sexuality portion of this table suggests otherwise. Issues relating to identity development in gay, lesbian, bisexual, and transgendered youth are detailed in Tables 2.12 through 2.15. Also, not all adolescents will want to marry, but decisions regarding commitment and long-term relationships are salient for all adolescents.

Adapted from Johnson RL. Adolescent growth and development. In: Hofman A, Greydanus D, eds. *Adolescent Medicine*. Norwalk, CT: Appleton and Lange; 1989:13.

Table 2.13
Identity

Gender identity	Personal sense of being male or female, established by age 3 y
Sex roles	Social and cultural expectations, attitudes (eg, stereotypes), and beliefs of male and female behavior, usually established between the ages of 3 and 7 y
Sexual orientation	Pattern of physical behavior and emotional-erotic attraction to others, believed to be established by early childhood
Homosexuality	Same-sex attraction
Heterosexuality	Opposite-sex attraction
Bisexuality	Attraction to both sexes

Identity is comprised of gender identity, sex (or gender) role, sexual orientation and personality. Consolidating adult identity is a primary developmental task of adolescence.
Adapted from Ryan C, Futterman D. Lesbian and gay youth: care and counseling. *Adolesc Med*. 1997;8(2):213, 256.

Table 2.14
Stages of lesbian/gay identity development

Stage 1: sensitization	Before puberty, children experience feelings of being "different" from peers based on gender-neutral or atypical gender role choices or behaviors; few see themselves as sexually different before age 12 y
Stage 2: identity confusion	After puberty, adolescents become aware of same-sex thoughts and feelings
	Negative stereotypes of homosexuality lead to cognitive dissonance and confusion as adolescents struggle to make sense of their emerging identity; lack of accurate information about homosexuality or positive lesbian/gay role models increases isolation and confusion; adolescents respond by developing coping behaviors and usually hide their sexual identity or may adopt a bisexual identity
Stage 3: identity assumption	During midadolescence to late adolescence or early adulthood, youth begin to self-identify and disclose their identity (come out) to other gay people; over a period of several years, they interact with lesbian and gay peers; positive experiences strengthen self-esteem and dispel negative stereotypes; access to an organized lesbian/gay community provides opportunities for socialization and for developing relationships and finding positive role models; youth learn a variety of strategies to manage their stigmatized identity
Stage 4: commitment	Serf-acceptance generally culminates with incorporating sexual identity into all aspects of one's life, usually during adulthood; sexual identity is shared increasingly with nongay friends and close family members; however, not all lesbians and gay males consolidate identity; integration depends on various factors, including access to support and positive role models, personal strengths and vulnerabilities, and experiences with discrimination

Adapted from Troiden RR. The formation of homosexual identities. *J Homosex.* 1989;17(1–2):43–73.

Table 2.15
Transgender identity

Gender bender	Crossing the gender line in dress and behavior to make a political statement, to feel more comfortable, to express difference from conventional society (eg, "queer" identity), or to provide entertainment (eg, drag queens)
Transvestite	Cross-dressing (wear clothes of the opposite sex) for emotional comfort or erotic fulfillment
Androgyne	Blending masculine and feminine characteristics for sense of emotional completeness
Transsexual	Feeling "trapped in the wrong body"; anatomical gender does not match internal sense of being male or female
Nonsurgical	Choosing to live as the opposite sex without sex-reassignment surgery; may or may not use hormones to enhance development of secondary sex characteristics
Preoperative and postoperative	Choosing to have sex-reassignment surgery; generally seeking assistance from gender-identity clinics, which recommend counseling and living full-time for at least 1 y as the opposite sex before initiating surgery

Transgender covers a broad range of gender-nonconforming identities and behaviors. Transgendered persons may be heterosexual, homosexual, bisexual, or asexual. Providers should not assume that all transgendered people experience gender dysphoria.

Adapted from Ryan C, Futterman D. Lesbian and gay youth: care and counseling. *Adolesc Med.* 1997;8(2):213, 256.

FORMULA FOR PREDICTING ADOLESCENTS' ADULT HEIGHT ON THE BASIS OF PARENTAL HEIGHTS

For girls: (father's height + mother's height)/2 − (6.5 cm or 2.5 in)

For boys: (father's height + mother's height)/2 + (6.5 cm or 2.5 in)

MOSTELLER'S FORMULA FOR CALCULATING BODY SURFACE AREA

Surface area (m^2) = $\sqrt{(\text{weight [kg]} \times \text{height [cm]})/3600}$

Reference: Mosteller RD. Simplified calculation of body-surface area. *N Engl J Med.* 1987;317(17):1098.

Search INSTITUTE — Practical research benefiting children and youth

40 Developmental Assets™

Search Institute[SM] has identified the following building blocks of healthy development that help young people grow up healthy, caring, and responsible.

HEALTHY COMMUNITIES • HEALTHY YOUTH®

	Category	Asset Name and Definition
External Assets	Support	1. **Family Support**-Family life provides high levels of love and support. 2. **Positive Family Communication**-Young person and her or his parent(s) communicate positively, and young person is willing to seek advice and counsel from parents. 3. **Other Adult Relationships**-Young person receives support from three or more nonparent adults. 4. **Caring Neighborhood**-Young person experiences caring neighbors. 5. **Caring School Climate**-School provides a caring, encouraging environment. 6. **Parent Involvement in Schooling**-Parent(s) are actively involved in helping young person succeed in school.
	Empowerment	7. **Community Values Youth**-Young person perceives that adults in the community value youth. 8. **Youth as Resources**-Young people are given useful roles in the community. 9. **Service to Others**-Young person serves in the community one hour or more per week. 10. **Safety**-Young person feels safe at home, school, and in the neighborhood.
	Boundaries & Expectations	11. **Family Boundaries**-Family has clear rules and consequences and monitors the young person's whereabouts. 12. **School Boundaries**-School provides clear rules and consequences. 13. **Neighborhood Boundaries**-Neighbors take responsibility for monitoring young people's behavior. 14. **Adult Role Models**-Parent(s) and other adults model positive, responsible behavior. 15. **Positive Peer Influence**-Young person's best friends model responsible behavior. 16. **High Expectations**-Both parent(s) and teachers encourage the young person to do well.
	Constructive Use of Time	17. **Creative Activities**-Young person spends three or more hours per week in lessons or practice in music, theater, or other arts. 18. **Youth Programs**-Young person spends three or more hours per week in sports, clubs, or organizations at school and/or in the community. 19. **Religious Community**-Young person spends one or more hours per week in activities in a religious institution. 20. **Time at Home**-Young person is out with friends "with nothing special to do" two or fewer nights per week.
Internal Assets	Commitment to Learning	21. **Achievement Motivation**-Young person is motivated to do well in school. 22. **School Engagement**-Young person is actively engaged in learning. 23. **Homework**-Young person reports doing at least one hour of homework every school day. 24. **Bonding to School**-Young person cares about her or his school. 25. **Reading for Pleasure**-Young person reads for pleasure three or more hours per week.
	Positive Values	26. **Caring**-Young person places high value on helping other people. 27. **Equality and Social Justice**-Young person places high value on promoting equality and reducing hunger and poverty. 28. **Integrity**-Young person acts on convictions and stands up for her or his beliefs. 29. **Honesty**-Young person "tells the truth even when it is not easy." 30. **Responsibility**-Young person accepts and takes personal responsibility. 31. **Restraint**-Young person believes it is important not to be sexually active or to use alcohol or other drugs.
	Social Competencies	32. **Planning and Decision Making**-Young person knows how to plan ahead and make choices. 33. **Interpersonal Competence**-Young person has empathy, sensitivity, and friendship skills. 34. **Cultural Competence**-Young person has knowledge of and comfort with people of different cultural/racial/ethnic backgrounds. 35. **Resistance Skills**-Young person can resist negative peer pressure and dangerous situations. 36. **Peaceful Conflict Resolution**-Young person seeks to resolve conflict nonviolently.
	Positive Identity	37. **Personal Power**-Young person feels he or she has control over "things that happen to me." 38. **Self-Esteem**-Young person reports having a high self-esteem. 39. **Sense of Purpose**-Young person reports that "my life has a purpose." 40. **Positive View of Personal Future**-Young person is optimistic about her or his personal future.

Fig 2.17. Forty developmental assets for adolescents (aged 12–18 years). (Reproduced with permission from www.search-institute.org/system/files/40AssetsList.pdf. Accessed April 24, 2009).

Adolesc Med 20 (2009) 386–415

3. The Adolescent Office Visit

Alain Joffe, MD, MPH.
E-mail address: ajoffe@jhu.edu.

 ISSN 1934-4287

Table 3.1
Comparisons among recommendations for adolescent preventive services developed by national organizations

	AAFP	AAP	AMA	BF	USPSTF
Immunizations					
ACIP recommendations	Yes	Yes	Yes	Yes	Yes
Health guidance for teenagers					
Normal development[a,b]	Yes	Yes	Yes	Yes	No
Injury prevention[a,c]	Yes	Yes	Yes	Yes	Yes
Nutrition[a]	Yes	Yes	Yes	Yes	Yes
Physical activity[a]	Yes	Yes	Yes	Yes	Yes
Dental health[a]	Yes	Yes	No	Yes	Yes
Breast or testicular self-examination[a]	Yes	Yes	No	Yes	No
Skin protection[a]	Yes	Yes	Yes	Yes	Yes
Health guidance for parents[a]	No	Yes	Yes	Yes	No
Screening/counseling[d]					
Obesity[a]	Yes	Yes	Yes	Yes	Yes
Contraception[e]	Yes	Yes	Yes	Yes	Yes
Tobacco use[a]	Yes	Yes	Yes	Yes	Yes
Alcohol use[a]	Yes	Yes	Yes	Yes	Yes
Substance use[a]	Yes	Yes	Yes	Yes	Yes
Hypertension[a]	Yes	Yes	Yes	Yes	Yes
Depression/suicide[a]	No	Yes	Yes	Yes	No
Eating disorders[a]	No	Yes	Yes	Yes	No
School problems[a]	No	Yes	Yes	Yes	No
Abuse[a]	No	Yes	Yes	Yes	No[f]
Hearing[a]	Yes	Yes	No	Yes	No
Vision[a]	No	Yes	No	Yes	No
Tests					
Tuberculosis[e]	Yes	Yes	Yes	Yes	Yes
Papanicolaou test[e]	Yes	Yes	Yes	Yes	Yes
HIV infection[e]	Yes	Yes	Yes	Yes	Yes
Sexually transmitted diseases[e]	Yes	Yes	Yes	Yes	Yes
Cholesterol[e]	Yes	Yes	Yes	Yes	No
Urinalysis[a]	No	Yes	No	No	No
Hematocrit[a]	No	Yes	No	No	No
Periodicity of visits	Tailored	Annual	Annual	Annual	Tailored
Target age range, y[g]	13–18	11–21	11–21	11–21	11–24

AAFP indicates American Academy of Family Physicians; AAP, American Academy of Pediatrics; AMA, American Medical Association (data are from Elster and Kuznets); BF, Bright Futures (data are from Green); and USPSTF, US Preventive Services Task Force; ACIP, Advisory Committee on Immunization Practices.

[a] The procedure is recommended for all adolescents/parents.

(*Continued*)

Table 3.1
(Continued)

[b] This includes providing adolescents with information on normal physical, psychosocial, and sexual development.
[c] This includes activities such as promoting the use of safety belts and safety helmets, placement of home fire alarms, and reducing the risk of injury from firearms and violence; organizations differ in the activities they include for injury prevention.
[d] The AAP recommends "developmental/behavioral assessment."
[e] Procedure is recommended for selected adolescents who are at high risk for the medical problem.
[f] Child abuse is not addressed as a separate screening topic but is included in the general screening for family violence.
[g] The American Academy of Pediatrics, American Medical Association, and Bright Futures make a distinction among developmental stages of adolescence.
Adapted from Elster AB. Comparison of recommendations for adolescent clinical preventive services developed by national organizations. *Arch Pediatr Adolesc Med.* 1998;152(2):193–198.

Figures 3.1 and 3.2 are found in the insert.

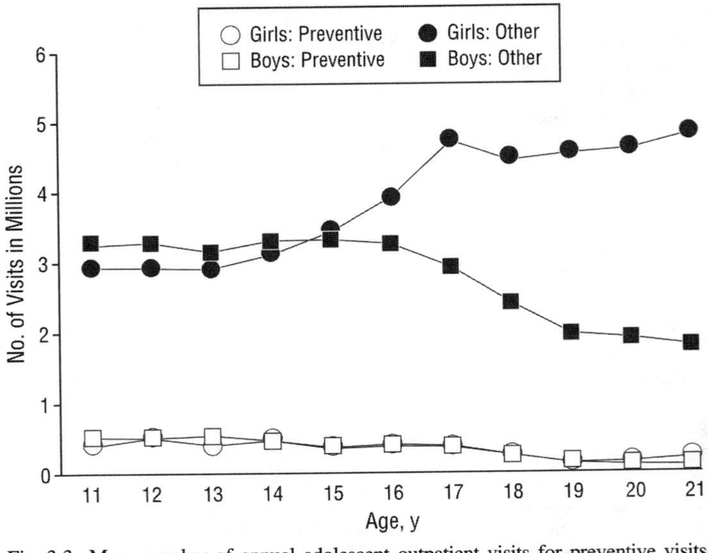

Fig 3.3. Mean number of annual adolescent outpatient visits for preventive visits versus other visits according to age and gender, 1994–2003, National Ambulatory Medical Care Survey and National Hospital Ambulatory Medical Care Survey. (Reproduced with permission from Rand CM, Shone LP, Albertin C. National health care visit patterns for adolescents. *Arch Pediatr Adolesc Med.* 2007;161[3]:252–259).

Table 3.2
Minors' access to contraceptive services

State	Explicitly Allows All Minors to Consent to Services	Explicitly Allows Certain Minors to Consent to Services					No Explicit Policy
		Health	Married	Parent	Pregnant or Ever Pregnant	Other	
Alabama			X[a]	X[a]	X[a]	High school graduate or 14 y[a]	
Alaska	X						
Arizona	X						
Arkansas	X						
California	X						
Colorado	X						
Connecticut			X[b]				
Delaware						12 y[c]	
District of Columbia	X						
Florida		X		X	X		
Georgia	X						
Hawaii						14 y[c]	
Idaho	X						
Illinois		X	X	X	X	Referral	
Indiana			X[b]				
Iowa	X						
Kansas						Mature minor	

(Continued)

Table 3.2
(Continued)

State	Explicitly Allows All Minors to Consent to Services	Explicitly Allows Certain Minors to Consent to Services					No Explicit Policy
		Health	Married	Parent	Pregnant or Ever Pregnant	Other	
Kentucky	X[c]						
Louisiana			X[b]				
Maine		X	X	X			
Maryland	X[c]						
Massachusetts	X[d]						
Michigan			X[b]				
Minnesota	X[c]						
Mississippi			X	X		Referral	
Missouri			X[b]				
Montana	X[c]						
Nebraska			X[b]				
Nevada			X[b]	X[a]		Mature minor[a]	
New Hampshire						Mature minor[a]	
New Jersey			X[a]		X[a]		
New Mexico	X						
New York	X[d]						
North Carolina	X						
North Dakota							X

(Continued)

Table 3.2
(Continued)

State	Explicitly Allows All Minors to Consent to Services	Explicitly Allows Certain Minors to Consent to Services					No Explicit Policy
		Health	Married	Parent	Pregnant or Ever Pregnant	Other	
Ohio							X
Oklahoma			X[c]		X[c]		
Oregon	X[c]						
Pennsylvania			X[a]		X[a]	High school graduate[a]	
Rhode Island							X
South Carolina			X[b]			16 y or mature minor	
South Dakota			X[b]				
Tennessee	X						
Texas			X[b]			[e]	
Utah			X[b]			[e]	
Vermont			X[b]				
Virginia	X						
Washington	X						
West Virginia			X[b]			Mature minor	
Wisconsin							X

(Continued)

Table 3.2
(Continued)

State	Explicitly Allows All Minors to Consent to Services	Explicitly Allows Certain Minors to Consent to Services					No Explicit Policy
		Health	Married	Parent	Pregnant or Ever Pregnant	Other	
Wyoming	X						
Total	21 + DC	3	21	6	6	11	4

[a] State policy does not specifically address contraceptive services but applies to medical care in general.
[b] State law confers the rights and responsibilities of adulthood to minors who are married.
[c] Physician may, but is not required to, inform the minor's parents.
[d] The state funds a statewide program that gives minors access to confidential contraceptive care.
[e] State funds may not be used to provide minors with confidential contraceptive services.

Adapted from Guttmacher Institute. State Policies in Brief: an overview of minors' consent law. Available at: www.guttmacher.org/statecenter/spibs/spib_OMCL.pdf. Accessed April 24, 2009.

Table 3.3
Minors' access to sexually transmitted infection services

State	Minors May Consent to STI Services	Consent to HIV Testing and Treatment Included	Physician May, but Is Not Required to, Inform Parents
Alabama	12 y	X	X
Alaska	X		
Arizona	X		
Arkansas	X		X
California	12 y	X	
Colorado	X	X[a]	
Connecticut	X	X	
Delaware	12 y	X	X
District of Columbia	X		
Florida	X	X	
Georgia	X		X
Hawaii	14 y		X
Idaho	14 y	X	
Illinois	12 y	X	X
Indiana	X		
Iowa	X	X[b]	
Kansas	X		X
Kentucky	X	X	X
Louisiana	X		X
Maine	X		X
Maryland	X		X
Massachusetts	X[c]		
Michigan	X	X	X
Minnesota	X		X
Mississippi	X	X[d]	
Missouri	X		X
Montana	X	X	X
Nebraska	X		
Nevada	X	X	
New Hampshire	14 y		
New Jersey	X	13 y	X
New Mexico	X	X[d]	
New York	X	X[d]	
North Carolina	X	X	
North Dakota	14 y	X	
Ohio	X	X[d]	
Oklahoma	X	X	X
Oregon	X	X	

(*Continued*)

Table 3.3
(Continued)

State	Minors May Consent to STI Services	Consent to HIV Testing and Treatment Included	Physician May, but Is Not Required to, Inform Parents
Pennsylvania	X	X	
Rhode Island	X	X	
South Carolina	16 y or mature minor	X	
South Dakota	X		
Tennessee	X	X	
Texas	X	X	X
Utah	X		
Vermont	12 y	X[d]	
Virginia	X	X	
Washington	14 y	X	
West Virginia	X		
Wisconsin	X		
Wyoming	X	X	
TOTAL	50 + DC	31	18

STI indicates sexually transmitted infection.
[a] Physician may inform parents of minor's decision to consent to HIV/AIDS services if the minor is younger than 16 years.
[b] A parent must be notified of a positive HIV test result.
[c] The state funds a statewide program that gives minors access to sexually transmitted infection services.
[d] Does not include the right to consent to HIV/AIDS treatment.
Adapted from Guttmacher Institute. State Policies in Brief: an overview of minors' consent law. Available at: www.guttmacher.org/statecenter/spibs/spib_OMCL.pdf. Accessed April 24, 2009.

Table 3.4
Parental involvement in minors' abortions

State	Required Parental Involvement			Alternatives		Exceptions	
	Consent Only	Notification and Consent	Notification Only	Judicial Bypass	Other Adult Relatives	Medical Emergency	Abuse, Assault, Incest or Neglect
Alabama	X			X		X	
Alaska	[a]						
Arizona	X			X		X	X
Arkansas	X			X		X	X
California	[a]						
Colorado			X	X		X	X
Delaware			X[b,c]	X[b,c]	X[c]	X[c]	
Florida			X	X		X	
Georgia			X	X		X	
Idaho	X			X		X	X
Illinois			[a]				
Indiana	X			X		X	
Iowa			X	X	X	X	X
Kansas			X	X		X	X
Kentucky	X			X		X	
Louisiana	X			X		X	
Massachusetts	X			X		X	
Michigan	X			X		X	
Minnesota			Both parents	X		X	X
Mississippi	Both parents			X		X	
Missouri	X			X			
Montana			[a]				
Nebraska			X	X		X	X
Nevada			[a]			X	
New Jersey			[a]			X	
New Mexico	[a]						
North Carolina	X			X	X	X	
North Dakota	Both parents			X		X	
Ohio	X			X			
Oklahoma		X		X		X	X
Pennsylvania	X			X		X	
Rhode Island	X			X			
South Carolina	X[c]			X[c]	X[c]	X[c]	X[c]
South Dakota			X	X		X	
Tennessee	X			X		X	X
Texas	X			X		X	
Utah		X		X[d]		X	X[e]
Virginia	X			X	X	X	X
West Virginia			X[b]	X[b]		X	
Wisconsin	X[b]			X[b]	X	X	X
Wyoming	X			X		X	
Total	22	2	10	34	6	33	14

Except where indicated, policies require the involvement of 1 parent.

[a] Enforcement permanently enjoined by court order; policy not in effect.

[b] Allows specified health professionals to waive parental involvement in limited circumstances.

[c] Although most states laws apply to all minors, Delaware's law applies to women younger than 16 years, and South Carolina's law applies to women younger than 17 years.

[d] The provision only applies to parental consent requirements.

[e] The provision only applies to the parental notice requirements.

Adapted from Guttmacher Institute. State Policies in Brief: an overview of minors' consent law. Available at: www.guttmacher.org/statecenter/spibs/spib_OMCL.pdf. Accessed April 24, 2009.

Table 3.5
What minors may consent to

State	Contraceptive Services	STI Services	Prenatal Care	Adoption	Medical Care for Minor's Child	Abortion Services
Alabama	All[a]	All[b]	All	All	All	Parental consent
Alaska	All	All	All		All	(Parental consent)[c]
Arizona	All	All		All		Parental consent
Arkansas	All	All[b]	All		All	Parental consent
California	All	All	All	All		(Parental consent)[c]
Colorado	All	All	All	All	All	Parental notice
Connecticut	Some	All		Legal counsel	All	All
Delaware	All[b]	All[b]	All[b]	All	All	Parental notice[d]
District of Columbia	All	All	All	All	All	All
Florida	Some	All	All		All	Parental notice
Georgia	All	All[b]	All	All	All	Parental notice
Hawaii	All[a,b]	All[a,b]	All[a,b]	All		
Idaho	All	All[a]	All	All	All	Parental consent
Illinois	Some	All[b]	All	All	All	(Parental notice)[c]
Indiana	Some	All		All		Parental consent
Iowa	All	All				Parental notice
Kansas	Some	All[b]	Some	All	All	Parental notice
Kentucky	All[b]	All[b]	All[b]	Legal counsel	All	Parental consent
Louisiana	Some	All[b]		Parental consent	All	Parental consent
Maine	Some	All[b]				All
Maryland	All[b]	All[b]	All[b]	All	All	All
Massachusetts	All	All	All		All	Parental consent
Michigan	Some	All[b]	All[b]	Parental consent	All	Parental consent
Minnesota	All[b]	All[b]	All[b]	Parental consent	All	Parental notice
Mississippi	Some	All	All	All	All	Parental consent
Missouri	Some	All[b]	All[b]	Legal counsel	All	Parental consent
Montana	All[b]	All[b]	All[b]	Legal counsel	All	(Parental notice)[c]
Nebraska	Some	All				Parental notice
Nevada	Some	All	Some	All	All	(Parental notice)[c]
New Hampshire	Some	All[a]	Some	All[e]		
New Jersey	Some	All[b]	All[b]	All	All	
New Mexico	All	All	All	All		(Parental consent)[c]
New York	All	All	All	All	All	
North Carolina	All	All	All			Parental consent
North Dakota		All[a,b]		All		Parental consent
Ohio		All		All		Parental consent
Oklahoma	Some	All[b]	All[b]	All[a]	All	Parental consent and notice
Oregon	All[b]	All	All[b,f]			
Pennsylvania	Some	All	All	Parental notice	All	Parental consent
Rhode Island		All		Parental consent	All	Parental consent
South Carolina	All[g]	All[g]	All[g]	All	All	Parental consent
South Dakota	Some	All				Parental notice
Tennessee	All	All	All	All	All	Parental consent

(*Continued*)

Table 3.5
(Continued)

State	Contraceptive Services	STI Services	Prenatal Care	Adoption	Medical Care for Minor's Child	Abortion Services
Texas	Some	All[b]	All[b]			Parental consent
Utah	Some	All	All	All	All	Parental consent and Notice
Vermont	Some	All		All		
Virginia	All	All	All	All	All	Parental consent
Washington	All	All[a]	All	Legal counsel		
West Virginia	Some	All	Some	All		Parental notice
Wisconsin		All				Parental consent
Wyoming	All	All		All		Parental consent
Total	25 + DC	50 + DC	32 + DC	28 + DC	30 + DC	3 + DC

"All" applies to minors aged 12 years and older unless otherwise noted; "some" applies to specified categories of minors (those who have a health issue, or are married, pregnant, mature, etc). The totals include only those states that allow all minors to consent. STI indicates sexually transmitted infection.

[a] Applies to minors aged 14 years and older.

[b] Physicians may, but are not required to, inform the minor's parents.

[c] Enforcement permanently or temporarily enjoined by a court order; policy not in effect.

[d] Applies to minors younger than 17 years.

[e] A court may require parental consent.

[f] Applies to minors aged 15 years and older.

[g] Applies to mature minors aged 15 years and younger and to minors aged 16 years and older.

Adapted from Guttmacher Institute. State Policies in Brief: an overview of minors' consent law. Available at: www.guttmacher.org/statecenter/spibs/spib_OMCL.pdf. Accessed April 24, 2009.

Table 3.6
Statutory rape laws

State	Age of Consent, y	Minimum Age of Victim, y	Age Differential Between the Victim and Defendant (if Victim Is Above Minimum Age), y	Minimum Age of Defendant to Prosecute, y
Alabama	16	12	2	16
Alaska	16	NA	3	NA
Arizona	18	15	2 (defendant must be in high school and <19)	NA
Arkansas	16	NA	3 (if victim is <14)	20 (if victim is = 14)
California	18	18	NA	NA
Colorado	17	NA	4 (if victim is <15), 10 (if victim is <17)	NA
Connecticut	16	NA[a]	2	NA
Delaware	18[b]	16	NA	NA
District of Columbia	16	NA	4	NA
Florida	18	16	NA	24 (if victim is = 16)
Georgia	16	16	NA	NA
Hawaii	16	14	5	NA
Idaho	18[c]	18	NA	NA
Illinois	17	17	NA	NA
Indiana	16	14	NA	18 (if victim is = 14)
Iowa	16	14	4	NA
Kansas	16	16	NA	NA
Kentucky	16	16	NA	NA
Louisiana	17	13	3 (if victim is <15), 2 (if victim is <17)	NA
Maine	16	14[d]	5	NA
Maryland	16	NA	4	NA
Massachusetts	16	16	NA	NA
Michigan	16	16[e]	NA	NA
Minnesota	16	NA	3 (if victim is <13), 2 (if victim is <16)	NA
Mississippi	16	NA	2 (if victim is <14), 3 (if victim is <16)	NA
Missouri	17	14	NA	21 (if victim is = 14)
Montana	16	16[f]	NA	NA
Nebraska	16	16[g]	NA	19
Nevada	16	16	NA	18
New Hampshire	16	16	NA	NA
New Jersey	16	13[h]	4	NA
New Mexico	16	13	4	18 (if victim is = 13)
New York	17	17	NA	NA
North Carolina	16	NA	4	12
North Dakota	18	15	NA	18 (if victim is = 15)
Ohio	16	13	NA	18 (if victim is = 13)
Oklahoma	16	14	NA	18 (if victim is >14)
Oregon	18	15	3	NA
Pennsylvania	16	13	4	NA
Rhode Island	16	14	NA	18 (if victim is = 14)

(*Continued*)

Table 3.6
(Continued)

State	Age of Consent, y	Minimum Age of Victim, y	Age Differential Between the Victim and Defendant (if Victim Is Above Minimum Age), y	Minimum Age of Defendant to Prosecute, y
South Carolina	16	14	Illegal if victim is 14 to 16 and defendant is older than victim	NA
South Dakota	16	10[i]	3	NA
Tennessee	18	13	4	NA
Texas	17	14	3	NA
Utah	18	16	10	NA
Vermont	16	16	NA	16
Virginia	18	15	NA	18 (if victim is = 15)
Washington	16	NA	2 (if victim is <12), 3 (if victim is <14), 4 (if victim is <16)	NA
West Virginia	16	NA	4 (if victim is = 11)	16, 14 (if victim is <11)
Wisconsin	18	18	NA	NA
Wyoming	16	NA	4	NA

Note that some states have marital exemptions; it is assumed here that the 2 parties are not married to one another. NA indicates not applicable.

[a] Engaging in sexual intercourse with someone who is <16 years of age is legal under certain circumstances. However, sexual contact with someone who is <15 years of age is illegal regardless of the age of the defendant.

[b] Sexual acts with individuals who are at least 16 years of age are only illegal if the defendant is ≥30 years of age.

[c] Intercourse with a girl who is <18 years of age is illegal regardless of the age of the defendant. However, sexual acts not amounting to penetration are legal under certain circumstances in cases where the victim is at least 16 years of age.

[d] It is illegal to engage in a sexual act with someone who is <14 years of age regardless of the age of the defendant. However, sexual contact or sexual touching with someone who is <14 years of age is legal under certain circumstances.

[e] It is illegal to engage in a sexual penetration with someone who is <16 years of age. However, sexual contact with someone who is at least 13 years of age is legal under certain circumstances.

[f] Sexual intercourse with someone who is <16 years of age is illegal regardless of the age of the defendant. However, sexual contact with someone who is at least 14 years of age is legal under certain circumstances.

[g] Under the offense "debauching a minor," it is illegal to debauch or deprave morals by lewdly inducing someone <17 years of age to carnally know any other person.

[h] It is illegal to engage in a sexual penetration with someone who is <13 years of age regardless of the age of the defendant. However, sexual contact with someone who is <13 years of age is legal under certain circumstances.

[i] Engaging in sexual penetration with someone who is at least 10 years of age and <16 years of age is legal under certain circumstances. However, sexual contact with someone who is <16 years of age is illegal regardless of the age of the defendant.

Adapted from Glosser A, Gardiner K, Fishman M; Lewin Group. Statutory rape: a guide to state laws and reporting requirements. Available at: www.lewin.com/content/publications/3068.pdf. Accessed April 24, 2009.

Table 3.7
Overlooked Clues in the Psychosocial History

Information about parents[a] or other family members

• Chronic of life-threatening disease	• Poor or complete lack of family communications
• Sibling with chronic illness or special health-care needs	• Significant events in parents' childhood
• Death of sibling (recent or remote)	• Marital[b] discord, blended families, separation, divorces
• Family member or sibling with disability	• Family violence
• Parents of same sex	• Social isolation
• Psychiatric illness	• Parental learning problems, lack of education, academic failure
• Alcohol or other drug abuse	• Incarceration or legal troubles
• Unemployment, financial concerns, poverty	• Teenage pregnancy (parent or sibling)

Information about the adolescent

- School problems including homework conflicts, conflicts with teachers, truancy
- Problems with peers (teasing, bullying)
- Lack of social skills or friends
- How the chief complaint presents in various settings (home, school, work, with friends) and at different times (weekdays, weekends, mornings, evenings)
- History of or current abuse (physical, verbal, sexual) or neglect by parent, family member, or school personnel
- Unwanted or forced sexual experiences (with peers, partners, boyfriend/girlfriend)
- Concerns about sexual identity
- History of or ongoing intimate partner violence
- Frequent foster home placements
- Disruptive moves
- Drug use
- Body image concerns
- Peer with serious illness or hospitalization, recent suicide attempt/suicide
- Recent romantic rejection (perceived or real)
- Lack of connection to any adult

Information about the parent-adolescent relationship

- Unrealistic parental expectations regarding adolescent's athletic, social, or academic capabilities
- Adolescent bears physical resemblance to absent, estranged, or dead parent
- Poor parental understanding of adolescent development
- Poor parental supervision
- Parental expectations not clearly communicated to adolescent
- Parent(s) not emotionally available to adolescent

(*Continued*)

Table 3.7
(Continued)

Neighborhood characteristics
- High levels of crime, drug use, violence
- Isolation (either secondary to above or because of geographic distance)
- Lack of community recreational opportunities

[a] The term parents is used broadly to include anyone with responsibility for the adolescent. This could include guardians, stepparents, domestic partners, etc.
[b] Marital discord is used here to included discord between any two people with responsibility for child rearing, regardless of whether they are legally married or of the same or opposite sex.
Adapted from: Green M, Sullivan P, Eichberg C. Avoid a "Swiss cheese" history when psychosocial complaints are on the menu. *Contemp Pediatr.* 2002;19: 115–125. Used by permission of Advanstar Communications, Inc.

MNEMONICS FOR CLINICAL PRACTICE

Global Evaluation of Adolescent Functioning

Table 3.8
HEADS/HEADSS

Home	Assess the adolescent's home life/living situation—family composition, living arrangements, relationships, who shares the home, etc.
Education	Current grade, school performance, absences, bullying at school, goals for the future, attitudes toward school (connectedness).
Activities	Peer relationships, hobbies, sports participation, exercise, driving, work experience.
Drugs	Current/past use of alcohol, tobacco, and other drugs; should include questions about use of illicit drugs, nonmedical use of prescription drugs, over-the-counter products, herbal remedies, nutritional supplements, etc; inquire about parental substance abuse.
Sexuality	Same/opposite-sex attractions, sexual behaviors (coital and noncoital), need for contraception (and contraceptive use if applicable); need for protection against sexually transmitted infections; history of current/past unwanted sex or intimate partner violence; sexual abuse.
Suicide/ depression	Assess for symptoms of depression (see SIGECAPS below); past/current history of suicidal thoughts/attempts; family history of mental health problems/suicide.

The original HEADS assessment is credited to Berman HS. Talking HEADS: interviewing adolescents. *HMO Pract.* 1987;1(1):3–11. HEADS was subsequently modified (to HEADSS) by Cohen to include an additional question about suicide/depression (Goldenring JM, Cohen E. Getting into adolescent heads. *Contemp Pediatr.* 1998;5[200]:75–90. Reprinted by permission of Advanstar Communications, Inc. All rights reserved).

HEADS/HEADSS has been modified by other clinicians to assess other key components of an adolescent's level of functioning or to draw out in greater detail areas that are covered in HEADS/HEADSS.

Table 3.9
HEADSS FIRST

Home	Same as original HEADS.
Education	Same as original HEADS.
Abuse	How do parents discipline the adolescent? Questions about any kind of abuse (physical, sexual, emotional, verbal), either directed toward the adolescent or perpetrated by him or her; assess for intimate partner violence.
Drugs	Same as original HEADS.
Safety	Pertains to all the adolescent's safety practices: use of seat belts, driving while intoxicated/high or riding with someone who is intoxicated/ high, use of protective equipment during sports, especially use of helmets while bicycling.
Sexuality	Same as original HEADS.
Family/friends	See original HEADS; covered under home (family) and activities (friends) in original HEADS.
Image	Assess adolescent's perceived body image; observe physical appearance; note tattoos/piercings.
Recreation	Covers adolescent's engagement in work, physical exercise, sports participation, media use (computer, video games, television, etc).
Spirituality	Questions relating to the role that religion/spirituality plays in the adolescent's life (church attendance, youth-group activities, religiosity).
Threats/violence	Questions regarding the adolescent's involvement in fighting, weapon carrying, self-injurious behavior (suicide, cutting), running away from home, legal problems, etc.

Dias PJ. Adolescent substance abuse: assessment in the office. *Pediatr Clin North Am.* 2002;49(2):269–300, with permission from Elsevier.

Alternatives to HEADS/HEADSS are SAFETIMES (Schubiner), SHADSSS (Clark), and SAFETEENS (Feldman). Each covers most of the topics listed above but may also add emphasis to certain areas or add new topics for discussion.

Table 3.10
SAFE TIMES

Sexuality	Questions pertaining to types of sexual activity, unwanted sexual activity, contraception, sexually transmitted diseases
Affect/Abuse	Questions pertaining to depression; suicidal thoughts or attempts; tobacco, alcohol, or drug experimentation or use; physical and/or emotional abuse
Family/Friends	Questions pertaining to adjustment and/or conflict
Exam/Exercise	Questions pertaining to self-exam (testes or breasts for older adolescents), exercise
Timing	Questions pertaining to timing of development, height, weight, and sexual maturity rating and any concerns about the adolescent's height, weight or level of development
Immunizations	Assessment of need for tetanus; mumps, measles, rubella (MMR); hepatitis B; meningococcal vaccine; tuberculin skin testing
Meals	Questions pertaining to meal pattern (regular, skipped), intake of calcium, fat, iron, fiber
Education	Questions pertaining to grades, difficulties, aspirations, and plans
Safety	Questions pertaining to use of seat belts or helmets, involvement in fights, carrying weapons, unsafe driving or swimming

In general, the interview is conducted in reverse order (starting with safety and ending with sexuality) to ask the least threatening (less personal or confidential) questions first.
From Schubiner H, Tzelepis A, Wright K, Podany E. The clinical utility of the safe times questionnaire. *J Adolesc Health*. 1994; 15(5): 374–382, with permission from Elsevier.

Table 3.11
SHADSSS

School
Home
Activities
Depression/Self esteem
Substance abuse
Sexuality
Safety

From Clark LR. Commentary: Lessons from a teendoc: the joys and challenges of adolescent medicine. *J Ped Psychol.* 1998;23:389–391. Reprinted by permission of Oxford University Press.

Table 3.12
SAFE TEENS

Sexuality
Accidents (injuries)
Firearms/homicide
Toxins (tobacco, alcohol, other drugs)
Exercise
Nutrition
Shots (immunizations)

From Gilchrist VJ. Preventive health care for the adolescent. *Am Fam Physician.* 1991;43(3): 877, with permission.

PACES

Another approach is use of the mnemonic PACES as follows (adapted from Kreipe RE. Introduction to interviewing: the art of communicating with adolescents. *Adolesc Med.* 2008;19[1]:1–17):

"To remind myself of the questions I want to ask all my teenaged patients, I use the word 'PACES' because each letter stand for something that can affect their health. Are you ready to go through the PACES for your health?

The 'P' stands for 'peers' and 'parents.' We'll start with peers, because if your peers have some health problems, you may have them too. What do you think are the main health problems for your peers, people your age, your friends?

The 'P' is also for parents. How is your father's health; your mother's? Does either of them take medicines or need to see the doctor often? Do they have any habits that make you worry about their health?

The 'A' in PACES stands for the major cause of death for young people your age—what do you think that is? [Accidents or alcohol is the correct answer; if the adolescent chooses another cause, steer back to accidents.] Have your friends or you ever had an accident? What do they (or you) do to prevent accidents? [For adolescents who reside in neighborhoods with high levels of violence, accidents can be reframed to "assaults."]

The 'C' in PACES stands for the leading 'cause' of sickness and death among adults but is a habit that usually starts before age 18. What do you think that might be? [Cigarettes is correct but may need to be broadened to cigars, snuff, or chew.] If adolescent answers 'cancer,' steer them back to cigarettes through its link to cancer.

The 'E' in PACES stands for a lot of things; can you think of something beginning with 'e' that can affect your health, either good or bad? [Items to be explored include exercise, eating, and emotions. For adolescents who may not see the link between emotions and health, ask about the second leading cause of death for adolescents. Adolescents usually are aware of the link between suicide and emotions.]

The 'S' in paces stands for 'school' and 'sexuality.' You probably know some ways sexual activity can affect an adolescent's health but school is also related to health. It helps to do well in school if you are healthy, and teens who are not in school sometimes are not as healthy as those who are."

Screening Adolescents for Substance Abuse

John Knight, at Children's Hospital Boston, developed a brief screening tool for adolescent substance abuse. In its current form, the CRAFFT questions are preceded by 3 screening questions:

Part A

During the PAST 12 MONTHS, did you:	No	Yes
1. Drink any alcohol (more than a few sips)?	☐	☐
2. Smoke any marijuana or hashish?	☐	☐
3. Use anything else to get high? "anything else" includes illegal drugs, over the counter and prescription drugs, and things that you sniff or "huff"	☐	☐

If the patient answered NO to ALL of the questions in Part A, ask the CAR question below only. If the patient answered YES to ANY of the questions in Part A, ask ALL SIX CRAFFT questions below.

Part B

	No	Yes
1. Have you ever ridden in a **CAR** driven by someone (including yourself) who was "high" or had been using alcohol or drugs?	☐	☐
2. Do you ever use alcohol or drugs to **RELAX**, feel better about yourself, or fit in?	☐	☐
3. Do you ever use alcohol or drugs while you are by yourself, or **ALONE**?	☐	☐
4. Do you ever **FORGET** things you did while using alcohol or drugs?	☐	☐
5. Do your **FAMILY** or **FRIENDS** ever tell you that you should cut down on your drinking or drug use?	☐	☐
6. Have you ever gotten into **TROUBLE** while you were using alcohol or drugs?	☐	☐

Adolescents who give "yes" answers to two of the six CRAFFT questions may have a significant drug and/or alcohol problem and require a more in-depth assessment of the adolescent's drug use.

Fig 3.4. CRAFFT Questions. © Children's Hospital Boston, 2009. (Reproduced with permission from the Center for Adolescent Substance Abuse Research, CeASAR. Children's Hospital Boston, 617-355-5433, or www.ceasar.org. See also: Knight JR, Sheritt L, Shrier LA, et al. Validity of the CRAFFT substance abuse screening test among selected adolescent clinic patients. Arch Pediatr Adolesc Med. 2002;156:607–614.)

Screening Adolescents for Depression

Table 3.13
SIGECAPS

Sleep	Sleep problems (too much sleep, too little sleep, difficulty staying asleep, early awakening).
Interests	Whether the adolescent reports loss of interest in usual activities (work, school, hobbies, sports), either solitary or with peers.
Guilty	Feeling guilty or worthless.
Energy	Adolescent reports decreased energy level (may be described as fatigue or feeling tired even after an adequate amount of sleep).
Concentration	The adolescent may report difficulty concentrating or paying attention at work, school, or home; parents, teachers, supervisors, or peers may note these behaviors in the adolescent.
Appetite	Appetite may be either increased or decreased.
Pleasure	Loss of pleasure from doing things that he or she previously enjoyed.
Suicidal	The adolescent may report suicidal feelings or thoughts and may have developed a plan.

A similar mnemonic is SPACE DIGS. The "P" refers to psychomotor agitation or retardation (the adolescent appears "wound up" or "wound down"). The "D" refers to depressed mood (the adolescent feels or acts "down") (see Kroenke K. A 75-year-old man with depression. *JAMA*. 2002;287[12]:1568 –1576).

Monitoring Complications From Use of Combined Hormonal Contraceptives: ACHES

Table 3.14
ACHES: the presence of any of the following could indicate a serious complication from use of hormonal contraception

Abdominal pain (severe)
Chest pain (especially if accompanied by difficulty breathing, shortness of breath, worse with breathing in)
Headaches (especially if different than usual headache or accompanied by numbness or weakness of extremities or slurred speech
Eye problems (any visual disturbance [eg, blurred vision or loss of vision])
Severe leg pain occurring in the calf or thigh

Adapted from Joffe A, Blythe M. The office visit. In: Joffe A, Blythe M, eds. Handbook of Adolescent Medicine. *Adolesc Med.* 2003;14:272.

Partnering With Adolescents to Effect Behavior Change

Table 3.15
FRAMES

Feedback	Ask the adolescent for permission to provide feedback. On the basis of information obtained during the history, indicate how a given behavior is affecting the adolescent's functioning (using the adolescent's own words if possible). Elicit feedback from the adolescent on your observations.
Responsibility	Emphasize that it is the adolescent's choice alone whether to change a given behavior(s) and that only the adolescent can make the change happen. Offer support (eg, "I'd like to work with you, but it's up to you to make the change").
Advice	Provide specific advice to the adolescent about the need to change (eg, "I believe the best thing for you would be to stop using drugs and alcohol"). If asked, offer advice about how to change.
Menu	Ask the adolescent to describe possible changes he or she could make. If none are offered, suggest changes (eg, "You could stop using completely, you could try to cut down, or I could refer you to a specialist"). Elicit the adolescent's feedback on any changes you suggest.
Empathy	Explain that you understand that change can be difficult and perhaps even scary. Offer support (eg, "I know that these things may be difficult to hear and making a change can be hard, but I am worried about you. I care about your health and your future").
Self-efficacy	Express your confidence in the teenager's ability to make a change(s) in his or her behavior (eg, "Although this may be difficult, I believe in you, and I know that you can do this if you try"). Review any past successes the adolescent may have had in making changes or accomplishing something that he or she thought would be difficult. Reframe past failures as important first steps to change and as providing valuable experience.

Adapted with permission from Miller WR, Sanchez VC. Motivating young adults for treatment and lifestyle change. In: Howard G, ed. *Issues in Alcohol Use and Misuse by Young Adults*. Notre Dame, IN: University of Notre Dame Press; 1993; and Jellinek M, Patel BP, Froehle MC, eds. 2002. *Bright Futures in Practice: Mental Health–Volume I: Practice Guide*. Arlington, VA: National Center for Education in Maternal and Child Health.

A. To assess an adolescent's readiness to make a behavior change or to start a new behavior, use the readiness ruler:

0___1___2___3___4___5___6___7___8___9___10
/ /
Least ready Most ready

Ask the adolescent to indicate on the ruler where he/she sees himself/herself in terms of making a change or adapting a new behavior. Your focus is on exploring the pros and cons of the current behavior or the pros and cons of making a change.

If the adolescent rates his/her readiness between 0 and 5, ask about the pros of staying the same (maintaining the current behavior). Probe until all pros are identified. Then ask about the cons of maintaining the behavior. Probe until all cons have been identified. Then review the list of pros and cons (presenting the cons first) to determine whether the adolescent wishes to maintain the old behavior or change.

If the adolescent indicates a score of 6-10, ask about the pros of making the change. Probe until all pros are identified. Then ask about the cons of making a change. Probe until all cons have been identified. Then review the list of pros and cons (presenting the pros first) to determine whether the adolescent wants to make the change.

B. To determine how important a change in behavior is to an adolescent and whether he/she feels he/she can make the change, use the importance/confidence rulers:

How important making this behavior change is to him/her?

0___1___2___3___4___5___6___7___8___9___10
/ /
Least important Most important

How confident he/she is he/she can make this change?

0___1___2___3___4___5___6___7___8___9___10
/ /
Least confident Most confident

If one number is significantly lower than the other, focus on the lower number first. If importance is $\leq$ 5 or if both confidence and importance levels are about equal, focus on importance first. If both are $\leq$ 3, explore whether the adolescent wishes to talk about the behavior.

If the focus is on importance, ask: "What made you choose [the number they chose] and not a lower number?" What makes changing this behavior important? Probe for more reasons. Then ask "What makes changing this behavior important right now?" Finally, ask "What would have to happen to make changing this behavior a little more important to you?"

If the focus is on confidence, ask: "What made you choose [the number they chose] and not a lower number?" What makes you feel this confident that you can change this behavior? Probe for more reasons. Then ask "What would have to happen to make you feel a little but more confident that you can change this behavior?"

Adapted from Gold MA, Delisi K. Motivational interviewing and sexual and contraceptive behaviors. *Adolesc Med*. 2008;19:69-82.

Fig 3.5. Motivational Interviewing: Using rulers/scales to help adolescents make decisions about behavior change.

INSTRUCTIONS FOR USE

Pediatric Symptom Checklist

The Pediatric Symptom Checklist is a psychosocial screen designed to facilitate the recognition of cognitive, emotional, and behavioral problems so that appropriate interventions can be initiated as early as possible. Included here are two versions, the parent-completed version (PSC) and the youth self-report (Y-PSC). The Y-PSC can be administered to adolescents ages 11 and up.

INSTRUCTIONS FOR SCORING

The PSC consists of 35 items that are rated as "Never," "Sometimes," or "Often" present and scored 0, 1, and 2, respectively. The total score is calculated by adding together the score for each of the 35 items. For children and adolescents ages 6 through 16, a cutoff score of 28 or higher indicates psychological impairment. For children ages 4 and 5, the PSC cutoff score is 24 or higher (Little et al., 1994; Pagano et al., 1996). The cutoff score for the Y-PSC is 30 or higher. Items that are left blank are simply ignored (i.e., score equals 0). If four or more items are left blank, the questionnaire is considered invalid.

HOW TO INTERPRET THE PSC OR Y-PSC

A positive score on the PSC or Y-PSC suggests the need for further evaluation by a qualified health (e.g., M.D., R.N.) or mental health (e.g., Ph.D., L.I.C.S.W.) professional. Both false positives and false negatives occur, and only an experienced health professional should interpret a positive PSC or Y-PSC score as anything other than a suggestion that further evaluation may be helpful. Data from past studies using the PSC and Y-PSC indicate that two out of three children and adolescents who screen positive on the PSC or Y-PSC will be correctly identified as having moderate to serious impairment in psychosocial functioning. The one child or adolescent "incorrectly" identified usually has at least mild impairment, although a small percentage of children and adolescents turn out to have very little or no impairment (e.g., an adequately functioning child or adolescent of an overly anxious parent). Data on PSC and Y-PSC negative screens indicate 95 percent accuracy, which, although statistically adequate, still means that 1 out of 20 children and adolescents rated as functioning adequately may actually be impaired. The inevitability of both false-positive and false-negative screens underscores the importance of experienced clinical judgment in interpreting PSC scores. Therefore, it is especially important for parents or other laypeople who administer the form to consult with a licensed professional if their child receives a PSC or Y-PSC positive score.

For more information, visit the Web site: http://psc.partners.org.

REFERENCES

Jellinek MS, Murphy JM, Little M, et al. 1999. Use of the Pediatric Symptom Checklist (PSC) to screen for psychosocial problems in pediatric primary care: A national feasability study. *Archives of Pediatric and Adolescent Medicine* 153(3):254–260.

Jellinek MS, Murphy JM, Robinson J, et al. 1988. Pediatric Symptom Checklist: Screening school-age children for psychosocial dysfunction. *Journal of Pediatrics* 112(2):201–209. Web site: http://psc.partners.org.

Little M, Murphy JM, Jellinek MS, et al. 1994. Screening 4- and 5-year-old children for psychosocial dysfunction: A preliminary study with the Pediatric Symptom Checklist. *Journal of Developmental and Behavioral Pediatrics* 15:191–197.

Pagano M, Murphy JM, Pedersen M, et al. 1996. Screening for psychosocial problems in 4–5 year olds during routine EPSDT examinations: Validity and reliability in a Mexican-American sample. *Clinical Pediatrics* 35(3):139–146.

Fig 3.6. Instructions for use: pediatric symptom checklist.

Pediatric Symptom Checklist (PSC)

Emotional and physical health go together in children. Because parents are often the first to notice a problem with their child's behavior, emotions, or learning, you may help your child get the best care possible by answering these questions. Please indicate which statement best describes your child.

Please mark under the heading that best describes your child:

		Never	Sometimes	Often
1. Complains of aches and pains	1	___	___	___
2. Spends more time alone	2	___	___	___
3. Tires easily, has little energy	3	___	___	___
4. Fidgety, unable to sit still	4	___	___	___
5. Has trouble with teacher	5	___	___	___
6. Less interested in school	6	___	___	___
7. Acts as if driven by a motor	7	___	___	___
8. Daydreams too much	8	___	___	___
9. Distracted easily	9	___	___	___
10. Is afraid of new situations	10	___	___	___
11. Feels sad, unhappy	11	___	___	___
12. Is irritable, angry	12	___	___	___
13. Feels hopeless	13	___	___	___
14. Has trouble concentrating	14	___	___	___
15. Less interested in friends	15	___	___	___
16. Fights with other children	16	___	___	___
17. Absent from school	17	___	___	___
18. School grades dropping	18	___	___	___
19. Is down on him or herself	19	___	___	___
20. Visits the doctor with doctor finding nothing wrong	20	___	___	___
21. Has trouble sleeping	21	___	___	___
22. Worries a lot	22	___	___	___
23. Wants to be with you more than before	23	___	___	___
24. Feels he or she is bad	24	___	___	___
25. Takes unnecessary risks	25	___	___	___
26. Gets hurt frequently	26	___	___	___
27. Seems to be having less fun	27	___	___	___
28. Acts younger than children his or her age	28	___	___	___
29. Does not listen to rules	29	___	___	___
30. Does not show feelings	30	___	___	___
31. Does not understand other people's feelings	31	___	___	___
32. Teases others	32	___	___	___
33. Blames others for his or her troubles	33	___	___	___
34. Takes things that do not belong to him or her	34	___	___	___
35. Refuses to share	35	___	___	___

Total score ___________

Does your child have any emotional or behavioral problems for which she or he needs help? ( ) N ( ) Y

Are there any services that you would like your child to receive for these problems? ( ) N ( ) Y

If yes, what services?___________________________________

Fig 3.6. (Continued)

Pediatric Symptom Checklist—Youth Report (Y-PSC)

Please mark under the heading that best fits you:

		Never	Sometimes	Often
1. Complain of aches or pains	1			
2. Spend more time alone	2			
3. Tire easily, little energy	3			
4. Fidgety, unable to sit still	4			
5. Have trouble with teacher	5			
6. Less interested in school	6			
7. Act as if driven by motor	7			
8. Daydream too much	8			
9. Distract easily	9			
10. Are afraid of new situations	10			
11. Feel sad, unhappy	11			
12. Are irritable, angry	12			
13. Feel hopeless	13			
14. Have trouble concentrating	14			
15. Less interested in friends	15			
16. Fight with other children	16			
17. Absent from school	17			
18. School grades dropping	18			
19. Down on yourself	19			
20. Visit doctor with doctor finding nothing wrong	20			
21. Have trouble sleeping	21			
22. Worry a lot	22			
23. Want to be with parent more than before	23			
24. Feel that you are bad	24			
25. Take unnecessary risks	25			
26. Get hurt frequently	26			
27. Seem to be having less fun	27			
28. Act younger than children your age	28			
29. Do not listen to rules	29			
30. Do not show feelings	30			
31. Do not understand other people's feelings	31			
32. Tease others	32			
33. Blame others for your troubles	33			
34. Take things that do not belong to you	34			
35. Refuse to share	35			

Fig 3.6. (Continued)

With permission from National Center for Education in Maternal and Child Health. 2002. Middle childhood checklist. In Jellinek M, Patel BP, Froehle MC, eds., *Bright Futures in Practice: Mental Health—Volume II. Tool Kit.* Arlington, VA: National Center for Education in Maternal and Child Health at Georgetown University.

Middle Childhood Checklist

The following list highlights key topics to consider in promoting mental health in middle childhood. These topics may be discussed selectively during office visits, depending on the needs of the child and family.

Self

- ❑ **Self-esteem, including**
  - ☐ Fostering success
  - ☐ Taking reasonable risks
  - ☐ Resilience and handling failure
  - ☐ Parental verbal abuse
  - ☐ Importance of supportive family and peer relationships to self-esteem
- ❑ **Self-image, including**
  - ☐ Body image
  - ☐ Prepubertal changes
  - ☐ Initiating discussions about sexuality and reproductive health

Family

- ❑ **What matters at home, including**
  - ☐ Expectations and limit setting
  - ☐ Family time together
  - ☐ Communication
  - ☐ Family responsibilities
  - ☐ Family transitions—divorce, blended families
  - ☐ Sibling relationships

Friends

- ❑ **Friendships, including**
  - ☐ Making friends
  - ☐ Aggression and bullying
  - ☐ Victims of bullying
  - ☐ Family support of friendships

Community

- ❑ **School, including**
  - ☐ Expectations for school performance
  - ☐ Homework
  - ☐ Child-teacher conflicts
- ❑ **High-risk behaviors and environments, including**
  - ☐ Absenteeism
  - ☐ Substance use (e.g., alcohol, tobacco, and other drugs)
  - ☐ Unsafe friendships
  - ☐ Unsafe community environments

Bridges

- ❑ **Opportunities for early identification, including**
  - ☐ Anxiety disorders
  - ☐ Attention deficit hyperactivity disorder
  - ☐ Child maltreatment
  - ☐ Domestic violence
  - ☐ Eating disorders
  - ☐ Learning problems and disorders
  - ☐ Mental retardation
  - ☐ Mood disorders: depressive disorders and bipolar disorder
  - ☐ Obesity
  - ☐ Oppositional and aggressive behaviors
  - ☐ Parental depression
  - ☐ Pervasive developmental disorders
  - ☐ Substance use disorders

Notes

____

____

____

____

____

____

____

With permission from National Center for Education in Maternal and Child Health. 2002. Middle childhood checklist. In Jellinek M, Patel BP, Froehle MC, eds., *Bright Futures in Practice: Mental Health—Volume II. Tool Kit.* Arlington, VA: National Center for Education in Maternal and Child Health at Georgetown University.

Fig 3.7. Middle childhood checklist.

Adolescence Checklist

The following list highlights key topics to consider in promoting mental health in adolescence. These topics may be discussed selectively during office visits, depending on the needs of the adolescent and family.

Self

- ☐ **Self-esteem, including**
  - ☐ Parental support
  - ☐ Peer influence
  - ☐ Resilience and handling failure
- ☐ **Mood, including**
  - ☐ Stability of moods
  - ☐ Depression
  - ☐ Suicidal ideation (suicidal thoughts) and behaviors
- ☐ **Body image, including**
  - ☐ Physical appearance
  - ☐ Weight
- ☐ **Sexuality, including**
  - ☐ Sexual development/puberty
  - ☐ Sexual behavior
  - ☐ Sexual identity
  - ☐ Parental expectations and communication
  - ☐ Prevention of sexually transmitted diseases, including HIV/AIDS
  - ☐ Pregnancy
  - ☐ Sexual abuse and rape

Family

- ☐ **Independence and responsibility, including**
  - ☐ Importance of family support in adolescence
  - ☐ Increased independence
  - ☐ Increased influence of peers
  - ☐ Parental expectations and limit setting
  - ☐ Family conflict

Friends

- ☐ **Peer relationships, including**
  - ☐ Peer support
  - ☐ Peer influence

Community

- ☐ **School, including**
  - ☐ Transition from middle school/junior high school to high school
  - ☐ Academic success
  - ☐ Homework
  - ☐ Extracurricular activities
  - ☐ Absenteeism, dropping out
  - ☐ Transition from high school to college or work
- ☐ **High-risk behaviors and risk factors, including**
  - ☐ Substance use
  - ☐ Violent behaviors
  - ☐ Firearm use
  - ☐ Exposure to violence

Bridges

- ☐ **Opportunities for early identification and intervention, including**
  - ☐ Anxiety problems and disorders
  - ☐ Attention deficit hyperactivity disorder
  - ☐ Child maltreatment
  - ☐ Eating disorders
  - ☐ Learning problems and disorders
  - ☐ Mental retardation
  - ☐ Mood disorders: depressive and bipolar disorders
  - ☐ Obesity
  - ☐ Oppositional and aggressive behavior
  - ☐ Pervasive developmental disorders
  - ☐ Substance use

Notes

____

____

With permission from National Center for Education in Maternal and Child Health. 2002. Adolescence checklist. In Jellinek M, Patel BP, Froehle MC, eds., *Bright Futures in Practice: Mental Health—Volume II. Tool Kit.* Arlington, VA: National Center for Education in Maternal and Child Health at Georgetown University.

Fig 3.8. Adolescence checklist.

Symptoms of Depression in Adolescents

The following symptoms may indicate depression in adolescents, particularly when they last for more than 2 weeks:

- Poor performance in school
- Withdrawal from friends and activities
- Feelings of sadness and hopelessness
- Lack of enthusiasm, energy, or motivation
- Lack of pleasure in performance of acts that would normally be pleasurable
- Feelings of anger and rage
- Overreaction to criticism
- Feelings of being unable to satisfy ideals
- Low self-esteem
- Feelings of guilt
- Indecision, lack of concentration, or forgetfulness
- Restlessness and agitation
- Changes in eating or sleeping patterns
- Substance abuse
- Problems with authority
- Suicidal ideation (suicidal thoughts) or actions

If symptoms of depression are present, talk with your health professional. Get help. You don't need to fight depression alone. Depression can get better with help.

Fig 3.9. Symptoms of depression in adolescents. Reproduced by Permission of Mental Health America. 2009. Depression in Teens [fact sheet]. Alexandria, VA: Mental Health America. www.mentalhealthamerica.net. Accessed July 16, 2009.

Adolesc Med 20 (2009) 416–456

4. Endocrine/Metabolic

A. DIABETES MELLITUS TYPES 1 AND 2

Table 4.1
American Diabetes Association Criteria for Diagnosis of Diabetes Mellitus

Normoglycemia	Prediabetes	Diabetes
FPG <100 mg/dL	FPG ≥100–125 mg/dL (IFG)	FPG ≥126 mg/dL
2-h OGTT <140 mg/dL	2-h OGTT ≥140–199 mg/dL (IGT)	2-h OGTT ≥200 mg/dL
		Symptoms of diabetes and casual plasma blood glucose concentration >200 mg/dL

FPG indicates fasting plasma glucose (fasting is no caloric intake for 8 h); IFG, impaired fasting glucose (prediabetes); IGT, impaired glucose tolerance (prediabetes); 2-h OGTT, 2-hour oral glucose-tolerance test requiring the use of 75 g of anhydrous glucose dissolved in water.
Adapted from Genuth S, Alberti KG, Bennett P, et al. Follow-up report on the diagnosis of diabetes mellitus. *Diabetes Care*. 2003;26(11):3160–3167.

Types of Diabetes

Type 1 diabetes results from β-cell destruction, usually leading to absolute insulin deficiency.

- Immune mediated
- Idiopathic

Type 2 diabetes

- Insulin resistance in peripheral tissue as muscle, fat, and liver
- Defective insulin secretion in response to glucose stimulation (hyperinsulinemia)

Margaret J. Blythe, MD.
E-mail address: mblythe@iupui.edu.

 ISSN 1934-4287

- Increased glucose production by the liver from diminished initial insulin and C-peptide results in excess glucagon, resulting in increased glucose output by the liver

Other specific types of diabetes from other causes:
- Genetic defects in β-cell function
- Genetic defects in insulin action
- Endocrinopathies
- Diseases of the exocrine pancreas (such as cystic fibrosis) and drug- or chemical-induced destruction of pancreas (such as in the treatment of AIDS or after organ transplantation)

Gestational diabetes mellitus (diabetes diagnosed during pregnancy).

Recommendations for Diagnosis of Diabetes

- Fasting plasma glucose test is the preferred test for diagnosing diabetes in children and nonpregnant women
- Use of the A1c alone for the diagnosis of diabetes is not recommended at this time

Reference: American Diabetes Association. Standards of medical care in diabetes: 2008. *Diabetes Care*. 2008;31(suppl 1):S12–S54.

Recommendations for Testing for Type 2 Diabetes in Children and Adolescents

Criteria.
- Overweight (BMI >85th percentile for age and gender and/or weight >120% of ideal for height)

Plus any 2 of the following risk factors.
- Family history of type 2 diabetes in first- or second-degree relative
- Race/ethnicity (eg, Native American, black, Latino, Asian American, and Pacific Islander)
- Signs of insulin resistance or conditions associated with insulin resistance (eg, acanthosis nigricans, hypertension, dyslipidemia, or polycystic ovary syndrome)
- Maternal history of diabetes or gestational diabetes mellitus

Age of initiation of testing: 10 years, or at onset of puberty if puberty occurs at a younger age.

Frequency: every 2 years.

Test: fasting plasma glucose preferred.

Reference: American Diabetes Association. Standards of medical care in diabetes: 2008 [Table 4]. *Diabetes Care*. 2008;31(suppl 1):S12–S54. Reprinted with permission from The American Diabetes Association.

Prevalence of impaired fasting glucose in a nationally representative sample of teenagers from the 1999–2000 National Health and Nutrition Examination Survey was 7% and higher in boys (10%) than girls (4%); for those with a BMI at ≥95th percentile, it was 17.8% (Williams DE, Cadwell BL, Cheng YJ, et al. Prevalence of impaired fasting glucose and its relationship with cardiovascular disease risk factors in US adolescents, 1999–2000. *Pediatrics*. 2005;116[5]:1122–1126).

Recommendations for Prevention of Diabetes Type 2

- Counsel patients with impaired glucose tolerance or impaired fasting glucose on weight loss to decrease 5% to 10% of body weight and to increase physical activity with moderate activity to at least 150 minutes/week (eg, 5 sessions of 30 minutes each)
- Follow-up counseling is important for success
- On the basis of potential cost savings of diabetes prevention, such counseling should be covered by third-party payers
- Metformin may be considered for those who are at very high risk for diabetes mellitus (as impaired fasting glucose and/or impaired glucose tolerance plus other risk factors) and who are obese (BMI >35 kg/m^2) and <60 years of age
- Monitoring for the development of diabetes in those with prediabetes should be performed every year

Reference: American Diabetes Association. Standards of medical care in diabetes: 2008. *Diabetes Care*. 2008;31(suppl 1):S12–S54.

Recommendations for Monitoring Those With Diabetes Mellitus

A1c

- Perform A1c test at least 2 times per year for patients who meet treatment goals with stable glycemic control
- Perform A1c test quarterly for patients whose therapy has changed or who are not meeting glycemic goals
- Use of point-of-care testing for A1c to allow for timely decisions on therapy changes, when needed

Self–Blood Glucose Monitoring

- Minimally 3 times per day if on insulin
- If not on insulin, optimal frequency is unknown but should facilitate reaching glycemic goals

Reference: American Diabetes Association. Standards of medical care in diabetes: 2008. *Diabetes Care*. 2008;31(suppl 1):S12–S54.

Summary of Glycemic Recommendations for Adolescents/ Adults With Diabetes

- A1c: <7.0% (for adolescents, consider nighttime testing before bed; want between 100 and 150 mg%)
- Preprandial capillary plasma glucose level: 70 to 130 mg/dL (3.9–7.2 mmol/L)
- Peak postprandial capillary plasma glucose level: <180 mg/dL (<10.0 mmol/L) (Postprandial glucose may be targeted if A1c goals are not met despite reaching preprandial glucose goals)

Key Concepts

- A1c is the primary target for glycemic control
- Goals should be individualized on the basis of
  - Duration of diabetes
  - Pregnancy status
  - Age/developmental level
  - Comorbid conditions
  - Hypoglycemia unawareness
  - Individual patient considerations/goals
  - More stringent glycemic goals (ie, a normal A1c level, <6%) may further reduce complications at the cost of increased risk of hypoglycemia

Reference: American Diabetes Association. Standards of medical care in diabetes: 2008 [Table 8]. *Diabetes Care*. 2008;31(suppl 1):S12–S54.

Guidelines for Glycemic Control

- Lowering A1c to an average of ~7% reduces microvascular and neuropathic complications of diabetes and, possibly, macrovascular disease
- Epidemiologic studies have suggested a small benefit to lowering A1c from 7% into the normal range (<6%); consider for selected individual patients without significant hypoglycemia
- Less stringent A1c goals may be appropriate for patients with a history of severe hypoglycemia, patients with limited life expectancies, children, individuals with comorbid conditions, and those with long-standing diabetes and minimal or stable microvascular complications

Reference: American Diabetes Association. Standards of medical care in diabetes: 2008. *Diabetes Care*. 2008;31(suppl 1):S12–S54.

Medications for Controlling Diabetes Types 1 and 2 (Table 4.2)

Table 4.2
Oral agents for treating type 2 diabetes in adults and adolescents

Agent	Class	Primary Action	Typical Dosage
Tolbutamide (Ornase); Tolazamide (Tolinase); Chlorpropamide (Diabinese)	Sulfonylureas (first generation)	Increases insulin production in the pancreas	Tolbutamide: 0.25–2.00 g/d in divided doses; max, 3 g/d; Tolazamide: 100–1000 mg/d in divided doses; max, 1 g/d; Chlorpropamide: 100–500 mg/d twice/d; max, 750 mg/d
Glyburide (Micronase, Diabeta, Glynase); Glipizide (Glucotrol, Glucotrol XL); Glimepiride (Amaryl)	Sulfonylureas (second generation)	Increases insulin production in the pancreas	Glyburide: 1.25–5 mg/once or twice/d; max, 20 mg/d; Glynase: 0.75–12.0 mg/d; max, 12 mg/d; glipizide: 2.5–20 mg 1 or 2 times/d; max, 40 mg/d; or XL[a] 2.5–10.0 mg 1 or 2 times/d; max, 20 mg/d; Glimepiride: 1–8 mg/d; max, 8 mg/d
Repaglinide (Prandin)	Meglitinide	Increases insulin release from pancreas	New diag or A1c <8%, 0.5 mg; A1c >8%, 1–2 mg, 15–30 min preprandial increase weekly until results are obtained; maximum, 16 mg/d
Nateglinide (Starlix)	Phenylalanine derivative	Increases insulin release from pancreas	60–120 mg preprandial

(*Continued*)

Table 4.2

Adverse Effects	Precautions	Critical Tests	Comments
Hypoglycemia, weight gain, hyperinsulinemia; disulfiram reaction with alcohol	Chlorpropamide active for up to 60 h; use extreme caution with elderly patients or patients with hepatic or renal dysfunction	All metabolized in liver; periodic evaluation of liver function is suggested	Not recommended unless the patient has a well-established history of taking them; second-generation sulfonylureas provide more predictable results with fewer adverse effects and more convenient dosing
Hypoglycemia, weight gain, hyperinsulinemia	Clearance may be diminished in patients with hepatic or renal impairment		Glipizide is preferred with renal impairment; doses of >15 mg should be divided; glimepiride indicated for use with insulin; shown to have some insulin-sensitizing effect
Hypoglycemia, weight gain, hyperinsulinemia	Use with caution on patients with hepatic or renal impairment		Instruct patients to take medication no more than 30 min before a meal; if meals are skipped or added, medication should be skipped or added; approved for use as monotherapy or combined with thiazolidinedione or metformin
Minimal risk of hypoglycemia	Currently no contraindications; use with caution with moderate-to-severe hepatic disease	Periodic evaluation of liver function tests	Approved as monotherapy or in combination with metformin or thiazolidinedione; has only a 2-h duration of action; if meals are skipped or added, medication should be skipped or added

(*Continued*)

Table 4.2
(Continued)

Agent	Class	Primary Action	Typical Dosage
Metformin (Fortamet, Glumetza, Glucophage)	Biguanide	Primarily decreases hepatic glucose production; minor increase in muscle glucose uptake; may improve insulin resistance	500 mg/d twice/d with meals, increase by 500 mg every 1–3 wk, 2 or 3 times/d; usually most effective at 2000 mg/d; maximum, 2550 mg/d; long-acting form Glucophage XR: 500 mg 1 time/d, maximum, 2000 mg once/d
Rosiglitazone (Avandia)	Thiazolidinedione	Decreases insulin resistance, increasing glucose uptake, fat redistribution; minor decrease in hepatic glucose output; preserves β-cell function; decreases vascular inflammation	Initially 4 mg/d in single or divided doses; increase to 8 mg/d in 12 wks, if needed; maximum, 8 mg/d with or without food
Pioglitazone (Actos)	Thiazolidinedione	Decreases insulin resistance, increasing glucose uptake, fat redistribution; minor decrease in hepatic glucose output; preserves β-cell function; decreases vascular inflammation	Initially 15 or 30 mg/d; maximum with or without food, 45 mg for monotherapy, 30 mg for combination therapy

(*Continued*)

Table 4.2
(Continued)

Adverse Effects	Precautions	Critical Tests	Comments
Nausea, diarrhea, metallic taste, possible lactic acidosis	Because of increased risk of lactic acidosis, do not use if frequent alcohol use, liver or kidney disease, or suspected CHF	Contraindicated if serum creatinine is >1.5 mg/dL in men or >1.4 mg/dL in women; do not use if creatinine clearance is abnormal; monitor hematological and renal function annually	Especially beneficial for obese patients because of potential for weight loss, improved lipid profile, and lack of potential for hypoglycemia requiring supplemental carbohydrate intake; discontinue for 48 h after contrast-dye procedures
Minor weight increase of 3–6 lb, edema	Do not use in patients with CHF or hepatic disease; can cause mild-to-moderate edema	Avoid initiation if ALT is >2.5× upper limit of normal; measure ALT periodically; discontinue if ALT is >3× upper limit of normal	Approved for use as monotherapy and in combination with metformin, sulfonylureas, or insulin; fewer interactions associated with CYP-450
Minor weight increase of 3–6 lb, edema	Do not use in patients with CHF or hepatic disease; can cause mild-to-moderate edema	Avoid initiation if ALT is >2.5× upper limit of normal; measure ALT periodically; discontinue if ALT is >3× upper limit of normal	Avoid initiation if ALT is >2.5× upper limit of normal; measure ALT periodically; discontinue if ALT is >3× upper limit of normal

(*Continued*)

Table 4.2
(Continued)

Agent	Class	Primary Action	Typical Dosage
Acarbose (Precose); Miglitol (Glyset)	α -Glucosidase inhibitor	Slows absorption of complex carbohydrate from gastrointestinal tract	25 mg/d; increase by 25 mg/d every 4–6 wk; maximum, split dose before meals (with first bite of food), 300 mg/d (150 mg/d for weight <60 kg)
Combinations			
Glucovance (glyburide and metformin)	Sulfonylureas and biguanide	Decreases hepatic glucose production; increases insulin secretion	Ratios of glyburide and metformin (in mg): 1.25/250, 2.5/500, 5/500; initial: 1.25/250 1 or 2 times/d, increased every 2 wks; second line: 2.5–5/500 2 times/d, increased every 1–2 wk; average dose 7.5/1500; maximum daily dose not to exceed 20 mg of glyburide/2000 mg of metformin
Metaglip (glipizide and metformin)	Sulfonylureas and biguanide	Decreases hepatic glucose production; increases insulin secretion	Ratios of glipizide and metformin (in mg): 2.5/250, 2.5/500, 5/500; initial: 2.5/250 1 or 2 times/d, increased every 2 wks; second line: 2.5–5/500 twice a day, increased every 1–2 wk; maximum daily dose not to exceed 20 mg of glipizide/ 2000 mg of metformin

(Continued)

Table 4.2
(Continued)

Adverse Effects	Precautions	Critical Tests	Comments
Gas and bloating, sometimes diarrhea for both drugs	Do not use if gastrointestinal disorders are concurrent	Avoid if serum creatinine is >2.0 mg/dL; monitor serum transaminase every 3 mo for first year of therapy	Approved for use as monotherapy and in combination with metformin, sulfonylureas, or insulin; if used with hypoglycemic agents such as sulfonylureas or insulin, treat hypoglycemia with glucose, not sucrose
Hypoglycemia, weight gain, lactic acidosis	Do not use if frequent alcohol use, liver or kidney disease, or CHF is suspected	Same caveats as individual components	Patients may frequently use 2 different-dose tablets to attain desired daily dosage and results; discontinue for 48 h after procedures using contrast dye
Hypoglycemia, weight gain, lactic acidosis	Do not use if frequent alcohol use, liver or kidney disease, or CHF is suspected	Same caveats as individual components	Patients may frequently use 2 different-dose tablets to attain desired daily dosage and results; discontinue for 48 h after procedures using contrast dye

(Continued)

Table 4.2
(Continued)

Agent	Class	Primary Action	Typical Dosage
Avandamet (rosiglitazone and metformin)	Thiazolidinedione and biguanide	Decreases hepatic glucose production, increases glucose uptake, decreases insulin resistance, preserves β-cell function	Ratios of rosiglitazone and metformin (in mg): 1/500, 2/500, 4/500, 2/1000, 4/1000 2 times/d; dosage based on individuals' current therapy; maximum, 8 mg/2000 mg/d
Actoplus Met (pioglitazone and metformin)	Thiazolidinedione and biguanide	Decreases hepatic glucose production, increases glucose uptake, decreases insulin	Ratios of pioglitazone and metformin (in mg): 15/500, 15/850
Avandaryl (Rosiglitazone and Glimepiride)	Thiazolidinedione and sulfonylurea	Decreases insulin resistance, increases insulin secretion	Ratios of rosiglitazone and glimepiride (in mg): 4/1, 4/1

(*Continued*)

Table 4.2
(Continued)

Adverse Effects	Precautions	Critical Tests	Comments
Edema, possible lactic acidosis	Do not use if frequent alcohol use, liver or kidney disease, or CHF is suspected	Same caveats as individual components	Less expensive than using agents separately; reported decrease in gastrointestinal upset associated with metformin and weight increase associated with rosiglitazone; discontinue for 48 h after procedures using contrast dye
Same caveats as individual components	Same caveats as individual components	Same caveats as individual components	Same caveats as individual components
Same caveats as individual components	Same caveats as individual components	Same caveats as individual components	Same caveats as individual components

[a] Agents in a class of medicines share mechanisms of action, require similar precautions, and generally have similar adverse effects.

For proper usage, please read label. Agents should not be used in patients with type 1 diabetes. A1c indicates glycated hemoglobin; ALT, alanine aminotransferase; CHF, congestive heart failure; CYP 450, cytochrome P 450. Reprinted with permission from The Diabetes Center, Old Saybrook, CT: Copyright © 2002.

Table 4.3
Insulin Facts

Insulin	Onset	Peak	Effective Duration	Maximal Duration	Comments
Glulisine (Apidra)	<15 min	0.5–1 hr	3 hr	3 hr	Should be given just prior to or just after eating
Lispro (Humalog)	<15 min	1–3 hr	3–5 hr	4–6 hr	
Aspart (Novolog)	<15 min	1–2 hr	2–4 hr	3–5 hr	
Regular	0.5–1 hr	2–4 hr	3–5 hr	4–8 hr	Best if dosed 30 min prior to meal
NPH	2–4 hr	4–10 hr	10–16 hr	14–18 hr	Bedtime dosing minimizes nocturnal hypoglycemia
Lente	3–4 hr	4–12 hr	12–18 hr	16–20 hr	Often used in pediatrics patients over NPH
Insulin Glargine (Lantus)	4–6 hr	none	24 hr	24+ hr	Not to be mixed with any other insulins. Not recommended for pre-filling syringes.
Insulin Detemir (Levemir)	3–4 hr	50% of effect in 3–4 hrs lasting up to 14	5.7–23 hr	Increases with dose	Very slow absorbtion from injection site with 98% of detemir in bloodstream bound to albumin. Can not be mixed with any other insulin.
Humulin/Novolin 70/30	0.5–1	2–10 hr	10–16 hr	14–18 hr	Can convert to Humalog 75/25 or Novolog Mix 70/30 dose per dose
Humalog Mix 70/30, Novolog Mix 75/25	<15 min	1–2 hr	10–16 hr	14–18 hr	Must be taken just prior to or just after eating

Table 4.4
Oral Agents

Medication	Blood Glucose Most Affected	SMBG* Testing to Recommend	Greatest Risk for Hypoglycemia
Sulfonylureas	Fasting and postprandial	2–3 times per day, especially fasting	4–6 hr after meal and fasting
Meglitinide phenylalanine derivative	Postprandial	2 hr after meal	2–3 hr after meal
Biguanide	Fasting	Fasting	None if used as single agent
Alpha-glucosidase inhibitor	Postprandial	2 hr after meal	None if used as single agent
Thiazolidinedione	Fasting and postprandial	2–3 times per day, especially fasting	After exercise when used with sulfonylureas or insulin
Glucovance	Fasting and postprandial	2–3 times per day, especially fasting	4–6 hr after meal and fasting

*SMBG, self-monitoring of blood glucose.
Testing frequency and times may vary on the basis of individual assessment.
(See Table 4.2 for specific drugs.)
Reprinted with permission from The Diabetes Center. Old Saybrook, CT: Copyright © 2002.

Approach to Insulin Treatment of Type 1 Diabetes Mellitus

Typical Insulin Dosage Hints

For an average adolescent with a total daily insulin dose of ~1 U/kg,

- 1 U of short-/rapid-acting insulin will usually lower blood glucose level by 50 to 100 mg/dL
- 8 to 15 g of carbohydrate will require ~1 U of short-/rapid-acting insulin
- 10 to 15 g of dietary carbohydrate will usually change blood glucose level by 40 to 60 mg

Reference: Orr DP. Contemporary management of adolescents with diabetes mellitus. Part 1: type 1 diabetes. *Adolesc Health Update.* 2000;12(2):8.

*Intensive Insulin Regimens**

1. Basal Coverage (~40%–45% of Total Daily Dose [TDD])

a. Long-acting insulin preparation as glargine insulin as a single injection once daily or detemir insulin as twice daily at breakfast and bedtime; or

b. Continuous subcutaneous insulin infusion (pump)

Table 4.5
Recommended insulin storage

Insulin Type	Refrigerated (36°F–46°F)		Room Temperature (59°F–86°F)	
	Opened	Unopened	Opened	Unopened
Vial				
Humalog, Novolog, Humulin, Novolin, Apidra	28 d	Until expiration date	28 d	28 d
Lantus (10 mL)	28 d	Until expiration date	28 d	28 d
Detemir (Levemir)	42 d	Until expiration date	42 d	42 d
Pens/cartridges	Not in use		In use	
Humalog	Until expiration date		28 d	
Humulin R (available in cartridge only)	Until expiration date		28 d	
Humulin N	Until expiration date		14 d	
Humulin 70/30	Until expiration date		10 d	
Humalog Mix 75/25	Until expiration date		10 d	
Novolog	Until expiration date		28 d	
Novolog Mix 70/30	Until expiration date		14 d	
Novolin R (prefilled and 1.5-mL cartridge)	Until expiration date		30 d	
Novolin R (3-mL cartridge)	Until expiration date		28 d	
Novolin N (prefilled and 1.5-mL cartridge)	Until expiration date		7 d	
Novolin N (3-mL cartridge)	Until expiration date		14 d	
Novolin 70/30 (prefilled and 1.5-mL cartridge)	Until expiration date		7 d	
Novolin 70/30 (3-mL cartridge)	Until expiration date		10 d	
Detemir (Levemir)	Until expiration date		42 d	
Apidra	Until expiration date		28 d	
Lantus	Until expiration date		28 d	
Self-filled syringes (not recommended for glargine)	14 d[a]		7 d	
Inhaled insulin	Not in use (unopened overwrap)		In use (unopened overwrap)	
Exubera (insulin blisters)	Room temperature (59–86°F)	Until expiration date	Room temperature (59–86°F)	90 d
Release unit	Do not refrigerate		Replace every 14 d	
Inhaler and chamber	Replace yearly (wash weekly)			

See color insert for Figure 4.1. Types of insulin storage pens and cartidges.

2. Meal Coverage

a. Short-acting insulin (regular or rapid-acting insulin) preparation based on premeal glucose level and carbohydrate consumption.
   - Define food dose: 1 U of rapid-acting insulin will cover 8 to 15 g of carbohydrates; to determine the amount of grams that each unit of insulin covers for an individual, divide 500 by the total daily dose (TDD) of units of insulin needed for control. Thus, food dose = number of grams of carbohydrate ingested/(carbohydrate/insulin)
   - Corrective dose: 1 U of rapid-acting insulin will usually lower blood glucose by 25 to 100 mg% depending on the individual's sensitivity factor. The sensitivity factor is calculated by dividing 1800 by the TDD. Corrective dose = measured blood glucose level − target blood glucose level divided by insulin sensitivity factor. For example, a 50-kg female who requires 1 unit/kg per day total insulin = 50 U/day

Long-acting insulin = 50 U/day × 40% = 20 U/day.

Short-acting insulin (rapid-acting [Lispro, Aspart, Glulisine]) to be given before each meal.

- Food dose: 500/50 = 10 g of carbohydrate per unit of insulin given
- Corrective dose: 1800/50 = 36 (sensitivity factor)
- Target blood glucose level = 120 mg%

Result: 20 U of long-acting insulin; then, before each meal test blood glucose level. For example, if blood glucose level = 280 before breakfast and will eat 40 g of carbohydrate for breakfast, then food dose + corrective dose = (40 g of carbohydrate/10 = 4.0) + [(280 − 120)/36 = 4.4], which means that 8 to 9 U of rapid-acting insulin are given at that meal.

*Meal coverage is based on 2 factors: food dose and corrective dose. If the patient is poorly controlled and TDD >1.4 U/kg, reduce TDD by 20%.

Reference: Orr DP. Diabetes mellitus. In: Neinstein LS, Gordon CM, Katzman DK, Rosen DS, Woods ER, eds. *Adolescent Health Care: A Practical Guide*. 5th ed. Philadelphia, PA: Wolters Kluwer/Lippincott, Williams & Wilkins; 2007:170–179.

Conventional Insulin Regimens

1. Two thirds of the TDD given at breakfast and one third of the TDD given in the evening with dinner and/or at bedtime.
   - Intermediate-acting insulin given at least twice a day at breakfast and dinner (or bedtime)
   - Rapid-acting insulin is given 2 to 3 times per day typically with breakfast NPH and then alone or with NPH at dinner or bedtime dose

Approach for Type 2 Diabetes

1. Lifestyle modification (diet and exercise).

2. Initial oral agent to be considered is metformin.

3. Addition medical therapies may be added as needed to achieve glycemic control.

Diabetic Ketoacidosis Protocol

Initial Management

Physical Examination

- Assess hydration: pulse, blood pressure, skin temperature
- Assess respiratory status: Kussmaul breathing
- Search for signs of an infection
- Assess mental status: documents current status and provides baseline for future

Laboratory Assessment

- Complete blood count with differential
- Lytes
- Serum urea nitrogen
- Creatinine
- Glucose
- Calcium
- PO_4
- Blood gas (arterial or venous)
- HbA1c
- Diabetes antibody panel for new diabetic patient
  - Anti-insulin antibodies
  - Anticytoplasmic islet cell antibodies
  - Glutamic acid decarboxylase antibodies

Fluids

- 0.9% normal saline, 10 mL/kg over 30 to 60 minutes as a bolus once

Insulin

- If serum bicarbonate level is <15 mEq/L, then use insulin drip
  - After fluid bolus, insulin drip should be started (1 U of insulin/mL)
  - Start 0.1 U/kg per hour (hourly rate equals 0.1 mL × weight in kg)
  - Ideally, blood glucose level should decrease 80 to 100 mg%/hour
- If serum bicarbonate level is ≥15 mEq/L, then start/use insulin subcutaneously rather than intravenously

Treatment

Examination

- Observe for neurologic changes and document mental status changes at least every 2 hours

- Abdominal pain should resolve when bicarbonate level is >10 mEq/L; consider pancreatitis for severe, unrelenting pain

Laboratory Tests

- Every 1 hour: blood glucose by meter
- Every 2 hours: lytes, serum urea nitrogen, creatinine, glucose
- Every 8 hours: calcium, PO_4
- Arterial blood gases (necessary only for severe acidosis or neurologic compromise)

Fluids After Initial Bolus

Rate

- 3000 to 3500 mL/m^2 every 24 hours or 2× maintenance† until intravenous fluids are no longer necessary; do not use urinary output as a guide for replacement of fluids

†Maintenance fluids

- 100 mL/kg per day for the first 10 kg of weight
- 50 mL/kg per day for the second 10 kg of weight
- 20 mL/kg per day for each additional kg of weight >20 kg

Fluids

- Use 0.9% normal saline for the first 4 to 6 hours and then switch to 0.45% normal saline
- Serum sodium artificially low with elevated glucose: corrected sodium = ([serum glucose − 100] × 0.016) + measured Na

Glucose

- Ideally, blood glucose should decrease 80 to 100 mg%/hour
- As glucose begins to approach 300 mg/dL, add 5% dextrose to the intravenous fluids
- If glucose falls below 200 mg/dL while acidosis persists, use 10% dextrose so that the insulin drip may continue
- Glucose should be maintained between 180 and 250 mg%

Potassium

Intracellular K^+ stores are always low; once insulin and fluids are started, serum K^+ will decrease rapidly.

- If serum K^+ >6 mEq/L, wait to add K^+ to intravenous fluids
- If serum K^+ <4.5 mEq/L, add 20 mEq/L KCl and 20 mEq/L KPO_4 to each 1000 mL of initial fluids administered
- If serum K^+ >4.5 mEq/L, but <6 mEq/L, add 15 mEq/L KCl and 15 mEq KPO_4 to each 1000 mL of initial fluids administered

Patient Intake

Should be nothing by mouth except for ice chips until acidosis improves significantly

Insulin

- Maintain insulin drip until acidosis resolves as measured by serum bicarbonate level or serum pH

- Serum bicarbonate level will often stabilize around 15 mEq/L until large amounts of Cl administered during initial therapy are excreted
- Once patient's bicarbonate level is >15 mEq/L, and adolescent has eaten, insulin may be switched to subcutaneous insulin

Anion gap = Na + K-Cl-HCO_3 (normal = 13–16) mEq/L (or mmol/L)

Cerebral Edema

- Occurs usually early in treatment within the first 24 hours
- Decline in neurologic status appears similar to hypoglycemia: recheck blood glucose levels
- For declining neurologic status, 1 g/kg of mannitol given rapidly over 15 to 20 minutes should result in rapid improvement
- Mannitol may need to be repeated in another 1 to 3 hours

Adapted from Endocrinology. In: *Pocket Pediatric Manual*. Indianapolis: Indiana University School of Medicine; 2001–2002:17.

B. ABNORMALITIES OF GROWTH AND DEVELOPMENT

Observation and need for assessment depends on the following.

Reliability of Measurements

Absolute Height

- For example, a teenager whose height is 3 SDs below the mean is more likely to have a pathologic condition than is a teenager whose height is only 1 SD below the mean; most teenagers whose heights are below the lowest percentile (3rd or 5th) do not have pathologic conditions

Growth Velocity

- Accurate determination of growth velocity requires at least 3 and preferably 6 months of observation

Weight-for-Height Ratio

- Endocrine disorders (including growth or thyroid hormone deficiency or glucocorticoid excess) usually are associated with relatively preserved weight gain or frank obesity in a short child
- In contrast, most "systemic" disorders that result in poor linear growth are associated with greater impairment of weight gain than linear growth, and affected children tend to be thin for their short stature

Additional Measurements

Predicted Height

- Boys: (father's height [cm] + [mother's height (cm) + 13])/2
- Girls: ([father's height (cm) − 13] + mother's height (cm)]/2

Bone Age

- Appearance of epiphyseal centers obtained on radiography is compared with age-appropriate published standards; examines epiphyseal maturation of the hand and wrist
- Conditions that cause poor linear growth also cause a delay in skeletal maturation and a retarded bone age
- Bone age not delayed in a short teenager is of much greater concern and may, in fact, be of some diagnostic value under certain circumstances; shortened metacarpals, "coned" epiphyses, or rachitic changes may point toward specific diagnoses including syndromes, chondrodysplasias, or rickets

Measurement of Upper-/Lower-Body Segment

- Arm span is approximately equal to height in children ≥8 years of age
- Arm span can be measured as the distance from left fingertips to right fingertips in a patient standing, arms spread, against a wall
- Arm span can be used as a surrogate for height measurement and for monitoring growth velocity in children who have scoliosis, spina bifida, or leg contractures or after spinal irradiation

Key Points

- Rapid linear growth velocity declines progressively after birth to ~25, 12, and 8 cm/year during the first 3 postnatal years, respectively
- Abnormal growth velocity documented after 3 years of age, regardless of absolute height, almost always is abnormal and requires careful evaluation and investigation
- Until the onset of puberty, linear growth occurs at a relatively constant rate of 4 to 7 cm/year and weight gain occurs at ~2.5 kg/year in both genders
- A small linear growth deceleration often is seen before the onset of puberty
- Pubertal growth spurt in girls occurs ~2 years earlier than in boys, usually at pubertal stage 3 for breast development in girls and pubertal stage 4 in boys
- Peak height velocity is slower in girls (8.3 cm/year) than in boys (9.5 cm/year)
- This factor, combined with a 2-year longer duration of growth in boys, results in an average 13-cm difference in adult height between the 2 genders
- Growth ultimately ceases after puberty, a result of estrogen-induced epiphyseal maturation and closure in both genders

- During puberty, children again may cross growth channels (either up or down), depending on when the particular child begins his or her pubertal growth spurt relative to that of the normal reference population

Growth deserves to be evaluated:

- if height is >3 SDs below the mean;
- if patient's height percent is >2 SDs different from that predicted by parents' heights;
- if deceleration with changing growth channels; or
- if linear growth is <4 to 5 cm/year

Adapted from Rose SR, Vogiatzi MG, Copeland KC. A general pediatric approach to evaluating a short child. *Pediatr Rev*. 2005;26(11):410–420. Additional reference: Mansfield JM, Neinstein LM. Abnormal growth and development. In: Neinstein LS, Gordon CM, Katzman DK, Rosen DS, Woods ER, eds. *Adolescent Health Care: A Practical Guide*. 5th ed. Philadelphia, PA: Wolters Kluwer/Lippincott, Williams & Wilkins; 2008:135–156.

Constitutional Delay of Growth and Adolescence

- Slowing growth velocity during the first 3 years after birth, typically with both weight and height crossing growth percentiles downward
- A normal or near-normal growth velocity, with height below but parallel to the 5th percentile during prepubertal years
- Delayed bone age and pubertal maturation; boys usually fail to achieve Sexual Maturity Rating (SMR) G2 (genital growth) by 14 years of age, and girls fail to achieve SMR B2 (breast development) by 13 years of age
- Family history is usually present in the father or male relatives
- Predicted adult height is usually within the normal range, although occasionally lower than expected for parental height
- Screening laboratory test results are normal, including those for thyroid, blood count, sedimentation rate, electrolytes and serum urea nitrogen, urinalysis, liver function, and serum creatinine

Additional Screens to Consider

- Screens for celiac disease: antiendomysial antibodies, immunoglobulin A (IgA) and antitransglutaminase IgG, transglutaminase antibodies, and anti-gliadin IgG titers
- Consider obtaining karyotype if bone age is normal and patient is extremely short
- Perform central imaging studies if tumor is suspected
- Endocrine studies may include insulin growth factor I and insulin growth factor–binding protein 3 as screens and growth hormone–stimulation test by an endocrinologist

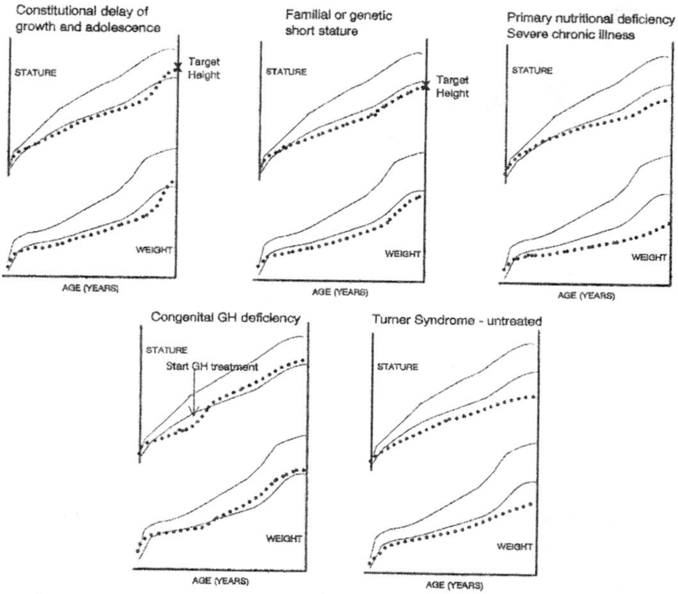

Fig 4.2. Schematic demonstration of height and weight growth curves in various conditions associated with short stature. (Reprinted from Rose SR, Vogiatzi MG, Copeland KC. A general pediatric approach to evaluating a short child [figure 2]. *Pediatr Rev.* 2005;26(11):410–420).

References: Rose SR, Vogiatzi MG, Copeland KC. A general pediatric approach to evaluating a short child. *Pediatr Rev.* 2005;26(11):410–420; and Mansfield JM, Neinstein LM. Abnormal growth and development. In: Neinstein LS, Gordon CM, Katzman DK, Rosen DS, Woods ER, eds. *Adolescent Health Care: A Practical Guide*. 5th ed. Philadelphia, PA: Wolters Kluwer/Lippincott, Williams & Wilkins; 2008:135–156.

Genetic or Familial Short Stature

- Similar growth pattern to constitutional delay
- No evidence of an endocrine or systemic disorder
- Family history of short stature
- Normal weight and length at birth, crossing linear growth percentiles downward during the first 3 years after birth until genetic-appropriate linear growth percentile is reached
- Experience steady growth below but parallel to the normal linear growth curves
- Bone age is typically not delayed and is consistent with chronological age
- Onset of puberty and its rate of progression are normal for chronological age; adult height is short but, by definition, appropriate for parental heights

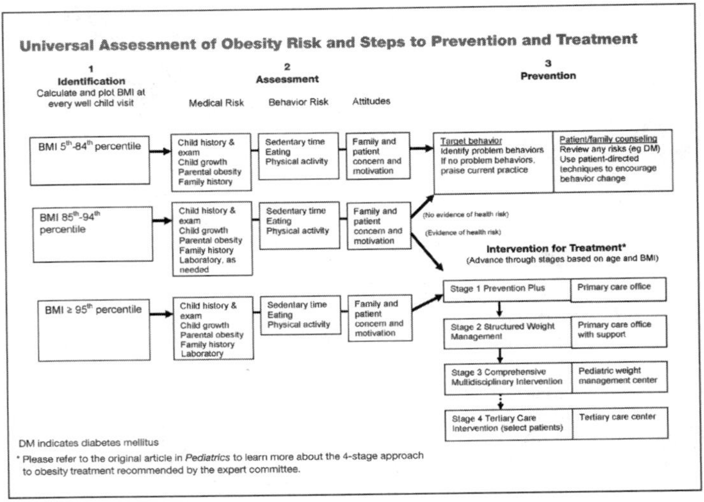

Fig 4.3. Universal assessment of obesity risk and step to prevention and treatment. [Reproduced from Barlow SE, Expert Committee. Expert committee recommendations regarding the prevention, assessment, and treatment of child and adolescent overweight and obesity; summary report. *Pediatrics.* 2007;120(suppl):S164–S192].

Clinical Presentations That Would Indicate Further Evaluation

Short Stature With Increased Weight-for-Height Ratio and Normal Upper- to Lower-Body Proportion

Differential.

- Hypothyroidism (acquired hypothyroidism in childhood usually is an autoimmune condition [lymphocytic or Hashimoto thyroiditis])
- Glucocorticoid excess (iatrogenic, caused by pharmacologic treatment of a concurrent disease such as renal or connective tissue disease or cancer; rarely, it may be caused by endogenous steroid production because of an adrenal tumor or corticotropin-secreting pituitary adenoma)
- Growth hormone deficiency (acquired growth hormone deficiency occurs most commonly as an idiopathic diagnosis but may result from tumors [craniopharyngioma, glioma, germinoma], traumatic head injury, central nervous system infection or irradiation, or surgical damage to the pituitary and hypothalamus)

Short Stature With Decreased Weight-for-Height Ratio and Normal Upper- to Lower-Body Proportion

Differential: variety of systemic diseases, most notably resulting in undernutrition or even malnutrition (eg, type 1 diabetes mellitus, inflammatory bowel disease, celiac disease, anorexia, kidney diseases as renal tubular acidosis or nephrogenic diabetes insipidus, other chronic diseases such as heart, pulmonary, immunologic, connective tissue, neurologic).

Abnormal Upper- to Lower-Body Proportion With Dysmorphic Features: Genetic or Syndromic Causes of Short Stature

Skeletal Dysplasias

- Chromosomal disorders: Turner, Down, and Prader-Willi syndromes
- Small for gestational age: dysmorphic features (eg, fetal alcohol, Russell-Silver, Prader- Willi, Down, and Cornelia de Lange syndromes)

Initial evaluation should include complete blood count with differential and platelets, sedimentation rate, electrolytes, serum urea nitrogen, creatinine, liver function, urinalysis, free thyroxine, thyrotropin.

Other screens.

- Screens for celiac disease antiendomysial antibodies, IgA and antitrans-glutaminase IgG, transglutaminase antibodies, and antigliadin IgG titers
- Consider obtaining karyotype if bone age is normal and patient is extremely short
- Perform central imaging studies if tumor is suspected
- Endocrine studies may include insulin growth factor I and insulin growth factor–binding protein 3 as screens and growth hormone–stimulation test by an endocrinologist

Reference: Rapaport R. Clinical aspects of growth and growth disorders. In: Pescovitz O, Eugster E, eds. *Pediatric Endocrinology: Mechanisms, Manifestations, and Management*. Philadelphia, PA: Lippincott, Williams & Wilkins; 2004.

C. SYNDROMES ASSOCIATED WITH GROWTH AND DEVELOPMENT ABNORMALITY

Prader-Willi Syndrome

- Characteristics: childhood hyperphagia; obesity; childhood hypotonia and lethargy; hypogonadism secondary to hypothalamic dysfunction with cryptorchidism and micropenis; short stature; mild-to-moderate mental retardation and behavioral difficulties
- Inheritance: rarely familial, with abnormality of long arm of chromosome 15 in region of q11-q13 thought secondary to paternal deletion
- Prevalence: 1 in 20 000

Laurence-Moon, Bardet-Biedl, and Biemond Syndromes

- Laurence-Moon and Bardet-Biedl syndromes: autosomal recessive retinitis pigmentosa; hypogonadism; developmental delay
- Laurence-Moon syndrome: additionally spastic paraplegia
- Bardet-Biedl syndrome: additionally polydactyly, obesity
- Biemond syndrome: iris coloboma, hypogonadism, obesity, polydactyly, developmental delay

Kallman Syndrome

- Luteinizing hormone-releasing hormone deficiency: absent or arrested puberty
- Arrested migration of luteinizing hormone-releasing hormone neurosecretory neurons from olfactory area to medial basal hypothalamus
- Anosmia or hyposmia: aplasia or hypoplasia of olfactory bulb and sulcus
- Characteristics: microphallus or cryptorchidism noted in infancy; normal stature and growth; normal adrenarche; eunuchoid proportions
- Associated midline defects: cleft lip, cleft plate, midline cranial anomalies
- MRI: aplasia or hypoplasia of olfactory bulbs and/or sulci
- Inheritance: X-linked recessive, X chromosome deficiency or autosomal dominant or recessive
- Prevalence: 1 in 7500 males and 1 in 50 000 females

Turner Syndrome (45,X)

- Facies: micrognathia, epicanthal folds, low-set ears, narrow high-arched plate, ptosis, and strabismus
- Chest: square and shield-like with microthelia, inverted nipples that are often wide-spaced
- Neck: short and broad with low hairline and webbing of neck
- Cardiovascular abnormalities: present in 20% to 50% with coarctation most common (10%) with bicuspid aortic valves, mitral valve prolapse, anomalous venous drainage, hypoplastic left heart, and aortic root dilatation are reported; aortic root dilatation has led to aortic rupture
- Renal abnormalities: rotation of the kidney, horseshoe kidney, duplication of the renal pelvis and ureter, and hydronephrosis secondary to ureteropelvic obstruction
- Short stature
- Sexual immaturity
- Associated abnormalities: autoimmune thyroiditis, insulin resistance, otitis media with conductive hearing loss, and sensorineural deafness

D. CAUSES OF DELAYED PUBERTY

Box 4.1 Definitions and causes of delayed puberty

Definitions
- Delayed puberty: no increase in testicular volume (ie, <4 mL) by the age of 14 y in boys and no breast development by the age of 13.5 y in girls
- Primary amenorrhea: lack of menstruation by the age of 16 y
- Pubertal arrest: no progress in puberty over 2 y

Causes
- Common (~90%)
  - Constitutional delay, affecting both growth and puberty; much more common (~10-fold) in boys than girls and may be familial; by definition, investigations are normal
- Rare (~10%)
  - Hypogonadotropic hypogonadism
    - Gonadotropin-releasing hormone deficiency, may be isolated or associated with other features (eg, anosmia [Kallman syndrome], cognitive impairment, and dysmorphic features [Prader-Willi syndrome])
    - Gonadotrophin deficiency, may be isolated (fertile eunuch resulting from luteinizing hormone deficiency) or more commonly associated with any form of hypopituitarism
  - Hypergonadotropic hypogonadism
    - Sex chromosome abnormality (eg, Klinefelter syndrome in boys [47,XXY and variants], Turner syndrome in girls [45,X0])
    - Gonadal dysgenesis with normal karyotype
    - Gonadal damage: viral (eg, mumps orchitis), iatrogenic (surgical, chemotherapy, or radiotherapy), autoimmune (often associated with Addison disease); gametes are generally more sensitive to damage that steroid-secreting cells
    - Loss-of-function mutation in the β -luteinizing hormone subunit; reduced luteinizing hormone bioactivity but elevated concentrations of luteinizing hormone in immunoassay
    - Loss-of-function mutation in gonadotrophin receptors: resistant ovary syndrome

A temporary delay in pubertal development is very common in the presence of any serious illness (eg, renal failure, bowel or liver disease). Progress depends on the course of the underlying disease. Endocrine causes of temporary delay include hypothyroidism, growth hormone deficiency, and excess glucocorticoids of whatever cause. Please also review the gynecology chapter in this book.

Adapted from Achermann JC. Delayed puberty [Table 22-1]. In: Pescovitz O, Eugster E, eds. *Pediatric Endocrinology: Mechanisms, Manifestations, and Management.* Philadelphia, PA; Lippincott, Williams & Wilkins: 2004:335.

E. OBESITY

Measurement of Obesity*

*See chapter on Biologic and Psychosocial Growth and Development for BMI Charts.

Table 4.6
Age and gender-based BMI cut-offs (kg/m^2)

Age, y	Male >85%	Female >85%	Male >95%	Female >95%
13	21.8	22.6	25.2	26.2
14	22.6	23.4	26.0	27.2
15	23.4	24.0	26.8	28.0
16	24.2	24.6	27.6	28.8
17	24.9	25.0	28.2	29.6

Please see biological and psychosocial growth chapter in this book for BMI charts. Adapted from Love-Osborne K. An approach to obesity management in primary care: yes, we can make a difference. *Adolesc Med State Art Rev*. 2009;20(1):91–108, ix; see also: Centers for Disease Control and Prevention. 2000 CDC growth charts: United States. Available at: www.cdc.gov/growthcharts. Accessed August 4, 2009.

Triceps Measurement

Calipers placed 1 cm above the midpoint between the acromion and olecranon process on the posterior of a relaxed right arm and measured 3 times using the average.

Table 4.7
95th percentiles of triceps skinfold thickness for National Health and Nutrition Examination Survey I subjects

Male Age, y	95th Percentile, mm	Female Age, y	95th Percentile
6–6.9	14	6–6.9	16
7–7.9	16	7–7.9	18
8–8.9	17	8–8.9	20
9–9.9	19	9–9.9	22
10–10.9	21	10–10.9	24
11–11.9	22	11–11.9	26
12–12.9	23	12–12.9	28
13–13.9	24	13–13.9	30
14–14.9	23	14–14.9	31
15–15.9	22	15–15.9	32
16–16.9	22	16–16.9	33
17–17.9	22	17–17.9	34
18–18.9	22	18–18.9	34
19–19.9	22	19–19.9	35

Triceps skinfold measurement: determine the midpoint between the acromion and olecranon process on the posterior surface of the right arm and mark it. With the patient's arm relaxed, grasp the skinfold ~1 cm above the midpoint, taking care to exclude muscle from the grasp. Measure skinfold thickness with calipers at the midpoint. Repeat the measure 2 to 3 times. Adapted from AMERICAN JOURNAL OF CLINICAL NUTRITION by Must, Dallal, Dietz. Copyright 1991 by American Society for Nutrition. Reproduced with permission of American Society for Nutrition via Copyright Clearance Center.

Waist Circumference

Table 4.8
Ninetieth percentile for waist circumference (in cm) according to age and demographic

Age, y	Black Boys	Black Girls	Hispanic Boys	Hispanic Girls	White Boys	White Girls
8	69	72	74	73	71	70
9	73	76	78	76	74	73
10	76	80	81	79	78	76
11	79	83	85	82	81	78
12	82	87	88	85	85	81
13	85	91	92	89	88	84
14	89	94	95	92	91	87
15	92	98	98	95	95	90
16	95	102	102	98	98	93
17	98	105	105	101	102	96
18	101	109	109	104	105	98

Reprinted from Love-Osborne K. An approach to obesity management in primary care: yes, we can make a difference. *Adolesc Med.* 2009;20:97.

Visceral abdominal fat is an independent risk factor for cardiovascular disease in adults.

National Health and Nutrition Examination Survey III for children and adolescents used midpoint between the bottom of rib cage and above the top of the iliac crest at minimal respiration; they defined abnormal as >90th percentile for age and gender of the sample population.

Definition of Metabolic Syndrome*

Definition of pediatric metabolic syndrome is modified from Adult National Cholesterol Education Program defined by an expert panel definition on detection, evaluation and treatment of high blood cholesterol in adults (Adult Treatment Panel III).

---

*Review the cardiorespiratory chapter in this book to obtain abnormal adolescent values for hypertension and lipids.

Table 4.9
Pediatric definitions of "metabolic syndrome"

	Cook et al[a]	Cruz et al[b]	Caprio[c]	Jolliffe and Janssen[d]
Abdominal obesity	WC ≥90th percentile for age/gender[e]	WC ≥90th percentile for age/gender/race[f]	BMI z ≥2.0	WC ≥92nd percentile for age/boys; WC ≥72nd percentile for age/girls
Elevated blood pressure	SBP or DBP ≥90th percentile[g]	≥95th percentile[g]	≥95th percentile[g]	SBP ≥92nd percentile or DBP ≥97th percentile for age/boys; SBP ≥93rd percentile or DBP ≥99th percentile for age/girls
High triglycerides	≥110 mg/dL	≥95th percentile for age and gender	≥95th percentile for age, gender, and race	Triglycerides ≥89th percentile for age/boys; triglycerides ≥89th percentile for age/girls
Low HDL cholesterol	≤40 mg/dL	HDL ≤5th percentile for age/gender	HDL ≤5th percentile for age/gender/race	HDL ≤26th percentile for age/boys; HDL ≤43rd percentile for age/girls
Impaired fasting glucose metabolism/elevated glucose	≥100 mg/dL	Impaired glucose tolerance: >140 but <200 mg/dL at 2 h	Impaired glucose tolerance: >140 but <200 mg/dL at 2 h	≥100 mg/dL

WC indicates waist circumference; DBP, diastolic blood pressure; SBP, systolic blood pressure; HDL, high-density lipoprotein.
Pediatric definitions of "metabolic syndrome" are modified from the adult National Cholesterol Education Program definition commonly reported in the literature (defined as the presence of ≥3 of the risk determinants in column 1).

[a] Cook S, et al. *J Pediatr.* 2008;152:165–170.
[b] Cruz ML, et al. *J Clin Endocrinol Metab.* 2004;89:108–113.
[c] Caprio S. *Int J Obesity.* 2005:29(suppl 2):S24–S25.
[d] Joliffe CJ, et al. *J Am Coll Cardiol.* 2007;49:891–898.
[e] Li C, et al. *Pediatrics.* 2006;152:165–170.
[f] Fernandez JR, et al. *J Pediatr.* 2004;145:439–444.
[g] National High Blood Pressure Education Program Working Group on High Blood Pressure in Children and Adolescents 2004. Please see the resource/reading list on page 8 for citations.

Adapted from Gabel M, Cook S. Obesity in adolescence. Part 2: cardiometabolic risks. *Adolesc Health Update*. 2009;21(2):1–10.

Table 4.10
Comparing 2 adaptations of the diagnostic criteria for the metabolic syndrome for pediatrics with Adult Treatment Panel III criteria

Risk Factor	Defining Level per the NCEP ATPIII[a]	Defining Level per Cook et al[b]	Defining Level per Weiss et al[c]
Central obesity	Men: >102 cm; women: >88 cm	Waist circumference >90th percentile for age and gender from sample population	BMI ≥97th percentile for age and gender
Triglycerides	≥150 mg/dL	≥110 mg/dL	≥95th percentile for age and gender
HDL cholesterol	Men: <40 mg/dL; women: <50 mg/dL	≤40 mg/dL	≤5th percentile for age and gender
Blood pressure	≥130/≥85 mm Hg	≥90th percentile for age, gender, and height	≥95th percentile for age, gender, and height
Fasting glucose	≥110 mg/dL	≥110 mg/dL	Impaired glucose tolerance

NCEP indicates Adult National Cholesterol Education Program; ATPIII, Adult Treatment Panel III; HDL, high-density lipoprotein.

[a] National High Blood Pressure Education Program Working Group on High Blood Pressure in Children and Adolescents. The fourth report on the diagnosis, evaluation, and treatment of high blood pressure in children and adolescents. *Pediatrics*. 2004;114(2 suppl 4th report): 555–576; and Daniels SR, Greer FR; Committee on Nutrition. Lipid screening and cardiovascular health in childhood. *Pediatrics*. 2008;122(1):198–208.

[b] Cook S, Weitzman M, Auinger P, Nguyen M, Dietz WH. Prevalence of a metabolic syndrome phenotype in adolescents: findings from the third National Health and Nutrition Examination Survey, 1988–1994. *Arch Pediatr Adolesc Med*. 2003;157(8):821–827.

[c] Weiss R, Dziura J, Burgert TS, et al. Obesity and the metabolic syndrome in children and adolescents. *N Engl J Med*. 2004;350(23):2362–2374.

Adapted from Biltoft CA, Muir A. The metabolic syndrome in children and adolescents: a clinician's guide. *Adolesc Med State Art Rev*. 2009;20(1):109–120.

Definition of Metabolic Syndrome (*Continued*)

Metabolic syndrome in adolescents is defined as ≥3 of the following:

- Elevated blood pressure for age/gender/height
- BMI at 95th percentile or waist circumference at >90th percentile
- Fasting triglyceride level of >110 mg%
- High-density lipoprotein cholesterol level of <40 mg%
- Impaired fasting glucose (100–125 mg%), impaired glucose-tolerance test (2-hour glucose = 140–199 mg%), or diabetes (fasting glucose ≥126 mg%; 2-hour glucose ≥200 mg%)

References: Cook S, Weitzman M, Auinger P, Nguyen M, Dietz WH. Prevalence of a metabolic syndrome phenotype in adolescents: findings from the third National Health and Nutrition Examination Survey, 1988–1994. *Arch Pediatr Adolesc Med.* 2003;157(8):821–827; and Love-Osborne K. An approach to obesity management in primary care: yes, we can make a difference. *Adolesc Med State Art Rev.* 2009;20(1):91–108, ix.

Assessment of Obesity and Approach to Treatment

Findings on Review of Systems in Obesity Assessment and Possible Causes (Table 4.11)

Table 4.11
Findings on review of systems in obesity assessment and possible causes

Symptom	Possible Causes
Anxiety, school avoidance, social isolation	Depression
Severe recurrent headaches	Pseudotumor cerebri
Shortness of breath, exercise intolerance	Asthma, lack of physical conditioning
Snoring, apnea, daytime sleepiness	Obstructive sleep apnea, obesity hypoventilation syndrome
Sleepiness or wakefulness	Depression
Abdominal pain	Gastroesophageal reflux disease, constipation, gallbladder disease, nonalcoholic fatty liver disease[a]
Hip pain, knee pain, walking pain	Slipped capital femoral epiphysis, musculoskeletal stress from weight (may be barrier to physical activity)
Foot pain	Musculoskeletal stress from weight (may be barrier to physical activity)
Irregular menses (<9 cycles per y)	Polycystic ovary syndrome; may be normal if recent menarche
Primary amenorrhea	Polycystic ovary syndrome, Prader-Willi syndrome
Polyuria, polydipsia	Type 2 diabetes mellitus[a]
Unexpected weight loss	Type 2 diabetes mellitus[a]
Nocturnal enuresis	Obstructive sleep apnea
Tobacco use	Increased cardiovascular risk; may be used as form of weight control

[a] These conditions are often asymptomatic.

Adapted from Barlow SE; Expert Committee. Expert committee recommendations regarding the prevention, assessment, and treatment of child and adolescent overweight and obesity: summary report. *Pediatrics*. 2007;120(suppl):S164–S192.

Physical Examination Findings in Obesity Assessment and Possible Causes (Table 4.12)

Table 4.12
Physical examination findings in obesity assessment and possible causes

System	Findings	Possible Explanations
Anthropometric features	High BMI percentile	Overweight or obesity
	Short stature	Underlying endocrine or genetic condition
Vital signs	Elevated blood pressure	Hypertension if systolic or diastolic blood pressure at ≥95th percentile for age, gender, and height on ≥3 occasions
Skin	Acanthosis nigricans	Common in obese children, especially when skin is dark; increased risk of insulin resistance
	Excessive acne, hirsutism	Polycystic ovary syndrome
	Irritation, inflammation	Consequence of severe obesity
	Violaceous striae	Cushing syndrome
Eyes	Papilledema	Pseudotumor cerebri
	Cranial nerve VI paralysis	
Throat	Tonsillar hypertrophy	Obstructive sleep apnea
Neck	Goiter	Hypothyroidism
Chest	Wheezing	Asthma (may explain or contribute to exercise intolerance)
Abdomen	Tenderness	Gastroesophageal reflux disorder, gallbladder disease, nonalcoholic fatty liver disease[a]
	Hepatomegaly	Nonalcoholic fatty liver disease[a]
Reproductive system	Tanner stage	Premature puberty in <7-y-old white girls, <6-y-old black girls, and <9-y-old boys
	Apparent micropenis	May be normal penis that is buried in fat
	Undescended testes	Prader-Willi syndrome
Extremities	Abnormal gait, limited hip range of motion	Slipped capital femoral epiphysis
	Bowing of tibia	Blount disease
	Small hands and feet; polydactyly	Some genetic syndromes

[a] These conditions are usually without signs.
Adapted from Barlow SE; Expert Committee. Expert committee recommendations regarding the prevention, assessment, and treatment of child and adolescent overweight and obesity: summary report. *Pediatrics*. 2007;120(suppl):S164–S192.

Medical Screening (Table 4.13)

Table 4.13
Key features of cardiometabolic conditions related to obesity

	Clinical Features	Family History	Suggested Testing
NAFLD	Obesity, vague abdominal pain, hepatomegaly, acanthosis nigricans	NAFLD, obesity, type 2 DM	Laboratory: elevated AST/ALT, insulin resistance, and other diagnoses reasonably excluded; ultrasound: hyperechogenic liver; histology: steatosis, lobular inflammation, and ballooning degeneration
PCOS	Obesity or normal weight, oligomenorrhea or amenorrhea, hirsutism	PCOS, obesity, infertility	Laboratory: elevated free testosterone, insulin resistance; ultrasound: polycystic ovaries
OSAS	Obesity, history of snoring or apnea, hypertension, daytime sleepiness or hyperactivity, depression	OSAS, obesity	Positive polysomnography study
Type 2 DM	Obesity, polyuria, polydipsia, but also may be asymptomatic	Obesity, hypertension, hyperlipidemia, heart disease, type 2 DM	Fasting glucose (≥126 mg/dL is diagnostic, 100–125 mg/dL is impaired fasting glucose); oral glucose-tolerance testing
Hypertension (essential)	Usually none	Obesity, hypertension, heart disease, type 2 DM	Laboratory: urinalysis, serum SUN, creatinine; ambulatory BP monitoring, cardiac echo; rule out other etiology of hypertension as indicated by history and physical

(*Continued*)

Table 4.13
(Continued)

	Clinical Features	Family History	Suggested Testing
Hyperlipidemia	Usually none	Hypercholesterolemia, premature heart disease, obesity	Fasting lipid panel: high triglycerides, low HDL described with obesity; very high levels of total and LDL cholesterol more suggestive of genetic/familial origin but the prevalence of obesity could lead to unrelated co-occurrences

NAFLD indicates nonalcoholic fatty liver disease; DM, diabetes mellitus; AST/ALT, aspartate aminotransferase/alanine aminotransferase; PCOS, polycystic ovary syndrome; OSAS, obstructive sleep apnea syndrome; SUN, serum urea nitrogen; BP, blood pressure; HDL, high-density lipoprotein; LDL, low-density lipoprotein
Data excerpted and modified from Barlow SE; Expert Committee. Expert committee recommendations regarding the prevention, assessment, and treatment of child and adolescent overweight and obesity: summary report. *Pediatrics*. 2007;120(suppl):S164–S192.

Diagnostic ICD-9 Codes

Table 4.14
Diagnostic ICD-9 codes useful for obesity-related conditions

278.02	Overweight
278.00	Obesity
278.01	Morbid obesity
251.1	Hyperinsulinism/insulin resistance
783.1	Abnormal/excess weight gain
V85.53	BMI, pediatric, 85th to <95th percentile for age
V85.54	BMI, pediatric, greater than or equal to 95th percentile for age
796.2	Elevated blood pressure without hypertension
701.2	Acanthosis nigricans
272.2	Mixed hyperlipidemia
272.4	Other/unspecified hyperlipidemia
780.57	Unspecified sleep apnea

Adapted from Gabel M, Cook S. Obesity in adolescence. Part 2: cardiometabolic risks. *Adolesc Health Update*. 2009;21(2):1–10.

Medications and Surgical Approaches to Weight Loss in Adolescents (Table 4.15)

Table 4.15
Medications and surgical approaches[a] to weight loss in adolescents

Orlistat (Xenical, Alli), approved for patients ≥12 y of age
Gastrointestinal lipase inhibitor, blocks the uptake of approximately one third of ingested fat
Multicenter randomized, controlled study of teenagers using Orlistat 120 mg 3 times per day compared to placebo; both groups received hypocaloric diet, exercise prescriptions, and behavioral therapy; both groups lost weight with some increased efficacy when used with drug
Adverse effects: gastrointestinal (such as flatulence, abdominal pain, oily staining, and diarrhea)
Contraindications: malabsorption syndromes, cholestasis; costs are high for medication
Sibutramine (Merida), approved for patients ≥16 y of age
Works by inhibiting reuptake of serotonin and norepinephrine, thus decreasing appetite
Randomized, controlled studies suggest that medication at 10 mg/d along with behavioral and nutritional therapy is helpful
Adverse effects: mild tachycardia and elevations in blood pressure, insomnia, headaches, dry mouth, constipation
Contraindications: anorexia, cardiac disease (such as coronary artery disease, congestive heart failure), pregnancy and lactation; other serotonergic drugs
Metformin (Glucophage), approved for treatment of diabetes in children ≥8 y of age
Works primarily through its suppression of hepatic glucose production (hepatic gluconeogenesis); metformin increases insulin sensitivity, enhances peripheral glucose uptake, increases fatty acid oxidation, and decreases absorption of glucose from the gastrointestinal tract; increased peripheral utilization of glucose may be a result of improved insulin binding to insulin receptors
Studied in teenaged population using 500 mg twice daily to 2000 mg daily in divided doses; may be used with good efficacy along with behavioral and nutritional intervention
Adverse effects: gastrointestinal (such as nausea, stomach upset, diarrhea, flatulence, or a metallic taste in the mouth)

[a] Experience with the surgical approach in adolescent patients has suggested significant and sustained weight loss in adolescents. (See www.hta.hca.wa.gov/documents/pbsexecutivesummary.pdf. Accessed August 6, 2009).
From Love-Osborne K. An approach to obesity management in primary care: yes, we can make a difference. *Adolesc Med State Art Rev*. 2009;20(1):91–108, ix.

F. THYROID DISORDERS

Pearls

- Single most sensitive test for evaluating thyroid disorders is thyrotropin: normal levels rule out hyperthyroidism or hypothyroidism

- Low thyroglobulin in association with hyperthyroidism is a hallmark of exogenous thyroid intake referred to as thyrotoxicosis factitia; consider dietary supplements "to increase metabolism to help weight loss"; also use foods (kelp, shellfish) or medications (eg, amiodarone) with extra iodine
- Central thyroid disease (eg, pituitary tumor): must use free thyroxine, not thyrotropin, to monitor replacement
- Euthyroid disease: normal thyrotropin, mildly low free thyroxine, low total triiodothyronine, decreased peripheral conversion of thyroxine to triiodothyronine (eg, systemic disease, illness, trauma, anorexia nervosa)

Table 4.16
Symptoms and Signs of Hypothyroidism

Symptoms
Constipation
Fatigue
Hoarseness
Slowed mentation (lethargy and impaired school performance)
Menstrual dysfunction, sometimes as dysfunctional uterine bleeding
Signs
Abdominal distension
Bradycardia (decreased cardiac output)
Coarse facial features
Coarse, brittle, strawlike hair
Decreased systolic blood pressure and increased diastolic blood pressure
Dry, sallow skin
Delayed deep tendon reflexes
Dull facial expression
Fluid retention and weight gain (impaired renal free water clearance)
Goiter
Growth retardation
Hypothermia
Hyporeflexia with delayed relaxation, ataxia, or both
Jaundice
Loss of scalp hair, axillary hair, pubic hair, or combination
Macroglossia
Nonpitting edema (myxedema)
Pubertal disorders (delay or pseudoprecocity)
Pallor
Periorbital puffiness
Pericardial effusion
Pitting edema of lower extremities
Slowed speech and movements
Skeletal maturational delay

Huang SA, Neinstein LS. Thyroid Disease in Adolescents. In: Neinstein LS, Gordon CM, Katzman DK, Rosen DS, Woods ER (eds) *Adolescent Health Care. A Practical Guide.* 5th ed. Philadelphia, PA: Lippincott, Williams & Wilkins; 2002. Reprinted with permission.

Available Tests

- Total thyroxine (TT_4) (4 iodine atoms): released from thyroid gland
- Free thyroxine (free T_4): <1%; >99% bound to proteins as thyroxine-binding globulin, prealbumin, and albumin
- Triiodothyronine (TT_3): 20% by produced by thyroid gland; other 80% results from peripheral conversion of thyroxine to triiodothyronine
- Free triiodothyronine (free T_3): nonbound to protein
- Thyroglobulin (T_9): protein whose production is under the influence of thyrotropin
- Thyroid-stimulating hormone (TSH) (thyrotropin): released from pituitary under control of thyrotropin-releasing hormone from hypothalamus; use third-generation thyrotropin assay (normal now 0.5–4.1 mIU/mL)
- Thyroxine-binding globulin (TBG)
- Thyrotropin-receptor antibodies (TSHR Abs)
- Antithyroid peroxidase antibodies (anti TPO Abs) = antimicrosomal antibodies → more sensitive than antithyroid globulin antibodies for diagnosing autoimmune thyroiditis
- Antithyroglobulin antibodies (anti Tg Abs)

Reference: Lu R, Burman KD. *Women's Health in Primary Care*. 2006;July–August:31–42.

Table 4.17
Classification of Autoimmune Thyroiditis

Type 1 autoimmune thyroiditis (Hashimoto disease type 1)	
1A	Goitrous
1B	Nongoitrous
Status: euthyroid with normal TSH	
Type 2 autoimmune thyroiditis (Hashimoto disease type 2)	
2A	Goitrous (classic Hashimoto disease)
2B	Nongoitrous (primary myxedema, atrophic thyroiditis)
Status: persistent hypothyroidism with increased TSH	
2C	Transient aggravation of thyroiditis (eg, postpartum thyroiditis)
Status: may start as transient, low RAIU thyrotoxicosis, followed by transient hypothyroidism	
Type 3 autoimmune thyroiditis (Graves disease)	
3A	Hyperthyroid Graves disease
3B	Euthyroid Graves disease
Status: hyperthyroid or euthyroid with suppressed TSH; stimulatory autoantipodies to the TSH receptor are present (autoantibodies to thyroglobulin and TPO are also usually present)	
3C	Hypothyroid Graves disease
Status: orbitopathy with hypothyroidism; diagnostic levels of autoantibodies to the TSH receptor (blocking or stimulating) may be detected (autoantibodies to Tg and TPO are also usually present)	

Reprinted with permission from Davies TF, Amino N. A new classification for human autoimmune thyroid disease. *Thyroid* 1993;3(4):331–333. The publisher for this copyrighted material is Mary Ann Liebert, Inc. publishers.

Tests to assess hypothyroidism: free thyroxine, thyrotropin, triiodothyronine; titers of antithyroid globulin antibodies (36% sensitive) and antimicrosomal antibodies (antithyroid peroxidase antibodies levels (99% sensitive).

Tests to assess hyperthyroid: free thyroxine, thyrotropin, free triiodothyronine; if symptoms present for <8 weeks, an ^{123}I uptake test (rather than radioactive iodine-uptake test), the results of which will be high, should be ordered to differentiate from sporadic thyroiditis or painful subacute thyroiditis, with which ^{123}I uptake will be low; hyperfunctioning nodules will show uptake of ^{123}I but not in tissue surrounding nodule.

Table 4.18
Differential Diagnosis of Thyrotoxicosis

Causes of Thyrotoxicosis
Thyrotoxicosis associated with sustained hormone overproduction (hyperthyroidism):
High RAIU
Graves disease
Toxic multinodular goiter
Toxic adenoma
Increased TSH secretion
Thyrotoxicosis without associated hyperthyroidism:
Low RAIU
Thyrotoxicosis factitia
Subacute thyroiditis
Chronic thyroiditis with transient thyroiditis (painless thyroiditis, silent thyroiditis, postpartum thyroiditis)
Ectopic thyroid issue (struma ovarii, functioning metastatic thyroid cancer)

Adapted with permission from Davis TF. Thyrotoxicosis. In: Larsen PR, Melmed S, Polonsky KS, eds. *Williams Textbook of Endocrinology*, 10th ed. Philadelphia, PA: WB Saunders; 2003.

Characteristics of Thyroid Nodules

- Frequency of nodules: 5% to 10% in adults but 0.05% to 1.8% in children; cancer rate is 5% to 10% of nodules in adults, whereas for children it is 5% to 33%
- Cause: high-dose radiation of neck and genetic disorders and familial adenomatous polyposis
- Evaluate with thyroid studies as free thyroxine, thyrotropin titers, anti-thyroid globulin antibodies and antimicrosomal antibodies, thyroid ultrasound and biopsy

Reference: Huang SA, Neinstein LS. Thyroid disease in adolescents [Table 9-4]. In: Neinstein LS, Gordon CM, Katzman DK, Rosen DS, Woods ER, eds. *Adolescent Health Care: A Practical Guide*. 5th ed. Philadelphia, PA: Wolters Kluwer/Lippincott, Williams & Wilkins; 2008:166–167.

Table 4.19
Conditions That Increase Levothyroxine Requirements

Pregnancy	
Gastrointestinal disease	Mucosal diseases of the small bowel (eg, sprue)
	Jejunoiteal bypass and small bowel resection
	Diabetic diarrhea
Drugs which impair L-T4 absorption	Cholestyramine
	Sucralfate
	Aluminum hydroxide
	Calcium carbonate
	Ferrous sulfate
Drugs which may enhance CYP3A4 and thereby accelerate levothyroxine clearance	Rifampi
	Carbamazepine
	Estrogen
	Phenytoin
	Sertraline
	Statins
Drugs which impair T4 to T3 conversion	Amiodarone
Conditions which may block type 1 deiodinase	Selenium deficiency
	Cirrhosis

Experience with the surgical approach in adolescent patients has suggested significant and sustained weight loss in adolescents (see www.hta.hca.wa.gov/documents/pbs_executive-_summary.pdf). Adapted with permission from Larsen PR. Hypothyroidism and thyroiditis. In: Larsen PR, Melmed S, Polonsky KS, eds. *Williams Textbook of Endocrinology*, 10th ed. Philadelphia, PA: WB Saunders; 2003.

Adolesc Med 20 (2009) 457–483

5. Gynecology

DEFINITION OF NORMAL AND ABNORMAL MENSES

A. Normal Menstrual Cycle[1]

- Begins at a median age of 12.43 years, with 80% between the ages of 11 and 13.8 years; ~10% at <11 years of age
  - White girls, 12.9 years; Hispanic girls, 12.55 years; black girls, 12.06 years
  - 10% by 11.1 years, 90% by 13.75 years
  - Onset of menarche by a sexual maturity rating of 3 to 4

- Begins ~2.3 years after initiation of puberty, with a range of 1 to 3 years
- Becomes regular after 2 to 2.5 years
- Occurs every 28 days, with a range of 21 to 42 days (3–6 weeks)
- Lasts for 3 to 5 days, with a range of 2 to 7 days
- Results in average loss of 40 mL of blood per cycle, with a range of 25 to 70 mL
- Ovulatory cycles depend on age of menarche: with 67% of girls by 2 years post-menarche; cycle length: averages 31 days

Adapted from Chumlea WC, Schubert CM, Roche AF, et al. Age at menarche and racial comparisons in US girls. *Pediatrics*. 2003;111(1):110–113; and Sun SS, Schubert CM, Chumlea WC, et al. National estimates of the timing of sexual maturation and racial differences among US children. *Pediatrics*. 2002;110(5):911–919.

B. Menstrual Irregularities: Variations in Frequency

- Polymenorrhea: frequent regular or irregular bleeding at <21-day intervals ("I'm having too many periods")
- Oligomenorrhea: infrequent irregular bleeding at >42-day intervals ("My periods don't come often enough")
- Primary amenorrhea: no menstrual flow by the age of 15.5 years
- Secondary amenorrhea: absence of vaginal bleeding for >3 months("I haven't had a period in months")
- Irregular menses: bleeding frequency that varies, occurring at >21-day but <42-day intervals ("My periods never come at the same time of the month")

Margaret J. Blythe, MD
E-mail address: mblythe@iupui.edu

C. Menstrual Irregularities: Variations in Amount and Duration

- Metrorrhagia: intermenstrual irregular bleeding between regular periods ("I'm bleeding between my periods")
- Menorrhagia: excessive amount and increased duration of uterine bleeding occurring regularly ("My periods are too long and too heavy and come too often")
- Dysfunctional uterine bleeding (DUB): prolonged excessive menstrual bleeding associated with irregular periods, usually a result of anovulation in adolescence ("I've been bleeding for 3 straight weeks")

D. Menstrual Irregularities: Variations in Amount

- Hypomenorrhea: decreased menstrual flow occurring at regular intervals ("My periods are too light")
- Hypermenorrhea: profuse menstrual flow of normal duration and occurring at regular intervals ("My periods are too heavy")

EVALUATION OF MENSTRUAL DISORDERS

A. History: Components to Document

Menstrual-Specific

- Age at menarche
- Last normal menstrual period
- Frequency and duration of flow
- Symptoms associated with menses
- Quantity of pads/tampons per day and number of periods
- Disruption of normal activities
- Last menstrual period
- Past treatment

Past Medical

- Hospitalization
- Bleeding disorders (eg, epistaxis, hematuria, hematochezia)
- Surgery
- Serious infections
- Congenital problems (eg, hydrocephalus)
- Previous gynecological evaluation and treatment
- Chronic illness (ie, rheumatological, endocrinologic, oncological, gastrointestinal)
- Growth and development
- Tanner stage/sexual maturity rating

Family History of Gynecologic Problems

- Maternal menarche
- Ovarian cysts
- Dysmenorrhea/premenstrual syndrome (PMS)
- Bleeding disorders
- Endometriosis
- Surgical procedures
- Malignancy
- Fertility problems
- Virilization

Medications/Substance Use or Misuse

- Use of contraceptives
- Tobacco
- Steroids
- Marijuana
- Alcohol
- Cocaine
- Others (antianxiety agents, antidepressants, antipsychotic medications)

Related Health Issues

- Weight change
- Emotional symptoms
- Nutrition history
- Psychiatric disorders/depression
- Exercise/sports
- Eating disorders

Sexual Behavior

- Sexual activity/behaviors
- Births, abortions, miscarriages
- Use of contraceptives/condoms
- Sexually transmitted infections (STIs)
- Sexual molestations/abuse

B. Physical Examination: Specific Elements to Document

- Vital signs: weight, height, blood pressure, heart rate, BMI (weight [kg]/height [m]^2 or [weight (lb)/height (in)^2] $\times$ 703)
- Sexual maturity rating: B1 through B5, P1 through P5
- External Signs
  - Acne
  - Acanthosis nigricans

- Bruising/ecchymosis/petechiae
- Galactorrhea
- Hirsute/virilization/striae
- Thyroid size

- External genitalia and pelvic examination
  - Clitoromegaly (clitoral index = transverse diameter [3.4 ± 1.0 mm] × longitudinal diameter [5.1 ± 1.4 mm] = mean (18.52 mm^2) (see Verkauf BS, Von Thron J, O'Brien WF. Clitoral size in normal women. *Obstet Gynecol.* 1992;80[1]:41–44); enlarged ≥35 mm^2
  - Evidence of estrogen effect—external genitalia, vaginal epithelium (vaginal smears) (Table 5.1)
  - Vaginal growths, foreign bodies
  - Cervix—erythema, friability, mucopus, shape of os

Table 5.1
Evaluating Estrogen Status

Ratio of superficial cells to parabasal cells, %	Interpretation
<5	"poor" or no estrogen effect
5–10	slight estrogen effect
10–30	moderate estrogen effect
>30	marked estrogen effect

Adapted from Emans SJ. Office evaluation of the child and adolescent. In: Emans SJ, Laufer MR, Goldstein DP, eds. *Pediatric and Adolescent Gynecology*. 5th ed. Philadelphia, PA: Lippincott-Raven; 2005:36. Reprinted by permission of Wolters Kluwer Health.

C. Laboratory and Radiologic Tests: Menu to Evaluate Menstrual Disorders

Routine

- Complete blood count (CBC) with differential and indices and platelets
- Erythrocyte sedimentation rate*
- Comprehensive metabolic profile (liver, renal functions)*
- Urinalysis and urine culture*
- Serum or urine pregnancy test†
- Papanicolaou test if indicated†
- Screens for STIs†

*Only if history suggests.

†Only if the teenager is currently sexually active or has a past history of sexual activity; if sexually active for ≥3 years, Papanicolaou test should be performed;

if sexually active and immunosuppressed, Papanicolaou testing should begin with initiation of being sexually active.

Hormone Studies‡§

- Testosterone (free and total) (normal total: ≤40 ng/dL; normal free: <8.5 pg/mL: total of ≥200 ng/dL suggests tumor)‡
- Thyroid studies (free thyroxine, thyrotropin)
- Prolactin
- Luteinizing hormone (LH), follicle-stimulating hormone (FSH) (normal: 5–25 mIU/mL; ≥50 mIU/mL indicates ovarian failure)
- Estradiol

‡Normal values differ depending on laboratory and pubertal stage of patient.

§Tests ordered depend on the presenting problem.

Additional Hormone Studies for Hirsutism and/or Virilization||¶

- Dehydroepiandrosterone sulfate (DHEA-S) (normal: 100–400 μg/dL; >700 μg/dL suggests tumor)||
- 17-Hydroxyprogesterone (17-OHP) (early morning) (normal: 30–130 ng/dL ≥200 ng/dL suggests need for additional adrenal tests looking for late onset adrenal hyperplasia)||
- Cortisol (early morning) (normal: 5–25 μg/dL)

||Normal values differ depending on laboratory and pubertal stage of patient.

¶Tests ordered depend on the presenting problem.

Other Laboratory Tests#**

Iron Studies

- Total iron-binding capacity (TIBC) (normal: 330 ± 30 μg/dL)
- Iron level (normal: 115 ± 50 μg/dL)
- Saturation = iron/TIBC = 35% ± 15%
- Ferritin (normal: 100 ± 60 μg/dL; decreased: <20 μg/dL)
- Cell indices

Other Tests

- Antithyroglobulin antibodies
- Antiperoxidase antibodies
- Antiovarian antibodies
- Antinuclear antibody (ANA)
  - Antiphospholipid antibody
- Fasting serum glucose/insulin levels (ratio >3.0–4.5)
- Evaluation of sex chromosomes

*Clotting Studies#***

- Reticulocyte count
- Platelet count
- Activated partial thromboplastin time (aPTT), prothrombin time
- Von Willebrand panel: Von Willebrand factor††, factor VIII coagulant antigen, ristocetin cofactor activity, platelet-aggregation studies

#Normal values differ depending on laboratory and pubertal stage of patient.

**Tests ordered depend on the presenting problem

††May be elevated falsely, affected by being on estrogen; should be off at least 1 week; also, type of blood (ie, O type may give falsely low values).

Radiologic Studies‡‡

- Bone age
- Bone density studies: dual-energy radiograph absorptiometry (DEXA)
- Skeletal radiographs
- Bone scan
- Pelvic ultrasound: transabdominal, vaginal
- Flat plate and upright of abdomen
- Renal ultrasound

‡‡Tests ordered depend on the presenting problem.

SPECIFIC MENSTRUAL PROBLEMS

A. Too Frequent, Too Long, Too Much Bleeding: Polymenorrhea, DUB, Menorrhagia

Differential Diagnosis

- Missed pregnancy
- Sexually acquired infections
- Stress
- Depression
- Medication: drug use/abuse (prescribed, over-the-counter, illegal, or banned)
- Eating disorders: bulimia, obesity
- Immaturity of reproductive axis (within 2 years of menarche)
- Coagulation disorders: congenital, acquired

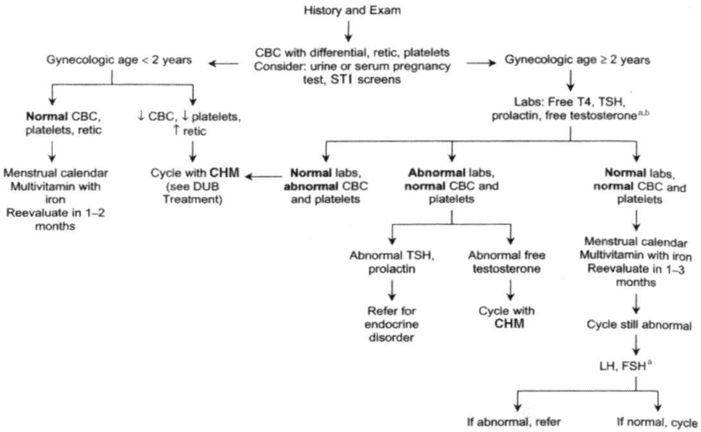

Fig 5.1. Evaluation: Too Frequent, Too Long, Too Much Bleeding CBC indicates complete blood count; T4, thyroxine; TSH, thyrotropin; CHM, combine hormone method. [a]Hirsutism or virilization: need DHEA-S, early-morning cortisol, and 17-OHP. [b]Consider renal/liver functions, sedimentation rate, and ANA. Combined-hormone method: oral contraceptives, patch, or ring.

- Endocrine disorders:
  - Functional ovarian hyperandrogenism
  - Excess adrenal androgen production
  - Thyroid disorders
  - Hyperprolactinemia

- Chronic/systemic diseases
- Vagina: foreign bodies/trauma/hemangiomas/polyps
- Premature ovarian failure
- Adrenal/ovarian hormone-producing tumors

B. Dysfunctional Uterine Bleeding

Definition

- Lack of positive feedback response by the hypothalamic pituitary system to estrogen
- Unopposed estrogen effect of the endometrium
- No dominant follicle with uncontrolled growth and atresia of many follicles, resulting in fluctuation of circulating estrogens
- Endometrial shedding dependant on amount of proliferative endometrium present

- Without ovulation, imbalance of the ratio of prostaglandins produced with the prostaglandin F2-α (vasoconstrictor) and prostaglandin E (vasodilator)

Differential for DUB

- Immature hypothalamic pituitary gonadal axis
- Drug use/abuse (prescribed, illegal or banned, tobacco)
- Chronic/systemic diseases
- Endocrine disorders
  - Anovulation
  - Functional ovarian hyperandrogenism
  - Thyroid disorders
  - Excess adrenal androgen production
  - Hyperprolactinemia

- Premature ovarian failure
- Adrenal/ovarian hormone-producing tumors

C. Too Infrequent, Too Short, Too Light Bleeding or not at All: Secondary Amenorrhea or Oligomenorrhea

Differential Diagnosis

- Pregnancy
- Immaturity of reproductive axis (within 2 years of menarche)
- Ovarian hyperandrogenism

Functional Hypothalamic Amenorrhea

- Stress
- Exercise
- Depression
- Eating disorders
  - Anorexia
  - Bulimia
  - Obesity

- Chronic illness (liver, kidney, diabetes, irritable bowel disorder) or history of past illness requiring chemotherapy and/or radiation
- Drugs: contraceptives, opiates, cannabis, tobacco

Table 5.2
Treatment of DUB with oral contraceptives

Mild	
Characteristics	Hematocrit >33% or hemoglobin >11 g/dL
Acute treatment	Menstrual calendar; iron supplementation; consider use of hormone method if patient wants more immediate control of periods and/or if sexually active and desires contraception
Long-term treatment	Monitor iron status (hemoglobin/hematocrit); follow-up at 1–2 mo
Moderate	
Characteristics	Hematocrit 27%–33% or hemoglobin 9–11 g/dL
Acute treatment	Begin: OCs (20- or 30-μg EE monophasic pill) + antiemetic if needed: 1 pill twice daily for 13–19 d, then allow withdraw bleed for 7 d
Long-term treatment	Next: cycle with OCs for 3 mo, using 1 pill per day the Sunday after withdrawal bleeding begins; length of use depends on when anemia resolves; maintain iron supplementation + OCs; monitor iron status; follow-up at 2–3 wk and then every 3 mo. Continue if contraception desired.
Severe	
Characteristics	Hematocrit <27% or hemoglobin <9 g/dL (or dropping)[a]
Acute treatment[b]	Begin: OCs (20- or 30-μg EE monophasic pill) + antiemetic if needed: 1 pill 4 times per day for 4 d, 1 pill 3 times per day for 4 d, and 1 pill twice per day for 13–19 days; allow withdrawal bleeding for 7 d
Long-term treatment	Next: cycle with OCs, 1 pill per day the Sunday after withdrawal bleeding begins; length of OC use depends on length of time needed for anemia to resolve; maintain iron supplementation; monitor iron status; follow-up at 2–3 wk and every 3 mo. Continue if contraception desired.

OC indicates oral contraceptive; EE, ethinyl estradiol.

[a] If hemoglobin <7 g/dL and actively bleeding and/or orthostatic signs are abnormal, consider admission to hospital for conjugated estrogens, 25 mg intravenously every 4 to 6 hours for 24 hours while simultaneously beginning OCs. Blood transfusion may be indicated after hydration, if it becomes apparent anemia is more profound.

[b] If not actively bleeding and hemoglobin is between 7 and 9 g/dL and orthostatic signs as measured by heart rate and blood pressure are normal, initial treatment may be limited to 1 pill twice per day for the next 2 to 3 weeks, followed by a withdrawal bleed.

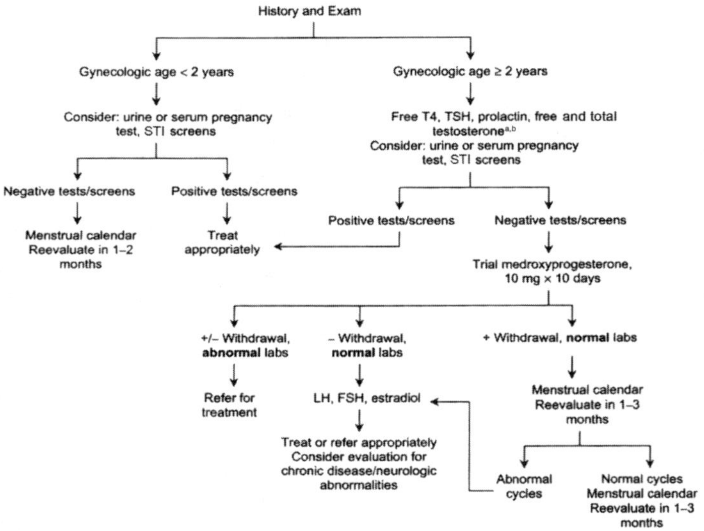

Fig 5.2. Evaluation: Too Short, Too Light Bleeding or Not at All. T4 indicates thyroxine; TSH, thyrotropin. [a]Hirsutism or virilization: need DHEA-S, early-morning cortisol, and 17-OHP. [b]Consider renal/liver functions, sedimentation rate, and ANA.

D. Features of Ovarian Hyperandrogenism

Rotterdam Consensus Conference:

Oligoovulation or anovulation

Clinical or biochemical signs of hyperandrogenism

Polycystic ovaries on ultrasound

Exclusion of congenital adrenal hyperplasia or Cushing syndrome or other causes of hyperandrogenism

Ultrasound Evidence

Presence of ≥12 follicles in each ovary measuring 2 to 9 mm in diameter and in periphery

Increased ovarian volume (>10 mL)

Transvaginal or transabdominal ultrasound 3 to 5 days after induced menses (see Rotterdam ESHRE/ASRM-Sponsored PCOS Consensus Workshop Group.

Revised 2003 consensus on diagnostic criteria and long-term health risks related to polycystic ovary syndrome. *Fertil Steril.* 2004;81[1]:19–25)

- Clinical findings: acne at early age
  - Other: hirsutism
- Irregular menses: (<21 days, >45 days) persistence of irregular pattern beyond 2 years after menarche
  - Menstrual cycle >90 days after first cycle

- Overweight or obese (BMI >85th percentile) present in approximately two thirds but not in one third
- Family history: polycystic ovary syndrome (PCOS), early hair loss, hirsutism, fertility problems, diabetes mellitus

Evaluation

- Serum testosterone (free and total)
- Thyrotropin
- LH/FSH
- Prolactin
- Pelvic ultrasound
- Urine pregnancy test (or serum pregnancy test)
- Fasting glucose and insulin (ratio abnormal if <4.5–3.0) (see Legro RS, Finegood D, Dunaif A. A fasting glucose to insulin ratio is a useful measure of insulin sensitivity in women with polycystic ovary syndrome. *J Clin Endocrinol Metab.* 1998;83[8]:2694–2698)

If overweight or obese, add:

- Fasting lipid profile
- Consider fasting and 2-hour oral glucose-tolerance test: examine glucose-to-insulin ratio at both tests.
- Consider A1c

If hirsutism/virilization is clinically present, add:

- DHEA-S
- Early-morning 17-OHP (if >200 ng/day, then corticotropin-stimulation test needs to be performed before treatment is initiated)
- Early-morning cortisol (dexamethasone suppression: 1 mg at 11 PM; measure cortisol at 8 AM: <6 μg/dL rules out Cushing syndrome)

Treatment With Combined-Hormone Method

- To treat menstrual irregularities; suppresses ovarian and adrenal production of androgens → net reduction in free and total testosterone
- For hyperandrogenic symptoms such as hirsuitism and acne:
  - Oral contraceptives increase hepatic production of sex hormone-binding globulin, which binds androgens and reduces bioavailability

    - Oral contraceptives inhibit enzyme 5α-reductase at the hair-follicle level resulting in lower levels of testosterone dihydrotestosterone produced
- To protect endometrium from development of endometrial hyperplasia

Other additional treatments:

- Antiandrogenic agents as spironolactone to treat the acne and hirsutism—competes at the hair-follicle level for the androgen receptor; cannot be used alone without combined-hormone method—contributes to irregular, prolonged menses
- Insulin-sensitizing agents as metformin, 500 to 2000 mg daily in divided doses
- Cosmetic measures: shaving, epilation (plucking, waxing), depilation (chemical that dissolves hair shaft), laser, electrolysis, topical (eflornithine [Vaniqa (SkinMedica, Inc, Carlsbad, CA)])

Long-term consequences of androgen excess:

- Acne
- Diabetes
- Adrenal hyperplasia
- Dyslipidemias
- Insulin resistance
- Alopecia
- Endometrial cancer
- PCOS
- Android obesity
- Hirsutism
- Cardiovascular disease
- Hypertension

E. Evaluation for the Adolescent With Hirsutism and Virilization

Causes of Hyperandrogenism in Adolescent Girls

Physical Examination in Hirsutism

F. Primary Amenorrhea

Primary Amenorrhea: Definitions

- No menarche by the age of 15.5 years in the presence of normal growth, breasts, and pubic hair
- Absence of menarche by 13 years in the absence of normal growth and breasts and with or without pubic hair
- No menarche by 2 to 5 years of achieving the B4 Tanner stage of breast development; absence of menarche by 4 years after initiation of puberty

Primary Amenorrhea: Etiologies

Chromosomal abnormalities: 50%

Hypothalamic hypogonadism: 20%

Absence of vagina, uterus, and/or cervix: 15%

Pituitary disease: 5%

Transverse vaginal septum or imperforate hymen: 5%

Other: <5%

See Reindollar RH, Byrd JR, McDonough PG. Delayed sexual development: a study of 252 patients. *Am J Obstet Gynecol*. 1981;140(4):371–380; and Iglesias EA, Coupey SM. Menstrual cycle abnormalities: diagnosis and management. *Adolesc Med*. 1999;10(2):255–273.

Table 5.3
Causes of hirsutism in adolescents

Ovarian disorders
PCOS
Hyperthecosis
Tumors
Enzyme deficiency
Adrenal disorders
Congenital adrenal hyperplasia (21-hydroxylase, 11β-hydroxylase, 3β-hydroxysteroid dehydrogenase deficiencies)
Cushing disease
Tumors
Idiopathic hirsutism
Drugs (phenytoin, danazol, diazoxide, minoxidil, glucocorticoid excess, androgens, valproate)
Pregnancy
Hypothyroidism
Central nervous system injury
Hyperprolactinemia
Stress
Anorexia nervosa, malnutrition
Peripheral tissue sensitivity
Male pseudohermaphroditism, mixed gonadal dysgenesis

Adapted from: Emans SJ. Androgen abnormalities in the adolescent girl [Table 9-1]. In: Emans SJ, Laufer MR, Goldstein DP, eds. *Pediatric and Adolescent Gynecology*. 5th ed. Philadelphia, PA: Lippincott-Raven; 2005:298. Reprinted by permission of Wolters Kluwer Health.

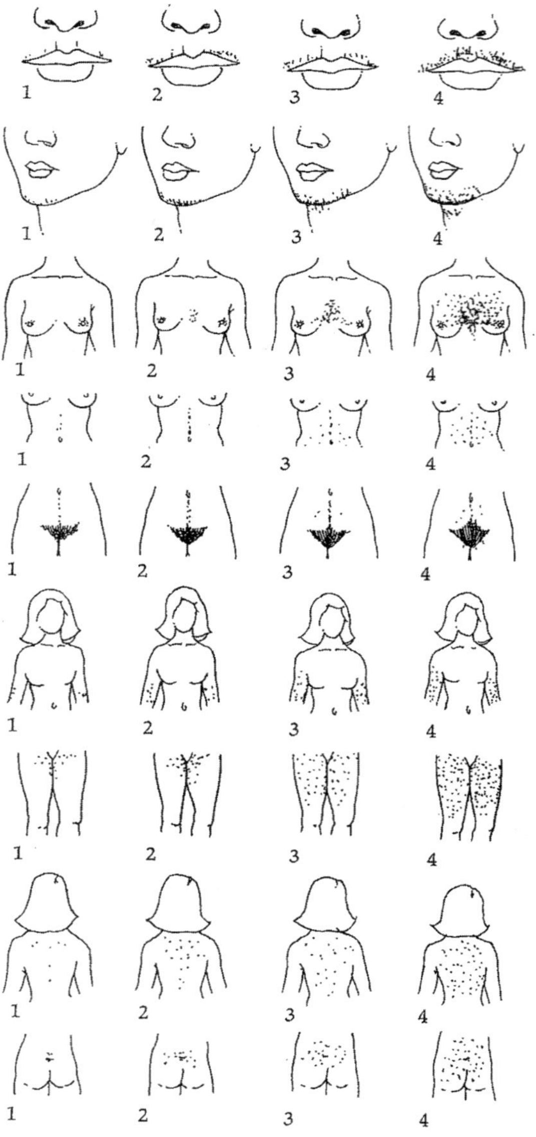

Fig 5.3. Evaluation of hirsutism. [(Top) Lorenzo E. Familial Study of Hirsutism. *J Clin Endocrinol Metab.* 1970;31(5):556–564. Copyright 1970, The Endocrine Society, with permission. (Bottom) Hatch R, Rosenfield RL, Kim MH, et al. Hirsutism: implications, etiology, and management. *Am J Obstet Gynecol.* 1981;140(7):815–830.]

Table 5.4
Hirsutism scoring sheet

Site	Grade	Definition
1. Upper Lip	1	A few hairs at outer margin
	2	A small moustache at outer margin
	3	A moustache extending halfway from outer margin
	4	A moustache extending to midline
2. Chin	1	A few scattered hairs
	2	Scattered hairs with small concentrations
	3 and 4	Complete cover, light and heavy
3. Chest	1	Circumareolar hairs
	2	With midline hair in addition
	3	Fusion of these areas, with three-quarter cover
	4	Complete cover
4. Upper back	1	A few scattered hairs
	2	Rather more, still scattered
	3 and 4	Complete cover, light and heavy
5. Lower back	1	A sacral tuft of hair
	2	With some lateral extension
	3	Three-quarter cover
	4	Complete cover
6. Upper abdomen	1	A few midline hairs
	2	Rather more, still midline
	3 and 4	Half and full cover
7. Lower abdomen	1	A few midline hairs
	2	A midline streak of hair
	3	A midline band of hair
	4	An inverted V-shaped growth
8. Arm	1	Sparse growth affecting not more than one quarter of the limb surface
	2	More than this; cover still incomplete
	3 and 4	Complete cover, light and heavy
9. Forearm	1–4	Complete cover of dorsal surface; 2 grades of light and 2 grades of heavy growth
10. Thigh	1–4	As for arm
11. Leg	1–4	As for arm

The Hirsutism scoring sheet: the Ferriman and Gallwey system for scoring hirsutism. A score of 0 at all sites indicates absence of terminal hair; a score of ≥8 indicates hirsutism
(From Ferriman D, Gallwey JC. Clinical assessment of body hair growth in women. *J Clin Endocrinol Metab.* 1961;21:1440–1447. Copyright 1961, The Endocrine Society, with permission.)

A

A. Clinical Scoring System for Acne Vulgaris*		
Score	Class	Lesions
	Microcomedones	Comedones, <2mm diameter
1	Minor	Comedones, 2 mm or greater (<10)
2	Mild	Comedones (10-20; pustular or nonpustular)
3	Moderate	Comedones (>20) or pustules (<20)
4	Severe	Pustules (>20)
5	Cystic	Inflammatory lesions >5 mm
*Face and trunk may be graded separately		

B

B. The Global Acne Grading System (GAGS)			
Location	Factor x Grade (0-4)* = Local score		
I Forehead	2		
II Right cheek	2		
III Left cheek	2		
IV Nose	1		
V Chin	1		
VI Chest and upper back	3		
	Global Score =		
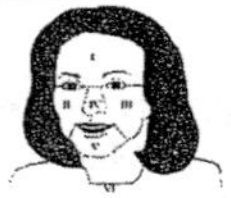	*Grade	Global score	
	0, No lesions	0	None
	1, ≥ one comedone	1-18	Mild
	2, ≥ one papule	19-30	Moderate
	3, ≥ one pustule	31-38	Severe
	4, ≥ one nodule	>39	Very Severe

Fig 5.4. Two acne scoring systems. A, Clinical scoring system for acne vulgaris. (Rosenfield RL. Pilosebaceous physiology in relation to hirsutism and acne. *Clin Endocrinol Metab*. 1986;15(2):341–362, with permission from Elsevier.) B, The 6 locations (I–VI) of the global acne grading system. (Reproduced with permission from Doshi A, Zaheer A, Stiller MJ. A comparison of current acne grading systems and proposal of a novel system. *Int J Dermatol*. 1997;36[6]:417).

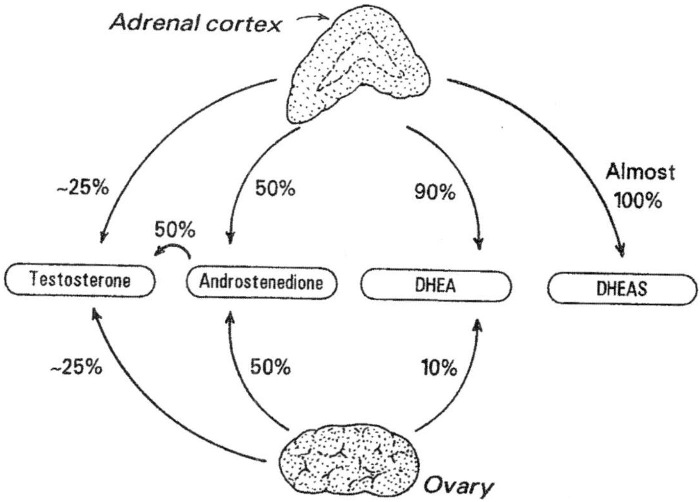

Fig 5.5. Source of androgens in adult women. (Reproduced from Emans SJ. Androgen abnormalities in the adolescent girl (Fig 9–11). In: Emans SJ, Laufer MR, Goldstein DP, eds. *Pediatric and Adolescent Gynecology*. 5th ed. Philadelphia, PA: Lippincott-Raven; 2005:312. Reprinted by permission of Wolters Kluwer Health.)

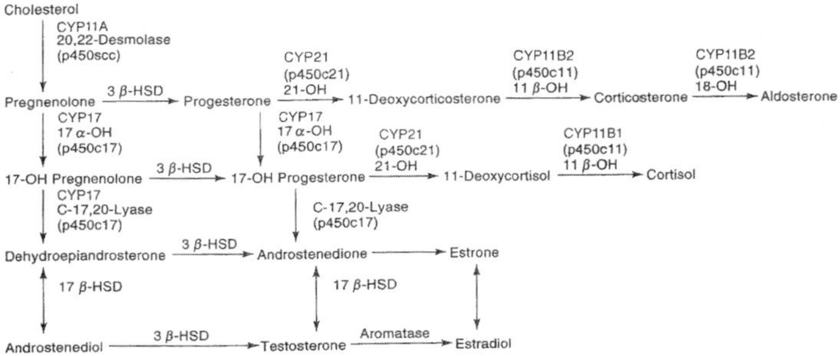

Fig 5.6. Major pathways of steroid biosynthesis. 21-OH indicates 21-hydroxylase; 11β-OH, 11β-hydroxylase; 18-OH, 18-hydroxylase; 3 β-HSD, 3-hydroxysteroid dehydrogenase; 17β-HSD, 17β-hydroxysteroid dehydrogenase. (Reproduced from Emans SJ. Androgen abnormalities in the adolescent girl (Fig 9–2). In: Emans SJ, Laufer MR, Goldstein DP, eds. *Pediatric and Adolescent Gynecology*. 5th ed. Philadelphia, PA: Lippincott-Raven; 2005: 309. Reprinted by permission of Wolters Kluwer Health.)

Table 5.5
Evaluation of a patient with hirsutism

- At time of clinic visit
  - FSH, LH, prolactin, thyrotropin
  - Testosterone, free testosterone (sex hormone-binding globulin)
  - DHEA-S
  - Cholesterol, high-density lipoprotein (or fasting lipid profile with cholesterol, high-density lipoprotein cholesterol, low-density lipoprotein cholesterol, triglycerides)
  - Random blood glucose
- If patient is obese and/or has acanthosis nigricans or all girls with PCOS
  - Fasting glucose and insulin level; 2-h glucose level after 75 g of oral glucose
  - American Diabetes Association criteria
    - Fasting glucose
      - Normal: <100 mg/dL
      - Impaired: 100–125 mg/dL
      - Diabetes: ≥126
    - Glucose 2 h, 75-g oral glucose tolerance
      - Normal: <140 mg/dL
      - Impaired: 140–199 mg/dL
      - Diabetes: ≥200 mg/dL
- If suspicious of late-onset congenital adrenal hyperplasia (high DHEA-S, clitoromegaly, premature pubarche, early onset) or all patients in some protocols
  - 17-Hydroxyprogesterone in follicular phase drawn between 7 and 8 AM
  - If 17-hydroxyprogesterone <200 ng/dL, unlikely to have 21-hydroxylase deficiency
    - 200–1000 ng/dL, perform 1-h corticotropin-stimulation test
    - >1000 ng/dL, 21-hydroxylase deficiency
- If pelvic examination is inadequate, testosterone level is high, or evaluation of ovarian morphology is desired
  - Pelvic ultrasound
- High suspicion of adrenal tumor
  - Computed tomography/MRI

Adapted from Emans SJ. Androgen abnormalities in the adolescent girl [Table 9-2]. In: Emans SJ, Laufer MR, Goldstein DP, eds. *Pediatric and Adolescent Gynecology*. 5th ed. Philadelphia, PA: Lippincott-Raven; 2005:309. Reprinted by permission of Wolters Kluwer Health.

Breast Development Absent/Uterus Present

- Constitutional delay of puberty
- Hypothalamic dysfunction
  - Stress/anxiety/depression
  - Intense exercise
  - Anorexia/eating disorders not otherwise specified/undernourishment
  - Chronic illness (eg, cystic fibrosis, inflammatory bowel disease)

- Pituitary failure (eg, craniopharyngioma)
- Gonadal dysgenesis (eg, Turner syndrome, mosaic, X or Y deletion)
- Deletion of arms of X: Xp gonads affected, Xq short stature
- Gonadal failure (eg, premature ovarian failure)
- Gonadotropin deficiency (eg, Kallman syndrome)

Breast Development Present/Uterus Present

- Pregnancy
- Hypothalamic dysfunction
  - Stress
  - Intense exercise
  - Anorexia
  - Chronic illness

- Hyperadrenogenic amenorrhea: endometrium deciduous or hyperplastic (eg, PCOS, late-onset 21-OH deficiency)
- Gonadal failure (eg, premature ovarian failure)
- Thyroid disease
- Hyperprolactinemia (eg, prescribed or street-drug induced, primary)
- Outflow tract obstructed-imperforate hymen; transverse vaginal septum, cervical stenosis; absence, hypoplasia of vagina (eg, Mullerian agenesis/anomalies)

Breast Development Present/Uterus Abnormal or Absent: Mullerian agenesis 1:5000 (Mayer-Rokitansky-Hauser Syndrome)

- No uterus, no upper two-thirds vagina
- Chromosomes: karyotype XX
- Testosterone low but normal for females
- Renal abnormalities in approximately one third

Mullerian Fusion Abnormalities: Characteristics

- Second most common cause of primary amenorrhea; affects 0.1% to 3.8% of the population
- Obstructive Mullerian Abnormalities: uterus normal → rudimentary
  - Imperforate hymen, transverse vaginal septum, longitudinal vaginal septum, bicornuate uterus
  - Uterus normal → rudimentary

- Female (46XX)
- Growth and development normal; normal hair distribution and breast development and growth
- Ten percent to 33% have urinary tract abnormalities: ectopic kidney, renal agenesis, horseshoe kidney, abnormal collecting system
- Three percent to 5% with spine abnormalities and rarely limb abnormalities
- VACTERL complex: vertebral, anal, cardiac, tracheoesophageal, renal, limb abnormalities

Breast Development Present/Uterus Abnormal or Absent: Androgen Insensitivity (Testicular Feminization)

- Peripheral androgen insensitivity (no androgen effects as pubic hair or acne)
- Normal breast development (peripheral conversion of androgens to estrogens) with blind pouch or dimple for vagina
- Chromosomes: karyotype XY (intra-abdominal gonads need to be removed)
- Testosterone levels high in normal range of pubertal male

Androgen Insensitivity: Characteristics

- Third most common cause of primary amenorrhea
- Male pseudohermaphrodite (46XY)
- Maternal X-linked recessive gene responsible for androgen intracellular receptor
- Prepubertal presentation may be inguinal hernia; 50% at puberty
- Growth and development normal; taller height
- Large breasts with small nipples, pale areolas
- Blind vaginal pouch with no uterus; presence of anti-Mullerian hormone
- Absent-to-sparse body hair
- Five percent of patients with this disorder will develop malignant gonad tumors: so remove at 16 to 18 years.
- May have renal abnormalities

Breast Development Absent/Uterus Abnormal or Absent: Syndrome of Vanishing Testes

- Chromosomes: karyotype XY
- Spontaneous regression of testes between 8 and 14 weeks' gestation
- Lack of testosterone results in failure of external and internal male organs
- Phenotype female but lacks ovaries, uterus, and upper vagina
- If regression of testes occurs later in pregnancy, results in phenotypic male but infantile genitalia (appears to be male with bilateral crypto-orchidism).

G. Primary and Secondary Dysmenorrhea

Definition

- Dysmenorrhea (primary): overall
    - Prevalence of 50% to 90%, painful menses with no identifiable pelvic pathology: mild, 27%; moderate, 41%; severe, 23%
- Dysmenorrhea (secondary): painful menses resulting from pelvic pathology
- Evaluation for Dysmenorrhea

H. Premenstrual Syndrome

Definition: Criteria for Premenstrual Dysphoric Disorder

A. Five or more of the symptoms are present most of the time during the last week of the luteal phase (week before period), began to remit within a few days after

(text continues on p. 478)

Table 5.6
Differential diagnosis of secondary dysmenorrhea

System	Common Possible Etiology
Reproductive organs	Endometriosis
	Genital tract malformations and/or obstruction
	Mittelschmerz
	Ovarian cyst
	Pelvic inflammatory disease (acute or chronic)
	Pelvic serositis
	Postoperative adhesions
Gastrointestinal	Constipation
	Irritable bowel
	Food intolerance
	Infections
	Inflammatory bowel disease
Urinary system	Infection
	Congenital/acquired obstruction
Musculoskeletal	Disk disease/malalignment
	Inflammation
	Neoplasms
	Stress fractures: pubis, vertebral body
Psychosomatic	

Table 5.7
Treatment of primary dysmenorrhea: common medications[a]

Drug	Usual Dose
Ibuprofen	200–800 mg qid (maximum: 3200 mg in 24 h)
Naproxen	500 mg initially, then 250–375 mg tid
Naproxen sodium	440 mg initially, then 440 mg tid

qid indicates four times per day; tid, three times per day.
[a] Not recommended for aspirin-sensitive patients with asthma, ulcers, or inflammatory bowel disease.

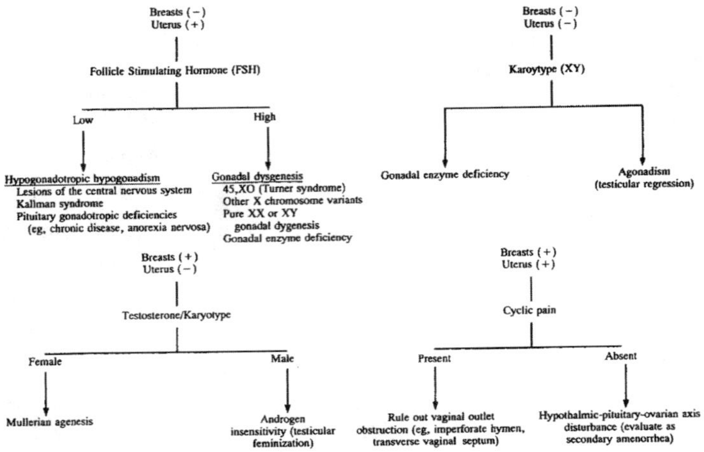

Fig 5.7. Evaluation of primary amenorrhea. (From Maschak CA, Kletzky OA, Davajan V, et al. Clinical and laboratory evaluation of patients with primary amenorrhea. *Obstet Gynecol.* 1981;57:715–721. Reprinted by permission of Wolters Kluwer Health.)

the onset of the follicular phase (menses), and absent in the week after menses. At least 1 of the 5 symptoms has to be 1 of the first 4:

1. Markedly depressed mood, feelings of hopelessness, or self-deprecating thoughts;
2. Marked anxiety, tension;
3. Marked mood lability;
4. Persistent and marked anger or irritability;
5. Decreased interest in usual activities;
6. Difficulty in concentrating;
7. Lethargy, easy fatigability, or marked lack of energy;
8. Marked change in appetite, overeating, or specific food cravings;
9. Hypersomnia or insomnia;
10. Sense of being overwhelmed or out of control;
11. Physical symptoms: breast tenderness or swelling, headaches, joint or muscle pain, a sensation of bloating, weight gain

B. The disturbance markedly interferes with work or school or with usual social activities and relationships with others;
C. The disturbance is not merely an exacerbation of the symptoms of another disorder (eg, major depressive disorder, panic disorder, dysthymic disorder, or a personality disorder)

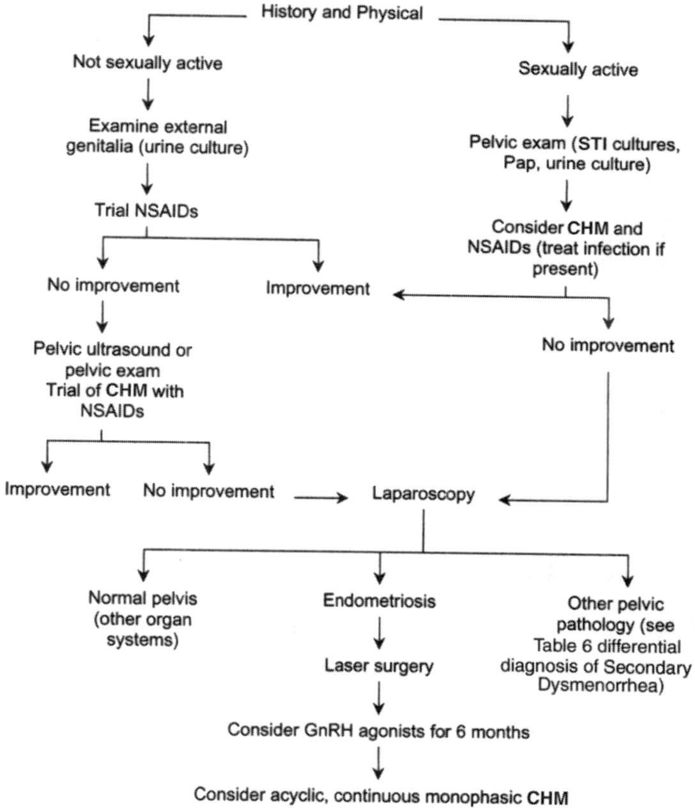

Fig 5.8. Evaluation and treatment of dysmenorrhea. Pap, Papanicolaou test; NSAID, nonsteroidal antiinflammatory drug; US, ultrasound; GnRH, gonadotropin-releasing hormone; CHM, combined hormone method.

Treatment for PMS

- Emphasize nutrition (eliminate caffeine, excess sugar; increase protein intake)
- Prescribe adequate vitamin B_6 and calcium supplements
- Prescribe exercise
- Discuss sleep requirements and habits
- Reevaluate use of prescribed and over-the-counter medications and supplements
- Evaluate use of tobacco and other substances

Table 5.8
Most common PMS symptoms reported by teenagers

Physical symptoms
Acne
Fatigue
Bloating
Cravings for sweets/food
Weight gain
Breast tenderness
Emotional symptoms
Depression
Anger
Moodiness/irritability
Crying
Intolerance/frustration
Nervousness

- Discuss possible causes of possible depression and anxiety and general stress
- Consider use of combined-hormone method (eg, monophasic pills)
- Consider use of selective serotonin reuptake inhibitors
- Consider other diagnoses

I. Cervical Cancer Screening Guidelines for Adolescents and Young Adults

Table 5.9
Cervical cancer screening guidelines for adolescents and adults younger than 30 years

Variable	ACOG	ACS	USPSTF
Age to begin screening	Within 3 y after first vaginal intercourse but no later than 21 y of age	Same as ACOG	Same as ACOG
Screening method	Conventional or liquid-based cytologic test	Same as ACOG	No specific recommendation
Frequency of screening with conventional Papanicolaou test	Annual	Annual	"No direct evidence that annual screening achieves better outcomes than screening every 3 years"
Frequency of screening with liquid-based cytologic test	Annual	Every 2 y	Insufficient evidence

ACOG indicates American College of Obstetricians and Gynecologists, ACS, American Cancer Society; USPSTF, US Preventive Services Task Force.
Adapted from Goldstein MA, Goodman A, del Carmen MG, Wilbur DC. Case records of the Massachusetts General Hospital: case 10-2009—a 23-year-old woman with an abnormal Papanicolaou smear. *N Engl J Med*. 2009;360(13):1339.

See color insert for Figure 5.9 a cytologic specimen of a Papanicolaou stain.

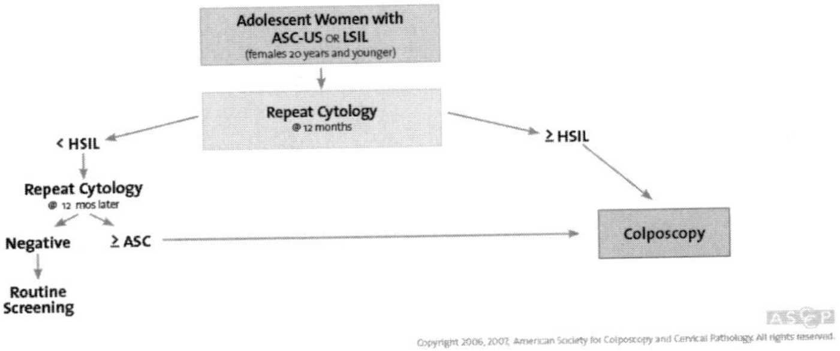

Fig 5.10. Management of adolescent women with either atypical squamous cells of undetermined significance (ASC-US) or low-grade squamous intraepithelial lesion (LSIL). HSIL indicates high-grade squamous intraepithelial lesion. (Reprinted from *The Journal of Lower Genital Tract Disease* Vol. 11 Issue 4, with the permission of ASCCP © American Society for Colposcopy and Cervical Pathology 2007. No copies of the algorithms may be made without the prior consent of ASCCP.)

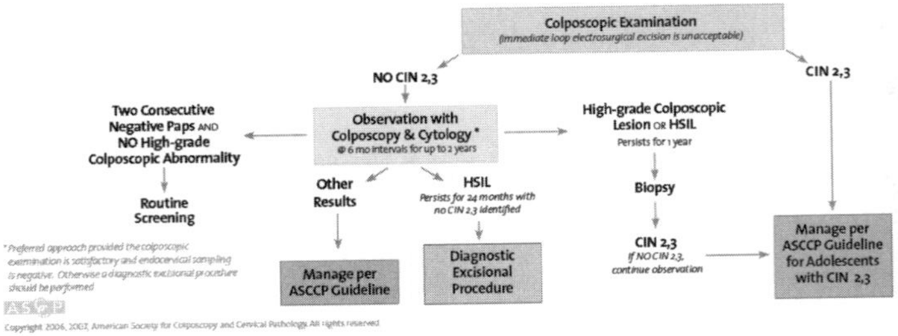

Fig 5.11. Management of adolescent women (20 years and younger) with high-grade squamous intraepithelial lesion (HSIL). Paps indicates Papanicolaou tests; $CIN_{2,3}$, cervical intraepithelial neoplasia 2/3; ASCCP, American Society for Colposcopy and Cervical Pathology. (Reprinted from *The Journal of Lower Genital Tract Disease* Vol. 11 Issue 4, with the permission of ASCCP © American Society for Colposcopy and Cervical Pathology 2007. No copies of the algorithms may be made without the prior consent of ASCCP.)

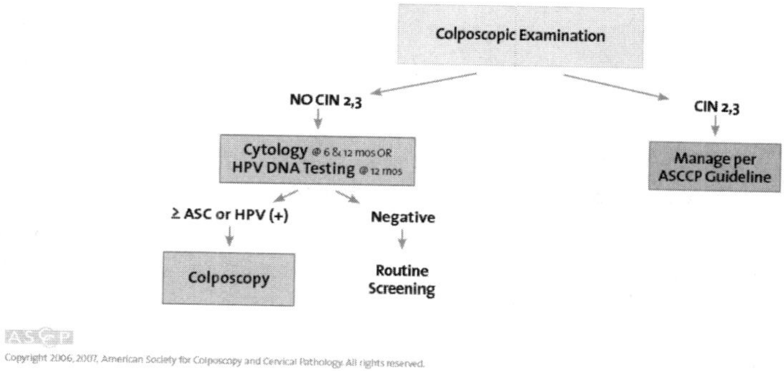

Fig 5.12. Management of adolescent women with atypical squamous cells: cannot exclude high-grade squamous intraepithelial lesion (ASC-H). $CIN_{2,3}$ indicates cervical intraepithelial neoplasia 2/3; HPV, human papillomavirus; ASCCP, American Society for Colposcopy and Cervical Pathology. (Reprinted from *The Journal of Lower Genital Tract Disease* Vol. 11 Issue 4, with the permission of ASCCP © American Society for Colposcopy and Cervical Pathology 2007. No copies of the algorithms may be made without the prior consent of ASCCP.)

Adolesc Med 20 (2009) 484–565

6. Contraception

A. CONTRACEPTIVES: YEAR METHODS APPROVED BY THE US FOOD AND DRUG ADMINISTRATION

1960: Combination oral contraceptive (OC) pills
1884: Copper T 380 (ParaGard)
1990: Levonorgestrel implants (Norplant)*
1992: Depo-medroxyprogesterone acetate (DMPA) injectable (Depo-Provera)
1993: Female condom
1977: Combination OCs (emergency contraception [EC])
1998: Combination pill (Preven)* (EC)
1999: Progestin-only pill (Plan B) (EC)
1999: Norplant II (Jadelle)*
2000: Medroxyprogesterone acetate/estradiol cypionate (Lunelle)*
2000: Levonorgestrel-releasing intrauterine device (Mirena)
2002: Vaginal ring (NuvaRing)
2002: Transdermal contraceptive system (Ortho Evra)
2003: Seasonale (3-month pill)
2006: Etonogestrel single-rod implant (Implanon)
2007: Lybrel (1-year pill)

* No longer available.

B. COMPARING ALL METHODS OF CONTRACEPTION

Margaret J. Blythe, MD
E-mail address: mblythe@iupui.edu

 ISSN 1934-4287

Table 6.1
Percentage of women experiencing an unintended pregnancy during the first year of typical use and the first year of perfect use of contraception and the percentage continuing use at the end of the first year, United States

Method	% of Women Experiencing an Unintended Pregnancy Within the First Year of Use		% of Women Continuing Use at 1 y
	Typical Use	Perfect Use	
No method	85	85	
Spermicides	29	18	42
Withdrawal	27	4	43
Fertility awareness–based methods	25		51
Standard-days method		5	
2-d method		4	
Ovulation method		3	
Sponge			
Parous women	32	20	46
Nulliparous women	16	9	57
Diaphragm	16	6	57
Condom			
Female (reality)	21	5	49
Male	15	2	53
Combined pill and progestin-only pill	8	0.3	68
Evra patch	8	0.3	68
NuvaRing	8	0.3	68
Depo-Provera	3	0.3	56
Intrauterine device			
ParaGard (copper T)	0.8	0.6	78
Mirena (levonorgestrel intrauterine system)	0.2	0.2	80
Implanon	0.05	0.05	84
Female sterilization	0.5	0.5	100
Male sterilization	0.15	0.10	100

EC pills: treatment initiated within 72 hours after unprotected intercourse reduces the risk of pregnancy by at least 75%. The lactational amenorrhea method is a highly effective, temporary method of contraception.

Adapted from Trussel J. Contraceptive efficacy. In: Hatcher RA, Trussell J, Nelson AL, et al, eds. *Contraceptive Technology*. 19th ed. New York, NY: Ardent Media; 2008:759.

C. WORLD HEALTH ORGANIZATION (WHO)

Medical Eligibility Criteria for Contraceptive Use, 2004

WHO classification 4: Use in adolescents and young adults absolutely contraindicated
WHO classification 3: Use in adolescents and young adults generally not recommended
WHO classification 2: Use in adolescents and young adults generally not limited
WHO classification 1: Condition for which where there is no restriction for use of method

Medical Eligibility Criteria for Contraceptive Use, Updates 2008

Table 6.2
Medical eligibility criteria for contraceptive use: 2008 update: summary of changes to the third edition of the *Medical Eligibility Criteria for Contraceptive Use* (changes are noted in bold)

Condition	COC/P/R	CIC	POP	DMPA NET-EN	LNG/ETG Implants	Cu-IUD	LNG-IUD	Clarification
Postpartum (breastfeeding or nonbreastfeeding women, including after cesarean delivery)								
a. < 48 h **including insertion immediately after delivery of the placenta**						1	**1 = not BF; 3 = BF**	
b. >48 h to <4 wk						3	3	
c. ≥4 wk						1	1	
d. Puerperal sepsis						4	4	
Obesity								
a. ≥30 kg/m² BMI	2	2	1	1	1	1	1	
b. **Menarche to <18 y and ≥30 kg/m² BMI**	2	2	1	**DMPA = 2; NET-EN = 1**[a]	1	1	1	There is no evidence of a differential weight gain between normal-weight and obese adolescents who use NET-EN; this condition is classified as category 1. However, the condition age <18 y is classified as category 2 because of evidence regarding potential effects of NET-EN on bone mineral density (see age condition).
DVT/PE								
a. History of DVT/PE	4	4	2	2	2	1	2	
b. Acute DVT/PE	4	4	3	3	3	1	3	
c. DVT/PE and established on anticoagulant therapy	4	4	2	2	2	1	2	

(Continued)

Table 6.2
(Continued)

Condition	COC/P/R	CIC	POP	DMPA NET-EN		LNG/ETG Implants	Cu-IUD		LNG-IUD	Clarification
d. Family history (first-degree relatives)	2	2	1	1		1	1		1	
e. Major surgery										
With prolonged immobilization	4	4	2	2		2	1		2	
Without prolonged immobilization	2	2	1	1		1	1		1	
f. Minor surgery without immobilization	1	1	1	1		1	1		1	
Rheumatic diseases				I	C		I	C		
SLE										
People with SLE are at increased risk of ischemic heart disease, stroke, and venous thromboembolism; categories assigned to such conditions in this guidance should be the same for women with SLE who present with these conditions; for all categories of SLE, classifications are based on the assumption that no other risk factors for cardiovascular disease are present; these classifications must be modified in the presence of such risk factors.										
a. **Positive (or unknown) antiphospholipid antibodies**	**4**	**4**	**3**	**3**	**3**	**3**	**1**	**1**	**3**	SLE and severe thrombocytopenia for IUDs: severe thrombocytopenia increases the risk of bleeding; the category should be assessed according to the severity of thrombocytopenia and its clinical manifestations. For women with very severe thrombocytopenia who are at risk for spontaneous bleeding, consultation with a specialist and certain pretreatments may be warranted.
b. **Severe thrombocytopenia**	**2**	**2**	**2**	**3**	**2**	**2**	**3**[a]	**2**[a]	**2**[a]	
c. **Immunosuppressive treatment**	**2**	**2**	**2**	**2**	**2**	**2**	**2**	**1**	**2**	
d. **None of the above**	**2**	**2**	**2**	**2**	**2**	**2**	**1**	**1**	**2**	
Gestational trophoblastic disease										
a. **Decreasing or undetectable β-hCG levels**	1	1	1	1		1	3		3	
b. **Persistently elevated β-hCG levels or malignant disease**	1	1	1	1		1	4		4	

(Continued)

Table 6.2
(Continued)

Condition	COC/P/R		CIC		POP	DMPA NET-EN	LNG/ETG Implants	Cu-IUD	LNG-IUD	Clarification
	I	C	I	C						
Viral hepatitis										
a. **Acute or flare**	3/4[a]	2	3	2	1		1	1	1	Viral hepatitis, acute or flare: the category should be assessed according to the severity of the condition.
b. **Carrier**	**1**	**1**	**1**	**1**	**1**	**1**	**1**	**1**	**1**	
c. **Chronic**	**1**	**1**	**1**	**1**	**1**	**1**	**1**	**1**	**1**	
Cirrhosis										
a. **Mild (compensated)**	**1**		**1**		**1**	**1**	**1**	**1**	**1**	
b. **Severe (decompensated)**	**4**		**3**		**3**	**3**	**3**	**1**	**3**	
Liver tumors										
a. **Benign**	**2**		**2**		**2**	**2**	**2**	**1**	**2**	
i. **Focal nodular hyperplasia**										
ii. **Hepatocellular adenoma**	4		3		3	3	3	1	3	
c. **Malignant (hepatoma)**	4		3/4		3	3	3	1	3	

(*Continued*)

Table 6.2
(Continued)

Condition	COC/P/R	CIC	POP	DMPA NET-EN	LNG/ETG Implants	Cu-IUD		LNG-IUD		Clarification
						I	C	I	C	
Drug interactions										
Antiretroviral therapy										
a. **NRTIs**	**1[a]**	**1**	**1**	**DMPA = 1; NET-EN = 1**	**1**	**2/3[a]**	**2[a]**	**2/3[a]**	**2[a]**	Antiretroviral therapy and hormonal contraception: Antiretroviral drugs have the potential to either decrease or increase the bioavailability of steroid hormones in hormonal contraceptives. Limited data suggest potential drug interactions between many antiretroviral drugs (particularly some non-NRTIs and ritonavir-boosted protease inhibitors) and hormonal contraceptives. These interactions may alter the safety and effectiveness of both the hormonal contraceptive and the antiretroviral drug. Thus, if a woman on antiretroviral treatment decides to initiate or continue hormonal contraceptive use, the consistent use of condoms is recommended. This is to both prevent HIV transmission and compensate for any possible reduction in the effectiveness of the hormonal contraceptive. When a COC is chosen, a preparation containing a minimum of 30 μg of EE should be used.
b. **Non-NRTIs**	**2[a]**	**2[a]**	**2[a]**	**DMPA = 1; NET-EN = 2[a]**	**2[a]**	**2/3[a]**	**2[a]**	**2/3[a]**	**2[a]**	Antiretroviral therapy and IUDs: there is no known interaction between antiretroviral therapy and IUD use. However, AIDS as a condition is classified as category 2 for continuation unless the woman is clinically well on antiretroviral therapy, in which case both insertion and continuation are classified as category 2 (see AIDS condition).
c. **Ritonavir-boosted protease inhibitors**	**3[a]**	**3[a]**	**3[a]**	**DMPA = 1; NET-EN = 2[a]**	**2[a]**	**2/3[a]**	**2[a]**	**2/3[a]**	**2[a]**	

(Continued)

Table 6.2
(Continued)

Condition	COC/P/R	CIC	POP	DMPA NET-EN	LNG/ETG Implants	Cu-IUD	LNG-IUD	Clarification
Anticonvulsant therapy								
a. Certain anticonvulsants (phenytoin, carbamazepine, barbiturates, primidone, topiramate, oxcarbazepine)	3[a]	2	3[a]	**DMPA = 1; NET-EN = 2[a]**	2[a]	1	1	Certain anticonvulsants and combined oral contraception: When a COC is chosen, a preparation containing a minimum of 30 μg of EE should be used. Certain anticonvulsants and progestogen-only contraception: although the interaction of certain anticonvulsants with POPs, NET-EN, and LNG/ETG implants is not harmful to women, it is likely to reduce the effectiveness of POPs, NET-EN, and LNG/ETG implants. Whether increasing the hormone dose of POPs alleviates this concern remains unclear. Use of other contraceptives should be encouraged for women who are long-term users of any of these drugs. Use of DMPA is a category 1, because its effectiveness is not decreased by the use of certain anticonvulsants
b. **Lamotrigine**	**3[a]**	**3**	**1**	**1**	**1**	**1**	**1**	When a COC is chosen, a preparation containing a minimum of 30 μg of EE should be used. The recommendation for lamotrigine applies only for situations in which lamotrigine monotherapy is taken concurrently with COCs. Anticonvulsant treatment regimens that combine lamotrigine and non–enzyme-inducing antiepileptic drugs (such as sodium valproate) do not interact with COCs.

(*Continued*)

Table 6.2
(Continued)

Condition	COC/P/R	CIC	POP	DMPA NET-EN	LNG/ETG Implants	Cu-IUD	LNG-IUD	Clarification
Antimicrobial therapy								
a. Broad-spectrum antibiotics	**1**	**1**	**1**	**1**	**1**	**1**	**1**	
b. Antifungal agents	**1**	**1**	**1**	**1**	**1**	**1**	**1**	
c. Antiparasitic agents	**1**	**1**	**1**	**1**	**1**	**1**	**1**	
d. Rifampicin or rifabutin therapy	**3[a]**	**2**	**3[a]**	**DMPA = 1; NET-EN = 2[a]**	**2[a]**	**1**	**1**	Rifampicin or rifabutin therapy and combined oral contraception: when a COC is chosen, a preparation containing a minimum of 30 μg EE should be used. Rifampicin or rifabutin therapy and progestogen-only contraception: although the interaction of rifampicin or rifabutin with POPs, NET-EN, and LNG/ETG implants is not harmful to women, it is likely to reduce the effectiveness of POPs, NET-EN, and LNG/ETG implants. Whether increasing the hormone dose of POPs alleviates this concern remains unclear. Use of other contraceptives should be encouraged for women who are long-term users of any of these drugs. Use of DMPA is a category 1 because its effectiveness is unlikely to be decreased by the use of rifampicin or rifabutin.

>P indicates patch contraceptive; R, ring contraceptive; CIC, combined injectable contraceptive; POP, progestin only pill; DMPA, depo-medroxyprogesterone acetate; NET-EN, norethisterone enantate; LNG/ETG, levonorgestrel/etonogestrel implants; Cu-IUD, copper intrauterine device; LNG-IUD, levonorgestrel intrauterine device; I, initiation; C, continuation; BF, breastfeeding; DVT, deep venous thrombosis; PE, pulmonary embolism; SLE, systemic lupus erythematosus; β-hCG; β-human chorionic gonadotropin; NRTI, nucleoside reverse-transcriptase inhibitors; EE, ethinyl estradiol.

[a] Consult the clarification column for this classification.

Adapted from World Health Organization, Reproductive Health and Research. Medical eligibility criteria for contraceptive use: 2008 update. Available at: www.who.int/reproductive-health/publications/mec/mec_update_2008.pdf. Accessed May 3, 2009.

Table 6.3
Low-dose combined OCs (COCs)

LOW-DOSE COMBINED ORAL CONTRACEPTIVES (COCs) ≤ 35 μg of ethinylestradiol	**COCs do not protect against STI/HIV. If there is risk of STI/HIV (including during pregnancy or postpartum), the correct and consistent use of condoms is recommended, either alone or with another contraceptive method. Male latex condoms are proven to protect against STI/HIV.**	
CONDITION	**CATEGORY** I=Initiation C=Continuation	**CLARIFICATIONS/EVIDENCE**
SMOKING		
a) Age < 35 years	2	**Evidence:** COC users who smoked were at increased risk of cardiovascular diseases, especially myocardial infarction, compared with those who did not smoke. Studies also showed an increased risk of myocardial infarction with increasing number of cigarettes smoked per day.
b) Age ≥ 35 years		
(i) <15 cigarettes/day	3	
(ii) ≥15 cigarettes/day	4	
OBESITY ≥ 30 kg/m² body mass index (BMI)	2	**Evidence:** Obese women who used COCs were at increased risk of VTE compared with non-users. The absolute risk of VTE remained small. Data are limited regarding the impact of obesity on COC effectiveness.
BLOOD PRESSURE MEASUREMENT UNAVAILABLE	NA	**Clarification:** It is desirable to have blood pressure measurements taken before initiation of COC use. However, in some settings blood pressure measurements are unavailable. In many of these settings pregnancy morbidity and mortality risks are high, and COCs are one of the few methods widely available. In such settings, women should not be denied use of COCs simply because their blood pressure cannot be measured.
CARDIOVASCULAR DISEASE		
MULTIPLE RISK FACTORS FOR ARTERIAL CARDIOVASCULAR DISEASE (such as older age, smoking, diabetes and hypertension)	3/4	**Clarification:** When a woman has multiple major risk factors, any of which alone would substantially increase the risk of cardiovascular disease, use of COCs may increase her risk to an unacceptable level. However, a simple addition of categories for multiple risk factors is not intended; for example, a combination of two risk factors assigned a category 2 may not necessarily warrant a higher category.
HYPERTENSION*		
For all categories of hypertension, classifications are based on the assumption that no other risk factors for cardiovascular disease exist. When multiple risk factors do exist, risk of cardiovascular disease may increase substantially. A single reading of blood pressure level is not sufficient to classify a woman as hypertensive.		
a) History of hypertension, where blood pressure CANNOT be evaluated (including hypertension in pregnancy)	3	**Clarification:** Evaluation of cause and level of hypertension is recommended, as soon as feasible. **Evidence:** Women who did not have a blood pressure check before COC use had an increased risk of acute myocardial infarction and stroke.

* See also additional comments at end of table

(Continued)

Table 6.3
(Continued)

LOW-DOSE COMBINED ORAL CONTRACEPTIVES (COCs) ≤ 35 μg of ethinylestradiol	**COCs do not protect against STI/HIV. If there is risk of STI/HIV (including during pregnancy or postpartum), the correct and consistent use of condoms is recommended, either alone or with another contraceptive method. Male latex condoms are proven to protect against STI/HIV.**	
CONDITION	**CATEGORY** I=Initiation C=Continuation	**CLARIFICATIONS/EVIDENCE**
HYPERTENSION (Cont'd)		
b) Adequately controlled hypertension, where blood pressure CAN be evaluated	3	**Clarification:** Women adequately treated for hypertension are at reduced risk of acute myocardial infarction and stroke as compared with untreated women. Although there are no data, COC users with adequately controlled and monitored hypertension should be at reduced risk of acute myocardial infarction and stroke compared with untreated hypertensive COC users.
c) Elevated blood pressure levels (properly taken measurements)		
(i) systolic 140-159 or diastolic 90-99	3	**Evidence:** Among women with hypertension, COC users were at increased risk of stroke, acute myocardial infarction, and peripheral arterial disease compared with non-users.
(ii) systolic ≥160 or diastolic ≥100	4	
d) Vascular disease	4	
HISTORY OF HIGH BLOOD PRESSURE DURING PREGNANCY (where current blood pressure is measurable and normal)	2	**Evidence:** Women who had a history of high blood pressure in pregnancy, who also used COCs, had an increased risk of myocardial infarction and venous thromboembolism, compared with COC users who did not have a history of high blood pressure during pregnancy. The absolute risks of acute myocardial infarction and venous thromboembolism in this population remained small.
DEEP VENOUS THROMBOSIS (DVT)/ PULMONARY EMBOLISM (PE)*		
a) History of DVT/PE	4	
b) Current DVT/PE	4	
c) Family history of DVT/PE (first-degree relatives)	2	
d) Major surgery		
(i) with prolonged immobilization	4	
(ii) without prolonged immobilization	2	
e) Minor surgery without immobilization	1	

(Continued)

Table 6.3
(Continued)

LOW-DOSE COMBINED ORAL CONTRACEPTIVES (COCs) ≤ 35 μg of ethinylestradiol	**COCs do not protect against STI/HIV. If there is risk of STI/HIV (including during pregnancy or postpartum), the correct and consistent use of condoms is recommended, either alone or with another contraceptive method. Male latex condoms are proven to protect against STI/HIV.**	
CONDITION	**CATEGORY** I=Initiation C=Continuation	**CLARIFICATIONS/EVIDENCE**
KNOWN THROMBOGENIC MUTATIONS (e.g., Factor V Leiden; Prothrombin mutation; Protein S, Protein C, and Antithrombin deficiencies)	4	**Clarification**: Routine screening is not appropriate because of the rarity of the conditions and the high cost of screening. **Evidence:** Among women with thrombogenic mutations, COC users had a two to twenty-fold higher risk of thrombosis than nonusers.
SUPERFICIAL VENOUS THROMBOSIS*		
a) Varicose veins	1	
b) Superficial thrombophlebitis	2	
CURRENT AND HISTORY OF ISCHEMIC HEART DISEASE*	4	
STROKE* (history of cerebrovascular accident)	4	
KNOWN HYPERLIPIDEMIAS	2/3	**Clarification:** Routine screening is not appropriate because of the rarity of the conditions and the high cost of screening. While some types of hyperlipidaemias are risk factors for vascular disease, the category should be assessed according to the type, its severity, and the presence of other cardiovascular risk factors.
VALVULAR HEART DISEASE*		
a) Uncomplicated	2	
b) Complicated (pulmonary hypertension, risk of atrial fibrillation, history of subacute bacterial endocarditis)	4	

(*Continued*)

Table 6.3
(Continued)

LOW-DOSE COMBINED ORAL CONTRACEPTIVES (COCs) ≤ 35 µg of ethinylestradiol	COCs do not protect against STI/HIV. If there is risk of STI/HIV (including during pregnancy or postpartum), the correct and consistent use of condoms is recommended, either alone or with another contraceptive method. Male latex condoms are proven to protect against STI/HIV.		
CONDITION	**CATEGORY** I=Initiation C=Continuation		**CLARIFICATIONS/EVIDENCE**
NEUROLOGIC CONDITIONS			
HEADACHES*	I	C	
a) Non-migrainous (mild or severe)	1	2	**Clarification:** Classification depends on accurate diagnosis of those severe headaches that are migrainous and those that are not. Any new headaches or marked changes in headaches should be evaluated. Classification is for women without any other risk factors for stroke. Risk of stroke increases with age, hypertension and smoking.
b) Migraine			**Evidence:** Among women with migraine, women who also had aura had a higher risk of stroke than those without aura. Among women with migraine, those who used COCs had a 2 to 4-fold increased risk of stroke compared with women who did not use COCs.
(i) without aura			
Age < 35	2	3	
Age ≥ 35	3	4	
(ii) with aura, at any age	4	4	
EPILEPSY	1		**Clarification:** If a woman is taking anticonvulsants, refer to the section on drug interactions. Certain anticonvulsants lower COC effectiveness.
DEPRESSIVE DISORDERS			
DEPRESSIVE DISORDERS	1		**Clarification**: The classification is based on data for women with selected depressive disorders. No data on bipolar disorder or postpartum depression were available. There is a potential for drug interactions between certain antidepressant medications and hormonal contraceptives. **Evidence**: COC use did not increase depressive symptoms in women with depression compared to baseline or to non-users with depression.
REPRODUCTIVE TRACT INFECTIONS AND DISORDERS			
VAGINAL BLEEDING PATTERNS*			
a) Irregular pattern *without* heavy bleeding	1		
b) Heavy or prolonged bleeding (includes regular and irregular patterns)	1		**Clarification:** Unusually heavy bleeding should raise the suspicion of a serious underlying condition.

(Continued)

Table 6.3
(Continued)

LOW-DOSE COMBINED ORAL CONTRACEPTIVES (COCs) ≤ 35 µg of ethinylestradiol	**COCs do not protect against STI/HIV. If there is risk of STI/HIV (including during pregnancy or postpartum), the correct and consistent use of condoms is recommended, either alone or with another contraceptive method. Male latex condoms are proven to protect against STI/HIV.**	
CONDITION	**CATEGORY** I=Initiation C=Continuation	**CLARIFICATIONS/EVIDENCE**
UNEXPLAINED VAGINAL BLEEDING* (suspicious for serious condition)		
Before evaluation	2	**Clarification:** If pregnancy or an underlying pathological condition (such as pelvic malignancy) is suspected, it must be evaluated and the category adjusted after evaluation.
ENDOMETRIOSIS*	1	
BENIGN OVARIAN TUMORS (including cysts)	1	
SEVERE DYSMENORRHEA	1	**Evidence:** There was no increased risk of side-effects with COC use among women with dysmenorrhoea compared to women not using COCs. Some COC users had a reduction in pain and bleeding.
TROPHOBLAST DISEASE		
a) Benign gestational trophoblastic disease	1	**Evidence:** Among women with benign or malignant gestational trophoblastic disease, there was no difference in mean times to hCG normalization or incidence of postmolar trophoblastic disease for COC users compared to non-hormonal users.
b) Malignant gestational trophoblastic disease	1	
CERVICAL ECTROPION*	1	
CERVICAL INTRAEPITHELIAL NEOPLASIA (CIN)	2	**Evidence:** Among women with persistent HPV infection, long-term COC use (≥ 5 years) may increase the risk of carcinoma in situ and invasive carcinoma.
CERVICAL CANCER* (awaiting treatment)	2	
BREAST DISEASE*		
a) Undiagnosed mass	2	**Clarification:** Evaluation should be pursued as early as possible.
b) Benign breast disease	1	
c) Family history of cancer	1	**Evidence:** Among COC users with a family history of breast cancer, there was no increased risk of breast cancer compared with non-COC users with a family history of breast cancer. Among women with BRCA1 mutations, COC users may have a small increased risk of breast cancer compared with non-users.

(*Continued*)

Table 6.3
(Continued)

LOW-DOSE COMBINED ORAL CONTRACEPTIVES (COCs) ≤ 35 µg of ethinylestradiol	**COCs do not protect against STI/HIV. If there is risk of STI/HIV (including during pregnancy or postpartum), the correct and consistent use of condoms is recommended, either alone or with another contraceptive method. Male latex condoms are proven to protect against STI/HIV.**	
CONDITION	**CATEGORY** I=Initiation C=Continuation	**CLARIFICATIONS/EVIDENCE**
BREAST DISEASE (Cont'd)		
d) Breast cancer		
(i) current	4	
(ii) past and no evidence of current disease for 5 years	3	
ENDOMETRIAL CANCER*	1	
OVARIAN CANCER*	1	
UTERINE FIBROIDS*		
a) Without distortion of the uterine cavity	1	
b) With distortion of the uterine cavity	1	
PELVIC INFLAMMATORY DISEASE (PID)*		
a) Past PID (assuming no current risk factors for STIs)		
(i) with subsequent pregnancy	1	
(ii) without subsequent pregnancy	1	
b) PID - current	1	
STIs*		
a) Current purulent cervicitis or chlamydial infection or gonorrhoea	1	
b) Other STIs (excluding HIV and hepatitis)	1	

(*Continued*)

Table 6.3
(Continued)

LOW-DOSE COMBINED ORAL CONTRACEPTIVES (COCs) ≤ 35 μg of ethinylestradiol	COCs do not protect against STI/HIV. If there is risk of STI/HIV (including during pregnancy or postpartum), the correct and consistent use of condoms is recommended, either alone or with another contraceptive method. Male latex condoms are proven to protect against STI/HIV.	
CONDITION	**CATEGORY** I=Initiation C=Continuation	**CLARIFICATIONS/EVIDENCE**
STIs (Cont'd)		
c) Vaginitis (including trichomonas vaginalis and bacterial vaginosis)	1	
d) Increased risk of STIs	1	**Evidence:** Evidence suggests that there may be an increased risk of chlamydial cervicitis among COC users at high risk of STIs. For other STIs, there is either evidence of no association between COC use and STI acquisition or limited evidence to draw any conclusions.
HIV/AIDS		
HIGH RISK OF HIV*	1	**Evidence:** Overall, evidence is inconsistent regarding whether there is any increased risk of HIV acquisition among COC users compared with non-users.
HIV-INFECTED	1	**Evidence:** Limited evidence suggests no association between COC use and changes in RNA levels or CD4 counts among HIV-infected women. There is also limited evidence showing no association between COC use and female to male HIV transmission, and mixed results regarding increased risk of HIV and herpes simplex virus (HSV) shedding among HIV-infected women using hormonal contraception.
AIDS	1	
On ARV therapy	2	**Clarification**: If a woman is taking antiretroviral (ARV) therapy, refer to the section on drug interactions. Because there may be drug interactions between hormonal contraceptives and ARVs, AIDS with ARV therapy is classified as Category 2.
OTHER INFECTIONS		
SCHISTOSOMIASIS		
a) Uncomplicated	1	**Evidence:** Among women with uncomplicated schistosomiasis, COC use had no adverse effects on liver function.
b) Fibrosis of liver (if severe, see cirrhosis)	1	
TUBERCULOSIS		
a) Nonpelvic	1	**Clarification:** If a woman is taking rifampicin, refer to the section on drug interactions. Rifampicin is likely to decrease COC effectiveness.
b) Known pelvic	1	
MALARIA	1	

(Continued)

Table 6.3
(Continued)

LOW-DOSE COMBINED ORAL CONTRACEPTIVES (COCs) ≤ 35 μg of ethinylestradiol	COCs do not protect against STI/HIV. If there is risk of STI/HIV (including during pregnancy or postpartum), the correct and consistent use of condoms is recommended, either alone or with another contraceptive method. Male latex condoms are proven to protect against STI/HIV.	
CONDITION	**CATEGORY** I=Initiation C=Continuation	**CLARIFICATIONS/EVIDENCE**
ENDOCRINE CONDITIONS		
DIABETES*		
a) History of gestational disease	1	
b) Nonvascular disease		
(i) noninsulin dependent	2	
(ii) insulin dependent	2	
c) Nephropathy/ retinopathy/ neuropathy	3/4	**Clarification:** The category should be assessed according to the severity of the condition.
d) Other vascular disease or diabetes of > 20 years' duration	3/4	**Clarification:** The category should be assessed according to the severity of the condition.
THYROID DISORDERS		
a) Simple goiter	1	
b) Hyperthyroid	1	
c) Hypothyroid	1	
GASTROINTESTINAL CONDITIONS		
GALLBLADDER DISEASE*		
a) Symptomatic		
(i) treated by cholecystectomy	2	
(ii) medically treated	3	
(iii) current	3	
b) Asymptomatic	2	
HISTORY OF CHOLESTASIS*		
a) Pregnancy-related	2	
b) Past COC-related	3	
VIRAL HEPATITIS*		
a) Active	4	
b) Carrier	1	

(Continued)

Table 6.3
(Continued)

LOW-DOSE COMBINED ORAL CONTRACEPTIVES (COCs) ≤ 35 μg of ethinylestradiol	**COCs do not protect against STI/HIV. If there is risk of STI/HIV (including during pregnancy or postpartum), the correct and consistent use of condoms is recommended, either alone or with another contraceptive method. Male latex condoms are proven to protect against STI/HIV.**	
CONDITION	**CATEGORY** I=Initiation C=Continuation	**CLARIFICATIONS/EVIDENCE**
CIRRHOSIS*		
a) Mild (compensated)	3	
b) Severe (decompensated)	4	
LIVER TUMORS*		
a) Benign (adenoma)	4	
b) Malignant (hepatoma)	4	
ANEMIAS		
THALASSEMIA*	1	
SICKLE CELL DISEASE	2	
IRON-DEFICIENCY ANEMIA*	1	
DRUG INTERACTIONS		
DRUGS WHICH AFFECT LIVER ENZYMES		
a) Rifampicin	3	**Clarification:** Although the interaction of rifampicin or certain anticonvulsants with COCs is not harmful to women, it is likely to reduce the effectiveness of COCs. Use of other contraceptives should be encouraged for women who are long-term users of any of these drugs. Whether increasing the hormone dose of COCs is of benefit remains unclear. **Evidence:** Use of rifampicin and certain anticonvulsants decreased the contraceptive effectiveness of COCs.
b) Certain anticonvulsants (phenytoin, carbamazepine, barbiturates, primidone, topiramate, oxcarbazepine)	3	
ANTIBIOTICS (excluding rifampicin)		
a) Griseofulvin	2	
b) Other antibiotics	1	**Evidence:** The contraceptive effectiveness of COCs was not affected by coadministration of most broad-spectrum antibiotics.

(Continued)

Table 6.3
(Continued)

LOW-DOSE COMBINED ORAL CONTRACEPTIVES (COCs) ≤ 35 μg of ethinylestradiol	COCs do not protect against STI/HIV. If there is risk of STI/HIV (including during pregnancy or postpartum), the correct and consistent use of condoms is recommended, either alone or with another contraceptive method. Male latex condoms are proven to protect against STI/HIV.	
CONDITION	**CATEGORY** I=Initiation C=Continuation	**CLARIFICATIONS/EVIDENCE**
ANTIRETROVIRAL THERAPY	2	**Clarification**: It is important to note that antiretroviral drugs (ARV) have the potential to either decrease or increase the bioavailability of steroid hormones in hormonal contraceptives. The limited data available (outlined in Annex 1) suggest that potential drug interactions between many ARVs (particularly some non-nucleoside reverse transcriptase inhibitors (NNRTIs) and protease inhibitors (PIs)) and hormonal contraceptives may alter safety and effectiveness of both the hormonal contraceptives and the ARVs. It is not known whether the contraceptive effectiveness of progestogen-only injectable contraceptives (such as depot medroxyprogesterone acetate and norethisterone enantate) would be compromised, as these methods provide higher blood hormone levels than other progestogen-only hormonal contraceptives, as well as than combined oral contraceptives. Studies are underway to evaluate potential interactions between depot medroxyprogesterone acetate and selected PI and NNRTI drugs. Thus, if a woman on ARV treatment decides to initiate or continue hormonal contraceptive use, the consistent use of condoms is recommended for preventing HIV transmission and may also compensate for any possible reduction in the effectiveness of the hormonal contraceptive. **Evidence:** See Annex 1.

Adapted from World Health Organization, Reproductive Health and Research. Medical eligibility criteria for contraceptive use. Available at: www.who.int/reproductive-health/publications/mec/mec.pdf. Accessed May 3, 2009.

Additional comments

AGE

Menarche to < 40 years: Theoretical concerns about the use of combined hormonal contraceptives among young adolescents have not been substantiated.

≥ 40 years: The risk of cardiovascular disease increases with age and may also increase with combined hormonal contraceptive use. In the absence of other adverse clinical conditions, combined hormonal contraceptives can be used until menopause.

BREASTFEEDING

< 6 weeks postpartum: There is some theoretical concern that the neonate may be at risk due to exposure to steroid hormones during the first 6 weeks postpartum.

≥ 6 weeks to < 6 months (primarily breastfeeding): Use of COCs during breastfeeding diminishes the quantity of breast milk, decreases the duration of lactation, and may thereby adversely affect the growth of the infant.

POSTPARTUM

< 21 days: There is some theoretical concern regarding the association between combined hormonal contraceptive use up to 3 weeks postpartum and risk of thrombosis in the mother. Blood coagulation and fibrinolysis are essentially normalized by 3 weeks postpartum.

PAST ECTOPIC PREGNANCY

The risk of future ectopic pregnancy is increased among women who have had an ectopic pregnancy in the past. Combined hormonal contraceptives provide protection against pregnancy in general, including ectopic gestation.

HYPERTENSION

Vascular disease: Among women with underlying vascular disease, the increased risk of arterial thrombosis associated with combined hormonal contraceptive use should be avoided.

DEEP VENOUS THROMBOSIS (DVT)/ PULMONARY EMBOLISM (PE)

Family history of DVT/PE (first-degree relatives): Some conditions which increase the risk of DVT/PE are heritable.

(Continued)

Major surgery: The degree of risk of DVT/PE associated with major surgery varies depending on the length of time that a woman is immobilized. There is no need to stop combined hormonal contraceptives prior to female surgical sterilization.

SUPERFICIAL VENOUS THROMBOSIS

Varicose veins: Varicose veins are not risk factors for DVT/PE.

CURRENT AND HISTORY OF ISCHEMIC HEART DISEASE

Among women with underlying vascular disease, the increased risk of arterial thrombosis associated with combined hormonal contraceptive use should be avoided.

STROKE

Among women with underlying vascular disease, the increased risk of arterial thrombosis associated with combined hormonal contraceptive use should be avoided.

VALVULAR HEART DISEASE

Among women with valvular heart disease, combined hormonal contraceptive use may further increase the risk of arterial thrombosis; women with complicated valvular heart disease are at greatest risk.

HEADACHES

Aura is a specific focal neurologic symptom. For more information on this and other diagnostic criteria, see: Headache Classification Subcommittee of the International Headache Society. The International Classification of Headache Disorders, 2nd Edition. Cephalalgia. 2004; 24 (Suppl 1): 1- 150.
http://216.25.100.131/ihscommon/guidelines/pdfs/ihc_II_main_no_print.pdf

VAGINAL BLEEDING PATTERNS

Irregular menstrual bleeding patterns are common among healthy women.

UNEXPLAINED VAGINAL BLEEDING

There are no conditions that cause vaginal bleeding that will be worsened in the short term by use of combined hormonal contraceptives.

ENDOMETRIOSIS

Combined hormonal contraceptives do not worsen, and may alleviate, the symptoms of endometriosis.

CERVICAL ECTROPION

Cervical ectropion is not a risk factor for cervical cancer, and there is no need for restriction of combined hormonal contraceptive use.

CERVICAL CANCER (awaiting treatment)

There is some theoretical concern that combined hormonal contraceptive use may affect prognosis of the existing disease. While awaiting treatment, women may use combined hormonal contraceptives. In general, treatment of this condition renders a woman sterile.

BREAST DISEASE

Family history of cancer: Women with BRCA1 or BRCA2 mutations have a much higher baseline risk of breast cancer than women who do not have these mutations. Most women with a family history of breast cancer do not have these mutations.

Breast cancer: Breast cancer is a hormonally sensitive tumour, and the prognosis of women with current or recent breast cancer may worsen with combined hormonal contraceptive use.

ENDOMETRIAL CANCER

COC use reduces the risk of developing endometrial cancer. While awaiting treatment, women may use COCs. In general, treatment of this condition renders a woman sterile.

OVARIAN CANCER

COC use reduces the risk of developing ovarian cancer. While awaiting treatment, women may use COCs. In general, treatment of this condition renders a woman sterile.

UTERINE FIBROIDS

COCs do not appear to cause growth of uterine fibroids.

PELVIC INFLAMMATORY DISEASE (PID)

COCs may reduce the risk of PID among women with STIs, but do not protect against HIV or lower genital tract STIs.

STIs

COCs may reduce the risk of PID among women with STIs, but do not protect against HIV or lower genital tract STIs.

HIGH RISK OF HIV

COCs may reduce the risk of PID among women with STIs, but do not protect against HIV or lower genital tract STIs.

DIABETES

Although carbohydrate tolerance may change with combined hormonal contraceptive use, the major concerns are vascular disease due to diabetes and additional risk of arterial thrombosis due to combined hormonal contraceptive use.

GALL-BLADDER DISEASE

COCs may cause a small increased risk of gall-bladder disease. There is also concern that COCs may worsen existing gall-bladder disease.

HISTORY OF CHOLESTASIS

Pregnancy-related: History of pregnancy-related cholestasis may predict an increased risk of developing COC-associated cholestasis.

Past COC-related: History of COC-related cholestasis predicts an increased risk with subsequent COC use.

VIRAL HEPATITIS

Active: COCs are metabolized by the liver, and their use may adversely affect women whose liver function is compromised.

CIRRHOSIS

COCs are metabolized by the liver and their use may adversely affect women whose liver function is compromised.

LIVER TUMORS

COCs are metabolized by the liver and their use may adversely affect women whose liver function is compromised. In addition, COC use may enhance the growth of tumors.

THALASSEMIA

There is anecdotal evidence from countries where thalassaemia is prevalent that COC use does not worsen the condition.

IRON-DEFICIENCY ANEMIA

Combined hormonal contraceptive use may decrease menstrual blood loss.

WHO 2008 Summary

Use in Adolescents and Young Adults Absolutely Contraindicated for OCs and Other Forms of Combination Contraceptives: WHO Classification 4

- Systolic blood pressures of >160 mm Hg or diastolic blood pressures of >100 mm Hg
- History/current/therapy for diagnosis of deep vein thrombosis (DVT)/ pulmonary embolism
- Less than 6 weeks postpartum and breastfeeding
- Known diagnosis of thrombophilia (eg, protein S deficiency)
- Positive antiphospholipid antibodies
- Migraine headaches with aura
- Prolonged immobilization after surgery
- Acute/flare liver disease: infection, cancer, cirrhosis
- Diabetic complications of nephropathy, neuropathy, and retinopathy
- Complications of valvular heart disease: atrial fibrillation, pulmonary hypertension, subacute bacterial endocarditis

Classification 4 indicates that the patient has a condition that represents an unacceptable health risk if the contraceptive method is used.

Use in Adolescents and Young Adults Generally not Recommended for OCs and Other Forms of Combination Contraceptives: WHO Classification 3

- Systolic blood pressures of 140 to 159 mm Hg or diastolic blood pressures of 90 to 99 mm Hg
- Current or medically treated gallbladder disease
- Breastfeeding primarily between 6 weeks and 6 months postpartum
- Postpartum, <21 days, nonbreastfeeding
- Mild cirrhosis of the liver
- Use of drugs that affect the liver such as rifampicin and anticonvulsants such as barbiturates, phenytoin, carbamazepine, oxycarbamazepine, phenytoin, and topiramates

Classification 3 indicates that the patient has a condition with which theoretical or proven risks of the method generally outweigh advantages of using the method.

Table 6.4
Combined injectable contraceptives, patch, and ring

COMBINED INJECTABLE CONTRACEPTIVES (CICs), PATCH (P), RING (R)	**CICs, patch, and ring do not protect against STI/HIV. If there is risk of STI/HIV (including during pregnancy or postpartum), the correct and consistent use of condoms is recommended, either alone or with another contraceptive method. Male latex condoms are proven to protect against STI/HIV.**			
CONDITION	**CATEGORY** I=Initiation C=Continuation			**CLARIFICATIONS/EVIDENCE**
	CICs	**P**	**R**	
PAST ECTOPIC PREGNANCY*	1	1	1	
HISTORY OF PELVIC SURGERY	1	1	1	
SMOKING				
a) Age < 35 years	2	2	2	
b) Age ≥ 35 years				
(i) <15 cigarettes/day	2	3	3	
(ii) ≥15 cigarettes/day	3	4	4	
OBESITY ≥ 30 kg/m² body mass index (BMI)	2	2	2	**Evidence:** Limited evidence suggests the effectiveness of the patch may decline for women weighing 90kg or more.
BLOOD PRESSURE MEASUREMENT UNAVAILABLE	NA	NA	NA	**Clarification:** It is desirable to have blood pressure measurements taken before initiation of CIC, P, or R use. However, in some settings blood pressure measurements are unavailable. In many of these settings, pregnancy morbidity and mortality risks are high, and CICs, P, or R may be one of the few methods available. In such settings, women should not be denied use of CICs, P, or R simply because their blood pressure cannot be measured.
CARDIOVASCULAR DISEASE				
MULTIPLE RISK FACTORS FOR ARTERIAL CARDIOVASCULAR DISEASE (such as older age, smoking, diabetes and hypertension)	3/4	3/4	3/4	**Clarification:** When a woman has multiple major risk factors, any of which alone would substantially increase the risk of cardiovascular disease, use of CICs, P, or R may increase her risk to an unacceptable level. However, a simple addition of categories for multiple risk factors is not intended; for example, a combination of two risk factors assigned a category 2 may not necessarily warrant a higher category.

* See also additional comments at end of table

(*Continued*)

Table 6.4
(Continued)

COMBINED INJECTABLE CONTRACEPTIVES (CICs), PATCH (P), RING (R)	**CICs, patch, and ring do not protect against STI/HIV. If there is risk of STI/HIV (including during pregnancy or postpartum), the correct and consistent use of condoms is recommended, either alone or with another contraceptive method. Male latex condoms are proven to protect against STI/HIV.**			
CONDITION	**CATEGORY** I=Initiation C=Continuation			**CLARIFICATIONS/EVIDENCE**
	CICs	**P**	**R**	
HYPERTENSION*				
For all categories of hypertension, classifications are based on the assumption that no other risk factors for cardiovascular disease exist. When multiple risk factors do exist, risk of cardiovascular disease may increase substantially. A single reading of blood pressure level is not sufficient to classify a woman as hypertensive.				
a) History of hypertension, where blood pressure CANNOT be evaluated (including hypertension in pregnancy)	3	3	3	**Clarification:** Evaluation of cause and level of hypertension is recommended as soon as feasible.
b) Adequately controlled hypertension, where blood pressure CAN be evaluated	3	3	3	**Clarification:** Women adequately treated for hypertension are at reduced risk of acute myocardial infarction and stroke as compared with untreated women. Although there are no data, CIC, P, or R users with adequately controlled and monitored hypertension should be at reduced risk of acute myocardial infarction and stroke compared with untreated hypertensive CIC, P, or R users.
c) Elevated blood pressure levels (properly taken measurements)				
(i) systolic 140-159 or diastolic 90-99	3	3	3	
(ii) systolic ≥160 or diastolic ≥100	4	4	4	
d) Vascular disease	4	4	4	
HISTORY OF HIGH BLOOD PRESSURE DURING PREGNANCY (where current blood pressure is measurable and normal)	2	2	2	

(*Continued*)

Table 6.4
(Continued)

COMBINED INJECTABLE CONTRACEPTIVES (CICs), PATCH (P), RING (R)	**CICs, patch, and ring do not protect against STI/HIV. If there is risk of STI/HIV (including during pregnancy or postpartum), the correct and consistent use of condoms is recommended, either alone or with another contraceptive method. Male latex condoms are proven to protect against STI/HIV.**			
CONDITION	**CATEGORY** I=Initiation C=Continuation			**CLARIFICATIONS/EVIDENCE**
	CICs	**P**	**R**	
DEEP VENOUS THROMBOSIS (DVT)/ PULMONARY EMBOLISM (PE)*				
a) History of DVT/PE	4	4	4	
b) Current DVT/PE	4	4	4	
c) Family history of DVT/PE (first-degree relatives)	2	2	2	
d) Major surgery				
(i) with prolonged immobilization	4	4	4	
(ii) without prolonged immobilization	2	2	2	
e) Minor surgery without immobilization	1	1	1	
KNOWN THROMBOGENIC MUTATIONS (e.g., Factor V Leiden; Prothrombin mutation; Protein S, Protein C, and Antithrombin deficiencies)	4	4	4	**Clarification:** Routine screening is not appropriate because of the rarity of the conditions and the high cost of screening.
SUPERFICIAL VENOUS THROMBOSIS*				
a) Varicose veins	1	1	1	
b) Superficial thrombophlebitis	2	2	2	
CURRENT AND HISTORY OF ISCHEMIC HEART DISEASE*	4	4	4	
STROKE* (history of cerebrovascular accident)	4	4	4	

(Continued)

Table 6.4
(Continued)

COMBINED INJECTABLE CONTRACEPTIVES (CICs), PATCH (P), RING (R)	**CICs, patch, and ring do not protect against STI/HIV. If there is risk of STI/HIV (including during pregnancy or postpartum), the correct and consistent use of condoms is recommended, either alone or with another contraceptive method. Male latex condoms are proven to protect against STI/HIV.**						
CONDITION	**CATEGORY** I=Initiation C=Continuation						**CLARIFICATIONS/EVIDENCE**
	CICs		**P**		**R**		
KNOWN HYPERLIPIDEMIAS	2/3		2/3		2/3		**Clarification:** Routine screening is not appropriate because of the rarity of the conditions and the high cost of screening. While some types of hyperlipidaemias are risk factors for vascular disease, the category should be assessed according to the type, its severity, and the presence of other cardiovascular risk factors.
VALVULAR HEART DISEASE*							
a) Uncomplicated	2		2		2		
b) Complicated (pulmonary hypertension, risk of atrial fibrillation, history of subacute bacterial endocarditis)	4		4		4		
NEUROLOGIC CONDITIONS							
HEADACHES*	I	C	I	C	I	C	
a) Non-migrainous (mild or severe)	1	2	1	2	1	2	**Clarification:** Classification depends on accurate diagnosis of those severe headaches that are migrainous and those that are not. Any new headaches or marked changes in headaches should be evaluated. Classification is for women without any other risk factors for stroke. Risk of stroke increases with age, hypertension and smoking.
b) Migraine							
(i) without aura							
Age < 35	2	3	2	3	2	3	
Age ≥ 35	3	4	3	4	3	4	
(ii) with aura, at any age	4	4	4	4	4	4	
EPILEPSY	1		1		1		**Clarification:** If a woman is taking anticonvulsants, refer to the section on drug interactions. Certain anticonvulsants lower COC effectiveness. The extent to which CIC, P or R use are similar to COC use in this regard remains unclear.

(Continued)

Table 6.4
(Continued)

COMBINED INJECTABLE CONTRACEPTIVES (CICs), PATCH (P), RING (R)	**CICs, patch, and ring do not protect against STI/HIV. If there is risk of STI/HIV (including during pregnancy or postpartum), the correct and consistent use of condoms is recommended, either alone or with another contraceptive method. Male latex condoms are proven to protect against STI/HIV.**			
CONDITION	**CATEGORY** I=Initiation C=Continuation			**CLARIFICATIONS/EVIDENCE**
	CICs	**P**	**R**	
DEPRESSIVE DISORDERS				
DEPRESSIVE DISORDERS	1	1	1	**Clarification:** The classification is based on data for women with selected depressive disorders. No data on bipolar disorder or postpartum depression were available. There is a potential for drug interactions between certain antidepressant medications and hormonal contraceptives.
REPRODUCTIVE TRACT INFECTIONS AND DISORDERS				
VAGINAL BLEEDING PATTERNS*				
a) Irregular pattern *without* heavy bleeding	1	1	1	
b) Heavy or prolonged bleeding (includes regular and irregular patterns)	1	1	1	**Clarification:** Unusually heavy bleeding should raise the suspicion of a serious underlying condition.
UNEXPLAINED VAGINAL BLEEDING* (suspicious for serious condition)				
Before evaluation	2	2	2	**Clarification:** If pregnancy or an underlying pathological condition (such as pelvic malignancy) is suspected, it must be evaluated and the category adjusted after evaluation.
ENDOMETRIOSIS*	1	1	1	
BENIGN OVARIAN TUMORS (including cysts)	1	1	1	
SEVERE DYSMENORRHOEA	1	1	1	
TROPHOBLAST DISEASE				
a) Benign gestational trophoblastic disease	1	1	1	
b) Malignant gestational trophoblastic disease	1	1	1	
CERVICAL ECTROPION*	1	1	1	

(Continued)

Table 6.4
(Continued)

COMBINED INJECTABLE CONTRACEPTIVES (CICs), PATCH (P), RING (R)	CICs, patch, and ring do not protect against STI/HIV. If there is risk of STI/HIV (including during pregnancy or postpartum), the correct and consistent use of condoms is recommended, either alone or with another contraceptive method. Male latex condoms are proven to protect against STI/HIV.			
CONDITION	**CATEGORY** I=Initiation C=Continuation			**CLARIFICATIONS/EVIDENCE**
	CICs	**P**	**R**	
CERVICAL INTRAEPITHELIAL NEOPLASIA (CIN)	2	2	2	**Evidence:** Limited evidence on women with low-grade squamous intraepithelial lesions found use of the vaginal ring did not worsen the condition.
CERVICAL CANCER* (awaiting treatment)	2	2	2	
BREAST DISEASE*				
a) Undiagnosed mass	2	2	2	**Clarification:** Evaluation should be pursued as early as possible.
b) Benign breast disease	1	1	1	
c) Family history of cancer	1	1	1	
d) Breast cancer				
(i) current	4	4	4	
(ii) past and no evidence of current disease for 5 years	3	3	3	
ENDOMETRIAL CANCER*	1	1	1	
OVARIAN CANCER*	1	1	1	
UTERINE FIBROIDS*				
a) Without distortion of the uterine cavity	1	1	1	
b) With distortion of the uterine cavity	1	1	1	
PELVIC INFLAMMATORY DISEASE (PID)*				
a) Past PID (assuming no current risk factors for STIs)				
i) with subsequent pregnancy	1	1	1	
ii) without subsequent pregnancy	1	1	1	
b) PID - current	1	1	1	

(Continued)

Table 6.4
(Continued)

COMBINED INJECTABLE CONTRACEPTIVES (CICs), PATCH (P), RING (R)	CICs, patch, and ring do not protect against STI/HIV. If there is risk of STI/HIV (including during pregnancy or postpartum), the correct and consistent use of condoms is recommended, either alone or with another contraceptive method. Male latex condoms are proven to protect against STI/HIV.			
CONDITION	**CATEGORY** I=Initiation C=Continuation			**CLARIFICATIONS/EVIDENCE**
	CICs	**P**	**R**	
STIs*				
a) Current purulent cervicitis or chlamydial infection or gonorrhoea	1	1	1	
b) Other STIs (excluding HIV and hepatitis)	1	1	1	
c) Vaginitis (including trichomonas vaginalis and bacterial vaginosis)	1	1	1	
d) Increased risk of STIs	1	1	1	
HIV/AIDS				
HIGH RISK OF HIV*	1	1	1	
HIV-INFECTED	1	1	1	
AIDS	1	1	1	
On ARV therapy	2	2	2	**Clarification**: If a woman is taking antiretroviral (ARV) therapy, refer to the section on drug interactions. Because there may be drug interactions between hormonal contraceptives and ARVs, AIDS with ARV therapy is classified as Category 2.
OTHER INFECTIONS				
SCHISTOSOMIASIS				
a) Uncomplicated	1	1	1	
b) Fibrosis of liver (if severe, see cirrhosis)	1	1	1	
TUBERCULOSIS				
a) Non-pelvic	1	1	1	**Clarification:** If a woman is taking rifampicin, refer to the section on drug interactions. Rifampicin is likely to decrease COC effectiveness. The extent to which CIC, P, or R use is similar to COC use in this regard remains unclear.
b) Known pelvic	1	1	1	
MALARIA	1	1	1	

(Continued)

Table 6.4
(Continued)

COMBINED INJECTABLE CONTRACEPTIVES (CICs), PATCH (P), RING (R)	CICs, patch, and ring do not protect against STI/HIV. If there is risk of STI/HIV (including during pregnancy or postpartum), the correct and consistent use of condoms is recommended, either alone or with another contraceptive method. Male latex condoms are proven to protect against STI/HIV.			
CONDITION	**CATEGORY** I=Initiation C=Continuation			**CLARIFICATIONS/EVIDENCE**
	CICs	**P**	**R**	
ENDOCRINE CONDITIONS				
DIABETES*				
a) History of gestational disease	1	1	1	
b) Non-vascular disease				
(i) non-insulin dependent	2	2	2	
(ii) insulin dependent	2	2	2	
c) Nephropathy/ retinopathy/ neuropathy	3/4	3/4	3/4	**Clarification:** The category should be assessed according to the severity of the condition.
d) Other vascular disease or diabetes of >20 years' duration	3/4	3/4	3/4	**Clarification:** The category should be assessed according to the severity of the condition.
THYROID DISORDERS				
a) Simple goiter	1	1	1	
b) Hyperthyroid	1	1	1	
c) Hypothyroid	1	1	1	
GASTROINTESTINAL CONDITIONS				
GALLBLADDER DISEASE*				
a) Symptomatic				
(i) treated by cholecystectomy	2	2	2	
(ii) medically treated	2	3	3	
(iii) current	2	3	3	
b) Asymptomatic	2	2	2	
HISTORY OF CHOLESTASIS*				
a) Pregnancy-related	2	2	2	
b) Past COC or CIC related	2	3	3	

(Continued)

Table 6.4
(Continued)

COMBINED INJECTABLE CONTRACEPTIVES (CICs), PATCH (P), RING (R)	CICs, patch, and ring do not protect against STI/HIV. If there is risk of STI/HIV (including during pregnancy or postpartum), the correct and consistent use of condoms is recommended, either alone or with another contraceptive method. Male latex condoms are proven to protect against STI/HIV.			
CONDITION	**CATEGORY** I=Initiation C=Continuation			**CLARIFICATIONS/EVIDENCE**
	CICs	**P**	**R**	
VIRAL HEPATITIS*				
a) Active	3/4	4	4	**Clarification:** The category should be assessed according to the severity of the condition.
b) Carrier	1	1	1	**Clarification**: In women with symptomatic viral hepatitis, CICs, P and R should be withheld until liver function returns to normal or 3 months after the woman becomes asymptomatic, whichever occurs earlier.
CIRRHOSIS*				
a) Mild (compensated)	2	3	3	
b) Severe (decompensated)	3	4	4	
LIVER TUMORS *				
a) Benign (adenoma)	3	4	4	
b) Malignant (hepatoma)	3/4	4	4	
ANEMIAS				
THALASSEMIA	1	1	1	
SICKLE CELL DISEASE	2	2	2	
IRON-DEFICIENCY ANEMIA *	1	1	1	
DRUG INTERACTIONS				
DRUGS WHICH AFFECT LIVER ENZYMES				
a) Rifampicin	2	3	3	**Clarification:** Although the interaction of rifampicin or certain anticonvulsants with P or R use is not harmful to women, it is likely to reduce P or R effectiveness. Use of other contraceptives should be encouraged for women who are long-term users of any of these drugs.
b) Certain anticonvulsants (phenytoin, carbamazepine, barbiturates, primidone, topiramate, oxcarbazepine)	2	3	3	
ANTIBIOTICS (excluding rifampicin)				
a) Griseofulvin	1	2	2	
b) Other antibiotics	1	1	1	

(*Continued*)

Table 6.4
(Continued)

COMBINED INJECTABLE CONTRACEPTIVES (CICs), PATCH (P), RING (R)	**CICs, patch, and ring do not protect against STI/HIV. If there is risk of STI/HIV (including during pregnancy or postpartum), the correct and consistent use of condoms is recommended, either alone or with another contraceptive method. Male latex condoms are proven to protect against STI/HIV.**			
CONDITION	**CATEGORY** I=Initiation C=Continuation			**CLARIFICATIONS/EVIDENCE**
	CICs	**P**	**R**	
ANTIRETROVIRAL THERAPY	2	2	2	**Clarification:** It is important to note that antiretroviral drugs (ARV) have the potential to either decrease or increase the bioavailability of steroid hormones in hormonal contraceptives. The limited data available (outlined in Annex 1) suggest that potential drug interactions between many ARVs (particularly some non-nucleoside reverse transcriptase inhibitors (NNRTIs) and protease inhibitors (PIs)) and hormonal contraceptives may alter safety and effectiveness of both the hormonal contraceptives and the ARVs. It is not known whether the contraceptive effectiveness of progestogen-only injectable contraceptives (such as depot medroxyprogesterone acetate and norethisterone enantate) would be compromised, as these methods provide higher blood hormone levels than other progestogen-only hormonal contraceptives, as well as than combined oral contraceptives. Studies are underway to evaluate potential interactions between depot medroxyprogesterone acetate and selected PI and NNRTI drugs. Thus, if a woman on ARV treatment decides to initiate or continue hormonal contraceptive use, the consistent use of condoms is recommended for preventing HIV transmission and may also compensate for any possible reduction in the effectiveness of the hormonal contraceptive.

Adapted from World Health Organization, Reproductive Health and Research. Medical eligibility criteria for contraceptive use. Available at: www.who.int/reproductive-health/publications/mec/mec.pdf. Accessed May 3, 2009.

Additional comments

AGE

Menarche to < 40 years: Theoretical concerns about the use of combined hormonal contraceptives among young adolescents have not been substantiated.

≥ 40 years: The risk of cardiovascular disease increases with age and may also increase with combined hormonal contraceptive use. In the absence of other adverse clinical conditions, combined hormonal contraceptives can be used until menopause.

BREASTFEEDING

< 6 weeks postpartum: There is some theoretical concern that the neonate may be at risk due to exposure to steroid hormones during the first 6 weeks postpartum.

≥ 6 weeks to < 6 months (primarily breastfeeding): Use of combined hormonal contraceptives during breastfeeding diminishes the quantity of breast milk, decreases the duration of lactation, and may thereby adversely affect the growth of the infant.

POSTPARTUM

< 21 days: There is some theoretical concern regarding the association between combined hormonal contraceptive use up to 3 weeks postpartum and risk of thrombosis in the mother. Blood coagulation and fibrinolysis are essentially normalized by 3 weeks postpartum.

PAST ECTOPIC PREGNANCY

The risk of future ectopic pregnancy is increased among women who have had an ectopic pregnancy in the past. Combined hormonal contraceptives provide protection against pregnancy in general, including ectopic gestation.

HYPERTENSION

Vascular disease: Among women with underlying vascular disease, the increased risk of arterial thrombosis associated with combined hormonal contraceptive use should be avoided.

DEEP VENOUS THROMBOSIS (DVT)/ PULMONARY EMBOLISM (PE)

Family history of DVT/PE (first-degree relatives): Some conditions which increase the risk of DVT/PE are heritable.

Major surgery: The degree of risk of DVT/PE associated with major surgery varies depending on the length of time that a woman is immobilized. There is no need to stop combined hormonal contraceptives prior to female surgical sterilization.

SUPERFICIAL VENOUS THROMBOSIS

Varicose veins: Varicose veins are not risk factors for DVT/PE.

CURRENT AND HISTORY OF ISCHAEMIC HEART DISEASE

Among women with underlying vascular disease, the increased risk of arterial thrombosis associated with combined hormonal contraceptive use should be avoided.

STROKE

Among women with underlying vascular disease, the increased risk of arterial thrombosis associated with combined hormonal contraceptive use should be avoided.

VALVULAR HEART DISEASE

Among women with valvular heart disease, combined hormonal contraceptive use may further increase the risk of arterial thrombosis; women with complicated valvular heart disease are at greatest risk.

HEADACHES

Aura is a specific focal neurologic symptom. For more information on this and other diagnostic criteria, see: Headache Classification Subcommittee of the International Headache Society. The International Classification of Headache Disorders, 2nd Edition. Cephalalgia. 2004; 24 (Suppl 1): 1- 150.
http://216.25.100.131/ihscommon/guidelines/pdfs/ihc_II_main_no_print.pdf

VAGINAL BLEEDING PATTERNS

Irregular menstrual bleeding patterns are common among healthy women.

UNEXPLAINED VAGINAL BLEEDING

There are no conditions that cause vaginal bleeding that will be worsened in the short term by use of combined hormonal contraceptives.

ENDOMETRIOSIS

Combined hormonal contraceptives do not worsen, and may alleviate, the symptoms of endometriosis.

CERVICAL ECTROPION

Cervical ectropion is not a risk factor for cervical cancer, and there is no need for restriction of combined hormonal contraceptive use.

(Continued)

CERVICAL CANCER (awaiting treatment)
There is some theoretical concern that combined hormonal contraceptive use may affect prognosis of the existing disease. While awaiting treatment, women may use combined hormonal contraceptives. In general, treatment of this condition renders a woman sterile.

BREAST DISEASE
Family history of cancer: Women with BRCA1 or BRCA2 mutations have a much higher baseline risk of breast cancer than women who do not have these mutations. Most women with a family history of breast cancer do not have these mutations.

Breast cancer: Breast cancer is a hormonally sensitive tumour, and the prognosis of women with current or recent breast cancer may worsen with combined hormonal contraceptive use.

ENDOMETRIAL CANCER
It is not known whether CIC, P, or R use reduces the risk of developing endometrial cancer, as is the case with COCs. While awaiting treatment, women may use CICs, P or R. In general, treatment of this condition renders a woman sterile.

OVARIAN CANCER
It is not known whether CIC, P, or R use reduces the risk of developing ovarian cancer, as is the case with COCs. While awaiting treatment, women may use CICs, P, or R. In general, treatment of this condition renders a woman sterile.

UTERINE FIBROIDS
COCs do not appear to cause growth of uterine fibroids and CICs, P, or R are not expected to do either.

PELVIC INFLAMMATORY DISEASE (PID)
COCs may reduce the risk of PID among women with STIs, but do not protect against HIV or lower genital tract STIs. Whether CICs, P or R reduce the risk of PID among women with STIs is unknown, but they do not protect against HIV or lower genital tract STIs.

STIs
COCs may reduce the risk of PID among women with STIs, but do not protect against HIV or lower genital tract STIs. Whether CICs, P or R reduce the risk of PID among women with STIs is unknown, but they do not protect against HIV or lower genital tract STIs.

HIGH RISK OF HIV
COCs may reduce the risk of PID among women with STIs, but do not protect against HIV or lower genital tract STIs. Whether CICs, P or R reduce the risk of PID among women with STIs is unknown, but they do not protect against HIV or lower genital tract STIs.

DIABETES
Although carbohydrate tolerance may change with combined hormonal contraceptive use, the major concerns are vascular disease due to diabetes and additional risk of arterial thrombosis due to combined hormonal contraceptive use.

GALLBLADDER DISEASE
P or R, like COCs, may cause a small increased risk of gall-bladder disease. There is also concern that they may worsen existing gall-bladder disease. However, unlike COCs, CICs have been shown to have a minimal effect on liver function in healthy women, and have no first-pass effect on the liver.

HISTORY OF CHOLESTASIS
Pregnancy-related: History of pregnancy-related cholestasis may predict an increased risk of developing cholestasis associated with combined hormone therapy.

Past COC or CIC related: History of COC- or CIC-related cholestasis predicts an increased risk associated with P or R use. Unlike COCs, CICs have been shown to have a minimal effect on liver function in healthy women and have no first-pass effect on the liver.

VIRAL HEPATITIS
Active: Unlike COCs, CICs have been shown to have a minimal effect on liver function in healthy women and have no first-pass effect on the liver. However, because CICs are metabo lized by the liver, they could, in theory, lead to adverse effects in women whose liver function is already compromised.

CIRRHOSIS
Unlike COCs, CICs have been shown to have a minimal effect on liver function in healthy women and have no first-pass effect on the liver. However, because CICs are metabolized by the liver, they could, in theory, lead to adverse effects in women whose liver function is already compromised

(*Continued*)

LIVER TUMORS

Unlike COCs, CICs have been shown to have a minimal effect on liver function in healthy women and have no first-pass effect on the liver. However, because CICs are metabolized by the liver, they could, in theory, lead to adverse effects in women whose liver function is already compromised.

IRON-DEFICIENCY ANEMIA

Combined hormonal contraceptive use may decrease menstrual blood loss.

Use in Adolescents and Young Adults Generally not Limited for OCs and Other Forms of Combination Contraceptives: WHO Classification 2

- Sickle cell disease
- Smoking in <35-year-olds
- Use of drugs such as griseofulvin and antiretroviral therapy

Classification 2 indicates that the patient has a condition with which advantages of using the method generally outweigh theoretical or proven risks of using the method.

Classification 1 indicates that there is no restriction for use of the method.

D. LIST OF OC PILLS

Table 6.5
Combination OCs classified according to estrogen dose (excluding 50-μg pills)

Name	Progestin	Dose, mg
20-μg EE		
Alesse, LevLite, Aviane,[a] Lessina,[a] Lutera[a]	Levonorgestrel	0.1
Loestrin FE 1/20,[b] Junel FE 1/20; non-FE also available[b]	Norethindrone acetate	1.0 (21 d of hormone, 7 d of 75-mg ferrous fumarate)
Mircette, Kariva,[c] Azurette[c]	Desogestrel	0.15 (21 pills of hormone, 2 d of hormone-free pill, 5 d of 10-μg EE)
25-μg EE		
Cyclessa, Velivet[a] (triphasic)	Desogestrel	0.100/0.125/0.150
Ortho Tri-Cyclen Lo (triphasic)	Norgestimate	0.18/0.215/0.25
30-μg EE		
Desogen, Ortho-Cept Apri	Desogestrel	0.15
Levlen, Nordette, Levora, Portia 0.15/30	Levonorgestrel	0.15
Loestrin 21 1.5/30, Microgestin FE, or no FE 1.5/30; Junel or Junel FE	Norethindrone acetate	1.5
Lo Ovral Low-Ogestrel-28, Cryselle	Norgestrel	0.3
Yasmin	Drospirenone	3.0
35-μg EE		
Brevicon, Modicon, Nortrel[a]	Norethindrone	0.5
Demulen 1/35-28, Zovia 1/35E-28, Kelnor, Norinyl 1 + 35, 28-d; Ortho-Novum 1/35, 28-d	Ethynodiol diacetate	1.0
Necon[a] 1/35, 28-d, Nortrel,[a] 21- and 28 d, Norethin[a] 1/35E, 28-d	Norethindrone	1.0
Ortho-Cyclen, Sprintec,[a] Mononessa[a]	Norgestimate	0.25
Ortho-Novum 7/7/7, Necon 7/7/7, Nortrel 7/7/7	Norethindrone	0.5/0.75/1.0
Ortho-Novum 10/11 (biphasic), Necon 10/11 28-d	Norethindrone	0.5/1.0
Ortho Tri-Cyclen Tri Sprintec,[a] TriNessa[a] (triphasic)	Norgestimate	0.18/0.215/0.25
Ovcon 35	Norethindrone	0.4
Tri-Norinyl (triphasic)	Norethindrone	0.5/1.0/0.5
Multiple estrogen dose		
Estrostep (20/30/35-μg EE)	Norethindrone acetate	1.0
Jenest (35 μg)	Norethindrone	0.5 (for 7 d), then 1.0 (for 14 d)
Tri-Levlen (30/40/30-μg EE), Triphasil (30/40/ 30-μg EE)	Levonorgestrel	0.05/0.075/0.125
Trivora-28, Enpresse		
Prepackaged extended cycling with COCs		
Seasonale, Quasense[a] (30-μg EE)	Levonorgestrel	0.15 (84 pills, 7 hormone-free)
Seasonique (30-μg EE)	Levonorgestrel	0.15 (84 pills, 7 pills 10-μg EE)
Lybrel (20-μg EE)	Levonorgestrel	0.9 mg daily

EE indicates ethinyl estradiol; FE, Iron.

[a] Generic formulations are indicated by italics.

[b] Formulations are monophasic unless otherwise noted.

[c] Twenty-three days of hormone, 5 days of 10-μg ethinyl estradiol.

Adapted from Nelson AL. Combined oral contraceptives. In: Hatcher RA, Trussell J, Nelson AL, et al, eds. *Contraceptive Technology*. 19th ed. New York, NY: Ardent Media; 2008: 193–269.

E. COMBINATION OCS

Table 6.6
Combination OCs classified according to the androgenic activity of the progestin component

Name	EE, μg	Progestin	Dose, mg
No or minimal androgenic activity of progestin component			
Yasmin	30	Drospirenone[a]	3.0
Yaz	20	Drospirenone[a]	3.0
Ortho-Cyclen	35	Norgestimate	0.25
Ortho Tri-Cyclen	35	Norgestimate	0.18/0.215/0.25
Ortho Tri-Cyclen Lo	25	Norgestimate	0.18/0.215/0.25
Cyclessa	25	Desogestrel	0.100/0.125/0.150
Desogen, Ortho-Cept	30	Desogestrel	0.15
Mircette	20/10	Desogestrel	0.15
Ovcon 35	35	Norethindrone	0.4
Brevicon, Modicon	35	Norethindrone	0.5
Medium androgenic activity of progestin component			
Demulen 1/35	35	Ethynodiol diacetate	1.0
Tri-Norinyl	35	Norethindrone	0.5/1.0/0.5
Ortho-Novum 10/11, Jenest-28	35	Norethindrone	0.5/1.0
Ortho-Novum 7/7/7	35	Norethindrone	0.5/0.75/1.0
Norinyl 1 + 35, Ortho-Novum 1/35	35	Norethindrone	1.0
Estrostep	20/30/35	Norethindrone acetate	1.0
Loestrin 1/20	20	Norethindrone acetate	1.0
Tri-Levlen; Triphasil	30/40/30	Levonorgestrel	0.05/0.075/0.125
High androgenic activity of progestin component			
Loestrin 1.5/30	30	Norethindrone acetate	1.5
Levlen, Nordette	30	Levonorgestrel	0.15
Lo/Ovral	30	Norgestrel	0.3

Products are listed in order of increasing androgenic activity; the panel noted that there is little difference in androgenic activity within each section. The products are listed with only 1 name; cross reference with Table 6.7 for generic names. EE indicates ethinyl estradiol.
[a] Drospirenone is the only progestin claiming antiandrogenic activity.
Adapted from *Dialogues Contracept.* 2002;2(7):3.

F. LIST OF OC PILLS THAT MIGHT BE USED FOR EC IN THE UNITED STATES

Table 6.7
Twenty-three OCs that can be used for EC in the United States

Brand	Company	Pills per Dose[a]	Ethinyl Estradiol per Dose, μg	Levonorgestrel per Dose, mg[b]
Progestin-only pills: take 1 dose[a]				
Plan B	Barr/Duramed	2 white pills	0	1.5
Combined progestin and estrogen pills: take 2 doses 12 h apart				
Alesse	Wyeth-Ayerst	5 pink pills	100	0.50
Aviane	Barr/Duramed	5 orange pills	100	0.50
Cryselle	Barr/Duramed	4 white pills	120	0.60
Enpresse	Barr/Duramed	4 orange pills	120	0.50
Jolessa	Barr/Duramed	4 pink pills	120	0.60
Lessina	Barr/Duramed	5 pink pills	100	0.50
Levlen	Berlex	4 light-orange pills	120	0.60
Levlite	Berlex	5 pink pills	100	0.50
Levora	Watson	4 white pills	120	0.60
Lo/Ovral	Wyeth-Ayerst	4 white pills	120	0.60
Low-Ogestrel	Watson	4 white pills	120	0.60
Lutera	Watson	5 white pills	100	0.50
Nordette	Wyeth-Ayerst	4 light-orange pills	120	0.60
Ogestrel	Watson	2 white pills	100	0.50
Ovral	Wyeth-Ayerst	2 white pills	100	0.50
Portia	Barr/Duramed	4 pink pills	120	0.60
Quasense	Watson	4 white pills	120	0.60

(*Continued*)

Table 6.7
(Continued)

Brand	Company	Pills per Dose[a]	Ethinyl Estradiol per Dose, µg	Levonorgestrel per Dose, mg[b]
Seasonale	Barr/Duramed	4 pink pills	120	0.60
Seasonique	Barr/Duramed	4 light–blue-green pills	120	0.60
Tri-Levlen	Berlex	4 yellow pills	120	0.50
Triphasil	Wyeth-Ayerst	4 yellow pills	120	0.50
Trivora	Watson	4 pink pills	120	0.50

Plan B, Next Choice, Plan B One-Step are now 3 dedicated products specifically marketed for EC. All have the same generic medication levonorgestrel, in the same 1.5 mg dose, either as 2 tablets or 1 tablet. Alesse, Aviane, Cryselle, Enpresse, Jolessa, Lessina, Levlen, Levlite, Levora, Lo/Ovral, Low-Ogestrel, Lutera, Nordette, Ogestrel, Ovral, Portia, Quasense, Seasonale, Seasonique, Tri-Levlen, Triphasil, and Trivora have been declared safe and effective for use as EC products by the US Food and Drug Administration. Worldwide, ~50 EC products are specifically packaged, labeled, and marketed. For example, Gedeon Richter and HRAPharma are marketing in many countries the levonorgestrel-only products Postinor 2 and NorLevo, respectively, each consisting of a 2-pill strip with each pill containing 0.75 mg of levonorgestrel. Levonorgestrel-only EC products are available either over-the-counter or from a pharmacist without having to see a clinician in 43 countries.

[a] The label for Plan B says to take 1 pill within 72 hours after unprotected intercourse and another pill 12 hours later. However, recent research has found that both Plan B pills can be taken at the same time. Research has also shown that all of the brands listed here are effective when used within 120 hours after unprotected sex.

[b] The progestin in Cryselle, Lo/Ovral, Low-Ogestrel, Ogestrel, and Ovral is norgestrel, which contains 2 isomers, only 1 of which (levonorgestrel) is bioactive; the amount of norgestrel in each tablet is twice the amount of levonorgestrel.

Adapted from Stewart F, Trussell J, Van Look PFA. Emergency contraception. In: Hatcher RA, Trussell J, Nelson AL, et al, eds. *Contraceptive Technology*. 19th ed. New York, NY: Ardent Media; 2008:89.

Other resources: www.go2planB.com and 1-888-not-2 LATE.

Table 6.8
Progestogen-only contraceptives

PROGESTOGEN-ONLY CONTRACEPTIVES (POCs)	POCs do not protect against STI/HIV. If there is risk of STI/HIV (including during pregnancy or postpartum), the correct and consistent use of condoms is recommended, either alone or with another contraceptive method. Male latex condoms are proven to protect against STI/HIV.			
CONDITION	**CATEGORY** I=Initiation, C=Continuation			**CLARIFICATIONS/EVIDENCE**
	POP	D/NE	LNG/ETG	
PARITY				
a) Nulliparous	1	1	1	
b) Parous	1	1	1	
BREASTFEEDING				
a) < 6 weeks postpartum	3	3	3	**Clarification:** There is concern that the neonate may be at risk of exposure to steroid hormones during the first 6 weeks postpartum. However, in many settings pregnancy morbidity and mortality risks are high, and access to services is limited. In such settings, POCs may be one of the few types of methods widely available and accessible to breastfeeding women immediately postpartum. **Evidence:** Studies have shown that among breast-feeding women less than 6 weeks postpartum, progestogen-only contraceptives did not affect breast-feeding performance and infant health and growth. However, there are no data evaluating the effects of progestogen exposure via breast milk on brain and liver development.
b) ≥ 6 weeks to < 6 months postpartum (primarily breastfeeding)	1	1	1	
c) ≥ 6 months postpartum	1	1	1	
POSTPARTUM* (in non-breastfeeding women)				
a) < 21 days	1	1	1	
b) ≥ 21 days	1	1	1	
POSTABORTION				
a) First trimester	1	1	1	**Clarification:** POCs may be started immediately post-abortion. **Evidence:** Limited evidence suggests that there are no adverse side effects when Norplant or NET-EN are initiated after a first trimester abortion.
b) Second trimester	1	1	1	
c) Immediate post-septic abortion	1	1	1	

See also additional comments at end of table

(*Continued*)

Table 6.8
(Continued)

PROGESTOGEN-ONLY CONTRACEPTIVES (POCs)	POCs do not protect against STI/HIV. If there is risk of STI/HIV (including during pregnancy or postpartum), the correct and consistent use of condoms is recommended, either alone or with another contraceptive method. Male latex condoms are proven to protect against STI/HIV.			
CONDITION	**CATEGORY** I=Initiation, C=Continuation			**CLARIFICATIONS/EVIDENCE**
	POP	D/NE	LNG/ETG	
PAST ECTOPIC PREGNANCY*	2	1	1	
HISTORY OF PELVIC SURGERY	1	1	1	
SMOKING				
a) Age < 35 years	1	1	1	
b) Age ≥ 35 years				
i) <15 cigarettes/day	1	1	1	
ii) ≥15 cigarettes/day	1	1	1	
OBESITY ≥ 30 kg/m² body mass index (BMI)	1	1	1	**Evidence:** Studies provide conflicting evidence regarding whether obese women are at increased risk of weight gain and bleeding problems with DMPA use relative to nonobese women with DMPA use. Studies show that obese women do not experience decreased effectiveness when using Norplant soft capsules or Jadelle.
BLOOD PRESSURE MEASUREMENT UNAVAILABLE	NA	NA	NA	**Clarification:** It is desirable to have blood pressure measurements taken before initiation of POC use. However, in some settings blood pressure measurements are unavailable. In many of these settings, pregnancy morbidity and mortality risks are high, and POCs are one of the few types of methods widely available. In such settings, women should not be denied use of POCs simply because their blood pressure cannot be measured.
CARDIOVASCULAR DISEASE				
MULTIPLE RISK FACTORS FOR ARTERIAL CARDIOVASCULAR DISEASE (such as older age, smoking, diabetes and hypertension)	2	3	2	**Clarification:** When multiple major risk factors exist, risk of cardiovascular disease may increase substantially. Some POCs may increase the risk of thrombosis, although this increase is substantially less than with COCs. The effects of DMPA and NET-EN may persist for some time after discontinuation.

(Continued)

Table 6.8
(Continued)

PROGESTOGEN-ONLY CONTRACEPTIVES (POCs)	**POCs do not protect against STI/HIV. If there is risk of STI/HIV (including during pregnancy or postpartum), the correct and consistent use of condoms is recommended, either alone or with another contraceptive method. Male latex condoms are proven to protect against STI/HIV.**			
CONDITION	**CATEGORY** I=Initiation, C=Continuation			**CLARIFICATIONS/EVIDENCE**
	POP	D/NE	LNG/ETG	
HYPERTENSION*				
For all categories of hypertension, classifications are based on the assumption that no other risk factors for cardiovascular disease exist. When multiple risk factors do exist, risk of cardiovascular disease may increase substantially. A single reading of blood pressure level is not sufficient to classify a woman as hypertensive.				
a) History of hypertension where blood pressure CANNOT be evaluated (including hypertension in pregnancy)	2	2	2	**Clarification:** It is desirable to have blood pressure measurements taken before initiation of POC use. However, in some settings blood pressure measurements are unavailable. In many of these settings pregnancy morbidity and mortality risks are high, and POCs are one of the few types of methods widely available. In such settings, women should not be denied use of POCs simply because their blood pressure cannot be measured.
b) Adequately controlled hypertension where blood pressure CAN be evaluated	1	2	1	**Clarification:** Women adequately treated for hypertension are at reduced risk of acute myocardial infarction and stroke as compared with untreated women. Although there are no data, POC users with adequately controlled and monitored hypertension should be at reduced risk of acute myocardial infarction and stroke compared with untreated hypertensive POC users.
c) Elevated blood pressure levels (properly taken measurements)				**Evidence:** Limited evidence suggests that among women with hypertension, those who used POPs or progestogen-only injectables had a small increased risk of cardiovascular events compared with women who did not use these methods.
i) systolic140-159 or diastolic 90-99	1	2	1	
ii) systolic ≥ 160 or diastolic ≥ 100	2	3	2	
d) Vascular disease	2	3	2	
HISTORY OF HIGH BLOOD PRESSURE DURING PREGNANCY (where current blood pressure is measurable and normal)	1	1	1	

(Continued)

Table 6.8
(Continued)

PROGESTOGEN-ONLY CONTRACEPTIVES (POCs)	**POCs do not protect against STI/HIV. If there is risk of STI/HIV (including during pregnancy or postpartum), the correct and consistent use of condoms is recommended, either alone or with another contraceptive method. Male latex condoms are proven to protect against STI/HIV.**			
CONDITION	**CATEGORY** I=Initiation, C=Continuation			**CLARIFICATIONS/EVIDENCE**
	POP	D/NE	LNG/ETG	
DEEP VENOUS THROMBOSIS (DVT)/ PULMONARY EMBOLISM (PE)*				
a) History of DVT/PE	2	2	2	
b) Current DVT/PE	3	3	3	
c) Family history of DVT/PE (first-degree relatives)	1	1	1	
d) Major surgery				
i) with prolonged immobilization	2	2	2	
ii) without prolonged immobilization	1	1	1	
e) Minor surgery without immobilization	1	1	1	
KNOWN THROMBOGENIC MUTATIONS (e.g., Factor V Leiden; Prothrombin mutation; Protein S, Protein C, and Antithrombin deficiencies)	2	2	2	**Clarification:** Routine screening is not appropriate because of the rarity of the conditions and the high cost of screening.
SUPERFICIAL VENOUS THROMBOSIS				
a) Varicose veins	1	1	1	
b) Superficial thrombophlebitis	1	1	1	
CURRENT AND HISTORY OF ISCHAEMIC HEART DISEASE*	I: 2, C: 3	3	I: 2, C: 3	
STROKE* (history of cerebrovascular accident)	I: 2, C: 3	3	I: 2, C: 3	

(*Continued*)

Table 6.8
(Continued)

PROGESTOGEN-ONLY CONTRACEPTIVES (POCs)	POCs do not protect against STI/HIV. If there is risk of STI/HIV (including during pregnancy or postpartum), the correct and consistent use of condoms is recommended, either alone or with another contraceptive method. Male latex condoms are proven to protect against STI/HIV.						
CONDITION	**CATEGORY** I=Initiation, C=Continuation						**CLARIFICATIONS/EVIDENCE**
	POP		D/NE		LNG/ETG		
KNOWN HYPERLIPIDEMIA	2		2		2		**Clarification:** Routine screening is not appropriate because of the rarity of the conditions and the high cost of screening. Some types of hyperlipidemias are risk factors for vascular disease.
VALVULAR HEART DISEASE							
a) Uncomplicated	1		1		1		
b) Complicated (pulmonary hypertension, risk of atrial fibrillation, history of subacute bacterial endocarditis)	1		1		1		
NEUROLOGIC CONDITIONS							
HEADACHES*	I	C	I	C	I	C	
a) Non-migrainous (mild or severe)	1	1	1	1	1	1	**Clarification:** Classification depends on accurate diagnosis of those severe headaches that are migrainous and those that are not. Any new headaches or marked changes in headaches should be evaluated. Classification is for women without any other risk factors for stroke. Risk of stroke increases with age, hypertension, and smoking.
b) Migraine							
i) without aura							
Age < 35	1	2	2	2	2	2	
Age ≥ 35	1	2	2	2	2	2	
ii) with aura, at any age	2	3	2	3	2	3	
EPILEPSY	1		1		1		**Clarification:** If a woman is taking anticonvulsants, refer to the section on drug interactions. Certain anticonvulsants lower POC effectiveness.

(*Continued*)

Table 6.8
(Continued)

PROGESTOGEN-ONLY CONTRACEPTIVES (POCs)	**POCs do not protect against STI/HIV. If there is risk of STI/HIV (including during pregnancy or postpartum), the correct and consistent use of condoms is recommended, either alone or with another contraceptive method. Male latex condoms are proven to protect against STI/HIV.**			
CONDITION	**CATEGORY** I=Initiation, C=Continuation			**CLARIFICATIONS/EVIDENCE**
	POP	D/NE	LNG/ETG	
DEPRESSIVE DISORDERS				
DEPRESSIVE DISORDERS	1	1	1	**Clarification:** The classification is based on data for women with selected depressive disorders. No data on bipolar disorder or postpartum depression were available. There is a potential for drug interactions between certain antidepressant medications and hormonal contraceptives. **Evidence:** POCs did not increase depressive symptoms in women with depression compared to baseline.
REPRODUCTIVE TRACT INFECTIONS AND DISORDERS				
VAGINAL BLEEDING PATTERNS*				
a) Irregular pattern *without* heavy bleeding	2	2	2	
b) Heavy or prolonged bleeding (includes regular and irregular patterns)	2	2	2	**Clarification:** Unusually heavy bleeding should raise the suspicion of a serious underlying condition.
UNEXPLAINED VAGINAL BLEEDING* (suspicious for serious underlying condition)				
Before evaluation	2	3	3	**Clarification:** If pregnancy or an underlying pathological condition (such as pelvic malignancy) is suspected, it must be evaluated and the category adjusted after evaluation.
ENDOMETRIOSIS	1	1	1	
BENIGN OVARIAN TUMORS (including cysts)	1	1	1	
SEVERE DYSMENORRHEA	1	1	1	

(*Continued*)

Table 6.8
(Continued)

PROGESTOGEN-ONLY CONTRACEPTIVES (POCs)	**POCs do not protect against STI/HIV. If there is risk of STI/HIV (including during pregnancy or postpartum), the correct and consistent use of condoms is recommended, either alone or with another contraceptive method. Male latex condoms are proven to protect against STI/HIV.**			
CONDITION	**CATEGORY** I=Initiation, C=Continuation			**CLARIFICATIONS/EVIDENCE**
	POP	D/NE	LNG/ETG	
TROPHOBLAST DISEASE				
a) Benign gestational trophoblastic disease	1	1	1	
b) Malignant gestational trophoblastic disease	1	1	1	
CERVICAL ECTROPION	1	1	1	
CERVICAL INTRAEPITHELIAL NEOPLASIA (CIN)	1	2	2	**Evidence:** Among women with persistent HPV infection, long-term DMPA use (≥ 5 years) may increase the risk of carcinoma in situ and invasive carcinoma.
CERVICAL CANCER (awaiting treatment)*	1	2	2	
BREAST DISEASE*				
a) Undiagnosed mass	2	2	2	**Clarification:** Evaluation should be pursued as early as possible.
b) Benign breast disease	1	1	1	
c) Family history of cancer	1	1	1	
d) Breast cancer				
(i) current	4	4	4	
(ii) past and no evidence of current disease for 5 years	3	3	3	
ENDOMETRIAL CANCER*	1	1	1	
OVARIAN CANCER*	1	1	1	
UTERINE FIBROIDS*				
a) Without distortion of the uterine cavity	1	1	1	
b) With distortion of the uterine cavity	1	1	1	

(Continued)

Table 6.8
(Continued)

PROGESTOGEN-ONLY CONTRACEPTIVES (POCs)	POCs do not protect against STI/HIV. If there is risk of STI/HIV (including during pregnancy or postpartum), the correct and consistent use of condoms is recommended, either alone or with another contraceptive method. Male latex condoms are proven to protect against STI/HIV.			
CONDITION	CATEGORY I=Initiation, C=Continuation			CLARIFICATIONS/EVIDENCE
	POP	D/NE	LNG/ETG	
PELVIC INFLAMMATORY DISEASE (PID)*				
a) Past PID (assuming no current risk factors for STIs)				
(i) with subsequent pregnancy	1	1	1	
(ii) without subsequent pregnancy	1	1	1	
b) PID - current	1	1	1	
STIs*				
a) Current purulent cervicitis or chlamydial infection or gonorrhoea	1	1	1	**Evidence:** Limited evidence suggests that there may be an increased risk of chlamydial cervicitis among DMPA users at high risk of STIs. For other STIs, there is either evidence of no association between DMPA use and STI acquisition or too limited evidence to draw any conclusions. There is no evidence for other POCs.
b) Other STIs (excluding HIV and hepatitis)	1	1	1	
c) Vaginitis (including trichomonas vaginalis and bacterial vaginosis)	1	1	1	
d) Increased risk of STIs	1	1	1	
HIV/AIDS				
HIGH RISK OF HIV*	1	1	1	**Evidence:** Overall, evidence is inconsistent regarding whether there is any increased risk of HIV acquisition among POC users compared with non-users.
HIV-INFECTED	1	1	1	**Evidence:** Studies are conflicting regarding whether there is an increased risk of HIV and herpes simplex virus (HSV) shedding among HIV-infected women using DMPA.

(Continued)

Table 6.8
(Continued)

PROGESTOGEN-ONLY CONTRACEPTIVES (POCs)	POCs do not protect against STI/HIV. If there is risk of STI/HIV (including during pregnancy or postpartum), the correct and consistent use of condoms is recommended, either alone or with another contraceptive method. Male latex condoms are proven to protect against STI/HIV.			
CONDITION	**CATEGORY** I=Initiation, C=Continuation			**CLARIFICATIONS/EVIDENCE**
	POP	D/NE	LNG/ETG	
AIDS	1	1	1	
On ARV therapy	2	2	2	**Clarification:** If a woman is taking antiretroviral (ARV) therapy, refer to the section on drug interactions. Because there may be drug interactions between hormonal contraceptives and ARVs, AIDS with ARV therapy is classified as Category 2.
OTHER INFECTIONS				
SCHISTOSOMIASIS				
a) Uncomplicated	1	1	1	**Evidence:** Among women with uncomplicated schistosomiasis, limited evidence showed that DMPA use had no adverse effects on liver function.
b) Fibrosis of liver (if severe, see cirrhosis)	1	1	1	
TUBERCULOSIS				
a) Nonpelvic	1	1	1	**Clarification:** If a woman is taking rifampicin, refer to the section on drug interactions. Rifampicin is likely to decrease POC effectiveness.
b) Known pelvic	1	1	1	
MALARIA	1	1	1	
ENDOCRINE CONDITIONS				
DIABETES*				
a) History of gestational disease	1	1	1	
b) Nonvascular disease				
(i) noninsulin dependent	2	2	2	
(ii) insulin dependent	2	2	2	

(*Continued*)

Table 6.8
(Continued)

PROGESTOGEN-ONLY CONTRACEPTIVES (POCs)	POCs do not protect against STI/HIV. If there is risk of STI/HIV (including during pregnancy or postpartum), the correct and consistent use of condoms is recommended, either alone or with another contraceptive method. Male latex condoms are proven to protect against STI/HIV.			
CONDITION	**CATEGORY** I=Initiation, C=Continuation			**CLARIFICATIONS/EVIDENCE**
	POP	D/NE	LNG/ETG	
DIABETES (Cont'd)				
c) Nephropathy/ retinopathy/ neuropathy	2	3	2	
d) Other vascular disease or diabetes of >20 years' duration	2	3	2	
THYROID DISORDERS				
a) Simple goiter	1	1	1	
b) Hyperthyroid	1	1	1	
c) Hypothyroid	1	1	1	
GASTROINTESTINAL CONDITIONS				
GALLBLADDER DISEASE				
a) Symptomatic				
(i) treated by cholecystectomy	2	2	2	
(ii) medically treated	2	2	2	
(iii) current	2	2	2	
b) Asymptomatic	2	2	2	
HISTORY OF CHOLESTASIS*				
a) Pregnancy-related	1	1	1	
b) Past COC-related	2	2	2	
VIRAL HEPATITIS*				
a) Active	3	3	3	
b) Carrier	1	1	1	
CIRRHOSIS*				
a) Mild (compensated)	2	2	2	
b) Severe (decompensated)	3	3	3	

(Continued)

Table 6.8
(Continued)

PROGESTOGEN-ONLY CONTRACEPTIVES (POCs)	POCs do not protect against STI/HIV. If there is risk of STI/HIV (including during pregnancy or postpartum), the correct and consistent use of condoms is recommended, either alone or with another contraceptive method. Male latex condoms are proven to protect against STI/HIV.			
CONDITION	**CATEGORY** I=Initiation, C=Continuation			**CLARIFICATIONS/EVIDENCE**
	POP	D/NE	LNG/ETG	
LIVER TUMORS*				
a) Benign (adenoma)	3	3	3	
b) Malignant (hepatoma)	3	3	3	
ANEMIAS				
THALASSEMIA	1	1	1	
SICKLE CELL DISEASE	1	1	1	**Evidence:** Among women with sickle cell disease, POC use did not have adverse effects on haematological parameters and, in some studies, was beneficial with respect to clinical symptoms.
IRON-DEFICIENCY ANEMIA*	1	1	1	
DRUG INTERACTIONS				
DRUGS THAT AFFECT LIVER ENZYMES				
a) Rifampicin	3	2	3	**Clarification:** Although the interaction of rifampicin or certain anticonvulsants with POPs and LNG/ETG implants is not harmful to women, it is likely to reduce the effectiveness of POPs and LNG/ETG implants. Use of other contraceptives should be encouraged for women who are long-term users of any of these drugs. Whether increasing the hormone dose of POPs alleviates this concern remains unclear. **Evidence:** Use of certain anticonvulsants decreased the contraceptive effectiveness of POCs.
b) Certain anticonvulsants (phenytoin, carbamazepine, barbiturates, primidone, topiramate, oxcarbazepine)	3	2	3	
ANTIBIOTICS (excluding rifampicin)				
a) Griseofulvin	2	1	2	
b) Other antibiotics	1	1	1	

(*Continued*)

Table 6.8
(Continued)

PROGESTOGEN-ONLY CONTRACEPTIVES (POCs)	**POCs do not protect against STI/HIV. If there is risk of STI/HIV (including during pregnancy or postpartum), the correct and consistent use of condoms is recommended, either alone or with another contraceptive method. Male latex condoms are proven to protect against STI/HIV.**		
CONDITION	**CATEGORY** I=Initiation, C=Continuation			**CLARIFICATIONS/EVIDENCE**
	POP	D/NE	LNG/ETG	
ANTIRETROVIRAL THERAPY	2	2	2	**Clarification**: It is important to note that antiretroviral drugs (ARV) have the potential to either decrease or increase the bioavailability of steroid hormones in hormonal contraceptives. The limited data available (outlined in Annex 1) suggest that potential drug interactions between many ARVs (particularly some non-nucleoside reverse transcriptase inhibitors (NNRTIs) and protease inhibitors (PIs)) and hormonal contraceptives may alter safety and effectiveness of both the hormonal contraceptives and the ARVs. It is not known whether the contraceptive effectiveness of progestogen-only injectable contraceptives (such as depot medroxyprogesterone acetate and norethisterone enantate) would be compromised, as these methods provide higher blood hormone levels than other progestogen-only hormonal contraceptives, as well as than combined oral contraceptives. Studies are underway to evaluate potential interactions between depot medroxyprogesterone acetate and selected PI and NNRTI drugs. Thus, if a woman on ARV treatment decides to initiate or continue hormonal contraceptive use, the consistent use of condoms is recommended for preventing HIV transmission and may also compensate for any possible reduction in the effectiveness of the hormonal contraceptive.

Adapted from World Health Organization, Reproductive Health and Research. Medical eligibility criteria for contraceptive use. Available at: www.who.int/reproductive-health/publications/mec/mec.pdf. Accessed May 3, 2009.

Additional comments

AGE

Menarche to < 18 years: For women under 18 years of age, there are theoretical concerns regarding the hypo-estrogenic effects of DMPA use, including whether these women will achieve their appropriate peak bone mass.

> 45 years: For women greater than age 45, there are theoretical concerns regarding hypo-estrogenic effects of DMPA use, including whether these women will regain all lost bone mass after discontinuation of DMPA.

POSTPARTUM

< 21 days: POCs may be safely used by non-breastfeeding women immediately postpartum.

PAST ECTOPIC PREGNANCY

POPs have a higher absolute rate of ectopic pregnancy compared with other POCs, but still less than using no method.

HYPERTENSION

Vascular disease: There is concern regarding hypo-estrogenic effects and reduced HDL levels, particularly among users of DMPA and NET-EN. However, there is little concern about these effects with regard to POPs or LNG/ETG implants. The effects of DMPA and NET-EN may persist for some time after discontinuation.

DEEP VENOUS THROMBOSIS (DVT)/ PULMONARY EMBOLISM (PE)

Some POCs may increase the risk of venous thrombosis, although this increase is substantially less than with COCs.

CURRENT AND HISTORY OF ISCHAEMIC HEART DISEASE

There is concern regarding hypo-estrogenic effects and reduced HDL levels, particularly among users of DMPA and NET-EN. However, there is little concern about these effects with regard to POPs or LNG/ETG implants. The effects of DMPA and NET-EN may persist for some time after discontinuation.

STROKE

There is concern regarding hypo-estrogenic effects and reduced HDL levels, particularly among users of DMPA and NET-EN. However, there is little concern about these effects with regard to POPs or LNG/ETG implants. The effects of DMPA and NET-EN may persist for some time after discontinuation.

HEADACHES

Aura is a specific focal neurologic symptom. For more information on this and other diagnostic criteria, see: Headache Classification Subcommittee of the International Headache Society. The International Classification of Headache Disorders, 2nd Edition. Cephalalgia. 2004; 24 (Suppl 1): 1- 150.
http://216.25.100.131/ihscommon/guidelines/pdfs/ihc_II_main_no_print.pdf

There is concern that severe headaches may increase with use of NET-EN, DMPA and implants. The effects of NET-EN and DMPA may persist for some time after discontinuation.

VAGINAL BLEEDING PATTERNS

Irregular menstrual bleeding patterns are common among healthy women. POC use frequently induces an irregular bleeding pattern. Implant use may induce irregular bleeding patterns, especially during the first 3-6 months, but these patterns may persist longer. ETG users are more likely than LNG users to develop amenorrhoea.

UNEXPLAINED VAGINAL BLEEDING

POCs may cause irregular bleeding patterns which may mask symptoms of underlying pathology. The effects of DMPA and NET-EN may persist for some time after discontinuation.

CERVICAL CANCER (awaiting treatment)

There is some theoretical concern that POC use may affect prognosis of the existing disease. While awaiting treatment, women may use POCs. In general, treatment of this condition renders a woman sterile.

BREAST DISEASE

Breast cancer: Breast cancer is a hormonally sensitive tumour, and the prognosis of women with current or recent breast cancer may worsen with POC use.

ENDOMETRIAL CANCER

While awaiting treatment, women may use POCs. In general, the treatment of this condition renders a woman sterile.

OVARIAN CANCER

While awaiting treatment, women may use POCs. In general, the treatment of this condition renders a woman sterile.

UTERINE FIBROIDS

POCs do not appear to cause growth of uterine fibroids.

(Continued)

PELVIC INFLAMMATORY DISEASE (PID)

Whether POCs, like COCs, reduce the risk of PID among women with STIs is unknown, but they do not protect against HIV or lower genital tract STI.

STIs

Whether POCs, like COCs, reduce the risk of PID among women with STIs is unknown, but they do not protect against HIV or lower genital tract STI.

HIGH RISK OF HIV

Whether POCs, like COCs, reduce the risk of PID among women with STIs is unknown, but they do not protect against HIV or lower genital tract STI.

DIABETES

Non-vascular disease: POCs may alter carbohydrate metabolism.

Nephropathy, retinopathy, neuropathy: There is concern regarding hypo-estrogenic effects and reduced HDL levels, particularly among users of DMPA and NET-EN. The effects of DMPA and NET-EN may persist for some time after discontinuation. Some POCs may increase the risk of thrombosis, although this increase is substantially less than with COCs.

Other vascular disease or diabetes of > 20 years' duration: There is concern regarding hypo-estrogenic effects and reduced HDL levels, particularly among users of DMPA and NET-EN. The effects of DMPA and NET-EN may persist for some time after discontinuation. Some POCs may increase the risk of thrombosis, although this increase is substantially less than with COCs.

HISTORY OF CHOLESTASIS

Theoretically, a history of COC-related cholestasis may predict subsequent cholestasis with POC use. However, this has not been documented.

VIRAL HEPATITIS

Active: POCs are metabolized by the liver and their use may adversely affect women whose liver function is compromised. This concern is similar to, but less than, that with COCs.

CIRRHOSIS

POCs are metabolized by the liver and their use may adversely affect women whose liver function is compromised. This concern is similar to, but less than, that with COCs.

LIVER TUMORS

POCs are metabolized by the liver and their use may adversely affect women whose liver function is compromised. In addition, POC use may enhance the growth of tumours. This concern is similar to, but less than, that with COCs.

IRON-DEFICIENCY ANEMIA

Changes in the menstrual pattern associated with POC use have little effect on haemoglobin levels.

G. MEDICATIONS THAT MAY BE USED TO TREAT NAUSEA (PRESCRIPTION AND NONPRESCRIPTION)

Table 6.9
Antinausea treatment options

Drug	Dose	Timing of Administration
Nonprescription drugs		
Meclizine hydrochloride (Dramamine II, Bonine)	One or two 25-mg tablets	1 h before first EC dose; repeat if needed in 24 h
Diphenhydramine Hydrochloride (Benadryl)	One or two 25-mg tablets	1 h before first EC dose; repeat as needed every 4–6 h
Dimenhydrinate (Dramamine)	One or two 50-mg tablets or 4–8 tsp of liquid	30 min to 1 h before first EC dose; repeat as needed every 4–6 h
Cyclizine hydrochloride (Marezine)	One 50-mg tablet	30 min before first EC dose; repeat as needed every 4–6 h
Prescription drugs		
Meclizine hydrochloride (Antivert)	One or two 25-mg tablets	1 h before first EC dose; repeat if needed in 24 h
Trimethobenzamide hydrochloride (Tigan)	One 250-mg tablet or 200-mg suppository	1 h before first EC dose; repeat as needed every 6–8 h
Promethazine hydrochloride (Phenergan)	One 25-mg tablet or suppository	30 min to 1 h before first EC dose; repeat as needed every 8–12 h

Adapted from Stewart F, Trussell J, Van Look PFA. Emergency contraception. In: Hatcher RA, Trussell J, Nelson AL, et al, eds. *Contraceptive Technology*. 19th ed. New York, NY: Ardent Media; 2008:105.

H. ADVERSE EFFECTS RELATED TO HORMONE CONTENT

Table 6.10
Potential adverse effects related to hormone content in the adolescent/young adult woman

Estrogen	Progestin
Reproductive hormones	
Effect[a]	Effect[b]
Increased breast size/tenderness	Increased breast size/tenderness
Dysmenorrhea	Decreased libido
Increased menstrual flow	Decreased menstrual flow
Increased mucous vaginal discharge	Frequent yeast infections
Deficiency[a]	Deficiency[b]
Breakthrough bleeding, day 1–10 pills	Breakthrough bleeding, day 10–21 pills
Decreased menstrual flow	Increased menstrual flow
Vaginal dryness/lack of lubrication	
Nervousness/irritability	
Vasomotor symptoms	
General	
Adverse effect	
Melasma/cholasma[c]	Appetite increase/weight gain, fluid retention
Nausea/vomiting	Depression/mood swings
Headache	Fatigue
Weight gain, increase in adipose tissue	Acne
	Hirsutism
	Constipation, bloating-slowed peristalsis
Cardiovascular	
Thromboembolic disease[d]	Increased insulin resistance
Hypertension[e]	Increased cholesterol (low-density lipoprotein)
Telangiectasia[f]	
Increase cholesterol (high-density lipoprotein)	
Increase triglycerides	
Arterial thromboses-stroke[g]	
Hepatocellular adenoma (minimal risk in only those on ≥50-μg EE pills)	

EE indicates ethinyl estradiol.

[a] Indicates a need to adjust the estrogen dose.

[b] Indicates a need to either adjust the progestin dose as switching (eg, monophasic to triphasic to reduce the dose of progestin) or switching types of progestins.

[c] Increased melanocyte activity.

[d] Risk of DVT is 4 to 5 per 100 000 general population, 48 to 60 per 100 000 for pregnant women, 24 to 60 per 100 000 for women on COCs with ≥50-μg COCs, and 12 to 20 per 100 000 for women on COCs with <50 μg of COCs. Alone, a BMI of >30 increases risk of DVT by almost 3.5 times. Rates of DVT are higher in desogestrel-containing pills (53.5 per 100 000) compared with norgestrel (30.6 per 100 000), levonorgestrel (27.1 per 100 000), and pregnancy (123 per 100 000).

[e] Increase liver's production of renin → plasma angiotensinogen → angiotensin I → angiotensin II → aldosterone; estrogen, progestin → aldosterone → fluid retention.

[f] Fine dilated intracutaneous veins.

[g] Ischemic stroke risks: migraine with visual aura, hypertension, smoking, and increased age; hemorrhagic stroke risks: increased age, hypertension, smoking, obesity, and heavy alcohol use.

Adapted from Hatcher RA, Trussell J, Nelson AL, Cates W Jr, Stewart FH, Kowal D. Combined oral contraceptives. In: *Contraceptive Technology*. 19th ed. New York, NY: Ardent Media; 2008:214–224, 240–249.

Table 6.11
Intrauterine devices

Cu-IUD = Copper-bearing IUD
LNG-IUD = Levonorgestrel-releasing IUD (20 μg /24hours)

INTRAUTERINE DEVICES (IUDs)	**IUDs do not protect against STI/HIV. If there is risk of STI/HIV (including the postpartum period), the correct and consistent use of condoms is recommended, either alone or with another contraceptive method. Male latex condoms are proven to protect against STI/HIV.**		
CONDITION	**CATEGORY** I=Initiation, C=Continuation		**CLARIFICATIONS/EVIDENCE**
	Cu-IUD	**LNG-IUD**	
PERSONAL CHARACTERISTICS AND REPRODUCTIVE HISTORY			
PREGNANCY	4	4	**Clarification:** The IUD is not indicated during pregnancy and should not be used because of the risk of serious pelvic infection and septic spontaneous abortion.
AGE*			
a) Menarche to < 20 years	2	2	
b) ≥ 20 years	1	1	
PARITY*			
a) Nulliparous	2	2	**Evidence:** There are conflicting data regarding whether IUD use is associated with infertility among nulliparous women, although recent, well-conducted studies suggest no increased risk.
b) Parous	1	1	
POSTPARTUM* (breastfeeding or non breastfeeding, including postcaesarean section)			
a) < 48 hours	2	3	**Evidence:** There was some increase in expulsion rates with delayed postpartum insertion compared to immediate insertion and with immediate postpartum insertion compared to interval insertion.
b) 48 hours to < 4 weeks	3	3	
c) ≥ 4 weeks	1	1	
d) Puerperal sepsis	4	4	

* See also additional comments at end of table

(Continued)

Table 6.11
(Continued)

INTRAUTERINE DEVICES (IUDs)	IUDs do not protect against STI/HIV. If there is risk of STI/HIV (including the postpartum period), the correct and consistent use of condoms is recommended, either alone or with another contraceptive method. Male latex condoms are proven to protect against STI/HIV.		
CONDITION	**CATEGORY** I=Initiation, C=Continuation		**CLARIFICATIONS/EVIDENCE**
	Cu-IUD	**LNG-IUD**	
POST-ABORTION*			
a) First trimester	1	1	**Clarification:** IUDs can be inserted immediately after first-trimester, spontaneous or induced abortion. **Evidence:** There was no difference in risk of complications for immediate versus delayed insertion of an IUD after abortion. Expulsion was greater when an IUD was inserted following a second-trimester abortion versus following a first-trimester abortion. There were no differences in safety or expulsions for post-abortion insertion of an LNG-IUD compared with Cu-IUD.
b) Second trimester	2	2	
c) Immediate postseptic abortion	4	4	
PAST ECTOPIC PREGNANCY*	1	1	
HISTORY OF PELVIC SURGERY (see postpartum, including caesarean section)	1	1	
SMOKING			
a) Age < 35 years	1	1	
b) Age ≥ 35 years			
(i) < 15 cigarettes/day	1	1	
(ii) ≥ 15 cigarettes/day	1	1	
OBESITY ≥ 30 kg/m² body mass index (BMI)	1	1	
BLOOD PRESSURE MEASUREMENT UNAVAILABLE	NA	NA	**Clarification:** While a blood pressure measurement may be appropriate for good preventative health care, it is not materially related to safe and effective IUD use. Women should not be denied use of IUDs simply because their blood pressure cannot be measured.

(Continued)

Table 6.11
(Continued)

INTRAUTERINE DEVICES (IUDs)	**IUDs do not protect against STI/HIV. If there is risk of STI/HIV (including the postpartum period), the correct and consistent use of condoms is recommended, either alone or with another contraceptive method. Male latex condoms are proven to protect against STI/HIV.**		
CONDITION	**CATEGORY** I=Initiation, C=Continuation		**CLARIFICATIONS/EVIDENCE**
	Cu-IUD	**LNG-IUD**	
CARDIOVASCULAR DISEASE			
MULTIPLE RISK FACTORS FOR ARTERIAL CARDIOVASCULAR DISEASE (such as older age, smoking, diabetes and hypertension)	1	2	
HYPERTENSION*			
For all categories of hypertension, classifications are based on the assumption that no other risk factors for cardiovascular disease exist. When multiple risk factors do exist, risk of cardiovascular disease may increase substantially. A single reading of blood pressure level is not sufficient to classify a woman as hypertensive.			
a) History of hypertension where blood pressure CANNOT be evaluated (including hypertension in pregnancy)	1	2	
b) Adequately controlled hypertension where blood pressure CAN be evaluated	1	1	
c) Elevated blood pressure levels (properly taken measurements)			
(i) systolic 140-159 or diastolic 90-99	1	1	
(ii) systolic ≥ 160 or diastolic ≥ 100	1	2	
d) Vascular disease	1	2	
HISTORY OF HIGH BLOOD PRESSURE DURING PREGNANCY (where current blood pressure is measurable and normal)	1	1	

(Continued)

Table 6.11
(Continued)

INTRAUTERINE DEVICES (IUDs)	IUDs do not protect against STI/HIV. If there is risk of STI/HIV (including the postpartum period), the correct and consistent use of condoms is recommended, either alone or with another contraceptive method. Male latex condoms are proven to protect against STI/HIV.		
CONDITION	**CATEGORY** I=Initiation, C=Continuation		**CLARIFICATIONS/EVIDENCE**
	Cu-IUD	**LNG-IUD**	
DEEP VENOUS THROMBOSIS (DVT)/ PULMONARY EMBOLISM (PE)*			
a) History of DVT/PE	1	2	
b) Current DVT/PE	1	3	
c) Family history of DVT/PE (first-degree relatives)	1	1	
d) Major surgery			
(i) with prolonged immobilization	1	2	
(ii) without prolonged immobilization	1	1	
e) Minor surgery without immobilization	1	1	
KNOWN THROMBOGENIC MUTATIONS (e.g., Factor V Leiden; Prothrombin mutation; Protein S, Protein C, and Antithrombin deficiencies)	1	2	**Clarification:** Routine screening is not appropriate because of the rarity of the conditions and the high cost of screening.
SUPERFICIAL VENOUS THROMBOSIS			
a) Varicose veins	1	1	
b) Superficial thrombophlebitis	1	1	
CURRENT AND HISTORY OF ISCHEMIC HEART DISEASE*	1	I: 2, C: 3	
STROKE* (history of cerebrovascular accident)	1	2	

(*Continued*)

Table 6.11
(Continued)

INTRAUTERINE DEVICES (IUDs)	IUDs do not protect against STI/HIV. If there is risk of STI/HIV (including the postpartum period), the correct and consistent use of condoms is recommended, either alone or with another contraceptive method. Male latex condoms are proven to protect against STI/HIV.			
CONDITION	**CATEGORY** I=Initiation, C=Continuation			**CLARIFICATIONS/EVIDENCE**
	Cu-IUD	**LNG-IUD**		
KNOWN HYPERLIPIDEMIAS	1	2		**Clarification:** Routine screening is not appropriate because of the rarity of the conditions and the high cost of screening.
VALVULAR HEART DISEASE				
a) Uncomplicated	1	1		
b) Complicated (pulmonary hypertension, risk of atrial fibrillation, history of subacute bacterial endocarditis)	2	2		**Clarification:** Prophylactic antibiotics to prevent endocarditis are advised for insertion.
NEUROLOGIC CONDITIONS				
HEADACHES*		I	C	
a) Non-migrainous (mild or severe)	1	1	1	**Clarification:** Any new headaches or marked changes in headaches should be evaluated.
b) Migraine				
(i) without aura				
Age < 35	1	2	2	
Age ≥ 35	1	2	2	
(ii) with aura, at any age	1	2	3	
EPILEPSY	1	1		
DEPRESSIVE DISORDERS				
DEPRESSIVE DISORDERS	1	1		**Clarification**: The classification is based on data for women with selected depressive disorders. No data on bipolar disorder or postpartum depression were available. There is a potential for drug interactions between certain antidepressant medications and hormonal contraceptives.

(*Continued*)

Table 6.11
(Continued)

INTRAUTERINE DEVICES (IUDs)	**IUDs do not protect against STI/HIV. If there is risk of STI/HIV (including the postpartum period), the correct and consistent use of condoms is recommended, either alone or with another contraceptive method. Male latex condoms are proven to protect against STI/HIV.**				
CONDITION	**CATEGORY** I=Initiation, C=Continuation				**CLARIFICATIONS/EVIDENCE**
	Cu-IUD		**LNG-IUD**		
REPRODUCTIVE TRACT INFECTIONS AND DISORDERS					
VAGINAL BLEEDING PATTERNS*			I	C	
a) Irregular pattern *without* heavy bleeding	1		1	1	
b) Heavy or prolonged bleeding (includes regular and irregular patterns)	2		1	2	**Clarification:** Unusually heavy bleeding should raise the suspicion of a serious underlying condition. **Evidence:** Among women with heavy or prolonged bleeding, LNG-IUDs were beneficial in treating menorrhagia.
UNEXPLAINED VAGINAL BLEEDING (suspicion for serious condition)	I	C	I	C	**Clarification:** If pregnancy or an underlying pathological condition (such as pelvic malignancy) is suspected, it must be evaluated and the category adjusted after evaluation. There is no need to remove the IUD before evaluation.
Before evaluation	4	2	4	2	
ENDOMETRIOSIS*	2		1		**Evidence:** LNG-IUD use among women with endometriosis decreased dysmenorrhoea and pelvic pain.
BENIGN OVARIAN TUMORS (including cysts)	1		1		
SEVERE DYSMENORRHEA*	2		1		
TROPHOBLAST DISEASE*					
a) Benign gestational trophoblastic disease	3		3		
b) Malignant gestational trophoblastic disease	4		4		
CERVICAL ECTROPION	1		1		
CERVICAL INTRAEPITHELIAL NEOPLASIA (CIN)*	1		2		
CERVICAL CANCER* (awaiting treatment)	I	C	I	C	
	4	2	4	2	

(Continued)

Table 6.11
(Continued)

INTRAUTERINE DEVICES (IUDs)	IUDs do not protect against STI/HIV. If there is risk of STI/HIV (including the postpartum period), the correct and consistent use of condoms is recommended, either alone or with another contraceptive method. Male latex condoms are proven to protect against STI/HIV.				
CONDITION	**CATEGORY** I=Initiation, C=Continuation				**CLARIFICATIONS/EVIDENCE**
	Cu-IUD		**LNG-IUD**		
BREAST DISEASE*					
a) Undiagnosed mass	1		2		
b) Benign breast disease	1		1		
c) Family history of cancer	1		1		
d) Breast cancer:					
(i) current	1		4		
(ii) past and no evidence of current disease for 5 years	1		3		
ENDOMETRIAL CANCER*	I	C	I	C	
	4	2	4	2	
OVARIAN CANCER*	3	2	3	2	
UTERINE FIBROIDS*					
a) Without distortion of the uterine cavity	1		1		**Evidence:** Among women with fibroids, there were no adverse health events with LNG-IUD use and there was a decrease in symptoms and size of fibroids for some women.
b) With distortion of the uterine cavity	4		4		
ANATOMICAL ABNORMALITIES*					
a) Distorted uterine cavity (any congenital or acquired uterine abnormality distorting the uterine cavity in a manner that is incompatible with IUD insertion)	4		4		
b) Other abnormalities (including cervical stenosis or cervical lacerations) not distorting the uterine cavity or interfering with IUD insertion	2		2		

(*Continued*)

Table 6.11
(Continued)

INTRAUTERINE DEVICES (IUDs)	**IUDs do not protect against STI/HIV. If there is risk of STI/HIV (including the postpartum period), the correct and consistent use of condoms is recommended, either alone or with another contraceptive method. Male latex condoms are proven to protect against STI/HIV.**				
CONDITION	**CATEGORY** I=Initiation, C=Continuation				**CLARIFICATIONS/EVIDENCE**
	Cu-IUD		**LNG-IUD**		
PELVIC INFLAMMATORY DISEASE (PID)*	I	C	I	C	
a) Past PID (assuming no known current risk factors for STIs)					
(i) with subsequent pregnancy	1	1	1	1	
(ii) without subsequent pregnancy	2	2	2	2	
b) PID - current	4	2	4	2	**Clarification for continuation:** Treat the PID using appropriate antibiotics. There is usually no need for removal of the IUD if the client wishes to continue its use. (See *Selected Practice Recommendations for Contraceptive Use*. WHO: Geneva, 2002). Continued use of an IUD depends on the woman's informed choice and her current risk factors for STIs and PID. **Evidence:** Among IUD users treated for PID, there was no difference in clinical course if the IUD was removed or left in place.
STIs*	I	C	I	C	
a) Current purulent cervicitis or chlamydial infection or gonorrhoea	4	2	4	2	**Clarification for continuation:** Treat the STI using appropriate antibiotics. There is usually no need for removal of the IUD if the client wishes to continue its use. Continued use of an IUD depends on the woman's informed choice and her current risk factors for STIs and PID. **Evidence:** There is no evidence regarding whether IUD insertion among women with STIs increases the risk of PID compared with no IUD insertion. Among women who have an IUD inserted, the absolute risk of subsequent PID was low among women with STI at the time of insertion but greater than among women with no STI at the time of IUD insertion.
b) Other STIs (excluding HIV and hepatitis)	2	2	2	2	
c) Vaginitis (including trichomonas vaginalis and bacterial vaginosis)	2	2	2	2	

(Continued)

Table 6.11
(Continued)

INTRAUTERINE DEVICES (IUDs)	**IUDs do not protect against STI/HIV. If there is risk of STI/HIV (including the postpartum period), the correct and consistent use of condoms is recommended, either alone or with another contraceptive method. Male latex condoms are proven to protect against STI/HIV.**				
CONDITION	**CATEGORY** I=Initiation, C=Continuation				**CLARIFICATIONS/EVIDENCE**
	Cu-IUD		**LNG-IUD**		
STIs (Cont'd)					
d) Increased risk of STIs	2/3	2	2/3	2	**Clarification for initiation**: If a woman has a very high individual likelihood of exposure to gonorrhoea or chlamydial infection, the condition is a Category 3. **Evidence:** Using an algorithm to classify STI risk status among IUD users, one study reported that 11% of high STI-risk women experienced IUD-related complications compared with 5% of those not classified as high risk.
HIV/AIDS					
HIGH RISK OF HIV*	I	C	I	C	
	2	2	2	2	**Evidence:** Among women at risk of HIV, copper IUD use did not increase risk of HIV acquisition.
HIV-INFECTED	2	2	2	2	**Evidence:** Among IUD users, there is limited evidence showing no increased risk of overall complications or infection-related complications when comparing HIV-infected women with non-infected women. Furthermore, IUD use among HIV-infected women was not associated with increased risk of transmission to sexual partners.
AIDS	3	2	3	2	**Clarification for continuation:** IUD users with AIDS should be closely monitored for pelvic infection.
Clinically well on ARV therapy	2	2	2	2	
OTHER INFECTIONS					
SCHISTOSOMIASIS					
a) Uncomplicated	1		1		
b) Fibrosis of the liver (if severe, see cirrhosis)	1		1		
TUBERCULOSIS*	I	C	I	C	
a) Non-pelvic	1	1	1	1	
b) Known pelvic	4	3	4	3	

(*Continued*)

Table 6.11
(Continued)

INTRAUTERINE DEVICES (IUDs)	IUDs do not protect against STI/HIV. If there is risk of STI/HIV (including the postpartum period), the correct and consistent use of condoms is recommended, either alone or with another contraceptive method. Male latex condoms are proven to protect against STI/HIV.		
CONDITION	CATEGORY I=Initiation, C=Continuation		CLARIFICATIONS/EVIDENCE
	Cu-IUD	LNG-IUD	
MALARIA	1	1	
ENDOCRINE CONDITIONS			
DIABETES*			
a) History of gestational disease	1	1	
b) Nonvascular disease			
(i) noninsulin dependent	1	2	
(ii) insulin dependent	1	2	
c) Nephropathy/ retinopathy/ neuropathy	1	2	
d) Other vascular disease or diabetes of >20 years' duration	1	2	
THYROID DISORDERS			
a) Simple goiter	1	1	
b) Hyperthyroid	1	1	
c) Hypothyroid	1	1	
GASTROINTESTINAL CONDITIONS			
GALLBLADDER DISEASE			
a) Symptomatic			
(i) treated by cholecystectomy	1	2	
(ii) medically treated	1	2	
(iii) current	1	2	
b) Asymptomatic	1	2	
HISTORY OF CHOLESTASIS*			
a) Pregnancy-related	1	1	
b) Past COC-related	1	2	

(Continued)

Table 6.11
(Continued)

INTRAUTERINE DEVICES (IUDs)	IUDs do not protect against STI/HIV. If there is risk of STI/HIV (including the postpartum period), the correct and consistent use of condoms is recommended, either alone or with another contraceptive method. Male latex condoms are proven to protect against STI/HIV.		
CONDITION	**CATEGORY** I=Initiation, C=Continuation		**CLARIFICATIONS/EVIDENCE**
	Cu-IUD	**LNG-IUD**	
VIRAL HEPATITIS*			
a) Active	1	3	
b) Carrier	1	1	
CIRRHOSIS*			
a) Mild (compensated)	1	2	
b) Severe (decompensated)	1	3	
LIVER TUMORS*			
a) Benign (adenoma)	1	3	
b) Malignant (hepatoma)	1	3	
ANEMIAS			
THALASSEMIA*	2	1	
SICKLE CELL DISEASE*	2	1	
IRON-DEFICIENCY ANEMIA*	2	1	
DRUG INTERACTIONS			
DRUGS THAT AFFECT LIVER ENZYMES			
a) Rifampicin	1	1	**Evidence:** One study found that rifabutin, which is in the same class of drugs as rifampicin, has no impact on the effectiveness of LNG-IUD.
b) Certain anticonvulsants (phenytoin, carbamazepine, barbiturates, primidone, topiramate, oxcarbazepine)	1	1	
ANTIBIOTICS (excluding rifampicin)	1	1	
a) Griseofulvin	1	1	
b) Other antibiotics	1	1	

(Continued)

Table 6.11
(Continued)

INTRAUTERINE DEVICES (IUDs)	**IUDs do not protect against STI/HIV. If there is risk of STI/HIV (including the postpartum period), the correct and consistent use of condoms is recommended, either alone or with another contraceptive method. Male latex condoms are proven to protect against STI/HIV.**				
CONDITION	**CATEGORY** I=Initiation, C=Continuation				**CLARIFICATIONS/EVIDENCE**
	Cu-IUD		**LNG-IUD**		
ANTIRETROVIRAL THERAPY	I	C	I	C	
	2/3	2	2/3	2	**Clarification**: There is no known drug interaction between ARV therapy and IUD use. However, AIDS as a condition is classified as Category 3 for insertion and Category 2 for continuation unless the woman is clinically well on ARV therapy in which case, both insertion and continuation are classified as Category 2. (See AIDS condition above.)

Adapted from World Health Organization, Reproductive Health and Research. Medical eligibility criteria for contraceptive use. Available at: www.who.int/reproductive-health/publications/mec/mec.pdf. Accessed May 3, 2009.

Additional comments

AGE

Menarche to < 20 years: There is concern both about the risk of expulsion due to nulliparity and risk of STIs due to sexual behaviour in younger age groups.

PARITY

Nulliparous: Nulliparity is related to an increased risk of expulsion.

POSTPARTUM

< 48 hours, 48 hours to < 4 weeks, ≥ 4 weeks: Concern that the neonate may be at risk due to exposure to steroid hormones with LNG-IUD use during the first 6 weeks postpartum is the same as for other POCs.

Puerperal sepsis: Insertion of an IUD may substantially worsen the condition.

POST-ABORTION

Immediate post-septic abortion: Insertion of an IUD may substantially worsen the condition.

PAST ECTOPIC PREGNANCY

The absolute risk of ectopic pregnancy is extremely low due to the high effectiveness of IUDs. However, when a woman becomes pregnant during IUD use, the relative likelihood of ectopic pregnancy is greatly increased.

HYPERTENSION

There is theoretical concern about the effect of LNG on lipids. There is no restriction for copper IUDs.

DEEP VENOUS THROMBOSIS (DVT)/ PULMONARY EMBOLISM (PE)

Some progestogens may increase the risk of venous thrombosis, although this increase is substantially less than for COCs.

CURRENT AND HISTORY OF ISCHAEMIC HEART DISEASE

There is theoretical concern about the effect of LNG on lipids. There is no restriction for copper IUDs.

STROKE

There is theoretical concern about the effect of LNG on lipids. There is no restriction for copper IUDs.

HEADACHES

Aura is a specific focal neurologic symptom. For more information on this and other diagnostic criteria, see: Headache Classification Subcommittee of the International Headache Society. The International Classification of Headache Disorders, 2nd Edition. Cephalalgia. 2004; 24 (Suppl 1): 1- 150.
http://216.25.100.131/ihscommon/guidelines/pdfs/ihc_II_main_no_print.pdf

VAGINAL BLEEDING PATTERNS

LNG-IUD use frequently causes changes in menstrual bleeding patterns. Over time, LNG-IUD users are more likely than non-users to become amenorrhoeic, thus LNG-IUDs are sometimes used as a treatment to correct heavy bleeding.

ENDOMETRIOSIS

Copper IUD use may worsen dysmenorrhoea associated with the condition.

SEVERE DYSMENORRHEA

Dysmenorrhea may intensify with copper IUD use. LNG-IUD use has been associated with reduction of dysmenorrhoea.

TROPHOBLAST DISEASE

There is an increased risk of perforation since the treatment for the condition may require multiple uterine curettages.

CERVICAL INTRAEPITHELIAL NEOPLASIA (CIN)

There is some theoretical concern that LNG-IUDs may enhance progression of CIN.

CERVICAL CANCER (awaiting treatment)

There is concern about the increased risk of infection and bleeding at insertion. The IUD will likely need to be removed at the time of treatment but, until then, the woman is at risk of pregnancy.

BREAST DISEASE

Breast cancer: Breast cancer is a hormonally sensitive tumour. Concerns about progression of the disease may be less with LNG-IUDs than with COCs or higher-dose POCs.

ENDOMETRIAL CANCER

There is concern about the increased risk of infection, perforation and bleeding at insertion. The IUD will likely need to be removed at the time of treatment but, until then, the woman is at risk of pregnancy.

(Continued)

OVARIAN CANCER
The IUD will likely need to be removed at the time of treatment but, until then, the woman is at risk of pregnancy.

UTERINE FIBROIDS
Without distortion of the uterine cavity: Women with heavy or prolonged bleeding should be assigned the category for that condition.

With distortion of the uterine cavity: Pre-existing uterine fibroids that distort the uterine cavity may be incompatible with insertion and proper placement of the IUD.

ANATOMICAL ABNORMALITIES
Distorted uterine cavity: In the presence of an anatomic abnormality that distorts the uterine cavity, proper IUD placement may not be possible.

PELVIC INFLAMMATORY DISEASE (PID)
IUDs do not protect against STI/HIV/PID. In women at low risk of STIs, IUD insertion poses little risk of PID. Current risk of STIs and desire for future pregnancy are relevant considerations.

STIs
IUDs do not protect against STI/HIV/PID. Among women with chlamydial infection or gonorrhoea, the potential increased risk of PID with IUD insertions should be avoided. The concern is less for other STIs.

HIGH RISK OF HIV
IUDs do not protect against STI/HIV/PID.

TUBERCULOSIS
Known pelvic: Insertion of an IUD may substantially worsen known the condition.

DIABETES
Whether the amount of LNG released by the IUD may slightly influence carbohydrate and lipid metabolism is unclear. Some progestogens may increase the risk of thrombosis, although this increase is substantially less than for COCs.

HISTORY OF CHOLESTASIS
There is concern that a history of COC-related cholestasis may predict subsequent cholestasis with LNG use. Whether there is any risk with use of an LNG-IUD is unclear.

VIRAL HEPATITIS
Active: POCs are metabolized by the liver and their use may adversely affect women whose liver function is compromised. This concern is similar to, but less than, that with COCs.

CIRRHOSIS
POCs are metabolized by the liver and their use may adversely affect women whose liver function is compromised. This concern is similar to, but less than, that with COCs.

LIVER TUMORS
POCs are metabolized by the liver and their use may adversely affect women whose liver function is compromised. In addition, POC use may enhance the growth of tumours. This concern is similar to, but less than, that with COCs.

THALASSEMIA
There is concern about an increased risk of blood loss with copper IUDs.

SICKLE CELL DISEASE
There is concern about an increased risk of blood loss with copper IUDs.

IRON-DEFICIENCY ANEMIA
There is concern about an increased risk of blood loss with copper IUDs.

I. STARTING OCS

- First-day start: first day of next period
- Sunday start: Sunday after the next period begins, even if still bleeding†
- Quick start: same-day start, if it can be documented that the patient is not pregnant, with use of a back-up method (eg, condoms or abstinence) for the next 7 days to avoid pregnancy‡

†Suppression of ovulation does not occur until at least 7 days of hormonally active pills are taken.
‡Offer EC if indicated.

J. OTHER IMPORTANT ALTERATION OF LABORATORY TESTS AND CLINICAL/METABOLIC EFFECTS BY COMBINED HORMONE CONTRACEPTIVES FOR ADOLESCENTS AND YOUNG ADULTS

Scenario: Increase in liver's production of thyroxine-binding globulin.

Result: patient appears "chemically" hyperthyroid if total thyroxine is used to screen for hyperthyroidism; suggest measuring free thyroxine and thyrotropin in patients on OCs to assess thyroid status.

Scenario: Increase in liver's production of sex hormone–binding globulin.

Result: diminished free fraction of sex steroids available as free testosterone.

Scenario: Increase liver's production of transcortin, the cortisol-binding globulin.

Result: clinical or metabolic effect unknown.

Clotting

Clot formation → balance of clotting factors

- Proclotting: I (fibrinogen), VII, IX, and X
- Anti-clotting: antithrombin III, protein C, and protein S
- Clot organization: plasminogen and plasminogen activator inhibitor 1
- Factors that lyse clots: tissue plasminogen activator, antiplasmin
- Imbalance equals clots
- Increase risk in clot formation when relative deficiency, such as in genetic thrombogenic mutations
- Activated protein C deficiency (APC resistance or factor V Leiden mutation): mutation renders activated factor V relatively resistant to degradation by APC; prevalence is ~5.3% among white population, 2.2% among Hispanic population, 1.2% among black population, and 0.45% among Asian American population in the US
- Other clotting problems: protein C deficiency, protein S deficiency, antithrombin III deficiency, and presence of antiphospholipid antibodies

K. HEALTH BENEFITS OF OCS

- Control menstrual function/disorders (eg, dysmenorrhea, dysfunctional uterine bleeding, menorrhagia, menstrual-related premenstrual syndrome symptoms, midcycle pain, polycystic ovary syndrome, premenstrual dysphoric disorder)
- Pain from endometriosis

- Reduce risk of ovulatory or postovulatory ovarian cysts
- Acne, hirsutism treatment
- Diminish iron loss with decreased risk of anemia
- Improve and/or stabilize bone mineral density
- Menstrual control for young women with developmental, physical disabilities
- Reduce risk for pelvic inflammatory disease associated with gonorrhea but not chlamydial infection
- Reduce risk for ectopic pregnancy
- Decrease risks of episodes of menstrual-related exacerbations of sickle cell disease, seizures, porphyria, and asthma
- Protective effect against endometrial cancer and ovarian cancer

L. REPRODUCTIVE CANCERS AND USE OF COCS

Breast (Second Most Common Cancer in Women)

- Incidence of breast cancer for women aged <35 years is ~1:250 (17 per 10 000 nonusers and 26 per 10 000 users); current users of pills are at a slight increased risk of breast cancer (relative risk: 1.2) because of earlier detection (in care) and/or promotion of already present cancer cells
- From ages 35 to 54 years, the diagnosis of breast cancer is not increased for women with a history of current or past use of COCs; 10 years after discontinuing pills, no increased risk
- Use of OCs in women with a strong family history of *BRCA1* or *BRCA2* mutations do not increase their risk by being on COCs

Cervical (Third Most Common Cancer in Women)

- More studies are needed to evaluate the use of OCs and their relationship to the incidence of cervical cancer
- Studies of several populations suggest increased risk with longer duration of COC use and infection with human papillomavirus (relative risk of 1.1 after 5 years of use, 1.6 after 5–10 years, and 2.2 after >10 years of use)

Endometrial (Fourth Most Common Cancer in Women)

- Ever use of low- or moderate-dose pills ≥30 μg is protective against endometrial cancer
- After 1 year of use, 20% reduction in risk; after 4 years, 60% reduction in risk
- Long-term use of COCs for >10 years provides 80% reduction in risk with protection lasting 30 years after discontinuation

Ovarian (Sixth Most Common Cancer in Women)

- Ever use of even low-dose COCs reduces risk of epithelial cancers by 34%; estimates are 50% protection after 5 years of use
- Long-term use of COCs for >10 years provides 80% reduction in the risk, with protection lasting for 30 years after discontinuation
- Studies of carriers of the *BRCA* genetic mutations indicate similar protection from ovarian cancer for those on COCs

References: Hatcher RA, Trussell J, Nelson AL, Cates W Jr, Stewart FH, Kowal D. Combined oral contraceptives. In: *Contraceptive Technology*. 19th ed. New York, NY: Ardent Media; 2008:201–224; and Bridging the Gap Communications. Managing contraception. Available at: www.managingcontraception.com. Accessed May 3, 2009.

M. DRUGS THAT INTERFERE WITH THE EFFICACY OF OCS

- Antibiotics: rifampin
- Anticonvulsant medications: carbamazepine, ethosuximide, felbamate, oxcarbazepine, phenobarbital, phenytoin, primidone, and topiramate
- Antidepressants: hypericum (St John's wort)
- Antifungal agents: griseofulvin
- Anti-HIV drugs: protease inhibitors (eg, amprenavir, indinavir, lopinavir/ritonavir, nelfinavir, and saquinavir)
- Nonnucleoside reverse transcriptase inhibitors (eg, nevirapine)

Note that some drugs may decrease the clearance of OCs and potentially increase estrogen side levels/adverse effects:

- Adverse effects: nausea, vomiting, breast tenderness, migraine headaches, and thromboembolic events
- Drugs: antidepressants (selective serotonin reuptake inhibitors or others such as nefazodone), antiviral agents (ritonavir), antifungal agents (ketoconazole), and calcium channel blockers (diltiazem)

The coadministration of OCs and some drugs may effectively increase the concentration of the drug:

- Oral corticosteroids
- Chlorpromazine
- Benzodiazepines (eg, alprazolam, diazepine, lorazepam, clonazepam, and clorazepate dipotassium)
- Theophylline

The coadministration of OCs and some drugs may effectively increase efficacy or concentration of the drug:

- Lamotrigine (Lamictal)
- Tricyclic antidepressants
- Aspirin
- Acetaminophen

Other herbal remedies with the potential to decrease efficacy of OCs:

- Milk thistle
- Agelica dahurica
- Ginseng
- Garlic preparations
- Danshen
- Liqorice

N. MISSED-PILL INSTRUCTIONS FOR SEXUALLY ACTIVE TEENAGERS

For those using <30-μg pills:

- Miss 1 pill: take pill as soon as it is remembered. Take same-day pill at the regular time. No back-up method is considered necessary. Consider EC if pills missed first week of new pack and unprotected intercourse
- Miss ≥2 pills: take pill as soon as it is remembered. Take same-day pill at the regular time. Consider EC if pills missed first week of new pack and unprotected intercourse. Use condoms or abstain from intercourse until active pills for at least 7 days in a row

For those using ≥30 μg pills:

- Miss 1 or 2 pills: take pill as soon as it is remembered. Take same-day pill at the regular time. No back-up method is considered necessary. Consider EC if pills missed first week of new pack and unprotected intercourse
- Miss ≥3 pills during first 2 weeks of pill pack: take pill as soon as it is remembered. Take same-day pill at the regular time. Consider EC if pills missed first week of new pack and unprotected intercourse. Use condoms or abstain from intercourse until active pills taken for at least 7 days in a row
- Miss ≥3 pills during third week of pill pack: finish active pills in pill pack and start new pack

O. CONDOM DOS AND DON'TS

Reference: Centers for Disease Control and Prevention. Male latex condoms and sexually transmitted diseases. Available at: www.cdc.gov/nchstp/od/condoms.pdf. Accessed May 3, 2009.

Condom Materials

- Natural rubber (latex)
- Polyurethane (plastic)
- Natural skin (lamb membrane) (natural skin is not recommended)

"Common" Condom Errors

- Failure to use condoms with every act of intercourse (inconsistent use)
- Failure to use condoms throughout intercourse (incorrect use)
- Improper lubricant use with latex condoms
  - Safe: spermicides, lubricants (Aqua Lube, Astroglide, Gynol II, H-R lubricating jelly, K-Y Jelly, Wet, egg whites, glycerin, saliva, and water)
  - Unsafe: baby oil, cold cream, edible oils (eg, olive, peanut, corn, sunflower), hand and body lotions, massage oils, petroleum jelly, rubbing alcohol, suntan oil or lotion, mineral oil, vaginal lubricants that contain mineral oil, and vaginal yeast infection medication (cream or suppositories)
- Incorrect placement of the condom on the penis (incorrect use)
- Incorrect withdrawal technique (inconsistent use)

Condom Instructions

- Open condom package carefully to avoid damaging it with fingernails, teeth, or other sharp objects
- Put on the condom before the penis comes in contact with the partner's mouth, anus, or vagina. If the penis is uncircumcised, pull the foreskin back before putting on the condom. Keep the condom on the penis until after intercourse or ejaculation
- Unroll the condom a short distance to make sure the condom is being unrolled in the right direction. The rolled ring should be on the outside. Then, hold the tip of the condom and unroll it down to the base of the erect penis. If the condom does not unroll easily, it is on upside-down and may expose the partner to infectious organisms contained in the preejaculate. Discard it and begin with a new condom
- Adequate lubrication is important. For latex condoms, use only water-based lubricants (such as water, lubricating jellies [eg, K-Y jelly]) or spermicidal cream, jellies, foam, or suppositories. Avoid oil-based lubricants such as cold cream, mineral oil, cooking oil, petroleum jelly, body lotions, massage oil, and baby oil, which can damage latex condoms. For polyurethane condoms, any type of lubricant may be used
- If the condom breaks or falls off during intercourse but before ejaculation, stop and put on a new condom. A new condom can also be used when you have prolonged intercourse or different types of intercourse within a single session (eg, vaginal and anal)
- After ejaculation, withdraw the penis while it is still erect. Hold the condom firmly against the base of the penis to prevent slippage and leakage of semen
- Check the condom for visible damage such as holes, then wrap it in tissue and discard; do not flush the condom in a toilet

- If the condom tears, breaks, or falls off, apply vaginal spermicide foam immediately and start EC as soon as possible. Seek medical care for concerns about sexually transmitted diseases

Reference: Hatcher RA, Nelson Al, Zieman M, et al. *Pocket Guide to Managing Contraception*. Tiger, GA: Bridging the Gap Foundation; 2002:53.

P. EXTENDED CYCLING

Table 6.12
Extended cycling with COCs

Progestin/Estrogen	Product Name	Progestin	Estrogen	No. of pills
Prepackaged extended cycling with COCs: levonorgestrel/EE	Seasonale[a]	0.15 mg	30 μg	84
		0 mg	0 μg	7
	Seasonique[a]	0.15 mg	30 μg	84
		0 mg	10 μg	7
	Lybrel[b]	0.09 mg	20 μg	28
Extended cycling with monophasic COCs[c]				
Norethindrone/EE	Brevicon	0.5 mg	35 μg	
	Norinyl 1 + 35, Nortrel 1/35, Ortho-Novum 1/35	1 mg	35 μg	
	Nortrel 0.5/35	0.5 mg	35 μg	
	Ovcon-35	0.4 mg	35 μg	
	Ovcon-50	1 mg	50 μg	
Norethindrone acetate/EE	Junel 21 1/20, Loestrin 1/20	1 mg	20 μg	
	Junel 21 1.5/30, Loestrin 1.5/30	1.5 mg	30 μg	
Levonorgestrel/EE	Alesse, Aviane, Lessina, Levlite	0.1 mg	20 μg	
	Levlen, Nordette	0.15 mg	30 μg	
Norgestrel/EE	Cryselle, Lo/Ovral	0.3 mg	30 μg	
	Ovral	0.5 mg	50 μg	
Ethynodiol diacetate/EE	Demulen 1/35, Kelnor 1/35	1 mg	35 μg	
	Demulen 1/50	1 mg	50 μg	
Norethindrone/mestranol	Norinyl 1 + 50, Ortho-Novum 1/50	1 mg	50 μg	

(*Continued*)

Table 6.12
(Continued)

Progestin/Estrogen	Product Name	Progestin	Estrogen	No. of pills
Desogestrel/EE	Apri, Desogen, Ortho-Cept	0.15 mg	30 μg	
Drospirenone/EE	Yasmin	3 mg	30 μg	
	Yaz	3 mg	20 μg	
Norgestimate/EE	Ortho-Cyclen, Sprintec	0.25 mg	35 μg	
Extended cycling with combined transdermal contraceptives				
Norelgestromin/EE	Ortho Evra[d]	0.15 mg/d	20 μg/d	
Extended cycling with combined intravaginal contraceptives				
Etonorgestrel/EE	NuvaRing[e]	0.12 mg/d	15 μg/d	

EE indicates ethinyl estradiol.

[a] Seasonale and Seasonique have sufficient medication in each dispensed pack for 3 months of daily pills and to allow menstruation every 3 months.

[b] Lybrel packs contain only a 1-month supply and are intended to suppress menstruation completely.

[c] Each pill pack contains 21 active hormone pills and 7 placebo pills. Eliminate the placebo pills in consecutive pill packs so that the patient takes 21 (1 pill pack), 42 (2 pill packs), 63 (3 pill packs), or 84 (4 pill packs) hormone-containing pills before a placebo week. Cycle length can be incrementally extended over time by adding a pill pack to the cycle length every 2 to 3 cycles, or the patient can start extended cycling at any of these intervals.

[d] Ortho Evra is dispensed in boxes of 3 active hormone patches that can be worn for up to 9 days each. The patient can wear each patch for 7 to 9 days for 3, 6, 9, or 12 consecutive patches followed by 1 week patch-free, during which menstruation begins. Cycle length can be extended incrementally over time by adding 3 patches to the cycle length every 2 to 3 cycles, or the patient can start extended cycling at any of these intervals.

[e] Each NuvaRing is dispensed individually and can be worn for up to 35 days. The patient can wear each ring for 28 to 35 days for 1, 2, 3, or 4 consecutive rings followed by 1 week ring-free, during which menstruation begins. Cycle length can be extended incrementally over time by adding 1 ring to the cycle length every 2 to 3 cycles, or the patient can start extended cycling at any of these intervals.

Adapted from Williams RL, Blythe MJ. Demystifying extended menstrual cycling. *Contemp Pediatr.* 2008;25(8):64–70.

Q. INJECTABLE CONTRACEPTIVE: DEPO-MEDROXYPROGESTERONE ACETATE (DMPA)

Description

- Formulation: inject 1 mL of 150 mg/mL every 11 to 13 weeks intramuscularly into the deltoid or gluteus muscle or 1 mL of 104 mg/mL every 11 to 13 weeks subcutaneously (described as less painful, with potential for self-administration)

- Mechanism: suppresses gonadotropin-releasing hormone and, thus, luteinizing hormone and follicle-stimulating hormone surges, thickens cervical mucous, slows tubal and endometrial mobility, and causes thinning of endometrium, preventing implantation
- Perfect-use failure rate in the first year: 0.3%; typical-use failure rate in the first year: 3%; discontinuation rates in the first year: 26% to 53%
- Absolute contraindications: undiagnosed vaginal bleeding, breast cancer, allergy to DMPA, current pregnancy, current venous thromboembolism, liver dysfunction, or history of myocardial infarction or stroke
- Drug interaction: concurrent administration of Cytadren (aminoglutethimide, adrenal corticosteroid synthesis blocker used to treat hypercorticalism) decreases DMPA effectiveness

Adverse Effects/Risks of DMPA

- Menstrual irregularities: 40% to 50% have amenorrhea in 1 year, 80% in 5 years (number 1 reason for discontinuation)
- Weight gain: average of 9 lb/year in teenagers; weight gain in first 3 months predicts additional weight gain; more common in black teenagers
- May contribute to risk of mood disorders such as depression, anxiety, and irritability
- Gives no protection from cervical or vaginal sexually transmitted infections
- Headaches, acne, and hirsutism may develop or become more apparent; hair loss, bloating, breast tenderness, and vasomotor symptoms have been reported
- Potential for decreasing bone mineral density if used for prolonged period of time; suggestions of studies indicate loss of bone mineral density with DMPA for teenagers, but after discontinuation, rapid and significant gain of bone mineral density back to values same as controls in 24 months has been noted
- Return to baseline fertility takes, on average, 10 months
- Potential negative impact on glucose, low-density lipoproteins, and high-density lipoproteins
- WHO category 2 or 3 for patients with diabetes mellitus for >20 years or with documented damage to vision, kidneys, or nervous system

Advantages of DMPA

- Less menstrual blood loss or anemia or fewer corpus luteum cysts
- 50% are amenorrheic after 1 year, and 80% are amenorrheic after 5 years
- Decrease in menstrual cramp and midcycle pain
- Significant reduction in endometrial cancer risks and perhaps a decrease in the risk of ovarian cancer
- Method of choice for women with chronic disorders/diseases such as epilepsy, hypertriglyceridemia, severe migraine headaches, systemic lupus erythematosus associated with antiphospholipid antibody, sickle cell disease, and thrombophilia and some developmentally or physically disabled teens

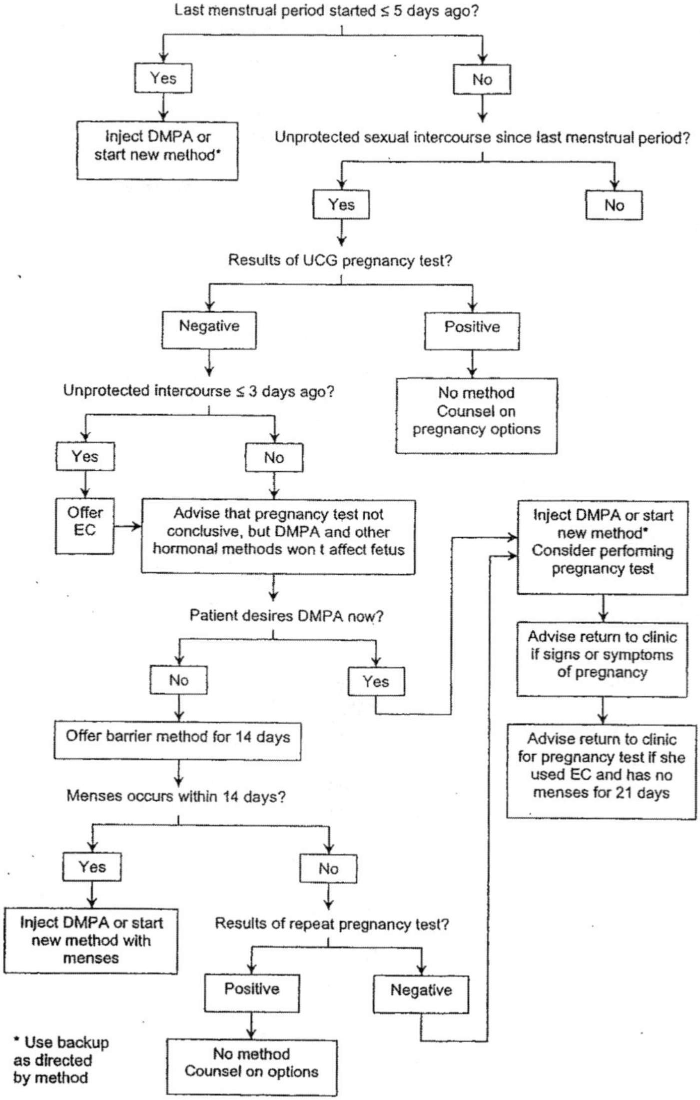

Fig 1. Initial injection of late reinjection (>13 weeks since last injection) of DMPA or switching from DMPA to COCs or another hormonal method. UCG indicates urine chorionic gonadotrophin. (Adapted from Hatcher RA, Nelson A, Zieman M, et al. *Pocket Guide to Managing Contraception*. Tiger, GA: Bridging the Gap Foundation; 2002:126).

- Method of choice when adverse effects of estrogen (such as nausea) are to be avoided
- Method of choice when compliance with a daily regimen is problematic

Instructions for DMPA

- Return in 11 to 13 weeks for next injection
- Watch caloric intake carefully, and increase exercise
- Between dietary intake/supplements, make sure that 1200 to 1500 mg of calcium is taken per day
- Call for heavy bleeding to rule out pregnancy and cervical infection: may treat with nonsteroidal antiinflammatory drugs (800 mg of ibuprofen every 6 hours, maximum of 2400 mg per day) or low-dose estrogen supplements as conjugated estrogen (eg, Premarin, 0.625, 1.25, or 2.5 mg by mouth daily) (may be used indefinitely and as frequently as necessary)

R. OTHER METHODS OF CONTRACEPTION

Transdermal Contraceptive Patch (Ortho Evra)

- 4.5-cm^2, 3-layer patch, applied to lower abdomen/buttocks or upper arm/upper torso
- Delivers norelgestromin (150 μg) and ethinyl estradiol (20 μg) daily
- Made from polyester; safe for women with latex allergies
- New 7-day patch applied same day each week for 3 sequential weeks at alternating sites (eg, left upper back, right upper back, then left upper back the third week)
- Compliance for sexually active women between the ages of 18 and 45 years for the patch was reported as 88%, whereas for the pill it was 77%
- 3319 women with 22 155 cycles over 6 to 13 cycles experienced 15 pregnancies; thus, the method failure or pearl index was 0.8%
- 33% of the pregnancies occurred in the 3% of women who were >198 pounds, suggesting decreased efficacy; this does not mean this group may not use the patch, but they should be more cautious and careful about using condoms
- Breakthrough bleeding occurred in the first cycle for approximately one fifth of the users and decreased in frequency with each subsequent cycle
- Partial or full detachment in ~5% of participants: 3% partial detachment and 2% complete detachment
- The most common adverse effects reported by ~20% of the users included headache, nausea, site reactions, and breast discomfort
- Skin irritation resulted in discontinuation for 2%, nausea occurred in 2%, moodiness occurred in 1.5%, and headache occurred in 1.1%
- Hormone levels remain therapeutic for at least 9 days in each patch
- Does not cause weight gain, with ~80% of participants remaining within 5 lb of their baseline weight

- Risk of estrogen-related thromboembolic events similar to those related to use of the 35-μg ethinyl estradiol/norgestimate pill
- Extended use of the patch has been tested, with fewer bleeding days on the extended patches

References: Stewart FH, Kaunitz AM, Laguardia KD, Karvois DL, Fisher AC, Friedman AJ. Extended use of transdermal norelgestromin/ethinyl estradiol: a randomized trial. *Obstet Gynecol.* 2005;105(6):1389–1396; Audet MC, Moreau M, Koltun WD, et al; Ortho Evra/Evra 004 Study Group. *JAMA.* 2001;285(18):2347–2354; and Hatcher RA, Trussell J, Nelson AL, Cates W Jr, Stewart FH, Kowal D. Contraceptive patch and vaginal contraceptive ring. In: *Contraceptive Technology.* 19th ed. New York, NY: Ardent Media; 2008:271–282.

Instructions for Ortho Evra Patch

If patch left on beyond 7 days

Week 1

- What to do: apply the first patch of new cycle as soon as remembered; patch-change day: first patch day of new cycle becomes new day 1; backup contraception (condoms or abstinence): must be used for the first 7 days of the new cycle

Week 2 (Day 8)/Week 3 (Day 15)

- For <48 hours
  - What to do: remove old patch and apply new patch immediately; patch-change day: remains the same; backup contraception (condoms or abstinence): not needed
- For ≥48 hours
  - What to do: remove old patch and apply new patch immediately; patch-change day: new patch day becomes new change day; backup contraception (condoms or abstinence): must be used for the first 7 days of the new cycle

At End of Cycle (Week 4/Day 22)

- What to do: remove patch as soon as remembered; patch-change day: remains the same; backup contraception (condoms or abstinence): not needed

If patch becomes loose or falls off

For <1 Day (Up to 24 Hours)

- What to do: try to reapply to the same place or replace with a new patch immediately; patch-change day: remains the same; backup contraception (condoms or abstinence): not needed

For >1 Day (≥24 Hours)

- What to do: remove old patch and replace with a new patch immediately; patch-change day: new patch day becomes new change day; backup contraception (condoms or abstinence): must be used for the first 7 days of the new cycle

Vaginal Ring (NuvaRing)

- Soft, flexible, transparent ring of ethylene vinyl acetate copolymer 2 inches in diameter and ⅛ inch in cross-section
- Worn intravaginally, releasing 15 μg of ethinyl estradiol and 120 μg of etonogestrel (metabolite of desogestrel)
- Inserted on day 5 of menses and worn for 3 weeks; remove and then insert a new one in 1 week
- Not a barrier for sexually transmitted diseases
- Irregular bleeding in 2.6% to 6.4% of cycles
- Pregnancy rate was 2 to 5 pregnancies per woman-year use
- May be felt by users or partners in 25% to 42% but did not affect acceptability
- Hormone levels remain therapeutic for at least 35 days
- Estrogen levels at least twofold lower than those of pills, threefold lower than those of the patch
- No weight effects noted in trials
- May be used in latex-allergic women
- May be out for 3 hours without affecting levels of hormone; if out longer, use backup contraception over the next 7 days and evaluate for needs or EC
- Most common adverse effect: headache (6%); vaginal symptoms as vaginal wetness, discomfort, expulsion; nausea; breast tenderness; and loss of libido
- May do first-day (of menses) start, first-Sunday (after menses) start, or quick start; with either first-Sunday or quick start, use 7 days of additional contraception (such as condoms or abstinence)

Reference: Hatcher RA, Trussell J, Nelson AL, Cates W Jr, Stewart FH, Kowal D. Contraceptive patch and vaginal contraceptive ring. In: *Contraceptive Technology*. 19th ed. New York, NY: Ardent Media; 2008: 282–292

Levonorgestrel-Releasing Intrauterine System (IUS) (Mirena)

- T-shaped 32-mm polyethylene device with a 52-mg levonorgestrel steroid reservoir
- Reservoir covered by silicone membrane, contains radiopaque material
- Releases 20 μg/day initially and less than half of that dose by 5 years
- First-year failure rate: 0.1%
- Adverse effects of irregular menstrual bleeding, usually in the first 3 to 6 months, but by 12 months 90% reduction of menstrual flow, with 20% having no periods
- Contraceptive effects: inhibition of ovulation, thickened cervical mucus, inhibition of sperm, and alteration of endometrium
- Low risk of pelvic inflammatory disease even for populations in which there is a high prevalence of sexually transmitted infections (see Hatcher RA, Trussell J, Nelson AL, Cates W Jr, Stewart FH, Kowal D. Intra-

uterine devices (IUDs). In: *Contraceptive Technology*. 19th ed. New York, NY: Ardent Media; 2008:117–143)
- Other adverse effects: 10% have abdominal pain, and 2% to 3% have acne, back pain, breast tenderness, and headache; spontaneous expulsion; perforation

Single Etonogestrel Implant (Implanon)

- Single implant is 4 cm long and 2 mm in diameter, with membrane of ethylene vinyl acetate copolymer and core of 68 mg of etonogestrel (3-keto-desogestrel), releasing 60 μg/day
- Placed in upper arm, with effective life of 3 years
- Thickens cervical mucus within 24 hours of placement, inhibits ovulation, and results in atrophic endometrium
- Advantages: decreased menstrual and midcycle pain; highly effective, with no pregnancies reported in trials; less complicated insertions and removal than previous insertable method; no adverse effect on acne
- Disadvantages: irregular menses with amenorrhea in 20% of users, no sexually transmitted infection protection, weight gain, or headaches
- Specific concerns: breastfeeding for <6 weeks, drug interactions similar to those of COC methods, active liver disease, unexplained vaginal bleeding, current diagnosis of breast cancer, past breast cancer by <5 years

Reference: Hatcher RA, Trussell J, Nelson AL, Cates W Jr, Stewart FH, Kowal D. Contraceptive implants. In: *Contraceptive Technology*. 19th ed. New York, NY: Ardent Media; 2008:145–156.

S. WEB SITE FOR HANDOUTS FOR TEENAGERS REGARDING METHOD OF BIRTH CONTROL

Washington State Department of Health. Choosing the method that's right for you. Available at: www.doh.wa.gov/cfh/FPRH/BirthControl.htm. Accessed May 3, 2009

T. OTHER TOPICS WITH WEB SITES AND REFERENCES

Minors' right to reproductive health care by state

- Guttmacher Institute. Adolescents: policies in brief. Available at: www.guttmacher.org/sections/adolescents.php?pub=spib. Accessed May 3, 2009
- Guttmacher Institute. Minors' access to contraceptive services. Available at: www.guttmacher.org/statecenter/spibs/spib_MACS.pdf. Accessed May 3, 2009

Approach to the sexual assault victim

- American Academy of Pediatrics, Committee on Adolescence. Care of the adolescent sexual assault victim. Available at: http://aappolicy.

aappublications.org/cgi/reprint/pediatrics;122/2/462.pdf. Accessed May 3, 2009

- World Health Organization. Guidelines for medico-legal care for victims of sexual violence. Available at: www.who.int/violence_injury_prevention/publications/violence/med_leg_guidelines/en. Accessed May 3, 2009
- Welch J, Mason F. Rape and sexual assault. *BMJ*. 2007;334(7604): 1154–334

HIV/AIDS Prophylaxis

No accurate data exist on the number of victims of sexual violence who become infected with HIV as a result of an assault. The risk of contracting HIV from sexual violence is estimated to be relatively low but depends on several factors.

- Facts that may be known by the evaluation
  - Type of assault (ie, vaginal, oral, anal)
  - Vaginal or anal trauma (including bleeding)
  - Frequency of assaults
  - Number of perpetrators
  - Use of barrier contraceptive method
  - High prevalence of HIV in the area
  - Whether and where on, or in, the body ejaculation occurred
- Facts that may or may not be known about the perpetrator(s)
  - HIV status
  - Viral load of ejaculate
  - Presence of sexually transmitted infections
  - Presence of genital lesions on either the victim or perpetrator
  - Intravenous drug use by perpetrator

Abortion statistics

- Guttmacher Institute. An overview of abortion in the United States. Available at: www.guttmacher.org/media/presskits/2005/06/28/abortionoverview.html. Accessed May 03, 2009

Contraception

- Stevens-Simon C, Adams Hillard PJ. An adolescent girl's first gynecologic visit and what she should know about contraception. Available at: www.contraceptiononline.org/monographs/adolescent-visit/adolescent_visit.pdf. Accessed May 03, 2009
- Creinin M, Cwiak C, Darney P, et al. *A Pocket Guide to Managing Contraception*. Tiger, GA: Bridging the Gap Foundation; 2007. Available at: www.managingcontraception.com/shopping/product.php?productid=16134&cat=0&bestseller=Y. Accessed May 03, 2009

Adolesc Med 20 (2009) 566–636

7. Infectious Diseases

Table 7.1
Sexually Transmitted Diseases Treatment Guidelines, 2006

Chlamydial infection in adolescents and adults

Treatment

Treatment of infected patients prevents transmission to sex partners, and for infected pregnant women, treatment usually prevents transmission of *Chlamydia trachomatis* to infants during birth. Treatment of sex partners helps to prevent reinfection of the index patient and infection of other partners.

Coinfection with *C trachomatis* often occurs among patients who have gonococcal infection; therefore, presumptive treatment of such patients for chlamydia is appropriate (see "Gonococcal Infection," "Dual Therapy for Gonococcal," and "Chlamydial Infections" in this table). The following recommended treatment regimens and alternative regimens cure infection and usually relieve symptoms.

Recommended regimens

- Azithromycin, 1 g orally in a single dose; or
- Doxycycline, 100 mg orally 2 times per day for 7 d

Alternative regimens

- Erythromycin base, 500 mg orally 4 times per day for 7 d; or
- Erythromycin ethylsuccinate, 800 mg orally 4 times per day for 7 d; or
- Ofloxacin, 300 mg orally 2 times per day for 7 d; or
- Levofloxacin, 500 mg orally once daily for 7 d

A recent meta-analysis of 12 randomized clinical trials of azithromycin vs doxycycline demonstrated that the 2 treatments were equally efficacious, with cure rates of 97% and 98%, respectively. These investigations were conducted primarily in populations in which follow-up was encouraged, adherence to a 7-d regimen was effective, and culture or enzyme immunoassay (rather than NAATs) were used to determine microbiological outcome. Azithromycin should always be available to treat patients for whom compliance with multiday dosing is questionable.

(*Continued*)

Alain Joffe, MD, MPH.
E-mail address: ajoffe@jhu.edu.

Table 7.1
(Continued)

In populations with erratic health care–seeking behavior, poor compliance with treatment, or unpredictable follow-up, azithromycin may be more cost-effective because it offers single-dose, directly observed therapy. However, doxycycline costs less than azithromycin and has no greater risk of adverse events. Erythromycin might be less efficacious than either azithromycin and doxycycline, mainly because the adverse gastrointestinal effects frequently discourage patients from complying with this regimen. Ofloxacin and levofloxacin are effective treatment alternatives but are more expensive and offer no advantage with regard to the dosage regimen. Other quinolones either are not reliably effective against chlamydial infection or have not been adequately evaluated.
To maximize compliance with recommended therapies, medications for chlamydial infections should be dispensed on site, and the first dose should be directly observed. To minimize further transmission of infection, patients treated for chlamydia should be instructed to abstain from sexual intercourse for 7 d after single-dose therapy or until completion of a 7-day regimen. Patients should also be instructed to abstain from sexual intercourse until all of their sex partners are treated to minimize the risk for reinfection.
Follow-up
Except for pregnant women, patients do not need to be retested for chlamydia after completing treatment with the recommended or alternative regimens unless compliance is in question, symptoms persist, or reinfection is suspected. False-negative results might occur because of small numbers of chlamydial organisms. In addition, NAAT conducted <3 wk after completion of therapy for patients who were treated successfully could yield false-positive results because of the continued presence of dead organisms.
Studies have demonstrated high rates of infection among women retested several months after treatment, presumably because of reinfection by an untreated sex partner; infection from a new partner with chlamydia is also possible. Repeat infections confer an increased risk for PID and other complications compared to the initial infection. Clinicians should consider advising all women with chlamydial infection to be retested ~3 mo after treatment. Clinicians are strongly encouraged to retest all women treated for *C trachomatis* whenever they next seek medical care in the next 3–12 mo, regardless of whether the woman believes her sex partner(s) was treated.
Management of sex partners
Patients should be instructed to refer partners for evaluation and treatment. The following recommendations on exposure intervals are based on limited evaluation. Sex partners should be evaluated, tested, and treated if they had sexual contact with the patient during the 60 d preceding onset of symptoms in the patient or diagnosis of chlamydia. The most recent sex partner should be evaluated and treated even if the time of the last sexual contact was >60 d before symptom onset or diagnosis.

(*Continued*)

Table 7.1
(Continued)

Patients should be instructed to abstain from sexual intercourse until they and their sex partner(s) have completed treatment. Abstinence should be continued until 7 d after a single-dose regimen or after completion of a 7-day regimen.

Pregnancy

Doxycycline, ofloxacin, and levofloxacin are contraindicated during pregnancy. Clinical experience and studies have suggested that azithromycin is safe and effective. Repeat testing (preferably by NAAT) 3 wk after completion of therapy with the following regimens is recommended for all pregnant women to ensure cure. The frequent adverse gastrointestinal effects associated with erythromycin might decrease patient compliance with the alternative regimens.

Recommended regimens

Azithromycin, 1 g in a single does; or

Amoxicillin, 500 mg orally 3 times per day for 7 d

Alternative regimens

Erythromycin base, 500 mg orally 4 times per day for 7 d; or

Erythromycin base, 250 mg orally 4 times per day for 14 d; or

Erythromycin ethylsuccinate, 800 mg orally 4 times per day for 7 d; or

Erythromycin ethylsuccinate, 400 mg orally 4 times per day for 14 d

Erythromycin estolate is contraindicated during pregnancy (hepatotoxicity). The lower-dose 14-d regimens may be considered if gastrointestinal tolerance is a concern.

Gonococcal infection in adolescents and adults

Dual therapy for gonococcal and chlamydial infections

Patients infected with *Neisseria gonorrhoeae* often are coinfected with *C trachomatis*; this finding led to the recommendation that patients treated for gonococcal infection also be treated routinely with a regimen effective against uncomplicated genital *C trachomatis* infection. Because most gonococci in the United States are susceptible to doxycycline and azithromycin, routine cotreatment might hinder the development of antimicrobial-resistant *N gonorrhoeae.*

Because of the high sensitivity of NAATs for chlamydial infection, patients with a negative chlamydial NAAT result at the time of treatment for gonorrhea do not need to be treated for chlamydia as well. However, if test results for chlamydia are not available or a non-NAAT was negative for chlamydia, patients should be treated for both chlamydia and gonorrhea.

Quinolone-resistant *N gonorrhoeae*

Because the prevalence of fluoroquinolone resistance among *N gonorrhoeae* isolates in the United States has increased and become widespread, the CDC no longer recommends the use of fluoroquinolones for the treatment of gonococcal infections and associated conditions such as PID (www.cdc.gov/STD/treatment/2006/GonUpdateApril2007.pdf).

(*Continued*)

Table 7.1
(Continued)

Uncomplicated gonococcal infections of the cervix, urethra, and rectum (this regimen is recommended for all adult and adolescent patients regardless of travel history or sexual behavior)

Recommended regimens

Ceftriaxone, 125 mg IM in a single dose; or

Cefixime, 400 mg orally in a single dose; plus

Treatment for chlamydia if chlamydial infection is not ruled out

Ceftriaxone in a single injection of 125 mg provides sustained, high bactericidal levels in the blood. Extensive clinical experience indicates that ceftriaxone is safe and effective for the treatment of uncomplicated gonorrhea at all anatomic sites, curing 98.9% of uncomplicated urogenital and anorectal infections in published clinical trials.

Cefixime has an antimicrobial spectrum similar to that of ceftriaxone, but the 400-mg oral dose does not provide as high, or as sustained, a bactericidal level as that provided by the 125-mg dose of ceftriaxone. In published clinical trials, the 400-mg dose cured 97.4% of uncomplicated urogenital and anorectal gonococcal infections. The advantage of cefixime is that it can be administered orally. Cefixime may not be available in many areas; the CDC or state health departments can provide updates on its availability.

Alternative regimens

Spectinomycin, 2 g IM in a single dose; or

Single-dose cephalosporin regimens

Spectinomycin is expensive and must be injected; however, it has been effective in published clinical trials, curing 98.2% of uncomplicated urogenital and anorectal gonococcal infections. Spectinomycin is useful for treatment of patients who cannot tolerate cephalosporins and quinolones. Spectinomycin is not currently available in the United States.

Single-dose cephalosporin regimens other than ceftriaxone 125 mg IM and cefixime 400 mg orally that are safe and highly effective against uncomplicated urogenital and anorectal gonococcal infections include: (*a*) ceftizoxime 500 mg IM; (*b*) cefoxitin 2 g IM with probenecid 1 g orally; and (*c*) cefotaxime 500 mg IM. None of the injectable cephalosporins offer any advantage over ceftriaxone. Some evidence indicates that cefpodoxime 400 mg and cefuroxime axetil 1 g might be oral alternatives. (Additional information on alternative oral regimens are available at www.cdc.gov/std).

Uncomplicated gonococcal infections of the pharynx (this regimen is recommended for all adult and adolescent patients regardless of travel history or sexual behavior)

Gonococcal infections of the pharynx are more difficult to eradicate than infections at urogenital and anorectal sites. Few antimicrobial regimens can reliably cure such infections >90% of the time. Although chlamydial coinfection of the pharynx is unusual, coinfection at genital sites sometimes occurs. Therefore, treatment for both gonorrhea and chlamydia is suggested.

(*Continued*)

Table 7.1
(Continued)

Recommended regimens

Ceftriaxone, 125 mg IM in a single dose plus

Treatment for chlamydia if chlamydial infection is not ruled out

Follow-up

Patients who have uncomplicated gonorrhea and are treated with any of the recommended or alternative regimens do not need a test of cure. Patients who have symptoms that persist after treatment should be evaluated with culture for *N gonorrhoeae*, and any gonococci isolated should be tested for antimicrobial susceptibility. Persistent urethritis, cervicitis, or proctitis also might be caused by *C trachomatis* or other organisms.

A high prevalence of *N gonorrhoeae* is observed in patients who have had gonorrhea in the preceding several months. The majority of infections identified after treatment with a recommended regimen are caused by reinfection rather than treatment failure. Repeat infection might confer an elevated risk for PID and other complications when compared with the initial infection. Clinicians should consider advising all patients with gonorrhea to be retested 3 mo after treatment, and those not seeking retesting in 3 mo should be tested when they next seek medical care in the ensuing 12 mo.

Management of sex partners

Patients should be instructed to refer sex partners for evaluation and treatment. Sex partners of patients with *N gonorrhoeae* infection whose last sexual contact with the patient was within 60 d of onset of symptoms or diagnosis in the patient should be evaluated and treated for *N gonorrhoeae* and *C trachomatis* infections. If a patient's last sexual intercourse was >60 d before onset of symptoms or diagnosis, the patient's most recent sex partner should be treated. Patients should be instructed to avoid sexual intercourse until therapy is completed and until they and their sex partner(s) no longer have symptoms.

Disseminated gonococcal infection

DGI results from gonococcal bacteremia. DGI often results in petechial or pustular acral skin lesions, asymmetrical arthralgia, tenosynovitis, or septic arthritis. The infection is complicated occasionally by perihepatitis and rarely by endocarditis or meningitis. Some strains of *N gonorrhoeae* that cause DGI may cause minimal genital inflammation.

No studies on the treatment of DGI have been published since the publication of the last CDC STD treatment guidelines. The following recommendations reflect the opinions of consultants; no treatment failures have been reported with these regimens.

(Continued)

Table 7.1
(Continued)

Treatment

Hospitalization is recommended for initial therapy, especially for patients who cannot be relied on to comply with treatment, for those in whom the diagnosis is uncertain, and for those who have purulent synovial effusions or other complications. Patients should be examined for clinical evidence of endocarditis and meningitis. Patients treated for DGI should be treated presumptively for concurrent *C trachomatis* infection unless appropriate testing excludes this infection.

Recommended regimen

Ceftriaxone, 1 g IM or IV every 24 h

Alternative regimens

Cefotaxime, 1 g IV every 8 h; or

Ceftizoxime, 1 g IV every 8 h; or

Spectinomycin, 2 g IM every 12 h (spectinomycin is not currently available in the United States)

All regimens should be continued for 24–48 h after improvement begins, at which time therapy may be switched to 1 of the following regimens to complete at least 1 wk of antimicrobial therapy.

Cefixime, 400 mg orally 2 times per day; or

Cefixime suspension, 500 mg twice daily orally (25 mL daily); or

Cefpodoxime, 400 mg orally twice daily

Fluoroquinolones may be an alternative treatment option if antimicrobial susceptibility can be documented by culture.

As with uncomplicated gonococcal infections, patients should be instructed to refer their sex partners for evaluation and treatment.

HPV infection: genital warts

Treatment

The primary goal of treating visible genital warts is the removal of the warts. In most patients, treatment can induce wart-free periods. Left untreated, visible warts may resolve, may remain unchanged, or may increase in size or number. Treatment possibly reduces, but does not eliminate, HPV infection. Current evidence indicates that presently available treatments might reduce, but probably do not eradicate, HPV infectivity. Whether the reduction in HPV viral DNA resulting from treatment impacts future transmission remains unclear. No evidence indicates that the presence of genital warts or their treatment is associated with the development of cervical cancer.

Regimens

Treatment of genital warts should be guided by the preference of the patient, the available resources, and the experience of the health care provider. No definitive evidence suggests that any of the available treatments are superior to other treatments, and no single treatment is ideal for all patients or all warts. Because of the uncertainty regarding the effect of treatment on future transmission of HPV and the possibility of spontaneous resolution, an acceptable alternative for some people is to forego treatment and wait for spontaneous resolution.

(*Continued*)

Table 7.1
(Continued)

The available treatments for visible genital warts are patient-applied (ie, podofilox and imiquimod) and provider-administered (ie, cryotherapy, podophyllin resin, TCA, BCA, interferon, and surgery) therapies. Most patients have <10 genital warts (with a total wart area of 0.5–1.0 cm^2), which are responsive to various treatment modalities. Factors that might influence selection of treatment include wart size, wart number, anatomical site of wart, wart morphology, patient preference, cost of treatment, convenience, adverse effects, and provider experience. Having a treatment plan or protocol is important, because the majority of patients require a course of therapy rather than a single treatment. In general, warts located on moist surfaces and/or in intertriginous areas respond better to topical treatment (eg, TCA, podophyllin, podofilox, and imiquimod) than do warts on drier surfaces.

The treatment modality should be changed if a patient has not improved substantially. The majority of genital warts respond within 3 mo of therapy. The response to treatment and its adverse effects should be evaluated throughout the course of therapy.

Complications rarely occur if treatments for warts are employed properly. Patients should be warned that persistent hypopigmentation or hyperpigmentation is common with ablative modalities. Depressed or hypertrophic scars are rare but can occur, especially if the patient has had insufficient time to heal between treatments. Treatment can result rarely in disabling chronic pain syndromes (eg, vulvodynia or analdynia, and hyperesthesia of the treatment site), or in the case of rectal warts, painful defecation or fistulas. A limited number of case reports of severe systemic effects from podophyllin resin and interferon have been documented.

Patient-applied treatments are preferred by some patients because they can be administered in the privacy of one's home. For these treatments to be effective, patients must be able to comply with the treatment regimen and be able to identify and reach all genital warts.

Recommended regimens for external genital warts

Patient-applied

Podofilox 0.5% solution or gel. Patients should apply podofilox solution with a cotton swab, or podofilox gel with a finger, to visible genital warts 2 times per day for 3 d, followed by 4 d of no therapy. This cycle may be repeated as necessary for up to 4 cycles. The total wart area treated should not exceed 10 cm^2, and the total volume of podofilox should not exceed 0.5 mL per day. If possible, the health care provider should apply the initial treatment to demonstrate the proper application technique and identify which warts should be treated. The safety of podofilox during pregnancy has not been established; or

Imiquimod 5% cream. Patients should apply imiquimod cream once daily at bedtime, 3 times per week for up to 16 wk. The treatment area should be washed with mild soap and water 6–10 h after the application. The safety of imiquimod during pregnancy has not been established.

(*Continued*)

Table 7.1
(Continued)

Provider-administered

- Cryotherapy with liquid nitrogen or cryoprobe. Repeat applications every 1–2 wk; or
- Podophyllin resin 10%–25% in compound tincture of benzoin. A small amount should be applied to each wart and allowed to air dry. The treatment can be repeated weekly if necessary. To avoid the possibility of complications associated with systemic absorption and toxicity, 2 important guidelines should be followed: (*a*) application should be limited to <0.5 mL of podophyllin or an area <10 cm^2 of warts per session; and (*b*) no open lesions or wounds should exist in the area to which the treatment is to be applied. Some experts suggest that the preparation should be thoroughly washed off 1–4 h after application to reduce local irritation. The safety of podophyllin during pregnancy has not been established; or
- TCA or BCA 80%–90%. Apply a small amount only to warts and allow to dry, at which time a white "frosting" develops. Powder with talc, sodium bicarbonate (ie, baking soda), or liquid soap to remove unreacted acid if an excess amount is applied. Repeat weekly if necessary; or
- Surgical removal either by tangential scissor excision, tangential shave excision, curettage, or electrosurgery.

Alternative treatments

- Intralesional interferon; or
- Laser surgery
- Podofilox 0.5% solution or gel is relatively inexpensive, easy to use, safe, and self-applied by patients. Podofilox is an antimitotic drug that results in destruction of warts. Most patients experience mild/moderate pain or local irritation after treatment. Imiquimod is a topically active immune enhancer that stimulates production of interferon and other cytokines. Local inflammatory reactions are common; these reactions include redness and irritation and are usually mild to moderate. Traditionally, follow-up visits are not usually recommended for patients using self-administered treatments, but they may be useful several weeks into therapy to determine if the treatment is being applied correctly and to measure the response to treatment.
- Cryotherapy destroys warts by thermal-induced cytolysis. Clinicians must be trained in the proper use of this treatment, because overtreatment or undertreatment can result in complications or low efficacy. Pain after application of the liquid nitrogen, followed by necrosis and sometimes blistering, are not unusual. Local anesthesia (topical or injected) might facilitate treatment if there are warts in many areas or if the area of warts is large.

(*Continued*)

Table 7.1
(Continued)

Podophyllin resin contains a number of compounds, including the podophyllin lignans that are antimitotic. The resin is most frequently compounded at 10%–25% in tincture of benzoin. However, podophyllin resin preparations differ in the concentration of active components and contaminants. The shelf life and stability of podophyllin preparations are unknown. It is important to apply a thin layer of podophyllin resin to the warts and allow it to air dry before the treated area comes into contact with clothing. Overapplication or failure to air dry can result in local irritation caused by spread of the compound to adjacent areas.

Both TCA and BCA are caustic agents that destroy warts by chemical coagulation of proteins. Although these preparations are widely used, they have not been investigated thoroughly. TCA solutions have a low viscosity comparable to water and can spread rapidly if applied excessively, thus damaging adjacent normal tissue. Both TCA and BCA should be applied sparingly and allowed to dry before the patient sits or stands. If pain is intense, the acid can be neutralized with soap or sodium bicarbonate (ie, baking soda).

Because of the shortcomings of available treatments, some clinics employ combination therapy (ie, the simultaneous use of ≥2 modalities on the same wart at the same time). No data support the use of >1 therapy at a time to improve the efficacy of treatment, and some specialists believe that combining modalities may increase complications.

Recommended regimens for cervical warts

- For women who have exophytic cervical warts, high-grade squamous intraepithelial lesions must be excluded before treatment is begun. Management of exophytic cervical warts should include consultation with an expert.

Recommended regimens for vaginal warts

- Cryotherapy with liquid nitrogen. The use of a cryoprobe in the vagina is not recommended because of the risk for vaginal perforation and fistula formation; or
- TCA or BCA 80%–90% applied to warts. Apply a small amount only to warts and allow to dry, at which time a white "frosting" develops; powder with talc or sodium bicarbonate (ie, baking soda) or with liquid soap preparations to remove unreacted acid if an excess amount is applied. Repeat weekly if necessary.

Recommended regimens for urethral meatus warts

- Cryotherapy with liquid nitrogen; or
- Podophyllin 10%–25% in compound tincture of benzoin. The treatment area must be dry before contact with normal mucosa. Podophyllin can be applied weekly if necessary. The safety of podophyllin during pregnancy has not been established. Although data evaluating the use of podofilox and imiquimod for the treatment of distal meatal warts are limited, some specialists recommend their use in some patients.

(*Continued*)

Table 7.1
(Continued)

Recommended regimen for anal warts

Cryotherapy with liquid nitrogen; or

TCA or BCA 80%–90% applied to warts. Apply a small amount only to warts and allow to dry, at which time a white "frosting" develops; powder with talc or sodium bicarbonate (ie, baking soda) or with liquid soap preparations to remove unreacted acid if an excess amount is applied. Repeat weekly if necessary; or

Surgical removal

Warts on the rectal mucosa should be managed in consultation with a specialist. Many individuals with anal warts also have warts on the rectal mucosa, so these patients can benefit from inspection of the rectal mucosa by digital examination or anoscopy.

Follow-up

After visible genital warts have cleared, a follow-up evaluation may be helpful. Patients should be cautioned to watch for recurrences, which occur most frequently during the first 3 mo. Because it may be difficult to identify external warts, it may be useful for patients to have a follow-up evaluation 3 mo after treatment. Earlier follow-up visits also may be useful to (*a*) document a wart-free state, (*b*) monitor for or treat complications of therapy, and (*c*) provide the opportunity for patient education and counseling. Women should be counseled regarding the need for regular Papanicolaou testing as recommended for women without genital warts.

Management of sex partners

Examination of sex partners is not necessary for the management of genital warts, because no data indicate that reinfection plays a role in recurrences. Also, providing treatment solely for the purpose of preventing future transmission cannot be recommended, because the value of treatment in reducing infectivity is unknown. However, sex partners of patients who have genital warts might benefit from counseling and examination to assess the presence of genital warts and other sexually transmitted infections. Female sex partners of patients who have genital warts should be reminded that cytological screening for cervical cancer is recommended for all sexually active women (see Papanicolaou test guidelines the gynecology chapter).

Genital HSV infection

Genital herpes is a chronic, lifelong viral infection. The majority of cases of recurrent genital herpes are caused by HSV-2, although HSV-1 might become more common as a cause of first-episode genital herpes. The majority of people with HSV-2 have not been diagnosed; many of them have mild or unrecognized disease but shed virus intermittently in the genital tract. The majority of genital herpes infections are transmitted by people who do not know they are infected or who are asymptomatic at the time transmission occurs.

(*Continued*)

Table 7.1
(Continued)

The classic painful multiple vesicular or ulcerative lesions are absent in many infected people. Up to 50% of first-episode cases of genital herpes are caused by HSV-1, but recurrences and subclinical shedding are much less frequent with genital HSV-1 infection than genital HSV-2 infection. Therefore, the clinical diagnosis of genital herpes should be confirmed by laboratory testing.
First clinical episode of genital herpes
Many patients with first-episode herpes have mild clinical manifestations but later develop severe or prolonged symptoms. Therefore, patients with initial genital herpes should receive antiviral therapy.
Recommended regimens
Acyclovir, 400 mg orally 3 times per day for 7–10 d; or
Acyclovir, 200 mg orally 5 times per day for 7–10 d; or
Famciclovir, 250 mg orally 3 times per day for 7–10 d; or
Valacyclovir, 1 g orally 2 times per day for 7–10 d
Treatment may be extended if healing is incomplete after 10 d of therapy.
Established HSV-2 infection
The majority of patients with symptomatic, first-episode genital HSV-2 infection will have recurrent episodes of genital lesions; recurrences are less frequent after initial genital HSV-1 infection. Intermittent asymptomatic shedding occurs in persons with genital HSV-2 infection, even in those with long-standing or clinically silent infection. Antiviral therapy for recurrent disease can be administered either episodically to ameliorate or shorten the duration of lesions or continuously as suppressive therapy to reduce the frequency of recurrences. Many persons, even those with mild or infrequent outbreaks, benefit from antiviral therapy; therefore, options for treatment should be discussed. Some persons may prefer suppressive therapy, which has the additional advantage of decreasing the risk of genital HSV-2 transmission to susceptible partners.
Daily suppressive therapy reduces the frequency of genital herpes recurrences by 70%–80% in patients who have frequent recurrences (ie, ≥6 recurrences per year). Treatment is also effective in patients with less frequent recurrences. Safety and efficacy have been documented among patients receiving daily therapy with acyclovir for as long as 6 y and with valacyclovir or famciclovir for 1 y. The frequency of recurrences diminishes over time in many patients, and the patient's psychological adjustment to disease might change. Therefore, periodically (eg, once per year), clinicians should discuss the need to continue suppressive therapy with the patient.
Suppressive therapy with valacyclovir 500 mg daily decreases the rate of HSV-2 transmission in discordant, heterosexual couples in which the source partner has a history of genital HSV-2 infection. Suppressive antiviral therapy probably reduces transmission when used by persons who have multiple partners (including men who have sex with men) and by those who are HSV-2 seropositive without a history of genital herpes.

(*Continued*)

Table 7.1
(Continued)

Recommended regimens for daily suppressive therapy
Acyclovir, 400 mg orally 2 times per day; or
Famciclovir, 250 mg orally 2 times per day; or
Valacyclovir, 500 mg orally once a day; or
Valacyclovir, 1.0 g orally once a day
Valacyclovir, 500 mg once a day may be less effective than other valacyclovir or acyclovir dosing regimens in patients who have very frequent recurrences (ie, at least 10 episodes per year). Several studies have compared valacyclovir or famciclovir with acyclovir. The results of these studies suggest that valacyclovir and famciclovir are comparable to acyclovir in clinical outcome. However, ease of administration and cost also are important considerations for prolonged treatment.

Episodic therapy for recurrent genital herpes
Effective episodic therapy of recurrent herpes requires initiation of therapy within 1 d of lesion onset or during the prodrome that precedes some outbreaks. The patient should be provided with a supply of drug or a prescription for the medication with instructions to initiate treatment as soon as symptoms begin.
Recommended regimens
Acyclovir, 400 mg orally 3 times per day for 5 d; or
Acyclovir, 800 mg orally 2 times per day for 5 d; or
Acyclovir, 800 mg orally 3 times per day for 2 d; or
Famciclovir, 125 mg orally 2 times per day for 5 d; or
Famciclovir, 1000 mg orally twice daily for 1 day; or
Valacyclovir, 500 mg orally 2 times per day for 3 d; or
Valacyclovir, 1.0 g once a day for 5 d

Primary and secondary syphilis

Treatment
Parenteral penicillin G is the preferred drug for treatment of all stages of syphilis. The preparation(s) used (ie, benzathine, aqueous procaine, or aqueous crystalline), the dosage, and the length of treatment depend on the stage and clinical manifestations of the disease.
Recommended regimen for adults
Adults who have primary or secondary syphilis should be treated with the following regimen:
Benzathine penicillin G, 2.4 million U IM in a single dose
Recommended regimen for children
Benzathine penicillin G, 50 000 U/kg IM, up to the adult dose of 2.4 million U in a single dose (a child/adolescent weighing ≥48 kg would receive the adult dose)

Other management considerations
All patients who have syphilis should be tested for HIV infection. In geographic areas in which the prevalence of HIV is high, patients who have primary syphilis should be retested for HIV after 3 mo if results of the first HIV test result were negative.

(*Continued*)

Table 7.1
(Continued)

Patients who have syphilis and symptoms or signs suggesting neurologic disease (eg, meningitis) or ophthalmic disease (eg, uveitis, iritis, neuroretinitis, or optic neuritis) should be evaluated fully for neurosyphilis and syphilitic eye disease; this evaluation should include CSF analysis and ocular slit-lamp examination. Such patients should be treated appropriately according to the results of this evaluation.
Invasion of CSF by *Treponema pallidum* accompanied by CSF abnormalities is common among adults who have primary or secondary syphilis. However, neurosyphilis develops in only a few patients after treatment with the regimens described here. Therefore, unless clinical signs or symptoms of neurologic or ophthalmic involvement are present, lumbar puncture is not recommended for routine evaluation of patients who have primary or secondary syphilis.
Follow-up
Treatment failure can occur with any regimen. However, assessing response to treatment often is difficult, and no definitive criteria for cure or failure have been established. Nontreponemal test titers may decline more slowly for patients who previously had syphilis. Patients should be reexamined clinically and serologically 6 and 12 mo after treatment; more frequent evaluation may be prudent if follow-up is uncertain.
Patients who have signs or symptoms that persist or recur or who have a sustained fourfold increase in nontreponemal test titer (ie, compared with the maximum or baseline titer at time of treatment) probably encountered treatment failure or were reinfected. These patients should be retreated and reevaluated for HIV infection. Because treatment failure usually cannot be reliably distinguished from reinfection with *T pallidum*, a lumbar puncture also should be performed. Clinical trial data have demonstrated that 15% of patients with early syphilis treated with recommended therapy will not achieve a 2 dilution decline in nontreponemal titer used to define response 1 y after treatment.
Failure of nontreponemal test titers to decline fourfold within 6 mo after therapy for primary or secondary syphilis might be indicative of probable treatment failure. Persons whose titers remain serofast should be reevaluated for HIV infection. Optimal management of such patients is unclear. At a minimum, these patients should have additional clinical and serologic follow-up. HIV-infected patients should be evaluated more frequently (ie, at 3-mo intervals instead of 6-mo intervals). If additional follow-up cannot be ensured, retreatment is recommended. Because treatment failure might be the result of unrecognized central nervous system infection, many specialists recommend CSF examination in such situations. For retreatment, most experts recommend weekly injections of benzathine penicillin G 2.4 million U IM for 3 wk, unless CSF examination indicates that neurosyphilis is present.

(*Continued*)

Table 7.1
(Continued)

Latent syphilis

Latent syphilis is defined as syphilis characterized by seroreactivity without other evidence of disease. Patients who have latent syphilis and who acquired syphilis within the preceding year are classified as having early latent syphilis. Patients can be diagnosed as having early latent syphilis if, within the year preceding the evaluation, they had (*a*) a documented seroconversion or fourfold or greater increase in titer of a nontreponemal test, (*b*) unequivocal symptoms of primary or secondary syphilis, (*c*) a sex partner documented to have primary, secondary, or early latent syphilis, or (*d*) reactive nontreponemal and treponemal tests whose only possible exposure occurred within the previous 12 mo. Nontreponemal serological titers usually are higher during early latent syphilis than late latent syphilis. However, early latent syphilis cannot be reliably distinguished from late latent syphilis solely on the basis of nontreponemal titers. All patients with latent syphilis should have careful examination of all accessible mucosal surfaces (oral cavity, perineum in women, perianal area, and underneath the foreskin in uncircumcised men) to evaluate for internal mucosal lesions. All patients who have syphilis should be tested for HIV infection.

Treatment

Treatment of latent syphilis usually does not affect transmission and is intended to prevent late complications. Although clinical experience supports the effectiveness of penicillin in achieving this goal, limited evidence is available for guidance in choosing specific regimens.

Recommended regimens for adults; the following regimens are recommended for nonallergic patients who have normal CSF examination (if performed)

Early latent syphilis

Benzathine penicillin G 2.4 million U IM in a single dose

Late latent syphilis or latent syphilis of unknown duration

Benzathine penicillin G 7.2 million U total, administered as 3 doses of 2.4 million U IM each at 1-wk intervals

Recommended regimens for children

Older children with acquired latent syphilis should be evaluated as described for adults and treated using the following pediatric regimens; these regimens are for penicillin-nonallergic children with acquired syphilis who have normal CSF examination results.

Early latent syphilis

Benzathine penicillin G, 50 000 U/kg IM, up to the adult doe of 2.4 million U, in a single dose (a child/adolescent who weighs ≥48 kg would receive the adult dose).

Late latent syphilis or latent syphilis of unknown duration

Benzathine penicillin G, 50 000 U/kg IM, up to the adult dose of 2.4 million U, administered as 3 doses at 1-wk intervals (total 150 000 U/kg up to the adult dose of 7.2 million U) (a child/adolescent who weighs ≥48 kg would receive the adult dose).

(*Continued*)

Table 7.1
(Continued)

Other management considerations

All patients who have latent syphilis should be evaluated clinically for evidence of tertiary disease (eg, aortitis and gumma) and syphilitic ocular disease (eg, iritis and uveitis). Patients with syphilis who demonstrate any of the following should have a prompt CSF examination: (*a*) neurologic or ophthalmic signs or symptoms; (*b*) evidence of active tertiary syphilis (eg, aortitis or gumma); (*c*) treatment failure; or (*d*) HIV infection with late latent syphilis or syphilis of unknown duration.

Some specialists recommend performing a CSF examination on all patients who have latent syphilis and a nontreponemal serologic test of ≥1:32 or if the patient is HIV infected with a CD4 count of ≤350. However, the likelihood of neurosyphilis in this circumstance is unknown. If the CSF examination demonstrates abnormalities consistent with neurosyphilis, the patient should be treated for neurosyphilis.

Follow-up

Quantitative nontreponemal serologic tests should be repeated at 6, 12, and 24 mo. Patients with a normal CSF examination should be retreated for latent syphilis if (*a*) titers increase fourfold, (*b*) an initially high titer (at least 1:32) fails to decline at least fourfold (ie, 2 dilutions) within 12–24 mo, or (*c*) signs or symptoms attributable to syphilis develop.

Pelvic inflammatory disease

PID comprises a spectrum of inflammatory disorders of the upper female genital tract, including any combination of endometritis, salpingitis, tubo-ovarian abscess, and pelvic peritonitis. Sexually transmitted organisms, especially *N gonorrhoeae* and *C trachomatis*, are implicated in many cases; however, microorganisms that comprise the vaginal flora (eg, anaerobes, *Gardnerella vaginalis*, *Haemophilus influenzae*, enteric Gram-negative rods, and *Streptococcus agalactiae*) also have been associated with PID. In addition, cytomegalovirus, *Mycoplasma hominis*, *Ureaplasma urealyticum*, and *Mycoplasma genitalium* might be associated with some cases of PID. All women who are diagnosed with acute PID should be tested for *N gonorrhoeae* and *C trachomatis* and screened for HIV infection.

Acute PID is difficult to diagnose because of the wide variation in the symptoms and signs. Many women with PID have subtle or mild symptoms. Delay in diagnosis and treatment probably contributes to inflammatory sequelae in the upper reproductive tract. Laparoscopy can be performed to obtain a more accurate diagnosis of salpingitis and a more complete bacteriological diagnosis. However, this diagnostic tool often is not readily available, and its use is not easy to justify when symptoms are mild or vague. Moreover, laparoscopy will not detect endometritis and may not detect subtle inflammation of the fallopian tubes. Consequently, a diagnosis of PID is usually based on clinical findings.

(*Continued*)

Table 7.1
(Continued)

The clinical diagnosis of acute PID is imprecise. Data indicate that a clinical diagnosis of symptomatic PID has a positive predictive value of 65%–90% for salpingitis in comparison with laparoscopy. The positive predictive value of a clinical diagnosis of acute PID differs depending on epidemiological characteristics of the population, with higher positive predictive values among sexually active young (especially adolescent) women, among patients attending STD clinics, or in settings where rates of gonorrhea or chlamydia are high. In all settings, however, no single historical, physical, or laboratory finding is both sensitive and specific for the diagnosis of acute PID (ie, can be used both to detect all cases of PID and to exclude all women without PID). Combinations of diagnostic findings that improve either sensitivity (ie, detect more women who have PID) or specificity (ie, exclude more women who do not have PID) do so only at the expense of the other. For example, requiring ≥2 findings excludes more women who do not have PID but also reduces the number of women with PID who are identified.
Many episodes of PID go unrecognized. Although some cases are asymptomatic, others are undiagnosed because the patient or the health care provider fails to recognize the implications of mild or nonspecific symptoms or signs (eg, abnormal bleeding, dyspareunia, or vaginal discharge). Because of the difficulty of diagnosis and the potential for damage to the reproductive health of women, even by apparently mild or subclinical PID, health care providers should maintain a low threshold for the diagnosis of PID.
The optimal treatment regimen and long-term outcome of women with asymptomatic or subclinical PID are unknown. The following suggestions for diagnosing PID are intended to help health care providers recognize when PID should be suspected and when they need to obtain additional information to increase diagnostic certainty. Diagnosis and management of other common causes of lower abdominal pain (eg, ectopic pregnancy, acute appendicitis, functional pain) are unlikely to be impaired by initiating empiric antimicrobial therapy for PID.
Empiric treatment of PID should be initiated in sexually active young women and others at risk for STDs if they are experiencing pelvic or lower abdominal pain, if no other cause for the illness other than PID can be identified, and if ≥1 of the following minimum criteria are present on pelvic examination:
Cervical motion tenderness; or
Uterine tenderness; or
Adnexal tenderness
Requiring that all 3 of the minimum criteria listed above be present before initiating antibiotic treatment could result in insufficient sensitivity for diagnosing PID. The presence of signs of lower genital tract involvement, in addition to 1 of the minimum criteria, increases the specificity of diagnosis. Clinicians should also consider the risk profile of the patient for STDs.

(Continued)

Table 7.1
(Continued)

More elaborate diagnostic evaluation is frequently needed because incorrect diagnosis and management might cause unnecessary morbidity. Additional criteria that can be used to enhance the specificity of the minimum criteria and support a diagnosis of PID include the following:
Oral temperature of >101°F (>38.3°C).
Abnormal cervical or vaginal mucopurulent discharge
Presence of abundant numbers of white blood cells on saline microscopy of vaginal secretions
Increased erythrocyte sedimentation rate
Increased levels of C-reactive protein
Laboratory documentation of cervical infection with *N gonorrhoeae* or *C trachomatis*
The majority of women with PID have either mucopurulent cervical discharge or evidence of white blood cells on a microscopic evaluation of a saline preparation of vaginal fluid. If the cervical discharge appears normal and no white blood cells are observed on the wet prep, the diagnosis if PID is unlikely, and alternative causes of pain should be investigated.
Treatment
PID treatment regimens must provide empiric, broad-spectrum coverage of likely pathogens. All regimens should be effective against *N gonorrhoeae* and *C trachomatis*, because negative endocervical screening results for these organisms does not preclude upper reproductive tract infection. The need to eradicate anaerobes from women who have PID has not been demonstrated definitively. Anaerobic bacteria have been isolated from the upper reproductive tract of women who have PID, and data from in vitro studies have revealed that some anaerobes (eg, *Bacteroides fragilis*) can cause tubal and epithelial destruction. In addition, bacterial vaginosis also is diagnosed in many women who have PID. Until treatment regimens that do not adequately cover these microbes have been shown to prevent sequelae as successfully as the regimens that are effective against these microbes, the use of regimens with anaerobic activity should be considered. Treatment should be initiated as soon as the presumptive diagnosis has been made, because prevention of long-term sequelae depends on immediate administration of appropriate antibiotics. When selecting a treatment regimen, health care providers should consider availability, cost, patient acceptance, and antimicrobial susceptibility.
Some specialists have recommended that all women with PID be hospitalized. However, in women with mild or moderate clinical severity, outpatient therapy can provide short- and long-term clinical outcomes similar to inpatient therapy. Limited data support the use of outpatient therapy in women with more severe clinical presentations. The decision to hospitalize should be based on the discretion of the health-care provider.

(*Continued*)

Table 7.1
(Continued)

The following criteria for hospitalization are suggested

Surgical emergencies (eg, appendicitis) cannot be ruled out

The patient is pregnant

The patient does not respond clinically to oral antimicrobial therapy

The patient is unable to tolerate or follow an outpatient oral regimen

The patient has severe illness, nausea and vomiting, or high fever; and

The patient has a tubo-ovarian abscess.

Many practitioners have preferred to hospitalize adolescents whose condition is diagnosed as PID. No evidence is available suggesting that adolescents benefit from hospitalization for treatment of PID. Younger women with mild-to-moderate acute PID have similar outcomes with either outpatient or inpatient therapy. In addition, clinical response to outpatient therapy is similar among younger and older women. The decision to hospitalize adolescents with acute PID should be based on the same criteria used for older women.

Parenteral treatment

For women with mild-to-moderate PID, parenteral and oral therapy seem to have similar clinical efficacy. Many randomized trials have demonstrated the efficacy of both parenteral and oral regimens. In the majority of clinical trials, parenteral treatment for at least 48 h has been used after the patient has demonstrated substantial clinical improvement. Clinical experience should guide decisions regarding transition to oral therapy, which usually can be initiated within 24 h of clinical improvement. The majority of clinicians recommend at least 24 h of direct inpatient observation for patients who have a tubo-ovarian abscess.

Recommended parenteral regimen A

Cefotetan, 2 g IV every 12 h; or

Cefoxitin, 2 g IV every 6 h; plus

Doxycycline, 100 mg orally or IV every 12 h

Because of pain associated with infusion, doxycycline should be administered orally when possible, even when the patient is hospitalized. Oral and IV administration of doxycycline provide similar bioavailability. Parenteral therapy may be discontinued 24 h after a patient improves clinically, and oral therapy with doxycycline (100 mg 2 times per day) should continue for a total of 14 d. When tubo-ovarian abscess is present, many health care providers use clindamycin or metronidazole with doxycycline for continued therapy rather than doxycycline alone, because they provide more effective anaerobic coverage.

Clinical data are limited regarding the use of other second- or third-generation cephalosporins (eg, ceftizoxime, cefotaxime, and ceftriaxone), which also might be effective therapy for PID and might replace cefotetan or cefoxitin. However, they are less active than cefotetan or cefoxitin against anaerobic bacteria.

(*Continued*)

Table 7.1
(Continued)

- Recommended parenteral regimen B
  - Clindamycin, 900 mg IV every 8 h; plus
  - Gentamicin, loading dose IV or IM (2 mg/kg of body weight), followed by a maintenance dose (1.5 mg/kg) every 8 h. Single daily dosing may be substituted.
  - Although use of a single daily dose of gentamicin has not been evaluated for the treatment of PID, it is efficacious in analogous situations. Parenteral therapy may be discontinued 24 h after a patient improves clinically; continuing oral therapy should consist of doxycycline 100 mg orally 2 times per day or clindamycin 450 mg orally 4 times per day to complete a total of 14 d of therapy. When tubo-ovarian abscess is present, many health care providers use clindamycin for continued therapy rather than doxycycline, because clindamycin provides more effective anaerobic coverage.
- Alternative parenteral regimens
  - Ampicillin/sulbactam, 3 g IV every 6 h; plus
  - Doxycycline, 100 mg orally or IV every 12 h

Oral treatment

- Oral therapy can be considered for women with mildly to moderately severe acute PID, because the clinical outcomes among women treated with oral therapy are similar to those treated with parenteral therapy. The following regimens provide coverage against the frequent etiological agents of PID. Patients who do not respond to oral therapy within 72 h should be reevaluated to confirm the diagnosis and should be administered parenteral therapy on either an outpatient or inpatient basis.
  - Recommended oral regimen
    - Ceftriaxone, 250 mg IM in a single dose; plus
    - Doxycycline, 100 mg orally 2 times per day for 14 d; with or without
    - Metronidazole, 500 mg orally 2 times per day for 14 d; or
    - Cefoxitin, 2 g IM in a single dose and probenecid, 1 g orally administered concurrently; plus
    - Doxycycline, 100 mg orally 2 times per day for 14 d; with or without
    - Metronidazole, 500 mg orally 2 times per day for 14 d; or
    - Other parenteral third-generation cephalosporin (eg, ceftizoxime or cefotaxime); plus
    - Doxycycline, 100 mg orally 2 times per day for 14 d; with or without
    - Metronidazole, 500 mg orally 2 times per day for 14 d

(*Continued*)

Table 7.1
(Continued)

The optimal choice of a cephalosporin is unclear; although cefoxitin has better anaerobic coverage, ceftriaxone has better coverage against *N gonorrhoeae*. Clinical trials have demonstrated that a single dose of cefoxitin is effective in obtaining short-term clinical response in women who have PID; however, the theoretical limitations in its coverage of anaerobes may require the addition of metronidazole. Metronidazole also will effectively treat bacterial vaginosis, which is frequently associated with PID. No data have been published regarding the use of oral cephalosporins for the treatment of PID. Limited data suggest that the combination of oral metronidazole and doxycycline after primary parenteral therapy is safe and effective.

Alternative oral regimens

If parenteral cephalosporin therapy is not feasible, use of fluoroquinolones (levofloxacin 500 mg orally once daily or ofloxacin 400 mg orally twice daily for 14 d) with or without metronidazole (500 mg orally twice daily for 14 d) may be considered if the community prevalence and individual risk of gonorrhea is low. Tests for gonorrhea must be performed before instituting therapy and the patient managed as follows if the test is positive

If the NAAT result is positive, parenteral cephalosporin is recommended

If culture for gonorrhea is positive, treatment should be based on the results of antimicrobial susceptibility. If isolate is quinolone-resistant *N gonorrhoeae* or antimicrobial susceptibility can't be assessed, parenteral cephalosporin is recommended.

Although data are limited, amoxicillin/clavulanic acid and doxycycline or azithromycin with metronidazole has demonstrated short-term clinical cure.

Epididymitis

It is recommended that all patients receive ceftriaxone plus doxycycline for the initial treatment of epididymitis. Additional therapy may include a quinolone if acute epididymitis is not caused by gonorrhea (results from culture or NAAT are negative) or if the infection is most likely caused by enteric organisms.

Recommended regimens

For acute epididymitis most likely caused by gonococcal or chlamydial infection:

Ceftriaxone, 250 mg IM in a single dose; plus

Doxycycline, 100 mg orally 2 times per day for 10 d

For acute epididymitis most likely caused by enteric organisms or with negative gonococcal culture or NAAT or for patients allergic to cephalosporins and/or tetracyclines

Ofloxacin, 300 mg orally 2 times per day for 10 d; or

Levofloxacin, 500 mg orally once daily for 10 d

(*Continued*)

Table 7.1
(Continued)

Proctitis, proctocolitis, and enteritis
Sexually transmitted gastrointestinal syndromes include proctitis, proctocolitis, and enteritis. Evaluation should include appropriate diagnostic procedures (eg, anoscopy or sigmoidoscopy, stool examination, and culture).
Proctitis is inflammation of the rectum (the distal 10–12 cm) that may be associated with anorectal pain, tenesmus, or rectal discharge. *N gonorrhoeae*, *C trachomatis* (including LGV serovars), *T pallidum*, and HSV are the most common sexually transmitted pathogens involved. In patients coinfected with HIV, herpes proctitis may be especially severe. Proctitis occurs predominately among persons who participate in receptive anal intercourse.
Proctocolitis is associated with symptoms of proctitis plus diarrhea and/or abdominal cramps and inflammation of the colonic mucosa extending to 12 cm above the anus. Fecal leukocytes may be detected on stool examination depending on the pathogen. Pathogenic organisms include *Campylobacter* sp., *Shigella* sp., *Entamoeba histolytica*, and, rarely, LGV serovars of *C trachomatis*. Cytomegalovirus or other opportunistic agents may be involved in immunosuppressed HIV-infected patients. Proctocolitis can be acquired by the oral route or by oral-anal contact, depending on the pathogen.
Enteritis usually results in diarrhea and abdominal cramping without signs of proctitis or proctocolitis; it occurs among persons whose sexual practices include oral-anal contact. In otherwise healthy patients, *Giardia lamblia* is most frequently implicated. When outbreaks of gastrointestinal illness occur among social or sexual networks of men who have sex with men, clinicians should consider sexual transmission as a mode of spread. Among HIV-infected patients, other infections that usually are not sexually transmitted may occur, including those caused by cytomegalovirus, *Mycobacterium avium-intracellulare*, *Campylobacter* sp., *Shigella* sp., *Salmonella* sp., *Cryptosporidium*, *Microsporidium*, and *Isospora*. Multiple stool examinations may be necessary to detect *Giardia*, and special stool preparations are required to diagnose cryptosporidiosis and microsporidiosis. In addition, enteritis may be a primary effect of HIV infection.
When laboratory diagnostic capabilities are available, treatment should be based on the specific diagnosis. Diagnostic and treatment recommendations for all enteric infections are beyond the scope of these guidelines.
Treatment
Acute proctitis of recent onset among persons who have recently practiced receptive anal intercourse is most often sexually transmitted. Such patients should be examined by anoscopy and should be evaluated for infection with HSV, *N gonorrhoeae*, *C trachomatis*, and *T pallidum*. If an anorectal exudate is found on examination, or if polymorphonuclear leukocytes are found on a Gram-stained smear of anorectal secretions, the following therapy may be prescribed pending results of additional laboratory tests.

(Continued)

Table 7.1
(Continued)

Recommended regimen
Ceftriaxone, 125 mg IM (or another agent effective against rectal and genital gonorrhea); plus
Doxycycline, 100 mg orally 2 times per day for 7 d
Patients with suspected or documented herpes proctitis should be managed in the same manner as those with genital herpes. If painful perianal ulcers are present or mucosal ulcers are detected on anoscopy, presumptive therapy should include a regimen for treating genital herpes. In addition, LGV proctitis and proctocolitis also should be considered. Appropriate diagnostic testing for LGV should be conducted, and doxycycline therapy should be administered (100 mg orally twice daily for 3 wk).

Most of the information contained herein is reproduced verbatim from the 2006 sexually transmitted diseases treatment guidelines published by the Centers for Disease Control and Prevention (Centers for Disease Control and Prevention; Workowski KA, Berman SM. Sexually transmitted diseases treatment guidelines, 2006 [published correction appears in *MMWR Recomm Rep*. 2006;55[36]:997]. *MMWR Recomm Rep*. 2006;55(RR-11):1–94) and from the updated recommended treatment regimens for gonococcal infections (Centers for Disease Control and Prevention. Updated recommended treatment regimens for gonococcal infections and associated conditions: United States, April, 2007. Available at: www.cdc.gov/STD/treatment/2006/updated-regimens.htm. Accessed January 30, 2009). In some places, I have edited the text to condense the material, incorporating only the information most relevant to the care of adolescents and young adults. I take sole responsibility for any seeming deviations in meaning from the original sources. A slightly different version of this material appears in Joffe A. Sexually transmitted infections. In: McInerny TK, Adam HM, Campbell DE, Kamat DM, Kelleher KJ, eds. *American Academy of Pediatrics Textbook of Pediatric Care*. Elk Grove Village, IL: American Academy of Pediatrics; 2009:2509–2534.

NAAT indicates nucleic acid amplification test; PID, pelvic inflammatory disease; CDC, Centers for Disease Control and Prevention; IM, intramuscularly; DGI, disseminated gonococcal infection; STD, sexually transmitted disease; IV, intravenously; HPV, human papillomavirus; TCA, trichloroacetic acid; BCA, bichloroacetic acid; HSV, herpes simplex virus; CSF, cerebrospinal fluid; LGV, lymphogranuloma venereum.

Adapted with permission from Centers for Disease Control and Prevention; Workowski KA, Berman SM. Sexually transmitted diseases treatment guidelines, 2006 [published correction appears in *MMWR Recomm Rep*. 2006;55(36):997]. *MMWR Recomm Rep*. 2006;55(RR-11): 56–57.

Table 7.2
Comparisons of sensitivity, specificity, and Food and Drug Administration–approval status of diagnostic tests for *Chlamydia trachomatis* and *Neisseria gonorrhoeae*

Diagnostic Method	*C trachomatis*			*N gonorrhoeae*		
	Sensitivity, %	Specificity, %	FDA Cleared	Sensitivity, %	Specificity, %	FDA Cleared
Culture	70–85	100	Yes	80–95	100	NA
Gram-stain						
Males						
Symptomatic				90–95	95–100	NA
Asymptomatic				50–70	95–100	
Females				50–70	95–100	
Direct fluorescent antibody[a]	80–85	99	Yes			
Enzyme immunoassay[b]	53–76	95	Yes			
Hybridization[c]	65–83	99	Yes	92.1–96.4	98.8–99.1	Yes
Ligase chain reaction[d]				96.7–98.6	99.7–99.9	Yes
Cervical	94.4–96.4	99.5–100	Yes			
Urine, female	93–98	99–100	Yes			
Urine, male	96.4	94–100	Yes			
Polymerase chain reaction[e]						
Cervical	89.7	99.4	Yes	92.4	99.5	Yes
Urine, female	89.2	99.0	Yes	64.8	99.8	No
Urine, male	90.3	98.4	Yes			
Urine, male (symptomatic)				94.1	99.9	Yes
Urine, male (asymptomatic)				78.6[f]	99.9	Yes
Strand displacement amplification[g]						
Cervical	92.8	98.1	Yes	96.6	98.0–100	Yes
Urine, female	80.5	98.4	Yes	84.9	99.3–100	Yes
Urine, male	93.1	93.8	Yes	97.9	92.5–100	Yes
Urethral, male				98.5	91.9–100	Yes
Transcriptional mediated amplification[h]						
Cervical	94.2	97.6	Yes	99.2	98.7	Yes
Urine, female	94.7	98.9	Yes	91.3	99.3	Yes
Urethral, male	97.0	99.1	Yes	98.8	98.2	Yes
Urine, male	95.2	98.2	Yes	97.1	99.2	Yes

The data for this table were provided by Charlotte Gaydos, DrPH, MPH, personal communication, April 24, 2009.

[a] For example, MicroTrak (Syva, Palo Alto, CA).

[b] For example, Chlamydiazyme EIA (Abbott, North Chicago, IL).

[c] Pace2 (Gen-Probe, San Diego, CA).

[d] LCx (Abbott).

[e] COBAS Amplicor (Roche, Branchburg, NJ).

[f] Sensitivity may be lower (see Martin DH, Cammarata C, Van Der Pol B, et al. Multicenter evaluation of AMPLICOR and automated COBAS AMPLICOR CT/NG tests for *Neisseria gonorrhoeae*. *J Clin Microbiol*. 2000;38[10]:3544–3549).

[g] ProbeTec (Becton-Dickinson, Sparks, MD).

[h] APTIMA Combo 2 (Gen-Probe).

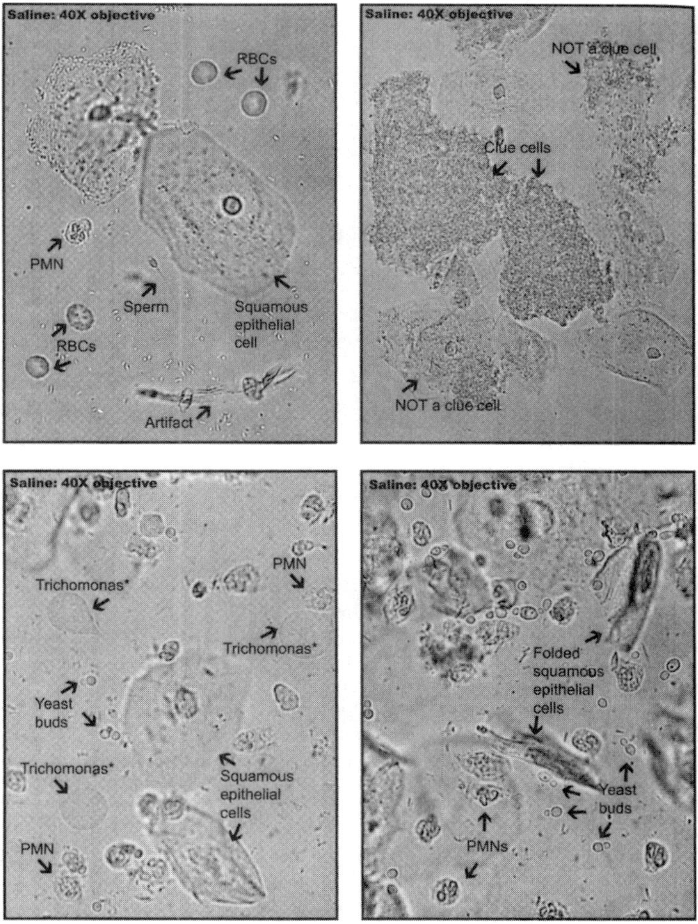

Fig 7.1. Normal and abnormal findings in vaginal wet preps. (Reproduced with permission from the Seattle STD/HIV Prevention Training Center and Cynthia Morrison, MA, ABS, Education Coordinator, Washington State Department of Health).

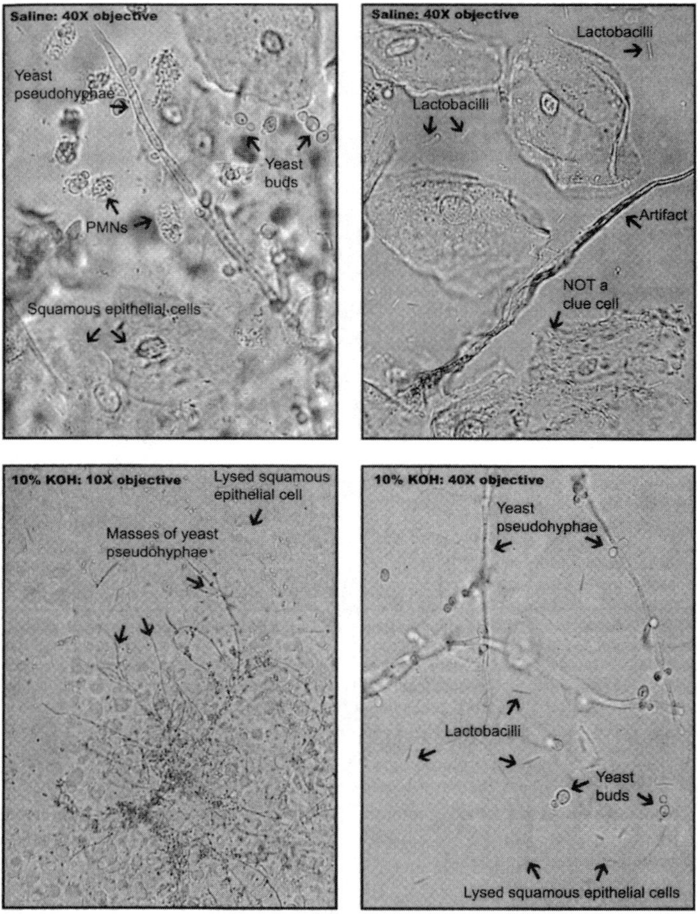

Fig 7.1. Continued.

Table 7.3
Diagnostic features of vaginal discharge

	Normal Vaginal Fluid	Vulvovaginal Candidiasis	Trichomonas Vaginitis	Bacterial Vaginosis
Causative organisms	Normal bacterial flora; *Lactobacillus* predominant	*Candida albicans*; other *Candida* sp. (*Candida glabrata* and other nonalbicans *Candida* species in recurrent infection)	*Trichomonas vaginalis*	Alteration of normal vaginal flora; decrease in *Lactobacillus*; increase in *Gardnerella vaginalis*, anaerobic organisms (*Bacteroides* and *Mobiluncus*), *Mycoplasma hominis*
Symptoms	None	Vulvar itching, burning, or irritation; dysuria; dyspareunia	Odor; dysuria; pruritis; dyspareunia or postcoital bleeding	Odor; slight pruritis; no dysuria
Discharge	None	Scant to moderate amounts; may be thick, curdy, or clumped; plaques adherent to vaginal wall	Profuse, homogeneous, yellow-green, gray, or white; bubbly or frothy	Moderate, white/gray discharge; homogeneous; adheres to vaginal wall
Inflammation of vulvar/vaginal epithelium	None	Erythema of external genitalia, introitus, and vaginal walls; may see satellite red papules on external genitalia	Erythema of vulvar and vaginal epithelium	None

(Continued)

Table 7.3
(Continued)

	Normal Vaginal Fluid	Vulvovaginal Candidiasis	Trichomonas Vaginitis	Bacterial Vaginosis
pH of vaginal fluid (obtained from lateral wall of vagina; avoid cervical secretions; not useful if blood is present)	≤4.5	≤4.5	>4.5 to 5.0 (occasionally may be normal)	>4.5[a]
Amine ("fishy") with 10% KOH	None	None	May be present	Present[a]
Microscopy (see Figs 1 and 2)	Predominance of lactobacilli; normal epithelial cells	Budding yeast, pseudohypha; some white cells may be present	Motile trichomonads (avoid drying of specimen); sensitivity only 60% compared to culture; white cells may be present (more than with *Candida*)	Motile curved rods (*Mobiluncus*); decreased lactobacilli; "clue" cells[a]
Other diagnostic tests		Culture	InPouch TV culture; Osom Trichomonas Rapid Test; Affirm VP III	Affirm VP III; Quickvue Advance pH and Amines test card; Quickvue Advance *G. vaginalis* test; Osom bacterial vaginosis blue

(*Continued*)

Table 7.3
(Continued)

	Normal Vaginal Fluid	Vulvovaginal Candidiasis	Trichomonas Vaginitis	Bacterial Vaginosis
Treatment of sex partner		Not usually; may be indicated if candidal dermatitis of penis is present	Yes	No

For treatment regimens, see Table 4.

[a] Amsel diagnostic criteria for bacterial vaginosis: must have three fourths of the following characteristics: vaginal pH >4.5; homogeneous discharge; "clue" cells; and positive "whiff" test.

Data sources: Holmes KK, Stamm WE. Lower genital tract infection syndromes in women. In: Holmes KK, Mardh PA, Sparling PF, et al, eds. *Sexually Transmitted Diseases*. 3rd ed. New York, NY: McGraw-Hill; 1999:768; Schwebke JR. Vaginal discharge. In: Klausner JD, Hook EW III, eds. *Current Diagnosis & Treatment of Sexually Transmitted Diseases*. New York, NY: McGraw-Hill; 2007. Available at: www.accessmedicine.com/content.aspx?aID=3025856. Accessed April 12, 2009; and Woods ER, Emans SJ. Vulvovaginal complaints in the adolescent. In: Emans SJ, Laufer MR, Goldstein DP, eds. *Pediatric and Adolescent Gynecology*. 5th ed. Philadelphia, PA: Lippincott, Williams & Wilkins; 2005:525–564.

Table 7.4
Recommended treatment for infections characterized by vaginal discharge

- Bacterial vaginosis
  - Recommended regimens
    - Metronidazole, 500 mg PO BID for 7 d; or
    - Metronidazole gel 0.75%, 1 full applicator (5 g) at bedtime intravaginally for 5 d; or
    - Clindamycin vaginal cream 2%, 1 full applicator (5 g) at bedtime intravaginally for 7 d[a]
  - Alternative regimens
    - Metronidazole, 2 g PO in a single dose; or
    - Clindamycin, 300 mg PO BID for 7 d; or
    - Clindamycin ovules, 100 g intravaginally once at bedtime for 3 d
  - During pregnancy
    - Metronidazole, 250 mg PO TID for 7 d; or
    - Clindamycin, 300 mg PO BID for 7 d
- Trichomoniasis
  - Recommended regimen (including treatment of sex partner)
    - Metronidazole, 2 g PO in a single dose
  - Alternative regimen (including treatment of sex partner)
    - Metronidazole, 500 mg PO BID for 7 d
    - If treatment failure occurs with the 2-g metronidazole dose and reinfection is excluded, treatment options are
      - Metronidazole, 500 mg PO BID for 7 d; or
      - Tinidazole, 2 g as a single dose
    - If either of these treatment regimens fail, clinicians should consider
      - Metronidazole, 2 g PO daily for 5 d; or
      - Tinidazole, 2 g PO daily for 5 d
- Vulvovaginal candidiasis
  - Recommended regimens[a]
    - Butoconazole 2% cream, 5g intravaginally for 3 d[b]; or
    - Butoconazole 2% cream, 5 g (butoconazole 1-sustained release), single intravaginal application; or
    - Clotrimazole 1% cream, 5g intravaginally for 7–14 d[b]; or
    - Clotrimazole, 100 mg vaginal tablets intravaginally daily for 7 d; or
    - Clotrimazole, 100 mg vaginal tablet, 2 tablets intravaginally daily for 3 d; or
    - Miconazole 2% cream, 5 g intravaginally for 7 d[b]; or
    - Miconazole, 100 mg vaginal suppository, 1 daily for 7 d[b]; or
    - Miconazole, 200 mg vaginal suppository, 1 daily for 3 d[b]; or
    - Miconazole, 1200 mg vaginal suppository, 1 suppository for 1 day[b]; or
    - Nystatin, 100 000-U vaginal tablet, 1 tablet intravaginally for 14 d; or
    - Tioconazole 6.5% ointment, 5 g intravaginally in a single application[b]; or
    - Terconazole 0.4% cream, 5 g intravaginally for 7 d; or
    - Terconazole 0.8% cream, 5g intravaginally for 3 d; or
    - Terconazole, 80-mg vaginal suppository, 1 suppository daily intravaginally for 3 d; or
    - Fluconazole, 150-mg oral tablet, 1 tablet in a single dose PO

PO, orally; BID indicates twice daily; TID, 3 times per day.

[a] The creams and suppositories recommended here are oil based and might weaken latex condoms and diaphragms. Refer to condom or clindamycin cream product labeling for further information.

[b] Over-the-counter treatment regimen.

Data source: Centers for Disease Control and Prevention; Workowski KA, Berman SM. Sexually transmitted diseases treatment guidelines, 2006 [published correction appears in *MMWR Recomm Rep*. 2006;55(36):997]. *MMWR Recomm Rep*. 2006;55(RR-11):1–94.

Table 7.5
Surveillance case definition for HIV infection among adults and adolescents (aged ≥13 years): United States, 2008

Stage	Laboratory Evidence[a]	Clinical Evidence
1	Laboratory confirmation of HIV infection and $CD4^+$ T-lymphocyte count of ≥500 cells per μ /L or $CD4^+$ T-lymphocyte percentage of ≥29	None required (but no AIDS-defining condition)
2	Laboratory confirmation of HIV infection and $CD4^+$ T-lymphocyte count of 200–499 cells per μ L or $CD4^+$ T-lymphocyte percentage of 14–28	None required (but no AIDS-defining condition)
3 (AIDS)	Laboratory confirmation of HIV infection and $CD4^+$ T-lymphocyte count of <200 cells per μ L or $CD4^+$ T-lymphocyte percentage of <14[b]	Or documentation of an AIDS-defining condition (with laboratory confirmation of HIV infection)[b]
Unknown[c]	Laboratory confirmation of HIV infection and no information on $CD4^+$ T-lymphocyte count or percentage	And no information on presence of AIDS-defining conditions

[a] The $CD4^+$ T-lymphocyte percentage is the percentage of total lymphocytes. If the $CD4^+$ T-lymphocyte count and percentage do not correspond to the same HIV infection stage, select the more severe stage.

[b] Documentation of an AIDS-defining condition (Table 6) supersedes a $CD4^+$ T-lymphocyte count of ≥200 cells per μL and a $CD4^+$ T-lymphocyte percentage of total lymphocytes of ≥14. Definitive diagnostic methods for these conditions are available in Appendix C of the 1993 revised HIV classification system and the expanded AIDS case definition (Centers for Disease Control and Prevention. 1993 revised classification system for HIV infection and expanded surveillance case definition for AIDS among adolescents and adults. *MMWR Recomm Rep*. 1992;41[RR-17]:1–19) and from the National Notifiable Diseases Surveillance System (available at www.cdc.gov/epo/dphsi/casedef/case_definitions.htm; accessed August 9, 2009).

[c] Although cases with no information on $CD4^+$ T-lymphocyte count or percentage or on the presence of AIDS-defining conditions can be classified as "stage unknown," every effort should be made to report $CD4^+$ T-lymphocyte counts or percentages and the presence of AIDS-defining conditions at the time of diagnosis. Additional $CD4^+$ T-lymphocyte counts or percentages and any identified AIDS-defining conditions can be reported as recommended (see Council of State and Territorial Epidemiologists. Laboratory reporting of clinical test results indicative of HIV infection: new standards for a new era of surveillance and prevention [position statement 04-ID-07]. Available at: www.cste.org/ps/2004pdf/04-ID-07-final.pdf. Accessed August 9, 2009).

Adapted from Schneider E, Whitmore S, Glynn KM, Dominguez K, Mitsch A, McKenna MT; Centers for Disease Control and Prevention. Revised surveillance case definitions for HIV infection among adults, adolescents, and children aged >18 months and for HIV infection and AIDS among children aged 18 months to <13 years: United States, 2008. *MMWR Recomm Rep*. 2008;57(RR-10):1–12. Available at: www.cdc.gov/mmwr/PDF/rr/rr5710.pdf. Accessed April 24, 2009.

Table 7.6
AIDS-defining conditions

Bacterial infections, multiple or recurrent[a]
Candidiasis of bronchi, trachea, or lungs
Candidiasis of esophagus[b]
Cervical cancer, invasive[c]
Coccidioidomycosis, disseminated or extrapulmonary
Cryptococcosis, extrapulmonary
Cryptosporidiosis, chronic intestinal (>1 mo duration)
Cytomegalovirus disease (other than liver, spleen, or nodes), onset at age >1 mo
Cytomegalovirus retinitis (with loss of vision)[b]
Encephalopathy, HIV related
Herpes simplex: chronic ulcers (>1 mo duration) or bronchitis, pneumonitis, or esophagitis (onset at age >1 mo)
Histoplasmosis, disseminated or extrapulmonary
Isosporiasis, chronic intestinal (>1 mo duration)
Kaposi sarcoma[b]
Lymphoid interstitial pneumonia or pulmonary lymphoid hyperplasia complex[a,b]
Lymphoma, Burkitt (or equivalent term)
Lymphoma, immunoblastic (or equivalent term)
Lymphoma, primary, of brain
Mycobacterium avium complex or *Mycobacterium kansasii,* disseminated or extrapulmonary[b]
Mycobacterium tuberculosis of any site, pulmonary,[b,c] disseminated,[b] or extrapulmonary[b]
Mycobacterium, other species or unidentified species, disseminated[b] or extrapulomary[b]
Pneumocystis jirovecii pneumonia[b]
Pneumonia, recurrent[b,c]
Progressive multifocal leukoencephalopathy
Salmonella septicemia, recurrent
Toxoplasmosis of brain, onset at age >1 mo[b]
Wasting syndrome attributed to HIV

[a] Only among children aged <13 years (Centers for Disease Control and Prevention. 1994 Revised classification system for human immunodeficiency virus infection in children <13 years of age. *MMWR Recomm Rep*. 1994;43[RR-12];1–10).

[b] Condition that might be diagnosed presumptively.

[c] Only among adults and adolescents aged ≥13 years (Centers for Disease Control and Prevention. 1993 revised classification system for HIV infection and expanded surveillance case definition for AIDS among adolescents and adults. *MMWR Recomm Rep*. 1992;41[RR-17]:1–19) and from the National Notifiable Diseases Surveillance System (available at www.cdc.gov/epo/dphsi/casedef/case_definitions.htm; accessed August 9, 2009).

Adapted from Schneider E, Whitmore S, Glynn KM, Dominguez K, Mitsch A, McKenna MT; Centers for Disease Control and Prevention. Revised surveillance case definitions for HIV infection among adults, adolescents, and children aged >18 months and for HIV infection and AIDS among children aged 18 months to <13 years: United States, 2008. *MMWR Recomm Rep*. 2008;57(RR-10):1–12. Available at: www.cdc.gov/mmwr/PDF/rr/rr5710.pdf. Accessed April 24, 2009.

Table 7.7
Prophylaxis to prevent first episode of opportunistic disease in HIV-infected adults and adolescents

Pathogen	Indication	First Choice	Alternative
Pneumocystis pneumonia	$CD4^+$ count <200 cells per μL (AI)* or oropharyngeal candidiasis (AII)*; $CD4^+$ <14% or history of AIDS-defining illness (BII)*; $CD4^+$ count >200 but <250 cells per μL if monitoring $CD4^+$ count every 1–3 mo is not possible (BII)*	TMP-SMX, 1 DS PO daily (AI)*; or 1 SS daily (AI)*	TMP-SMX 1 DS PO TIW (BI)*; or dapsone 100 mg PO daily or 50 mg PO BID (BI)*; or dapsone 50 mg PO daily + pyrimethamine 50 mg PO weekly + leucovorin 25 mg PO weekly (BI)*; or aerosolized pentamidine 300 mg via Respigard II nebulizer every month (BI)*; or atovaquone 1500 mg PO daily (BI)*; or atovaquone 1500 mg + pyrimethamine 25 mg + leucovorin 10 mg PO daily (CIII)*
Toxoplasma gondii encephalitis	Toxoplasma IgG-positive patients with $CD4^+$ count <100 cells per μL (AII)*; seronegative patients receiving *Pneumocystis* pneumonia prophylaxis not active against toxoplasmosis should have toxoplasma serology retested if $CD4^+$ count declines to <100 cells per μL (CIII)*; prophylaxis should be initiated if seroconversion occurred (AII)*	TMP-SMX, 1 DS PO daily (AII)*	TMP-SMX 1 DS PO TIW (BIII)*; or TMP-SMX 1 SS PO daily (BIII)*; dapsone 50 mg PO daily + pyrimethamine 50 mg PO weekly + leucovorin 25 mg PO weekly (BI)*; or (dapsone 200 mg + pyrimethamine 75 mg + leucovorin 25 mg) PO weekly (BI)*; (atovaquone 1500 mg ± pyrimethamine 25 mg + leucovorin 10 mg) PO daily (CIII)*

(Continued)

Table 7.7
(Continued)

Pathogen	Indication	First Choice	Alternative
Mycobacterium tuberculosis infection (TB) (treatment of LTBI)*	Positive diagnostic test for LTBI, no evidence of active TB, and no previous history of treatment for active or latent TB (AI)*; negative diagnostic test for LTBI but close contact with a person with infectious pulmonary TB and no evidence of active TB (AII)*; a history of untreated or inadequately treated, healed TB (ie, old fibrotic lesions) regardless of diagnostic tests for LTBI and no evidence of active TB (AII)*	Isoniazid 300 mg PO daily (AII)* or 900 mg PO BIW (BII)* for 9 mo—both plus pyridoxine 50 mg PO daily (BIII)*; or for persons exposed to drug-resistant TB, selection of drugs after consultation with public health authorities (AII)*	Rifampin 600 mg PO daily ×4 mo (BIII)*; or rifabutin (dose adjusted on the basis of concomitant ART) ×4 mo (BIII)*
Disseminated *Mycobacterium avium* complex disease	$CD4^+$ count <50 cells per μL, after ruling out active *M avium* complex infection (AI)*	Azithromycin 1200 mg PO once weekly (AI)*; or clarithromycin 500 mg PO BID (AI)*; or azithromycin 600 mg PO twice weekly (BIII)*	Rifabutin 300 mg PO daily (BI)* (dosage adjustment on the basis of drug-drug interactions with ART); rule out active TB before starting rifabutin
Streptococcus pneumoniae infection	$CD4^+$ count >200 cells per μL and no receipt of pneumococcal vaccine in the past 5 y (AII)*; $CD4^+$ count <200 cells per μL—vaccination can be offered (CIII)*; in patients who received PPV when $CD4^+$ count <200 cells per μL, but has increased to >200 cells per μL in response to ART (CIII)*	23-valent PPV 0.5 mL IM ×1 (BII)*; revaccination every 5 y may be considered (CIII)*	

(*Continued*)

Table 7.7
(Continued)

Pathogen	Indication	First Choice	Alternative
Influenza A and B virus infection	All HIV-infected patients (AIII)*	Inactivated influenza vaccine 0.5 mL IM annually (AIII)*	
Histoplasma capsulatum infection	$CD4^+$ count ≤150 cells per μL and at high risk because of occupational exposure or live in a community with a hyperendemic rate of histoplasmosis (>10 cases per 100 patient-years) (CI)*	Itraconazole 200 mg PO daily (CI)*	
Coccidioidomycosis	Positive IgM or IgG serologic test in a patient from a disease-endemic area; and $CD4^+$ count <250 cells per μL (CIII)*	Fluconazole 400 mg PO daily (CIII)*; itraconazole 200 mg PO BID (CIII)*	

(*Continued*)

Table 7.7
(Continued)

Pathogen	Indication	First Choice	Alternative
VZV infection	Preexposure prevention: patients with $CD4^+$ count ≥200 cells per μL who have not been vaccinated, have no history of varicella or herpes zoster, or who are seronegative for VZV (CIII)* (routine VZV serologic testing in HIV-infected adults is not recommended); postexposure—close contact with a person who has active varicella or herpes zoster: for susceptible patients (those who have no history of vaccination or of either condition, or are known to be VZV seronegative) (AIII)*	Preexposure prevention: primary varicella vaccination (Varivax), 2 doses (0.5 mL SQ) administered 3 mo apart (CIII)*; if vaccination results in disease because of vaccine virus, treatment with acyclovir is recommended (AIII)*; postexposure therapy: varicella-zoster immunoglobulin (VariZIG) 125 IU per 10 kg (maximum of 625 IU) IM, administered within 96 h after exposure to a person with active varicella or herpes zoster (AIII)* (as of June 2007, VariZIG can be obtained only under a treatment investigational new drug application [1-800-843-7477, FFF Enterprises])	VZV-susceptible household contacts of susceptible HIV-infected persons should be vaccinated to prevent potential transmission of VZV to their HIV-infected contacts (BIII)*; alternative postexposure therapy:postexposure varicella vaccine (Varivax) 0.5 mL SQ ×2 doses, 3 mo apart if $CD4^+$ count >200 cells per μL (CIII)*; or preemptive acyclovir 800 mg PO 5×/d for 5 d (CIII)*; these 2 alternatives have not been studied in the HIV population

(*Continued*)

Table 7.7
(Continued)

Pathogen	Indication	First Choice	Alternative
HPV infection	Women aged 15–26 y (CIII)*	HPV quadrivalent vaccine 0.5 mL IM months 0, 2, and 6 (CIII)*	
HAV infection	HAV-susceptible patients with chronic liver disease, or who are injection-drug users, or men who have sex with men (AII)*; certain specialists might delay vaccination until $CD4^+$ count >200 cells per μL (CIII)*	Hepatitis A vaccine 1 mL IM ×2 doses—at 0 and 6–12 mo (AII)*; IgG antibody response should be assessed 1 mo after vaccination; nonresponders should be revaccinated (BIII)*	
HBV infection	All patients with HIV without evidence of previous exposure to HBV should be vaccinated with HBV vaccine, including patients with $CD4^+$ count <200 cells per μL (AII)*; patients with isolated anti-HBc: (BII)* (consider screening for HBV DNA before vaccination to rule out occult chronic HBV infection); vaccine nonresponders: defined as anti-HBs <10 IU/mL 1 month after a vaccination series; for patients with low $CD4^+$ count at the time of first vaccination series, certain specialists might delay revaccination until after a sustained increase in $CD4^+$ count with ART	Hepatitis B vaccine IM (Engerix-B 20 μg/mL or Recombivax HB 10 μg/mL) at 0, 1, and 6 mo (AII)*; anti-HBs should be obtained 1 mo after completion of the vaccine series (BIII)*; revaccinate with a second vaccine series (BIII)*	Some experts recommend vaccinating with 40-μg doses of either vaccine (CIII)*; some experts recommend revaccinating with 40-μg doses of either vaccine (CIII)*

(Continued)

Table 7.7
(Continued)

Pathogen	Indication	First Choice	Alternative
Malaria	Travel to disease-endemic area	Recommendations are the same for HIV-infected and -uninfected patients; 1 of the following 3 drugs is usually recommended depending on location: atovaquone/proguanil, doxycycline, or mefloquine; refer to www.cdc.gov/malaria for the most recent recommendations based on region and drug susceptibility (AIII)*	

TMP-SMX indicates trimethoprim-sulfamethoxazole; DS, indicates double strength; SS, single strength; PO, by mouth; IgG, immunoglobulin G; BID, twice daily; TIW, 3 times weekly; TB, tuberculosis; LTBI, latent tuberculosis infection; BIW, 2 times weekly; SQ, subcutaneous; IM, intramuscular; ART, antiretroviral therapy; PPV, polysaccharide pneumococcal vaccination; IgM, immunoglobulin M; VZV, varicella-zoster virus; HPV, human papillomavirus; HAV, hepatitis A virus; HBV, hepatitis B virus. Strength of Recommendation Ratings: A, Both strong evidence for efficacy and substantial clinical benefit support recommendations; B, Moderate evidence for efficacy–or strong evidence for efficacy but only limited clinical benefit–supports recommendation for you. Should generally be offered; C, Evidence for efficacy is insufficient to support a recommendation for or against use. Or evidence for efficacy might not outweigh adverse consequences (eg, drug toxicity, drug interactions) or cost of the treatment or alternative approaches. Optional; D, Moderate evidence for lack of efficacy or for adverse outcome supports a recommendation against use. Should generally not be offered; E, Good evidence for lack of efficacy or for adverse outcome supports a recommendation against use. Should never be offered.

(*Continued*)

Table 7.7
(Continued)

Quality of the evidence supporting the recommendation: I, Evidence from at least one properly-designed randomized, controlled trial; II, Evidence from at least one well-designed clinical trial without randomization, from cohort or case-controlled analytic studies (preferably from more than one center), or from multiple time-series studies, or dramatic results from uncontrolled experiments; III, Evidence from opinions of respected authorities based on clinical experience, descriptive studies, or reports or expert committees.

Data source: Kaplan JE, Benson C, Holmes KH, Brooks JT, Pau A, Masur H; Centers for Disease Control and Prevention; National Institutes of Health; HIV Medicine Association of the Infectious Diseases Society of America. Guidelines for prevention and treatment of opportunistic infections in HIV-infected adults and adolescents: recommendations from CDC, the National Institutes of Health, and the HIV Medicine Association of the Infectious Diseases Society of America. *MMWR Recomm Rep*. 2009;58(RR-4):145–146. Available at: www.cdc.gov/mmwr/PDF/rr/rr5804.pdf. Accessed April 24, 2009.

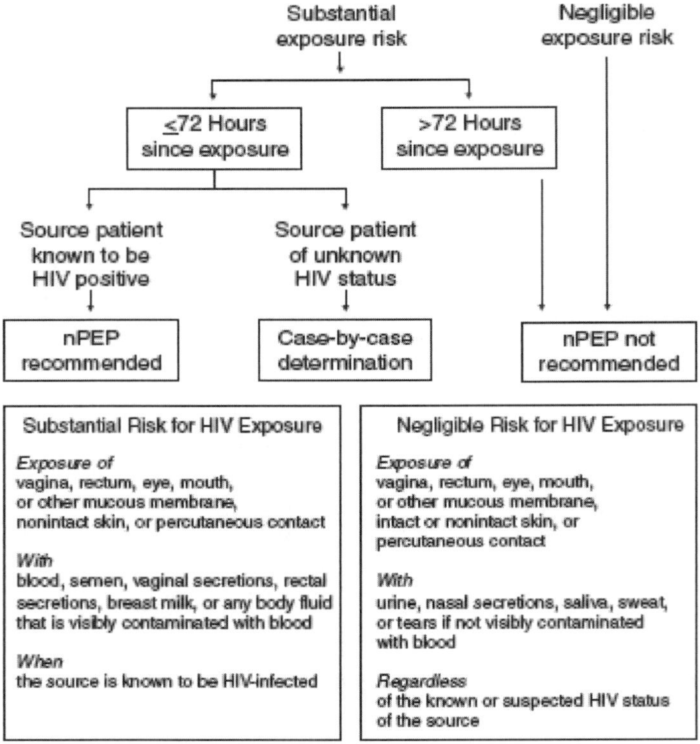

Fig 7.2. Algorithm for evaluation and treatment of possible nonoccupational HIV exposures. nPEP indicates nonoccupational postexposure prophylaxis. (Reproduced with permission from Smith DK, Grohskopf LA, Black RJ, et al; US Department of Health and Human Services. Antiretroviral postexposure prophylaxis after sexual, injection-drug use, or other nonoccupational exposure to HIV in the United States: recommendations from the US Department of Health and Human Services. *MMWR Recomm Rep*. 2005;54[RR-2]:8–13. Available at: www.cdc.gov/mmwr/PDF/rr/rr5402.pdf).

Table 7.8
Antiretroviral regimens for nonoccupational postexposure prophylaxis of HIV infection

Preferred regimens	
NNRTI-based	Efavirenz[a] plus (lamivudine or emtricitabine) plus (zidovudine or tenofovir)
PI-based	Lopinavir/ritonavir (coformulated as Kaletra) plus (lamivudine or emtricitabine) plus zidovudine
Alternative regimens	
NNRTI-based	Efavirenz plus (lamivudine or emtricitabine) plus abacavir or didanosine or stavudine[b]
PI-based	Atazanavir plus (lamivudine or emtricitabine) plus (zidovudine or stavudine or abacavir or didanosine) or (tenofovir plus ritonavir [100 mg/d])
	Fosamprenavir plus (lamivudine or emtricitabine) plus (zidovudine or stavudine) or (abacavir or tenofovir or didanosine)
	Fosamprenavir/ritonavir[c] plus (lamivudine or emtricitabine) plus (zidovudine or stavudine or abacavir or tenofovir or didanosine)
	Indinavir/ritonavir[c,d] plus (lamivudine or emtricitabine) plus (zidovudine or stavudine or abacavir or tenofovir or didanosine)
	Lopinavir/ritonavir (coformulated as Kaletra) plus (lamivudine or emtricitabine) plus (stavudine or abacavir or tenofovir or idanosine)
	Nelfinavir plus (lamivudine or emtricitabine) plus (zidovudine or stavudine or abacavir or tenofovir or didanosine)
	Saquinavir (hgc or sgc)/ritonavir plus (lamivudine or emtricitabine) plus (zidovudine or stavudine or abacavir or tenofovir or didanosine)
Triple NRTI	Abacavir plus lamivudine plus zidovudine (only when an NNRTI- or PI-based regimen cannot or should not be used)

NNRTI indicates nonnucleoside reverse transcriptase inhibitor; NRTI, nucleoside reverse transcriptase inhibitor; PI, protease inhibitor; sgc, soft-gel saquinavir capsule (Fortovase); hgc, hard-gel saquinavir capsule (Invirase).

[a] Efavirenz should be avoided in pregnant women and women of child-bearing potential.

[b] Higher incidence of lipoatrophy, hyperlipidemia, and mitochondrial toxicities associated with stavudine than with other nucleoside reverse transcriptase inhibitors.

[c] Low-dose (100–400 mg) ritonavir.

[d] Use of ritonavir with indinavir might increase risk for adverse renal events.

Adapted from Centers for Disease Control and Prevention. Antiretroviral postexposure prophylaxis after sexual, injection-drug use, or other nonoccupational exposure to HIV in the United States. *MMWR Recomm Rep*. 2005;54(RR-2):8–13. Available at: www.cdc.gov/mmwr/PDF/rr/rr5402.pdf. Accessed April 24, 2009.

Table 7.9
Recommended laboratory evaluation for nonoccupational postexposure prophylaxis of HIV infection

Test	Baseline	During nPEP[a]	4–6 wk After Exposure	3 mo After Exposure	6 mo After Exposure
HIV antibody testing	E, S[b]		E	E	E
Complete blood count with differential	E	E			
Serum liver enzymes	E	E			
Serum urea nitrogen/ creatinine	E	E			
Sexually transmitted disease screen (gonorrhea, chlamydia, syphilis)	E, S	E[c]	E[c]		
Hepatitis B serology	E, S		E[c]	E[c]	
Hepatitis C serology	E, S			E	E
Pregnancy test (for women of reproductive age)	E	E[c]	E[c]		
HIV viral load	S		E[d]	E[d]	E[d]
HIV resistance testing	S		E[d]	E[d]	E[d]
$CD4^+$ T-lymphocyte count	S		E[d]	E[d]	E[d]

nPEP indicates nonoccupational postexposure prophylaxis; E, exposed patient; S, source.
[a] Other specific tests might be indicated depending on the antiretroviral agents prescribed. Literature pertaining to individual agents should be consulted.
[b] HIV antibody testing of the source patient is indicated for source of unknown serostatus.
[c] Additional testing for pregnancy, sexually transmitted diseases, and hepatitis B should be performed as clinically indicated.
[d] If determined to be HIV-infected on follow-up testing; perform as clinically indicated once diagnosed.
Adapted from Centers for Disease Control and Prevention. Antiretroviral postexposure prophylaxis after sexual, injection-drug use, or other nonoccupational exposure to HIV in the United States. *MMWR Recomm Rep*. 2005;54(RR-2):8–13. Available at: www.cdc.gov/mmwr/PDF/rr/rr5402.pdf. Accessed April 24, 2009.

Table 7.10
Disease risk for contacts of people with meningococcal disease

High risk: chemoprophylaxis recommended (close contacts)
Household contact, especially children <2 y old
Child care or preschool contact at any time during 7 d before onset of illness
Direct exposure to index patient's secretions through kissing or through sharing toothbrushes or eating utensils, markers of close social contact, at any time during 7 d before onset of illness
Mouth-to-mouth resuscitation, unprotected contact during endotracheal intubation at any time 7 d before onset of illness
Frequently slept in same dwelling as index patient during 7 d before onset of illness
Passengers seated directly next to the index case during airline flights lasting >8 h
Low risk: chemoprophylaxis not recommended
Casual contact: no history of direct exposure to index patient's oral secretions (eg, school or work)
Indirect contact: only contact is with a high-risk contact, no direct contact with the index patient
Health care professionals without direct exposure to patient's oral secretions
In outbreak or cluster
Chemoprophylaxis for people other than people at high risk should be administered only after consultation with local public health authorities

American Academy of Pediatrics. Meningococcal Infections. In: Pickering LK, Baker CJ, Kimberlin DW, Long SS, eds. *Red Book: 2009 Report of the Committee on Infectious Diseases.* 28th ed. Elk Grove Village, IL: American Academy of Pediatrics; 2009:459.

Table 7.11
Recommended chemoprophylaxis regimens for high-risk contacts and people with invasive meningococcal disease

Age of Infants, Children, and Adults	Dose	Duration, d	Efficacy, %	Cautions
Rifampin[a]				
<1 mo	5 mg/kg, orally, every 12 h	2		
≥1 mo	10 mg/kg (maximum: 600 mg), orally, every 12 h	2	90–95	Can interfere with efficacy of oral contraceptives and some seizure and anticoagulant medications; can stain soft contact lenses
Ceftriaxone				
<15 y	125 mg, intramuscularly	Single dose	90–95	To decrease pain at injection site, dilute with 1% lidocaine
≥15 y	250 mg, intramuscularly	Single dose	90–95	To decrease pain at injection site, dilute with 1% lidocaine
Ciprofloxacin[a,b]				
≥1 mo	20 mg/kg (maximum 500 mg), orally	Single dose	90–95	Not recommended routinely for people <18 years of age; use may be justified after assessment of risks and benefits for the individual patient
Azithromycin	10 mg/kg (maximum 500 mg)	Single dose	90	Not recommended routinely; equivalent to rifampin for eradication of *Neisseria meningitidis* from nasopharynx in 1 study

[a] Not recommended for use in pregnant women.
[b] Use only if fluoroquinolone-resistant strains of *N meningitidis* have not been identified in the community (Centers for Disease Control and Prevention. Emergence of fluoroquinolone-resistant *Neisseria meningitidis*: Minnesota and North Dakota, 2007–2008. *MMWR Morb Mortal Wkly Rep*. 2008;57(7):173–175.

American Academy of Pediatrics. Meningococcal Infections. In: Pickering LK, Baker CJ, Kimberlin DW, Long SS, eds. *Red Book: 2009 Report of the Committee on Infectious Diseases*. 28th ed. Elk Grove Village, IL: American Academy of Pediatrics; 2009:460.

Table 7.12
How do I interpret some of the common hepatitis B panel results?

Test	Result	Interpretation	Vaccinate?
HBsAg Anti-HBc Anti-HBs	Negative Negative Negative	Susceptible	Vaccinate if indicated
HBsAg Anti-HBc Anti-HBs	Negative Negative Positive with ≥10 mIU/mL[a]	Immune because of vaccination	No vaccination necessary
HBsAg Anti-HBc Anti-HBs	Negative Positive Positive	Immune because of natural infection	No vaccination necessary
HBsAg Anti-HBc IgM anti-HBc Anti-HBs	Positive Positive Positive Negative	Acutely infected	No vaccination necessary
HBsAg Anti-HBc IgM anti-HBc Anti-HBs	Positive Positive Negative Negative	Chronically infected	No vaccination necessary (may need treatment)
HBsAg Anti-HBc Anti-HBs	Negative Positive Negative	4 interpretations possible[b]	Use clinical judgment

HBsAg indicates surface antigen of the hepatitis B virus; HBc, antibody to hepatitis B core antigen; IgM, immunoglobulin M; HBs, hepatitis B surface antibody.

[a] Postvaccination testing, when it is recommended, should be performed 1 to 2 months after dose 3.

[b] (1) May be recovering from acute hepatitis B virus infection; (2) may be distantly immune, and the test is not sensitive enough to detect a very low level of anti-HBs in serum; (3) may be susceptible with a false-positive anti-HBc; or (4) may be chronically infected and have an undetectable level of HBsAg present in the serum.

Adapted from Immunization Action Coalition. *Needle Tips*. 2002;12(1):21. Available at: www.immunize.org/nslt.d/n26/n26.pdf. Accessed April 24, 2009.

Table 7.13
Patterns of Epstein-Barr viral antibodies in Epstein-Barr virus infection

Infection Status	Heterophile	Anti-VCA IgM	Anti VCA IgG	Anti-EA(D)	Anti-EA(R)	Anti-EBNA
No previous infection	−	−	−	−	−	−
Acute infection	+	+	+	+/−	−	−
Recent infection	+/−	+/−	+	+/−	+/−	+/−
Past infection	−	−	+	+/−	−	+
Reactivation with immunodeficiency	−	−	+	+	+	+/−
Comment		Present at diagnosis; persist for 4–8 wk; other herpes viruses can induce IgM antibodies to cell lines that express EBV antigen	Present at diagnosis; lifelong persistence	Present in ~70% of patients with acute infection; titer correlates with severity and duration of illness; persist 3–6 mo	Few patients have EA(R); if present, may persist for >3 y after infection	Appear late in course of infection (6–12 wk after onset of symptoms); presence excludes active infection; persist for life

− indicates negative; +, positive; VCA, viral capsid antigen; EA(D); early antigen, diffuse staining of nucleus and cytoplasm; EA(R), early antigen, staining restricted to cytoplasm; EBNA, Epstein-Barr nuclear antigen; IgM, immunoglobulin M; EBV, Epstein-Barr virus.

Data sources: American Academy of Pediatrics. Epstein-Barr virus infections. In: Pickering LK, Baker CJ, Long SS, McMillan JA, eds. *Red Book: 2006 Report of the Committee on Infectious Diseases*. 27th ed. Elk Grove Village, IL: American Academy of Pediatrics; 2006:286–288; and Johannsen EC, Schooley RT, Kaye KM. Epstein-Barr virus (infectious mononucleosis). In: Mandell GL, Bennett JE, Dolin R, eds. *Principles and Practice of Infectious Diseases*. 6th ed. Philadelphia, PA: Churchill Livingstone; 2005:1801–1815.

Table 7.14
Definitions of positive tuberculin skin test results in infants, children, and adolescents[a]

Induration ≥5 mm
Children in close contact with known or suspected contagious people with tuberculosis disease
Children suspected to have tuberculosis disease
Findings on chest radiograph consistent with active or previous tuberculosis disease
Clinical evidence of tuberculosis disease[b]
Children receiving immunosuppressive therapy[c] or with immunosuppressive conditions, including HIV infection
Induration ≥10 mm
Children at increased risk of disseminated tuberculosis disease
Children <4 y of age
Children with other medical conditions, including Hodgkin disease, lymphoma, diabetes mellitus, chronic renal failure, or malnutrition
Children with likelihood of increased exposure to tuberculosis disease
Children born in high-prevalence regions of the world
Children frequently exposed to adults who are HIV infected, homeless, users of illicit drugs, residents of nursing homes, incarcerated or institutionalized, or migrant farm workers
Children who travel to high-prevalence regions of the world
Induration ≥15 mm
Children ≥4 y of age without any risk factors

[a] These definitions apply regardless of previous bacille Calmette-Guerin (BCG) immunization (see also Table 18); erythema alone at tuberculin skin test site does not indicate a positive test result. Tests should be read 48 to 72 hours after placement.

[b] Evidence by physical examination or laboratory assessment that would include tuberculosis in the working differential diagnosis (eg, meningitis).

[c] Including immunosuppressive doses of corticosteroids.

American Academy of Pediatrics. Tuberculosis. In: Pickering LK, Baker CJ, Kimberlin DW, Long SS, eds. *Red Book: 2009 Report of the Committee on Infectious Diseases.* 28th ed. Elk Grove Village, IL: American Academy of Pediatrics; 2009.

Table 7.15
Tuberculin skin test recommendations for infants, children, and adolescents[a]

Children for whom immediate TST or IGRA is indicated[b]
Contacts of people with confirmed or suspected contagious tuberculosis (contact investigation)
Children with radiographic or clinical findings suggesting tuberculosis disease
Children immigrating from countries with endemic infection (eg, Asia, Middle East, Africa, Latin America, countries of the former Soviet Union), including international adoptees
Children with travel histories to countries with endemic infection and substantial contact with indigenous people from such countries[c]
Children who should have annual TST or IGRA
Children infected with HIV infection (TST only)
Incarcerated adolescents
Children at increased risk of progression of LTBI to tuberculosis disease: children with other medical conditions, including diabetes mellitus, chronic renal failure, malnutrition, and congenital or acquired immunodeficiencies deserve special consideration; without recent exposure, these people are not at increased risk of acquiring tuberculosis infection; underlying immunodeficiencies associated with these conditions theoretically would enhance the possibility for progression to severe disease; initial histories of potential exposure to tuberculosis should be included for all of these patients; if these histories or local epidemiologic factors suggest a possibility of exposure, immediate and periodic TST or IGRA should be considered; an initial TST or IGRA should be performed before initiation of immunosuppressive therapy, including prolonged steroid administration, use of tumor necrosis factor α antagonists, or other immunosuppressive therapy in any child requiring these treatments

TST indicates tuberculin skin test; IGRA, interferon γ release assay; LTBI, latent tuberculosis infection.

[a] Bacille Calmette-Guerin immunization is not a contraindication to a tuberculin skin test.

[b] Beginning as early as 3 months of age.

[c] If the child is well, the tuberculin skin test or IGRA should be delayed for up to 10 weeks after return.

Table 7.16
Validated questions for determining risk of latent tuberculosis infection in children in the United States

Has a family member or contact had tuberculosis disease?
Has a family member had a positive tuberculin skin test result?
Was your child born in a high-risk country (countries other than the United States, Canada, Australia, New Zealand, or Western European countries)?
Has your child traveled (had contact with resident populations) to a high-risk country for >1 week?

Table 7.17
Interpretation of tuberculin skin test results in previous recipients of Bacille Calmette-Guérin vaccine

The size of the TST reaction (ie, millimeters of induration) attributable to BCG immunization depends on many factors
Age at BCG immunization
Quality and strain of BCG vaccine used
No. of doses of BCG vaccine received
Nutritional and immunologic status of the vaccine recipient
Frequency of TST administration
Time lapse between immunization and TST
Evidence that increases the probability that a positive TST result is attributable to LTBI includes
Known contact with a person with contagious tuberculosis
A family history of tuberculosis disease
A long interval (>5 y) since neonatal BCG immunization
TST reaction ≥15 mm
Tuberculosis disease should be suspected strongly in any symptomatic person regardless of a TST result and history of BCG immunization; when evaluating an asymptomatic child who has a positive TST result and who possibly received BCG vaccine, certain factors, such as documented receipt of multiple BCG immunizations (as evidenced by BCG scars), decrease the likelihood that the positive TST result is attributable to LTBI

TST indicates tuberculin skin test; BCG, Bacille Calmette-Guerin; LTBI, latent tuberculosis infection.
Adapted from: American Academy of Pediatrics. Tuberculosis. In: Pickering LK, Baker CJ, Kimberlin DW, Long SS, eds. *Red Book: 2009 Report of the Committee on Infectious Diseases.* 28th ed. Elk Grove Village, IL: American Academy of Pediatrics; 2009:685–686.

IMMUNIZATIONS

Changes Listed in the Recommendations Relevant for Teenagers

Routine annual influenza vaccination is recommended for all children aged 6 months through 18 years. Children aged younger than 9 years who are receiving influenza vaccine for the first time or who were vaccinated for the first time during the previous season but only received 1 dose should receive 2 doses of influenza vaccine at least 4 weeks apart. Healthy nonpregnant persons aged 2 through 49 years may receive either live attenuated influenza vaccine or inactivated influenza vaccine.

The minimum interval between tetanus and diphtheria toxoids (Td) and tetanus and diphtheria toxoids and acellular pertussis vaccine (TdaP) for persons aged 10 through 18 years is addressed. An interval of <5 years may be used if pertussis immunity is needed.

(Page 1 of 3)

Vaccine name and route	Schedule for routine vaccination and other guidelines (any vaccine can be given with another)	Schedule for catch-up vaccination and related issues	Contraindications and precautions (mild illness is not a contraindication)
Hepatitis B (HepB) *Give IM*	• Vaccinate all children age 0 through 18yrs. • Vaccinate all newborns with monovalent vaccine prior to hospital discharge. Give dose #2 at age 1–2m and the final dose at age 6–18m (the last dose in the infant series should not be given earlier than age 24wks). After the birth dose, the series may be completed using 2 doses of single-antigen vaccine or up to 3 doses of Comvax (ages 2m, 4m, 12–15m) or Pediarix (ages 2m, 4m, 6m), which may result in giving a total of 4 doses of hepatitis B vaccine. • **If mother is HBsAg-positive:** give the newborn HBIG + dose #1 within 12hrs of birth; complete series at age 6m or, if using Comvax, at age 12–15m. • **If mother's HBsAg status is unknown:** give the newborn dose #1 within 12hrs of birth. If mother is subsequently found to be HBsAg positive, give infant HBIG within 7d of birth and follow the schedule for infants born to HBsAg-positive mothers.	• Do not restart series, no matter how long since previous dose. • 3-dose series can be started at any age. • Minimum spacing between doses: 4wks between #1 and #2, 8wks between #2 and #3, and at least 16wks between #1 and #3 (e.g., 0-, 2-, 4m; 0-, 1-, 4m).	**Contraindication** Previous anaphylaxis to this vaccine or to any of its components. **Precaution** Moderate or severe acute illness.
		Special Notes on Hepatitis B Vaccine (HepB) **Dosing of HepB:** Vaccine brands are interchangeable. For persons age 0 through 19yrs, give 0.5 mL of either Engerix-B or Recombivax HB. **Alternative dosing schedule for unvaccinated adolescents age 11 through 15yrs:** Give 2 doses Recombivax HB 1.0 mL (adult formulation) spaced 4–6m apart. (Engerix-B is not licensed for a 2-dose schedule.) **For preterm infants:** Consult ACIP hepatitis B recommendations (*MMWR* 2005; 54 [RR-16]).*	
DTaP, DT (Diphtheria, tetanus, acellular pertussis) *Give IM*	• Give to children at ages 2m, 4m, 6m, 15–18m, 4–6yrs. • May give dose #1 as early as age 6wks. • May give #4 as early as age 12m if 6m have elapsed since #3 and the child is unlikely to return at age 15–18m. • Do not give DTaP/DT to children age 7yrs and older. • If possible, use the same DTaP product for all doses.	• #2 and #3 may be given 4wks after previous dose. • #4 may be given 6m after #3. • If #4 is given before 4th birthday, wait at least 6m for #5 (age 4–6yrs). • If #4 is given after 4th birthday, #5 is not needed.	**Contraindications** • Previous anaphylaxis to this vaccine or to any of its components. • For DTaP/Tdap only: encephalopathy within 7d after DTP/DTaP. **Precautions** • Moderate or severe acute illness. • History of Arthus reaction following a prior dose of tetanus- and/or diphtheria-toxoid-containing vaccine, including MCV. • Guillain-Barré syndrome within 6wks after previous dose of tetanus toxoid-containing vaccine. • For DTaP only: Any of these events following a previous dose of DTP/DTaP: 1) temperature of 105°F (40.5°C) or higher within 48hrs; 2) continuous crying for 3hrs or more within 48hrs; 3) collapse or shock-like state within 48hrs; 4) convulsion with or without fever within 3d. • For DTaP/Tdap only: Unstable neurologic disorder. **Note:** Use of Td or Tdap is not contraindicated in pregnancy. At the provider's discretion, either vaccine may be administered during the 2nd or 3rd trimester.
Td, Tdap (Tetanus, diphtheria, acellular pertussis) *Give IM*	• Give 1-time Tdap dose to adolescents age 11–12yrs if 5yrs have elapsed since last dose DTaP; then boost every 10yrs with Td. • Give 1-time dose of Tdap to all adolescents who have not received previous Tdap. Special efforts should be made to give Tdap to persons age 11yrs and older who are - in contact with infants younger than age 12m. - healthcare workers with direct patient contact. • In pregnancy, when indicated, give Td or Tdap in 2nd or 3rd trimester. If not administered during pregnancy, give Tdap in immediate postpartum period.	• If never vaccinated with tetanus- and diphtheria-containing vaccine: give Td dose #1 now, dose #2 4wks later, and dose #3 6m after #2, then give booster every 10yrs. A 1-time Tdap may be substituted for any dose in the series, preferably as dose #1. For persons who previously received a Td booster, an interval of 2yrs or less between Td and Tdap may be used.	
Polio (IPV) *Give SC or IM*	• Give to children at ages 2m, 4m, 6–18m, 4–6yrs. • May give dose #1 as early as age 6wks. • Not routinely recommended for U.S. residents age 18yrs and older (except certain travelers).	• All doses should be separated by at least 4wks. • If dose #3 is given after 4th birthday, dose #4 is not needed.	**Contraindication** Previous anaphylaxis to this vaccine or to any of its components. **Precautions** • Moderate or severe acute illness. • Pregnancy.
Human papilloma-virus (HPV) *Give IM*	• Give 3-dose series to girls at age 11–12yrs on a 0, 2, 6m schedule. (May be given as early as age 9yrs.) • Vaccinate all older girls and women (through age 26yrs) who were not previously vaccinated.	Minimum spacing between doses: 4wks between #1 and #2; 12 wks between #2 and #3. Overall, there must be at least 24wks between doses #1 and #3.	**Contraindication** Previous anaphylaxis to this vaccine or to any of its components. **Precautions** • Moderate or severe acute illness. • Pregnancy.

*This document was adapted from the recommendations of the Advisory Committee on Immunization Practices (ACIP). To obtain copies of the recommendations, call the CDC-INFO Contact Center at (800) 232-4636; visit CDC's website at www.cdc.gov/vaccines/pubs/ACIP-list.htm; or visit the Immunization Action Coalition (IAC) website at www.immunize.org/acip. This table is revised periodically. Visit IAC's website at www.immunize.org/childrules to make sure you have the most current version.

Technical content reviewed by the Centers for Disease Control and Prevention, November 2008.

www.immunize.org/catg.d/p2010.pdf • Item #P2010 (11/08)

Immunization Action Coalition • 1573 Selby Avenue • Saint Paul, MN 55104 • (651) 647-9009 • www.immunize.org • www.vaccineinformation.org • admin@immunize.org

Fig 7.3. Summary of recommendations for vaccines for children and adolescents including those with medical conditions. (Reprinted with permission from Immunization Action Coalition. Summary of recommendations for childhood and adolescent immunization. Available at: www.immunize.org/catg.d/p2010.pdf).

Catch-up vaccination with human papillomavirus (HPV) vaccine is clarified. Routine dosing intervals should be used for series catch-up (ie, the second and third doses should be administered 2 and 6 months after the first dose). The third dose should be given at least 24 weeks after the first dose.

Web Site for Immunizations

www.cdc.gov/vaccines/recs/schedules

(Page 2 of 3)

Vaccine name and route	Schedule for routine vaccination and other guidelines (any vaccine can be given with another)	Schedule for catch-up vaccine administration and related issues	Contraindications and precautions (mild illness is not a contraindication)
Varicella (Var) (Chickenpox) *Give SC*	• Give dose #1 at age 12–15m. • Give dose #2 at age 4–6yrs. Dose #2 may be given earlier if at least 3m since dose #1. • Give a second dose to all older children and adolescents with history of only 1 dose. • MMRV may be used in children age 12m through 12yrs.	• If younger than age 13yrs, space dose #1 and #2 at least 3m apart. If age 13yrs or older, space at least 4wks apart. • May use as postexposure prophylaxis if given within 5d. • If Var and either MMR, LAIV, and/or yellow fever vaccine are not given on the same day, space them at least 28d apart.	**Contraindications** • Previous anaphylaxis to this vaccine or to any of its components. • Pregnancy or possibility of pregnancy within 4wks. • Children on high-dose immunosuppressive therapy or who are immunocompromised because of malignancy and primary or acquired cellular immunodeficiency, including HIV/AIDS (although vaccination may be considered if CD4+ T-lymphocyte percentages are either 15% or greater in children ages 1 through 8yrs or 200 cells/mL or greater in children age 9yrs or older). **Precautions** • Moderate or severe acute illness. • If blood, plasma, and/or immune globulin (IG or VZIG) were given in past 11m, see ACIP statement *General Recommendations on Immunization** regarding time to wait before vaccinating. **Note:** For patients with humoral immunodeficiency or leukemia, see ACIP recommendations*.
MMR (Measles, mumps, rubella) *Give SC*	• Give dose #1 at age 12–15m. • Give dose #2 at age 4–6yrs. Dose #2 may be given earlier if at least 4wks since dose #1. • Give a second dose to all older children and teens with history of only 1 dose. • MMRV may be used in children age 12m through 12yrs.	• If MMR and either Var, LAIV, and/or yellow fever vaccine are not given on the same day, space them at least 28d apart. • When using MMR for both doses, minimum interval is 4wks. • When using MMRV for both doses, minimum interval is 3m. • Within 72hrs of measles exposure, give 1 dose of MMR as postexposure prophylaxis to susceptible healthy children age 12m and older.	**Contraindications** • Previous anaphylaxis to this vaccine or to any of its components. • Pregnancy or possibility of pregnancy within 4wks. • Severe immunodeficiency (e.g., hematologic and solid tumors; receiving chemotherapy; congenital immunodeficiency; long-term immunosuppressive therapy, or severely symptomatic HIV). Note: HIV infection is NOT a contraindication to MMR for children who are not severely immunocompromised (consult ACIP MMR recommendations [*MMWR* 1998;47 [RR-8] for details*). **Precautions** • Moderate or severe acute illness. • If blood, plasma, or immune globulin given in past 11m, see ACIP statement *General Recommendations on Immunization** regarding time to wait before vaccinating. • History of thrombocytopenia or thrombocytopenic purpura. **Note:** MMR is not contraindicated if a TST (tuberculosis skin test) was recently applied. If TST and MMR are not given on same day, delay TST for at least 4wks after MMR.
Influenza Trivalent inactivated influenza vaccine (TIV) *Give IM* — Live attenuated influenza vaccine (LAIV) *Give intranasally*	• Vaccinate all children and teens age 6m through 18yrs, as well as all household contacts of infants and children through age 59m (4yrs 11m). • Vaccinate persons age 19yrs and older who - have a risk factor (e.g., pregnancy, heart or lung disease, renal, hepatic, hematologic, or metabolic disorder [including diabetes], immunosuppression, or have a condition that compromises respiratory function or the handling of respiratory secretions or that can increase the risk of aspiration) or live in a chronic-care facility. - live or work with at-risk people as listed above. • All other persons who want to reduce the likelihood of becoming ill with influenza or of spreading it to others. • LAIV may be given to healthy, non-pregnant persons age 2–49yrs. • Give 2 doses to first-time vaccinees age 6m through 8yrs, spaced 4wks apart. • For TIV, give 0.25 mL dose to children age 6–35m and 0.5 mL dose if age 3yrs and older.		**Contraindications** • Previous anaphylaxis to this vaccine, to any of its components, or to eggs. • For LAIV only: Pregnancy, asthma, reactive airways disease, or other chronic disorder of the pulmonary or cardiovascular systems; an underlying medical condition, including metabolic diseases such as diabetes, renal dysfunction, and hemoglobinopathies; known or suspected immune deficiency diseases or immunosuppressed states; for children younger than age 5yrs, possible reactive airways disease (e.g., recurrent wheezing or a wheezing episode within the past 12m). **Precautions** • Moderate or severe acute illness. • History of Guillain-Barré syndrome within 6wks of a previous influenza vaccination. **Note:** If LAIV and either MMR, Var, and/or yellow fever vaccine are not given on the same day, space them at least 28d apart.
Rotavirus (RV) *Give orally*	• Rotarix (RV1): give at age 2m, 4m • RotaTeq (RV5): give at age 2m, 4m, 6m • May give dose #1 as early as age 6wks. • Give dose #3 no later than age 8m 0 days.	• Do not begin series in infants older than age 15wks 0 days. • Intervals between doses may be as short as 4wks. • If prior vaccination included use of different or unknown brand(s), a total of 3 doses should be given.	**Contraindication** Previous anaphylaxis to this vaccine or to any of its components, including latex for RV1. **Precautions** • Moderate or severe acute illness. • Altered immunocompetence. • Moderate to severe acute gastroenteritis or chronic gastrointestinal disease. • History of intussusception.

Fig 7.3. Continued.

Web Site for Vaccine Information Statements Required to Give to Patients and Families

www.cdc.gov/vaccines/pubs/vis/default.htm

Web Site for Reporting Vaccine Adverse Events

www.vaers.hhs.gov

(Page 3 of 3)

Vaccine name and route	Schedule for routine vaccination and other guidelines (any vaccine can be given with another)	Schedule for catch-up vaccination and related issues	Contraindications and precautions (mild illness is not a contraindication)
Hib (*Haemophilus influenzae* type b) *Give IM*	• ActHib (PRP-T): give at age 2m, 4m, 6m, 12–15m (booster dose). • PedvaxHIB or Comvax (containing PRP-OMP): give at age 2m, 4m, 12–15m (booster dose). • Dose #1 of Hib vaccine should not be given earlier than age 6wks. • The last dose (booster dose) is given no earlier than age 12m and a minimum of 8wks after the previous dose. • Hib vaccines are interchangeable; however, if different brands of Hib vaccines are administered for dose #1 and dose #2, a total of 3 doses are necessary to complete the primary series in infants. • Any Hib vaccine may be used for the booster dose. • Hib is not routinely given to children age 5yrs and older.	**All Hib vaccines:** • If #1 was given at 12–14m, give booster in 8wks. • Give only 1 dose to unvaccinated children from age 15 through 59m. **ActHib:** • #2 and #3 may be given 4wks after previous dose. • If #1 was given at age 7–11m, only 3 doses are needed; #2 is given 4–8wks after #1, then boost at age 12–15m (wait at least 8wks after dose #2). **PedvaxHIB and Comvax:** • #2 may be given 4wks after dose #1.	**Contraindications** • Previous anaphylaxis to this vaccine or to any of its components. • Age younger than 6wks. **Precaution** Moderate or severe acute illness.
Pneumo. conjugate (PCV) *Give IM*	• Give at ages 2m, 4m, 6m, 12–15m. • Dose #1 may be given as early as age 6wks. • Give 1 dose to unvaccinated healthy children age 24–59m. • For high-risk** children ages 24–59m, give 2 doses at least 8wks apart if previous vaccinations were fewer than 3 doses, or give 1 dose if previously received 3 doses. • PCV is not routinely given to children age 5yrs and older. ****High-risk:** Those with sickle cell disease; anatomic/functional asplenia; chronic cardiac, pulmonary, or renal disease; diabetes; cerebrospinal fluid leaks; HIV infection; immunosuppression; diseases associated with immunosuppressive and/or radiation therapy; or who have or will have a cochlear implant.	• For age 7–11m: If history of 0–2 doses, give additional doses 4wks apart with no more than 3 total doses by age 12m; then give booster 8wks later. • For age 12–23m: If 0–1 dose before age 12m, give 2 doses at least 8wks apart. If 2–3 doses before age 12m, give 1 dose at least 8wks after previous dose. • For age 24–59m: If patient has had no previous doses, or has a history of 1–3 doses given before age 12m but no booster dose, or has a history of only 1 dose given at age 12–23m, give 1 dose now.	**Contraindication** Previous anaphylaxis to this vaccine or to any of its components. **Precaution** Moderate or severe acute illness.
Pneumo. polysacch. (PPSV) *Give IM or SC*	• Give 1 dose at least 8wks after final dose of PCV to high-risk children age 2yrs and older. • For children who are immunocompromised or have sickle cell disease or functional or anatomic asplenia, give a 2nd dose of PPSV 5yrs after previous PPSV (consult ACIP PPSV recommendations at http://www.cdc.gov/vaccines/pubs/ACIP-list.htm*).		**Contraindication** Previous anaphylaxis to this vaccine or to any of its components. **Precaution** Moderate or severe acute illness.
Hepatitis A (HepA) *Give IM*	• Give 2 doses to all children at age 1yr (12–23m) spaced 6m apart. • Vaccinate all previously unvaccinated children and adolescents age 2 years and older who - Live in a state, county, or community with a routine vaccination program already in place for children age 2yrs and older. - Travel anywhere except U.S., W. Europe, N. Zealand, Australia, Canada, or Japan. - Wish to be protected from HAV infection. - Have chronic liver disease, clotting factor disorder, or are MSM adolescents. - Are injecting or non-injecting drug users.	• Minimum interval between doses is 6m. • Children who are not fully vaccinated by age 2yrs can be vaccinated at subsequent visits. • Consider routine vaccination of children age 2yrs and older in areas with no existing program. • Give 1 dose as postexposure prophylaxis to incompletely vaccinated children age 12m and older who have recently (during the past 2wks) been exposed to hepatitis A virus.	**Contraindication** Previous anaphylaxis to this vaccine or to any of its components. **Precautions** • Moderate or severe acute illness. • Pregnancy.
Meningococcal conjugate (MCV) *Give IM* **polysaccharide** (MPSV) *Give SC*	• Give 1-time dose of MCV to adolescents age 11 through 18yrs. • Vaccinate all college freshmen living in dorms who have not been vaccinated. • Vaccinate all children age 2yrs and older who have any of the following risk factors (MCV is preferable to MPSV): - Anatomic or functional asplenia, or terminal complement component deficiency. - Travel to or reside in countries in which meningococcal disease is hyperendemic or epidemic (e.g., the "meningitis belt" of Sub-Saharan Africa).	If previously vaccinated with MPSV and risk continues, give MCV 5yrs after MPSV.	**Contraindication** Previous anaphylaxis to this vaccine or to any of its components, including diphtheria toxoid (for MCV). **Precautions** • Moderate or severe acute illness. • For MCV only: history of Guillain-Barré syndrome (GBS).

Fig 7.3. Continued.

Recommended Immunizations for the Traveler

wwwn.cdc.gov/Travel/contentVaccinations.aspx

Recommended Immunization Schedule for Persons Aged 7 Through 18 Years—United States • 2009

For those who fall behind or start late, see the schedule below and the catch-up schedule

Vaccine ▼ Age ▶	7–10 years	11–12 years	13–18 years
Tetanus, Diphtheria, Pertussis[1]	*see footnote 1*	Tdap	Tdap
Human Papillomavirus[2]	*see footnote 2*	HPV (3 doses)	HPV Series
Meningococcal[3]	MCV	MCV	MCV
Influenza[4]		Influenza (Yearly)	
Pneumococcal[5]		PPSV	
Hepatitis A[6]		HepA Series	
Hepatitis B[7]		HepB Series	
Inactivated Poliovirus[8]		IPV Series	
Measles, Mumps, Rubella[9]		MMR Series	
Varicella[10]		Varicella Series	

Range of recommended ages

Catch-up immunization

Certain high-risk groups

This schedule indicates the recommended ages for routine administration of currently licensed vaccines, as of December 1, 2008, for children aged 7 through 18 years. Any dose not administered at the recommended age should be administered at a subsequent visit, when indicated and feasible. Licensed combination vaccines may be used whenever any component of the combination is indicated and other components are not contraindicated and if approved by the Food and Drug Administration for that dose of the series. Providers should consult the relevant Advisory Committee on Immunization Practices statement for detailed recommendations, including high-risk conditions: http://www.cdc.gov/vaccines/pubs/acip-list.htm. Clinically significant adverse events that follow immunization should be reported to the Vaccine Adverse Event Reporting System (VAERS). Guidance about how to obtain and complete a VAERS form is available at http://www.vaers.hhs.gov or by telephone, 800-822-7967.

1. **Tetanus and diphtheria toxoids and acellular pertussis vaccine (Tdap).** ***(Minimum age: 10 years for BOOSTRIX® and 11 years for ADACEL®)***
   - Administer at age 11 or 12 years for those who have completed the recommended childhood DTP/DTaP vaccination series and have not received a tetanus and diphtheria toxoid (Td) booster dose.
   - Persons aged 13 through 18 years who have not received Tdap should receive a dose.
   - A 5-year interval from the last Td dose is encouraged when Tdap is used as a booster dose; however, a shorter interval may be used if pertussis immunity is needed.
2. **Human papillomavirus vaccine (HPV).** ***(Minimum age: 9 years)***
   - Administer the first dose to females at age 11 or 12 years.
   - Administer the second dose 2 months after the first dose and the third dose 6 months after the first dose (at least 24 weeks after the first dose).
   - Administer the series to females at age 13 through 18 years if not previously vaccinated.
3. **Meningococcal conjugate vaccine (MCV).**
   - Administer at age 11 or 12 years, or at age 13 through 18 years if not previously vaccinated.
   - Administer to previously unvaccinated college freshmen living in a dormitory.
   - MCV is recommended for children aged 2 through 10 years with terminal complement component deficiency, anatomic or functional asplenia, and certain other groups at high risk. See *MMWR* 2005;54(No. RR-7).
   - Persons who received MPSV 5 or more years previously and remain at increased risk for meningococcal disease should be revaccinated with MCV.
4. **Influenza vaccine.**
   - Administer annually to children aged 6 months through 18 years.
   - For healthy nonpregnant persons (i.e., those who do not have underlying medical conditions that predispose them to influenza complications) aged 2 through 49 years, either LAIV or TIV may be used.
   - Administer 2 doses (separated by at least 4 weeks) to children aged younger than 9 years who are receiving influenza vaccine for the first time or who were vaccinated for the first time during the previous influenza season but only received 1 dose.
5. **Pneumococcal polysaccharide vaccine (PPSV).**
   - Administer to children with certain underlying medical conditions (see *MMWR* 1997;46[No. RR-8]), including a cochlear implant. A single revaccination should be administered to children with functional or anatomic asplenia or other immunocompromising condition after 5 years.
6. **Hepatitis A vaccine (HepA).**
   - Administer 2 doses at least 6 months apart.
   - HepA is recommended for children older than 1 year who live in areas where vaccination programs target older children or who are at increased risk of infection. See *MMWR* 2006;55(No. RR-7).
7. **Hepatitis B vaccine (HepB).**
   - Administer the 3-dose series to those not previously vaccinated.
   - A 2-dose series (separated by at least 4 months) of adult formulation Recombivax HB® is licensed for children aged 11 through 15 years.
8. **Inactivated poliovirus vaccine (IPV).**
   - For children who received an all-IPV or all-oral poliovirus (OPV) series, a fourth dose is not necessary if the third dose was administered at age 4 years or older.
   - If both OPV and IPV were administered as part of a series, a total of 4 doses should be administered, regardless of the child's current age.
9. **Measles, mumps, and rubella vaccine (MMR).**
   - If not previously vaccinated, administer 2 doses or the second dose for those who have received only 1 dose, with at least 28 days between doses.
10. **Varicella vaccine.**
    - For persons aged 7 through 18 years without evidence of immunity (see *MMWR* 2007;56[No. RR-4]), administer 2 doses if not previously vaccinated or the second dose if they have received only 1 dose.
    - For persons aged 7 through 12 years, the minimum interval between doses is 3 months. However, if the second dose was administered at least 28 days after the first dose, it can be accepted as valid.
    - For persons aged 13 years and older, the minimum interval between doses is 28 days.

The Recommended Immunization Schedules for Persons Aged 0 Through 18 Years are approved by the Advisory Committee on Immunization Practices (www.cdc.gov/vaccines/recs/acip), the American Academy of Pediatrics (http://www.aap.org), and the American Academy of Family Physicians (http://www.aafp.org).

DEPARTMENT OF HEALTH AND HUMAN SERVICES • CENTERS FOR DISEASE CONTROL AND PREVENTION

CS103164

Fig 7.4. Recommended Immunization Schedule for Persons Aged 7 Though 18 Years-United States, 2009. (Reproduced with permission from Centers for Disease Control and Prevention, Department of Health and Human Services. 2009. Available at: www.edc.gov/vaccines/recs/schedules/downloads/child/2009/09_7-18yrs_schedule_pss.pdf).

Table 7.18
Guide to tetanus prophylaxis in routine wound management in children 7 years of age and older and adolescents

History of Absorbed Tetanus Toxoid (Doses)	Clean, Minor Wounds		All Other Wounds[a]	
	Td or TdaP[b]	TIG[c]	Td or TdaP[b]	TIG[c]
<3 or unknown	Yes	No	Yes	Yes
≥3[d]	No[e]	No	No[f]	No

Td indicates adult-type diphtheria and tetanus toxoids vaccine; TdaP, booster tetanus toxoid, reduced diphtheria toxoid, and acellular pertussis; TIG, tetanus immunoglobulin (human).

[a] Such as, but not limited to, wounds contaminated with dirt, feces, soil, and saliva; puncture wounds; avulsions; and wounds resulting from missiles, crushing, burns, and frostbite.

[b] TdaP is preferred to Td vaccine for adolescents who never have received TdaP vaccine. Td is preferred to tetanus toxoid vaccine for adolescents who received TdaP vaccine previously or when TdaP vaccine is not available.

[c] Immunoglobulin intravenous should be used when TIG is not available.

[d] If only 3 doses of fluid toxoid have been received, a fourth dose of toxoid, preferably an adsorbed toxoid, should be given. Although licensed, fluid tetanus toxoid rarely is used.

[e] Yes, if ≥10 years since last tetanus-containing vaccine dose.

[f] Yes, if ≥5 years since last tetanus-containing vaccine dose. More frequent boosters are not needed and can accentuate adverse effects.

Table 7.19
Special situation recommendations for use of a single dose of TdaP in 11- to 18-year-old adolescents

Situation	Recommendations
Tetanus prophylaxis indicated for wound management	Should receive TdaP (if not previously given) instead of Td; should administer TdaP concurrently with MCV4 (Menactra), if feasible, in people not previously immunized; do not defer giving a tetanus-containing vaccine when indicated if TdaP, MCV4, or both are not available
Lack of availability of TdaP or MCV4	The available vaccine generally should be administered and the other administered when missed vaccine becomes available (also see below)
Use of Td when TdaP is not available	Should receive Td when TdaP is indicated but not available if the last DTP/DTaP/DT/Td was administered at least 10 y previously; if vaccine was administered <10 y previously, immunization can be deferred temporarily (awaiting TdaP) if follow-up is likely
History of pertussis	Should receive TdaP
History of receipt of DT or Td but incomplete pertussis immunization	Should receive catch-up dose of TdaP; a 2-y interval generally is used (also see above)
History of no DTP/DTaP/DT or Td immunization	Should receive catch-up doses of 3 Td-containing vaccines, one of which is TdaP
History of receipt of DTP/DTaP/DT or Td but incomplete records	Consider serologic testing; if tetanus or diphtheria antibody concentrations are ≥0.1 IU/mL, presume previous immunization and administer a single dose of TdaP (to be considered the adolescent booster dose)
Pregnancy	Pregnancy is not a contraindication to TdaP (or Td) immunization; pregnant adolescents should be given the same considerations for immunization as nonpregnant adolescents (see text)
Postpartum	Mothers of newborn infants should be given a dose of TdaP as soon as is feasible if they previously have not received TdaP; household contacts should have immunization status evaluated and should be given DTaP or TdaP if indicated as soon as is feasible[a]

(*Continued*)

Table 7.19
(Continued)

Situation	Recommendations
Children 7–10 y of age with history of incomplete childhood DTP/DTaP immunization	Neither TdaP vaccine is licensed for use in children <10 y of age; required series of Td should be given, with a single adolescent booster dose of Td in children who are 10 y of age
People >18 y of age	The safety and immunogenicity of TdaP as a single booster dose has been demonstrated for people 19–64 y of age; recommendations for use are available[b]

TdaP indicates tetanus toxoid, reduced diphtheria toxoid and acellular pertussis vaccine; Td, diphtheria and tetanus toxoids (for children aged ≥7 years and adults); MCV4, tetravalent meningococcal conjugate vaccine; DTP, diphtheria and tetanus toxoids and whole-cell pertussis vaccine; DT, diphtheria and tetanus toxoids vaccine (for children <7 years of age).

[a] Infants <12 months of age are at highest risk of pertussis-related complications and hospitalizations compared with older age groups; young infants have the highest risk of death from pertussis.

[b] Centers for Disease Control and Prevention. Preventing tetanus, diphtheria and pertussis among adults: use of tetanus toxoid, reduced diphtheria toxoid, and acellular pertussis vaccines—recommendations of the Advisory Committee on Immunization Practices (ACIP). *MMWR Recomm Rep.* 2006;55(RR-3):1–34.

Table 7.20
Contraindications and precautions for administration of TdaP in adolescents

Contraindications
- History of immediate anaphylactic reaction[a] after any component of the vaccine
- History of encephalopathy[b] within 7 d after a pertussis vaccine

Precautions
- History of Guillain-Barré syndrome within 6 wk of a dose of a tetanus toxoid vaccine[c]
- Progressive neurologic disorder, uncontrolled epilepsy, or progressive encephalopathy until the condition has stabilized[d]

[a] Because of the importance of tetanus immunization, people with a history of anaphylaxis to components should be referred to an allergist to determine whether they have a specific allergy to tetanus toxoid, can be desensitized to tetanus toxoid, and safely can receive tetanus toxoid immunization.
[b] This syndrome has been defined as a severe, acute central nervous system disorder unexplained by another cause, which may be manifested by major alterations of consciousness or by generalized or focal seizures that persist for more than a few hours without recovery within 24 hours. Prudence justifies considering such an illness occurring within 7 days of receipt of pertussis-containing vaccine as a contraindication to additional doses of pertussis vaccine, and DT vaccine should be substituted for each of the recommended subsequent doses of diphtheria and tetanus toxoid.
[c] If decision is made to continue tetanus toxoid, TdaP is preferred if indicated.
[d] This condition is a contraindication for DTaP but a precaution for TdaP. The precaution is for the pertussis component. If decision is made to withhold pertussis immunization, Td may be used.

Table 7.21
Recommended antimicrobial therapy and postexposure prophylaxis for pertussis in adolescents

Recommended
- Azithromycin, 500 mg as a single dose on day 1, then 250 mg as a single dose on day 2–5; or
- Erythromycin, 2 g/d in 4 divided doses for 14 d; or
- Clarithromycin, 1 g/d in 2 divided doses for 7 d

Alternative regimen
- Trimethoprim, 200 mg/d; sulfamethoxazole, 1600 mg/d in 2 divided doses for 14 d

Data source: Tiwari T, Murphy TV, Moran J; National Immunization Program, Centers for Disease Control and Prevention. Recommended antimicrobial agents for the treatment and postexposure prophylaxis of pertussis: 2005 CDC Guidelines. *MMWR Recomm Rep*. 2005; 54(RR-14):10. Available at: www.cdc.gov/mmwr/PDF/rr/rr5414.pdf. Accessed April 24, 2009.

Note: These recommendations *must* be read with the footnotes that follow containing number of doses, intervals between doses, and other important information.

Recommended adult immunization schedule, by vaccine and age group

VACCINE ▼ AGE GROUP ▶	19–26 years	27–49 years	50–59 years	60–64 years	≥65 years
Tetanus, diphtheria, pertussis (Td/Tdap)[1,*]	Substitute 1-time dose of Tdap for Td booster; then boost with Td every 10 yrs				Td booster every 10 yrs
Human papillomavirus (HPV)[2,*]	3 doses (females)				
Varicella[3,*]	2 doses				
Zoster[4]				1 dose	
Measles, mumps, rubella (MMR)[5,*]	1 or 2 doses		1 dose		
Influenza[6,*]	1 dose annually				
Pneumococcal (polysaccharide)[7,8]	1 or 2 doses				1 dose
Hepatitis A[9,*]	2 doses				
Hepatitis B[10,*]	3 doses				
Meningococcal[11,*]	1 or more doses				

*Covered by the Vaccine Injury Compensation Program.

Legend:
- (light shading) For all persons in this category who meet the age requirements and who lack evidence of immunity (e.g., lack documentation of vaccination or have no evidence of prior infection)
- (dark shading) Recommended if some other risk factor is present (e.g., on the basis of medical, occupational, lifestyle, or other indications)
- (blank) No recommendation

Report all clinically significant postvaccination reactions to the Vaccine Adverse Event Reporting System (VAERS). Reporting forms and instructions on filing a VAERS report are available at www.vaers.hhs.gov or by telephone, 800-822-7967.

Information on how to file a Vaccine Injury Compensation Program claim is available at www.hrsa.gov/vaccinecompensation or by telephone, 800-338-2382. To file a claim for vaccine injury, contact the U.S. Court of Federal Claims, 717 Madison Place, N.W., Washington, D.C. 20005; telephone, 202-357-6400.

Additional information about the vaccines in this schedule, extent of available data, and contraindications for vaccination is also available at www.cdc.gov/vaccines or from the CDC-INFO Contact Center at 800-CDC-INFO (800-232-4636) in English and Spanish, 24 hours a day, 7 days a week.

Use of trade names and commercial sources is for identification only and does not imply endorsement by the U.S. Department of Health and Human Services.

Fig 7.5. Recommended adult immunization schedule (United States, 2009) according to vaccine and age group. Note that these recommendations must be read with footnotes that follow (after Fig 6) containing number of doses, intervals between doses, and other important information. (Reproduced with permission from Centers for Disease Control and Prevention, Department of Health and Human Services. Recommended adult immunization schedule: United States, 2009. Available at: www.cdc.gov/vaccines/recs/schedules/downloads/adult/2009/adult-schedule.pdf).

VACCINE ▼ / INDICATION ▶	Pregnancy	Immuno-compromising conditions (excluding human immunodeficiency virus [HIV])[13]	HIV infection[3,12,13] CD4+ T lymphocyte count <200 cells/µL	HIV infection CD4+ T lymphocyte count ≥200 cells/µL	Diabetes, heart disease, chronic lung disease, chronic alcoholism	Asplenia[12] (including elective splenectomy and terminal complement component deficiencies)	Chronic liver disease	Kidney failure, end-stage renal disease, receipt of hemodialysis	Health-care personnel
Tetanus, diphtheria, pertussis (Td/Tdap)[1,*]	Td	Substitute 1-time dose of Tdap for Td booster; then boost with Td every 10 yrs							
Human papillomavirus (HPV)[2,*]		3 doses for females through age 26 yrs							
Varicella[3,*]	Contraindicated			2 doses					
Zoster[4]	Contraindicated				1 dose				
Measles, mumps, rubella (MMR)[5,*]	Contraindicated			1 or 2 doses					
Influenza[6,*]	1 dose TIV annually								1 dose TIV or LAIV annually
Pneumococcal (polysaccharide)[7,8]		1 or 2 doses							
Hepatitis A[9,*]					2 doses				
Hepatitis B[10,*]					3 doses				
Meningococcal[11,*]					1 or more doses				

*Covered by the Vaccine Injury Compensation Program.

For all persons in this category who meet the age requirements and who lack evidence of immunity (e.g., lack documentation of vaccination or have no evidence of prior infection)

Recommended if some other risk factor is present (e.g., on the basis of medical, occupational, lifestyle, or other indications)

No recommendation

These schedules indicate the recommended age groups and medical indications for which administration of currently licensed vaccines is commonly indicated for adults ages 19 years and older, as of January 1, 2009. Licensed combination vaccines may be used whenever any components of the combination are indicated and when the vaccine's other components are not contraindicated. For detailed recommendations on all vaccines, including those used primarily for travelers or that are issued during the year, consult the manufacturers' package inserts and the complete statements from the Advisory Committee on Immunization Practices (www.cdc.gov/vaccines/pubs/acip-list.htm).

The recommendations in this schedule were approved by the Centers for Disease Control and Prevention's (CDC) Advisory Committee on Immunization Practices (ACIP), the American Academy of Family Physicians (AAFP), the American College of Obstetricians and Gynecologists (ACOG), and the American College of Physicians (ACP).

DEPARTMENT OF HEALTH AND HUMAN SERVICES
CENTERS FOR DISEASE CONTROL AND PREVENTION

CS208484-A

Fig 7.6. Vaccines that might be indicated for adults on the basis of medical and other indications. Note that these recommendations must be read with footnotes that follow containing number of doses, intervals between doses, and other important information. (Reproduced with permission from Centers for Disease Control and Prevention, Department of Health and Human Services. Recommended adult immunization schedule: United States, 2009. Available at: www.cdc.gov/vaccines/recs/schedules/downloads/adult/2009/adult-schedule.pdf).

Footnotes

For complete statements by the Advisory Committee on Immunization Practices (ACIP), visit www.cdc.gov/vaccines/pubs/ACIP-list.htm.

1. Tetanus, diphtheria, and acellular pertussis (Td/Tdap) vaccination

Tdap should replace a single dose of Td for adults aged 19 through 64 years who have not received a dose of Tdap previously.

Adults with uncertain or incomplete history of primary vaccination series with tetanus and diphtheria toxoid-containing vaccines should begin or complete a primary vaccination series. A primary series for adults is 3 doses of tetanus and diphtheria toxoid-containing vaccines; administer the first 2 doses at least 4 weeks apart and the third dose 6–12 months after the second. However, Tdap can substitute for any one of the doses of Td in the 3-dose primary series. The booster dose of tetanus and diphtheria toxoid-containing vaccine should be administered to adults who have completed a primary series and if the last vaccination was received 10 or more years previously. Tdap or Td vaccine may be used, as indicated.

If a woman is pregnant and received the last Td vaccination 10 or more years previously, administer Td during the second or third trimester. If the woman received the last Td vaccination less than 10 years previously, administer Tdap during the immediate postpartum period. A dose of Tdap is recommended for postpartum women, close contacts of infants aged less than 12 months, and all health-care personnel with direct patient contact if they have not previously received Tdap. An interval as short as 2 years from the last Td is suggested; shorter intervals can be used. Td may be deferred during pregnancy and Tdap substituted in the immediate postpartum period, or Tdap may be administered instead of Td to a pregnant woman after an informed discussion with the woman.

Consult the ACIP statement for recommendations for administering Td as prophylaxis in wound management.

2. Human papillomavirus (HPV) vaccination

HPV vaccination is recommended for all females aged 11 through 26 years (and may begin at 9 years) who have not completed the vaccine series. History of genital warts, abnormal Papanicolaou test, or positive HPV DNA test is not evidence of prior infection with all vaccine HPV types; HPV vaccination is recommended for persons with such histories.

Ideally, vaccine should be administered before potential exposure to HPV through sexual activity; however, females who are sexually active should still be vaccinated consistent with age-based recommendations. Sexually active females who have not been infected with any of the four HPV vaccine types receive the full benefit of the vaccination. Vaccination is less beneficial for females who have already been infected with one or more of the HPV vaccine types.

A complete series consists of 3 doses. The second dose should be administered 2 months after the first dose; the third dose should be administered 6 months after the first dose.

HPV vaccination is not specifically recommended for females with the medical indications described in Figure 2, "Vaccines that might be indicated for adults based on medical and other indications." Because HPV vaccine is not a live-virus vaccine, it may be administered to persons with the medical indications described in Figure 2. However, the immune response and vaccine efficacy might be less for persons with the medical indications described in Figure 2 than in persons who do not have the medical indications described or who are immunocompetent. Health-care personnel are not at increased risk because of occupational exposure, and should be vaccinated consistent with age-based recommendations.

3. Varicella vaccination

All adults without evidence of immunity to varicella should receive 2 doses of single-antigen varicella vaccine if not previously vaccinated or the second dose if they have received only one dose unless they have a medical contraindication. Special consideration should be given to those who 1) have close contact with persons at high risk for severe disease (e.g., health-care personnel and family contacts of persons with immunocompromising conditions) or 2) are at high risk for exposure or transmission (e.g., teachers; child care employees; residents and staff members of institutional settings, including correctional institutions; college students; military personnel; adolescents and adults living in households with children; nonpregnant women of childbearing age; and international travelers).

Evidence of immunity to varicella in adults includes any of the following: 1) documentation of 2 doses of varicella vaccine at least 4 weeks apart; 2) U.S.-born before 1980 (although for health-care personnel and pregnant women, birth before 1980 should not be considered evidence of immunity); 3) history of varicella based on diagnosis or verification of varicella by a health-care provider (for a patient reporting a history of or presenting with an atypical case, a mild case, or both, health-care providers should seek either an epidemiologic link with a typical varicella case or to a laboratory-confirmed case or evidence of laboratory confirmation, if it was performed at the time of acute disease); 4) history of herpes zoster based on health-care provider diagnosis or verification of herpes zoster by a health-care provider; or 5) laboratory evidence of immunity or laboratory confirmation of disease.

Pregnant women should be assessed for evidence of varicella immunity. Women who do not have evidence of immunity should receive the first dose of varicella vaccine upon completion or termination of pregnancy and before discharge from the health-care facility. The second dose should be administered 4–8 weeks after the first dose.

4. Herpes zoster vaccination

A single dose of zoster vaccine is recommended for adults aged 60 years and older regardless of whether they report a prior episode of herpes zoster. Persons with chronic medical conditions may be vaccinated unless their condition constitutes a contraindication.

5. Measles, mumps, rubella (MMR) vaccination

Measles component: Adults born before 1957 generally are considered immune to measles. Adults born during or after 1957 should receive 1 or more doses of MMR unless they have a medical contraindication, documentation of 1 or more doses, history of measles based on health-care provider diagnosis, or laboratory evidence of immunity.

A second dose of MMR is recommended for adults who 1) have been recently exposed to measles or are in an outbreak setting; 2) have been vaccinated previously with killed measles vaccine; 3) have been vaccinated with an unknown type of measles vaccine during 1963–1967; 4) are students in postsecondary educational institutions; 5) work in a health-care facility; or 6) plan to travel internationally.

Mumps component: Adults born before 1957 generally are considered immune to mumps. Adults born during or after 1957 should receive 1 dose of MMR unless they have a medical contraindication, history of mumps based on health-care provider diagnosis, or laboratory evidence of immunity.

A second dose of MMR is recommended for adults who 1) live in a community experiencing a mumps outbreak and are in an affected age group; 2) are students in postsecondary educational institutions; 3) work in a health-care facility; or 4) plan to travel internationally. For unvaccinated health-care personnel born before 1957 who do not have other evidence of mumps immunity, administering 1 dose on a routine basis should be considered and administering a second dose during an outbreak should be strongly considered.

Rubella component: 1 dose of MMR vaccine is recommended for women whose rubella vaccination history is unreliable or who lack laboratory evidence of immunity. For women of childbearing age, regardless of birth year, rubella immunity should be determined and women should be counseled regarding congenital rubella syndrome. Women who do not have evidence of immunity should receive MMR upon completion or termination of pregnancy and before discharge from the health-care facility.

6. Influenza vaccination

Medical indications: Chronic disorders of the cardiovascular or pulmonary systems, including asthma; chronic metabolic diseases, including diabetes mellitus, renal or hepatic dysfunction, hemoglobinopathies, or immunocompromising conditions (including immunocompromising conditions caused by medications or human immunodeficiency virus [HIV]); any condition that compromises respiratory function or the handling of respiratory secretions or that can increase the risk of aspiration (e.g., cognitive dysfunction, spinal cord injury, or seizure disorder or other neuromuscular disorder); and pregnancy during the influenza season. No data exist on the risk for severe or complicated influenza disease among persons with asplenia; however, influenza is a risk factor for secondary bacterial infections that can cause severe disease among persons with asplenia.

Occupational indications: All health-care personnel, including those employed by long-term care and assisted-living facilities, and caregivers of children less than 5 years old.

Other indications: Residents of nursing homes and other long-term care and assisted-living facilities; persons likely to transmit influenza to persons at high risk (e.g., in-home household contacts and caregivers of children aged less than 5 years old, persons 65 years old and older and persons of all ages with high-risk condition[s]); and anyone who would like to decrease their risk of getting influenza. Healthy, nonpregnant adults aged less than 50 years without high-risk medical conditions who are not contacts of severely immunocompromised persons in special care units can receive either intranasally administered live, attenuated influenza vaccine (FluMist®) or inactivated vaccine. Other persons should receive the inactivated vaccine.

7. Pneumococcal polysaccharide (PPSV) vaccination

Medical indications: Chronic lung disease (including asthma); chronic cardiovascular diseases; diabetes mellitus; chronic liver diseases, cirrhosis; chronic alcoholism, chronic renal failure or nephrotic syndrome; functional or anatomic asplenia (e.g., sickle cell disease or splenectomy [if elective splenectomy is planned, vaccinate at least 2 weeks before surgery]); immunocompromising conditions; and cochlear implants and cerebrospinal fluid leaks. Vaccinate as close to HIV diagnosis as possible.

Other indications: Residents of nursing homes or long-term care facilities and persons who smoke cigarettes. Routine use of PPSV is not recommended for Alaska Native or American Indian persons younger than 65 years unless they have underlying medical conditions that are PPSV indications. However, public health authorities may consider recommending PPSV for Alaska Natives and American Indians aged 50 through 64 years who are living in areas in which the risk of invasive pneumococcal disease is increased.

8. Revaccination with PPSV

One-time revaccination after 5 years for persons with chronic renal failure or nephrotic syndrome; functional or anatomic asplenia (e.g., sickle cell disease or splenectomy); and for persons with immunocompromising conditions. For persons aged 65 years and older, one-time revaccination if they were vaccinated 5 or more years previously and were aged less than 65 years at the time of primary vaccination.

9. Hepatitis A vaccination

Medical indications: Persons with chronic liver disease and persons who receive clotting factor concentrates.

Behavioral indications: Men who have sex with men and persons who use illegal drugs.

Occupational indications: Persons working with hepatitis A virus (HAV)-infected primates or with HAV in a research laboratory setting.

Other indications: Persons traveling to or working in countries that have high or intermediate endemicity of hepatitis A (a list of countries is available at wwwn.cdc.gov/travel/contentdiseases.aspx) and any person seeking protection from HAV infection.

Single-antigen vaccine formulations should be administered in a 2-dose schedule at either 0 and 6–12 months (Havrix®), or 0 and 6–18 months (Vaqta®). If the combined hepatitis A and hepatitis B vaccine (Twinrix®) is used, administer 3 doses at 0, 1, and 6 months; alternatively, a 4-dose schedule, administered on days 0, 7 and 21 to 30 followed by a booster dose at month 12 may be used.

10. Hepatitis B vaccination

Medical indications: Persons with end-stage renal disease, including patients receiving hemodialysis; persons with HIV infection; and persons with chronic liver disease.

Occupational indications: Health-care personnel and public-safety workers who are exposed to blood or other potentially infectious body fluids.

Behavioral indications: Sexually active persons who are not in a long-term, mutually monogamous relationship (e.g., persons with more than 1 sex partner during the previous 6 months); persons seeking evaluation or treatment for a sexually transmitted disease (STD); current or recent injection-drug users; and men who have sex with men.

Other indications: Household contacts and sex partners of persons with chronic hepatitis B virus (HBV) infection; clients and staff members of institutions for persons with developmental disabilities; international travelers to countries with high or intermediate prevalence of chronic HBV infection (a list of countries is available at wwwn.cdc.gov/travel/contentdiseases.aspx); and any adult seeking protection from HBV infection.

Hepatitis B vaccination is recommended for all adults in the following settings: STD treatment facilities; HIV testing and treatment facilities; facilities providing drug-abuse treatment and prevention services; health-care settings targeting services to injection-drug users or men who have sex with men; correctional facilities; end-stage renal disease programs and facilities for chronic hemodialysis patients; and institutions and nonresidential daycare facilities for persons with developmental disabilities.

If the combined hepatitis A and hepatitis B vaccine (Twinrix®) is used, administer 3 doses at

Fig 7.6. Continued.

0, 1, and 6 months; alternatively, a 4-dose schedule, administered on days 0, 7 and 21 to 30 followed by a booster dose at month 12 may be used.

Special formulation indications: For adult patients receiving hemodialysis or with other immunocompromising conditions, 1 dose of 40 μg/mL (Recombivax HB®) administered on a 3-dose schedule or 2 doses of 20 μg/mL (Engerix-B®) administered simultaneously on a 4-dose schedule at 0, 1, 2 and 6 months.

11. Meningococcal vaccination

Medical indications: Adults with anatomic or functional asplenia, or terminal complement component deficiencies.

Other indications: First-year college students living in dormitories; microbiologists who are routinely exposed to isolates of *Neisseria meningitidis*; military recruits; and persons who travel to or live in countries in which meningococcal disease is hyperendemic or epidemic (e.g., the "meningitis belt" of sub-Saharan Africa during the dry season [December–June]), particularly if their contact with local populations will be prolonged. Vaccination is required by the government of Saudi Arabia for all travelers to Mecca during the annual Hajj.

Meningococcal conjugate (MCV) vaccine is preferred for adults with any of the preceding indications who are aged 55 years or younger, although meningococcal polysaccharide vaccine (MPSV) is an acceptable alternative. Revaccination with MCV after 5 years might be indicated for adults previously vaccinated with MPSV who remain at increased risk for infection (e.g., persons residing in areas in which disease is epidemic).

12. Selected conditions for which *Haemophilus influenzae* type b (Hib) vaccine may be used

Hib vaccine generally is not recommended for persons aged 5 years and older. No efficacy data are available on which to base a recommendation concerning use of Hib vaccine for older children and adults. However, studies suggest good immunogenicity in persons who have sickle cell disease, leukemia, or HIV infection or who have had a splenectomy; administering 1 dose of vaccine to these persons is not contraindicated.

13. Immunocompromising conditions

Inactivated vaccines generally are acceptable (e.g., pneumococcal, meningococcal, and influenza [trivalent inactivated influenza vaccine]), and live vaccines generally are avoided in persons with immune deficiencies or immunocompromising conditions. Information on specific conditions is available at www.cdc.gov/vaccines/pubs/acip-list.htm.

Fig 7.6. Continued.

The table below provides catch-up schedules and minimum intervals between doses for children whose vaccinations have been delayed. A vaccine series does not need to be restarted, regardless of the time that has elapsed between doses. Use the section appropriate for the child's age.

CATCH-UP SCHEDULE FOR PERSONS AGED 4 MONTHS THROUGH 6 YEARS

Vaccine	Minimum Age for Dose 1	Minimum Interval Between Doses			
		Dose 1 to Dose 2	Dose 2 to Dose 3	Dose 3 to Dose 4	Dose 4 to Dose 5
Hepatitis B[1]	Birth	4 weeks	8 weeks (and at least 16 weeks after first dose)		
Rotavirus[2]	6 wks	4 weeks	4 weeks[2]		
Diphtheria, Tetanus, Pertussis[3]	6 wks	4 weeks	4 weeks	6 months	6 months[3]
Haemophilus influenzae type b[4]	6 wks	**4 weeks** if first dose administered at younger than age 12 months **8 weeks** (as final dose) if first dose administered at age 12-14 months **No further doses needed** if first dose administered at age 15 months or older	**4 weeks**[4] if current age is younger than 12 months **8 weeks** (as final dose)[4] if current age is 12 months or older and second dose administered at younger than age 15 months **No further doses needed** if previous dose administered at age 15 months or older	**8 weeks** (as final dose) This dose only necessary for children aged 12 months through 59 months who received 3 doses before age 12 months	
Pneumococcal[5]	6 wks	**4 weeks** if first dose administered at younger than age 12 months **8 weeks** (as final dose for healthy children) if first dose administered at age 12 months or older or current age 24 through 59 months **No further doses needed** for healthy children if first dose administered at age 24 months or older	**4 weeks** if current age is younger than 12 months **8 weeks** (as final dose for healthy children) if current age is 12 months or older **No further doses needed** for healthy children if previous dose administered at age 24 months or older	**8 weeks** (as final dose) This dose only necessary for children aged 12 months through 59 months who received 3 doses before age 12 months or for high-risk children who received 3 doses at any age	
Inactivated Poliovirus[6]	6 wks	4 weeks	4 weeks	4 weeks[6]	
Measles, Mumps, Rubella[7]	12 mos	4 weeks			
Varicella[8]	12 mos	3 months			
Hepatitis A[9]	12 mos	6 months			

CATCH-UP SCHEDULE FOR PERSONS AGED 7 THROUGH 18 YEARS

Vaccine	Minimum Age for Dose 1	Dose 1 to Dose 2	Dose 2 to Dose 3	Dose 3 to Dose 4	Dose 4 to Dose 5
Tetanus, Diphtheria/ Tetanus, Diphtheria, Pertussis[10]	7 yrs[10]	4 weeks	**4 weeks** if first dose administered at younger than age 12 months **6 months** if first dose administered at age 12 months or older	**6 months** if first dose administered at younger than age 12 months	
Human Papillomavirus[11]	9 yrs	Routine dosing intervals are recommended[11]			
Hepatitis A[9]	12 mos	6 months			
Hepatitis B[1]	Birth	4 weeks	8 weeks (and at least 16 weeks after first dose)		
Inactivated Poliovirus[6]	6 wks	4 weeks	4 weeks	4 weeks[6]	
Measles, Mumps, Rubella[7]	12 mos	4 weeks			
Varicella[8]	12 mos	**3 months** if the person is younger than age 13 years **4 weeks** if the person is aged 13 years or older			

1. **Hepatitis B vaccine (HepB).**
   - Administer the 3-dose series to those not previously vaccinated.
   - A 2-dose series (separated by at least 4 months) of adult formulation Recombivax HB® is licensed for children aged 11 through 15 years.
2. **Rotavirus vaccine (RV).**
   - The maximum age for the first dose is 14 weeks 6 days. Vaccination should not be initiated for infants aged 15 weeks or older (i.e., 15 weeks 0 days or older).
   - Administer the final dose in the series by age 8 months 0 days.
   - If Rotarix® was administered for the first and second doses, a third dose is not indicated.
3. **Diphtheria and tetanus toxoids and acellular pertussis vaccine (DTaP).**
   - The fifth dose is not necessary if the fourth dose was administered at age 4 years or older.
4. ***Haemophilus influenzae* type b conjugate vaccine (Hib).**
   - Hib vaccine is not generally recommended for persons aged 5 years or older. No efficacy data are available on which to base a recommendation concerning use of Hib vaccine for older children and adults. However, studies suggest good immunogenicity in persons who have sickle cell disease, leukemia, or HIV infection, or who have had a splenectomy; administering 1 dose of Hib vaccine to these persons is not contraindicated.
   - If the first 2 doses were PRP-OMP (PedvaxHIB® or Comvax®), and administered at age 11 months or younger, the third (and final) dose should be administered at age 12 through 15 months and at least 8 weeks after the second dose.
   - If the first dose was administered at age 7 through 11 months, administer 2 doses separated by 4 weeks and a final dose at age 12 through 15 months.
5. **Pneumococcal vaccine.**
   - Administer 1 dose of pneumococcal conjugate vaccine (PCV) to all healthy children aged 24 through 59 months who have not received at least 1 dose of PCV on or after age 12 months.
   - For children aged 24 through 59 months with underlying medical conditions, administer 1 dose of PCV if 3 doses were received previously or administer 2 doses of PCV at least 8 weeks apart if fewer than 3 doses were received previously.
   - Administer pneumococcal polysaccharide vaccine (PPSV) to children aged 2 years or older with certain underlying medical conditions (see *MMWR* 2000;49[No. RR-9]), including a cochlear implant, at least 8 weeks after the last dose of PCV.
6. **Inactivated poliovirus vaccine (IPV).**
   - For children who received an all-IPV or all-oral poliovirus (OPV) series, a fourth dose is not necessary if the third dose was administered at age 4 years or older.
   - If both OPV and IPV were administered as part of a series, a total of 4 doses should be administered, regardless of the child's current age.
7. **Measles, mumps, and rubella vaccine (MMR).**
   - Administer the second dose at age 4 through 6 years. However, the second dose may be administered before age 4, provided at least 28 days have elapsed since the first dose.
   - If not previously vaccinated, administer 2 doses with at least 28 days between doses.
8. **Varicella vaccine.**
   - Administer the second dose at age 4 through 6 years. However, the second dose may be administered before age 4, provided at least 3 months have elapsed since the first dose.
   - For persons aged 12 months through 12 years, the minimum interval between doses is 3 months. However, if the second dose was administered at least 28 days after the first dose, it can be accepted as valid.
   - For persons aged 13 years and older, the minimum interval between doses is 28 days.
9. **Hepatitis A vaccine (HepA).**
   - HepA is recommended for children older than 1 year who live in areas where vaccination programs target older children or who are at increased risk of infection. See *MMWR* 2006;55(No. RR-7).
10. **Tetanus and diphtheria toxoids vaccine (Td) and tetanus and diphtheria toxoids and acellular pertussis vaccine (Tdap).**
    - Doses of DTaP are counted as part of the Td/Tdap series
    - Tdap should be substituted for a single dose of Td in the catch-up series or as a booster for children aged 10 through 18 years; use Td for other doses.
11. **Human papillomavirus vaccine (HPV).**
    - Administer the series to females at age 13 through 18 years if not previously vaccinated.
    - Use recommended routine dosing intervals for series catch-up (i.e., the second and third doses should be administered at 2 and 6 months after the first dose). However, the minimum interval between the first and second doses is 4 weeks. The minimum interval between the second and third doses is 12 weeks, and the third dose should be given at least 24 weeks after the first dose.

Information about reporting reactions after immunization is available online at http://www.vaers.hhs.gov or by telephone, 800-822-7967. Suspected cases of vaccine-preventable diseases should be reported to the state or local health department. Additional information, including precautions and contraindications for immunization, is available from the National Center for Immunization and Respiratory Diseases at http://www.cdc.gov/vaccines or telephone, 800-CDC-INFO (800-232-4636).

DEPARTMENT OF HEALTH AND HUMAN SERVICES • CENTERS FOR DISEASE CONTROL AND PREVENTION

CS113897

Fig 7.7. Catch-up immunization schedule for persons aged 4 months through 18 years who start late or who are more than 1 month behind: United states, 2009. (Reproduced with permission from Centers for Disease Control and Prevention, Department of Health and Human Services. 2009 child & adolescent immunization schedules. Available at: www.cdc.gov/vaccines/recs/schedules/child-schedule.htm#printable).

Risk for a developing fetus from vaccination of the mother during pregnancy primarily is theoretical. No evidence exists of risk from vaccinating pregnant women with inactivated virus or bacterial vaccines or toxoids. Live vaccines pose a theoretical risk to the fetus. Benefits of vaccinating pregnant women usually outweigh potential risks when the likelihood of disease exposure is high, when infection would pose a risk to the mother or fetus, and when the vaccine is unlikely to cause harm."[1]

Generally, live-virus vaccines are contraindicated for pregnant women because of the theoretical risk of transmission of the vaccine virus to the fetus. If a live-virus vaccine is inadvertently given to a pregnant woman, or if a woman becomes pregnant within 4 weeks after vaccination, she should be counseled about the potential effects on the fetus. But vaccination is not ordinarily an indication to terminate the pregnancy.

Whether live or inactivated vaccines are used, vaccination of pregnant women should be considered on the basis of risks versus benefits – i.e., the risk of the vaccination versus the benefits of protection in a particular circumstance. The following table may be used as a general guide.

	VACCINE	SHOULD BE CONSIDERED IF OTHERWISE INDICATED	CONTRAINDICATED DURING PREGNANCY	SPECIAL/CONDITIONAL RECOMMENDATION (SEE TEXT)
ROUTINE	Hepatitis A			(See page 1)
	Hepatitis B	X		
	Human Papillomavirus (HPV)			(See page 1)
	Influenza (Inactivated)	Recommended		
	Influenza (LAIV)*		X	
	Measles*		X	
	Meningococcal (MCV4)			(See page 2)
	Mumps*		X	
	Pneumococcal			(See page 2)
	Polio (IPV)			(See page 2)
	Rubella*		X	
	Tetanus-Diphtheria (Td)	X		
	Tetanus-Diphtheria-Pertussis (Tdap)			(See page 4)
	Varicella*		X	
TRAVEL & OTHER	Anthrax			(See page 5)
	BCG*		X	
	Japanese Encephalitis			(See page 5)
	Meningococcal (MPSV4)	X		
	Rabies	X		
	Typhoid (Parenteral & Oral*)			(See page 5)
	Vaccinia*		X	(See page 5)
	Yellow Fever*			(See page 6)
	Zoster*		X	

*Live attenuated vaccine

Passive Immunization during Pregnancy

"No known risk exists for the fetus from passive immunization of pregnant women with immune globulin preparations."[1]

Fig 7.8. Vaccination of pregnant women. (Reproduced with permission from Centers for Disease Control and Prevention, Advisory Committee on Immunization Practices. Guidelines for vaccinating pregnant women. Available at: www.cdc.gov/vaccines/pubs/downloads/b_preg_guide.pdf).

Guidelines for Vaccinating Pregnant Women

Abstracted from recommendations of the Advisory Committee on Immunization Practices (ACIP)

Hepatitis A	• The safety of hepatitis A vaccination during pregnancy has not been determined; however, because hepatitis A vaccine is produced from inactivated [hepatitis A virus], the theoretical risk to the developing fetus is expected to be low. **The risk associated with vaccination should be weighed against the risk for hepatitis A in pregnant women who may be at high risk for exposure to [hepatitis A virus].**[2]
Hepatitis B	• **Pregnancy is not a contraindication to vaccination.** Limited data indicate no apparent risk for adverse events to developing fetuses when hepatitis B vaccine is administered to pregnant women. Current vaccines contain noninfectious HBsAg and should cause no risk to the fetus.[3] • **Pregnant women who are identified as being at risk for HBV** infection during pregnancy (e.g., having more than one sex partner during the previous 6 months, been evaluated or treated for an STD, recent or current injection drug use, or having had an HBsAg-positive sex partner) **should be vaccinated.**[3]
Human Papillomavirus (HPV)	• **Quadrivalent HPV vaccine is not recommended for use in pregnancy.**[4] • The vaccine has not been causally associated with adverse outcomes of pregnancy or adverse events to the developing fetus. However, data on vaccination during pregnancy are limited. Until additional information is available, initiation of the vaccine series should be delayed until after completion of the pregnancy. If a woman is found to be pregnant after initiating the vaccination series, the remainder of the 3-dose regimen should be delayed until after completion of the pregnancy. If a vaccine dose has been administered during pregnancy, no intervention is needed.[4] • A vaccine in pregnancy registry has been established; patients and health-care providers should report any exposure to . . . HPV vaccine during pregnancy (telephone: 800-986-8999).[4]
Influenza (Inactivated)	• Vaccination with inactivated influenza vaccine is recommended for the following persons who are at increased risk for severe complications from influenza: . . . Women who will be pregnant during the influenza season.[5] • One study of influenza immunization of approximately 2,000 pregnant women demonstrated no adverse fetal effects associated with influenza vaccine; similar results were observed in a study of 252 pregnant women who received inactivated influenza vaccine within 6 months of delivery.[5]

Fig 7.8. Continued.

Influenza (LAIV)	• Persons who should not be vaccinated with LAIV . . . pregnant women. . . . These persons should receive inactivated influenza vaccine.[5]
Measles	• **Measles-mumps-rubella (MMR) vaccine and its component vaccines should not be administered to women known to be pregnant**. Because a risk to the fetus from administration of these live virus vaccines cannot be excluded for theoretical reasons, women should be counseled to avoid becoming pregnant for 28 days after vaccination with measles or mumps vaccines or MMR or other rubella-containing vaccines.[6] • If vaccination of an unknowingly pregnant woman occurs or if she becomes pregnant within 4 weeks after MMR . . . vaccination, she should be counseled about the theoretical basis of concern for the fetus; however, MMR . . . vaccination during pregnancy should not be regarded as a reason to terminate pregnancy.[1]
Meningococcal (MCV4) (conjugate)	• MCV4 is safe and immunogenic among nonpregnant persons aged 11-55 years, but no data are available on the safety of MCV4 during pregnancy. **Women of childbearing age who become aware that they were pregnant at the time of MCV4 vaccination should contact their health-care provider or the vaccine manufacturer**.[7]
Mumps	• **Measles-mumps-rubella (MMR) vaccine and its component vaccines should not be administered to women known to be pregnant**. Because a risk to the fetus from administration of these live virus vaccines cannot be excluded for theoretical reasons, women should be counseled to avoid becoming pregnant for 28 days after vaccination with measles or mumps vaccines or MMR or other rubella-containing vaccines.[6] • If vaccination of an unknowingly pregnant woman occurs or if she becomes pregnant within 4 weeks after MMR . . . vaccination, she should be counseled about the theoretical basis of concern for the fetus; however, MMR . . . vaccination during pregnancy should not be regarded as a reason to terminate pregnancy.[1]
Pneumococcal (PPV23) (polysaccharide)	• The safety of pneumococcal polysaccharide vaccine during the first trimester of pregnancy has not been evaluated, although no adverse consequences have been reported among newborns whose mothers were inadvertently vaccinated during pregnancy.[8]
Polio (IPV)	• Although no adverse effects of IPV have been documented among pregnant women or their fetuses, **vaccination of pregnant women should be avoided on theoretical grounds**. However, if a pregnant woman is at increased risk for infection and requires immediate protection against polio, IPV can be administered in accordance with the recommended schedules for adults.[9]

Fig 7.8. Continued.

Rubella	• **Measles-mumps-rubella (MMR) vaccine and its component vaccines should not be administered to women known to be pregnant.** Because a risk to the fetus from administration of these live virus vaccines cannot be excluded for theoretical reasons, women should be counseled to avoid becoming pregnant for 28 days after vaccination with measles or mumps vaccines or MMR or other rubella-containing vaccines.[6] • If vaccination of an unknowingly pregnant woman occurs or if she becomes pregnant within 4 weeks after MMR . . . vaccination, she should be counseled about the theoretical basis of concern for the fetus; however, MMR . . . vaccination during pregnancy should not be regarded as a reason to terminate pregnancy.[1] • Rubella-susceptible women who are not vaccinated because they state they are or may be pregnant should be counseled about the potential risk for CRS and the importance of being vaccinated as soon as they are no longer pregnant.[10] • A registry of susceptible women vaccinated with rubella vaccine between 3 months before and 3 months after conception – the "Vaccine in Pregnancy (VIP) Registry" – was kept between 1971 and 1989. No evidence of CRS occurred in the offspring of the 226 women who received the current RA 27/3 rubella vaccine and continued their pregnancy to term.[10]
Tetanus & Diphtheria (Td) **(See also Tdap)**	• **Pregnant women should receive Td vaccine if indicated.** Previously vaccinated pregnant women who have not received a Td vaccination within the last 10 years should receive a booster dose.[1] • Pregnant women who have not received three doses of a vaccine containing tetanus and diphtheria toxoids should complete a series of 3 vaccinations. Two doses of Td should be administered during pregnancy to ensure protection against maternal and neonatal tetanus. The preferred schedule in pregnant women is two doses of Td separated by 4 weeks, and a dose of Tdap 6 months after the second dose (post-partum). Health-care providers can choose to substitute a single dose of Tdap for a dose of Td during pregnancy.[11] • Although no evidence exists that tetanus and diphtheria toxoids are teratogenic, waiting until the second trimester of pregnancy to administer Td is a reasonable precaution for minimizing any concern about the theoretical possibility of such reactions.[12]

Fig 7.8. Continued.

Tetanus, Diphtheria, & Pertussis (Tdap)

- **Pregnancy is not a contraindication for use of Tdap.** Data on safety, immunogenicity and the outcomes of pregnancy are not available for pregnant women who receive Tdap. When Tdap is administered during pregnancy, transplacental maternal antibodies might protect the infant against pertussis in early life. They also could interfere with the infant's immune response to infant doses of DTaP, and leave the infant less well protected against pertussis.[11]
- ACIP recommends Td when tetanus and diphtheria protection is required during pregnancy. **In some situations*, health-care providers can choose to administer Tdap instead of Td to add protection against pertussis.** When Td or Tdap is administered during pregnancy, the second or third trimester is preferred.[11]
- Providers who choose to administer Tdap to pregnant women should discuss the lack of data with the pregnant women and are encouraged to report Tdap administrations regardless of the trimester, to the appropriate manufacturer's pregnancy registry: for Boostrix® to GlaxoSmithKline Biologicals at 1-888-825-5249, or for Adacel®, to sanofi pasteur at 800-822-2463.[11]

* "Situations with increased risk for pertussis: Health-care providers can choose to administer Tdap instead of Td to protect against pertussis in pregnant adolescents for routine or "catch-up" vaccination because the incidence of pertussis is high among adolescents, in pregnant health-care personnel and child care providers to prevent transmission to infants younger than 12 months of age and to other vulnerable persons, and in pregnant women employed in an institution or living in a community with increased pertussis activity.[11]

Varicella

- The effects of the varicella virus vaccine on the fetus are unknown; therefore, **pregnant women should not be vaccinated.** Nonpregnant women who are vaccinated should avoid becoming pregnant for 1 month following each injection. For susceptible persons, having a pregnant household member is not a contraindication to vaccination.[13]
- Because the virulence of the attenuated virus used in the vaccine is less than that of the wild-type virus, the risk to the fetus, if any, should be even lower.[13]
- If vaccination of an unknowingly pregnant woman occurs or if she becomes pregnant within 4 weeks after . . . varicella vaccination, she should be counseled about the theoretical basis of concern for the fetus; however, . . . varicella vaccination during pregnancy should not be regarded as a reason to terminate pregnancy.[1]
- VZIG [Varicella Zoster Immune Globulin] should be strongly considered for susceptible, pregnant women who have been exposed.[13]
- NOTE: The manufacturer and CDC have established a Varivax® Pregnancy Registry to monitor outcomes of women who received the vaccine 3 months before or any time during pregnancy. Call 800-986-8999.

Fig 7.8. Continued.

Anthrax	• No studies have been published regarding use of anthrax vaccine among pregnant women. **Pregnant women should be vaccinated against anthrax only if the potential benefits of vaccination outweigh the potential risks to the fetus.**[14]
BCG	• Although no harmful effects to the fetus have been associated with BCG vaccine, **its use is not recommended during pregnancy.**[15]
Japanese Encephalitis	• No specific information is available on the safety of JE vaccine in pregnancy. Vaccination poses an unknown but theoretical risk to the developing fetus, and **the vaccine should not be routinely administered during pregnancy.**[16] • Pregnant women who must travel to an area where risk of JE is high should be vaccinated when the theoretical risks of immunization are outweighed by the risk of infection to the mother and developing fetus.[16]
Meningococcal (MPSV4) (polysaccharide)	• Studies of vaccination with MPSV4 during pregnancy have not documented adverse effects among either pregnant women or newborns. On the basis of these data, **pregnancy should not preclude vaccination with MPSV4, if indicated.**[7]
Rabies	• Because of the potential consequences of inadequately treated rabies exposure, and because there is no indication that fetal abnormalities have been associated with rabies vaccination, **pregnancy is not considered a contraindication to postexposure prophylaxis.**[17] • **If the risk of exposure to rabies is substantial, preexposure prophylaxis might also be indicated during pregnancy.**[17]
Typhoid	• No data have been reported on the use of any of the three typhoid vaccines among pregnant women.[18]
Vaccinia (Smallpox)	• Live-viral vaccines are contraindicated during pregnancy; therefore, **vaccinia vaccine should not be administered to pregnant women for routine nonemergency indications.**[19] • However, vaccinia vaccine is not known to cause congenital malformations. Although <50 cases of fetal vaccinia infection have been reported, vaccinia virus has been reported to cause fetal infection on rare occasions, almost always after primary vaccination of the mother.[19] • **Pregnant women who have had a definite exposure to smallpox virus (i.e., face-to-face, household, or close-proximity contact with a smallpox patient) and are, therefore, at high risk for contracting the disease, should . . . be vaccinated.** Smallpox infection among pregnant women has been reported to result in a more severe infection than among nonpregnant women. Therefore the risks to the mother and fetus from experiencing clinical smallpox substantially outweigh any potential risks regarding vaccination. In addition, vaccinia virus has not been documented to be teratogenic, and the incidence of fetal vaccinia is low.[19] • When the level of exposure risk is undetermined, the decision to vaccinate should be made after assessment by the clinician and the patient of the potential risks versus the benefits of smallpox vaccination.[19]

Fig 7.8. Continued.

Yellow Fever

- The safety of yellow fever vaccination during pregnancy has not been established, and the **vaccine should be administered only if travel to an endemic area is unavoidable and if an increased risk for exposure exists.**[20]
- . . . infection of the fetus with YF17D apparently occurs at a low rate . . . and has not been associated with congenital anomalies.[20]
- If international travel requirements are the only reason to vaccinate a pregnant woman, rather than an increased risk of infection, efforts should be made to obtain a waiver letter from the traveler's physician.[20]
- Pregnant women who must travel to areas where the risk of yellow fever is high should be vaccinated and, despite the apparent safety of this vaccine, infants born to these women should be monitored closely for evidence of congenital infection and other possible adverse effects resulting from yellow fever vaccination.[20]
- If vaccination of a pregnant woman is deemed necessary, serologic testing to document an immune response to the vaccine can be considered, because the seroconversion rate for pregnant women in a developing nation has been reported to be substantially lower than that observed for other healthy adults and children. To discuss the need for serologic testing, the appropriate state health department or the Division of Vector-Borne Infectious Diseases (telephone: 970-221-6400) or the Division of Global Migration and Quarantine (telephone: 404-498-1600) at CDC should be contacted.[20]

Zoster (Shingles)

The ACIP has not yet issued recommendations on zoster vaccine. The manufacturer recommends not administering the vaccine during pregnancy:

- Contraindications: **Zostavax should not be administered to individuals . . . who are or may be pregnant.**[21]
- It is . . . not known whether Zostavax can cause fetal harm when administered to a pregnant woman or can affect reproduction capacity. However, naturally occurring VZV infection is known to sometimes cause fetal harm. Therefore, **Zostavax should not be administered to pregnant females**; furthermore, pregnancy should be avoided for three months following vaccination.[21]

Fig 7.8. Continued.

Prenatal Serologic Screening

The ACIP currently recommends prenatal screening for rubella and hepatitis B:

Rubella: "Prenatal serologic screening . . . is indicated for all pregnant women who lack acceptable evidence of rubella immunity. Upon completion or termination of their pregnancies, women who do not have serologic evidence of rubella immunity or documentation of rubella vaccination should be vaccinated with MMR before discharge from the hospital, birthing center, or abortion clinic."[10]

Hepatitis B: "All pregnant women should be routinely tested for HBsAg during an early prenatal visit (e.g., first trimester) in each pregnancy, even if they have been previously vaccinated or tested." "Women who are HBsAg positive should be referred to an appropriate case-management program to ensure that their infants receive timely postexposure prophylaxis and followup." "Women who are HBsAg positive should be provided with or referred for appropriate counseling and medical management." "When HBsAg testing of pregnant women is not feasible (i.e., in remote areas without access to a laboratory), all infants should receive hepatitis B vaccine ≤12 hours of birth and should complete the hepatitis B vaccine series according to a recommended schedule for infants born to HBsAg-positive mothers."[3] For more information, see Reference 3, p. 635.

Vaccinating Women Who Are Breastfeeding

"Neither inactivated nor live vaccines administered to a lactating woman affect the safety of breast-feeding for mothers or infants. Breast-feeding does not adversely affect immunization and is not a contraindication for any vaccine, with the exception of smallpox vaccine."[1]

The following applies to varicella vaccine, which was licensed after the ACIP General Recommendations were published: "Whether attenuated vaccine VZV is excreted in human milk and, if so, whether the infant could be infected are not known. Most live vaccines have not been demonstrated to be secreted in breast milk. Attenuated rubella vaccine virus has been detected in breast milk but has produced only asymptomatic infection in the nursing infant. Therefore, varicella vaccine may be considered for a nursing mother."[11]

Fig 7.8. Continued.

References

1. CDC. General recommendations on immunization: recommendations of the Advisory Committee on Immunization Practices (ACIP). *MMWR* 2006; 55 (No. RR-15): 32-33.
2. CDC. Prevention of hepatitis A through active or passive immunization: recommendations of the Advisory Committee on Immunization Practices (ACIP). *MMWR* 2006; 55 (No. RR-7): 15.
3. CDC. A comprehensive immunization strategy to eliminate transmission of hepatitis B virus infection in the United States: recommendations of the Advisory Committee on Immunization Practices (ACIP) part 1: immunization of infants, children, and adolescents. *MMWR* 2005; 54 (No. RR-16): 12, 14.
4. CDC. Quadrivalent human papillomavirus vaccine: recommendations of the Advisory Committee on Immunization Practices (ACIP). *MMWR* 2007; 56 (No. RR-2): 18.
5. CDC. Prevention and control of influenza: recommendations of the Advisory Committee on Immunization Practices (ACIP). *MMWR* 2006; 55 (No. RR-10): 11-12.
6. CDC. Notice to readers: revised ACIP recommendation for avoiding pregnancy after receiving a rubella-containing vaccine. *MMWR* 2001; 50 (No. 49): 1117.
7. CDC. Prevention and control of meningococcal disease: recommendations of the Advisory Committee on Immunization Practices (ACIP). *MMWR* 2005; 54 (No. RR-7): 15.
8. CDC. Prevention of pneumococcal disease: recommendations of the Advisory Committee on Immunization Practices (ACIP). *MMWR* 1997; 46 (No. RR-8): 6.
9. CDC. Poliomyelitis prevention in the United States: recommendations of the Advisory Committee on Immunization Practices (ACIP). *MMWR* 2000; 49 (No. RR-5): 14.
10. CDC. Measles, mumps, and rubella — vaccine use and strategies for elimination of measles, rubella, and congenital rubella syndrome and control of mumps: recommendations of the Advisory Committee on Immunization Practices (ACIP). *MMWR* 1998; 47 (No. RR-8): 18, 32-33.
11. CDC. Prevention of tetanus, diphtheria and pertussis among pregnant women: provisional ACIP recommendations for the use of Tdap vaccine, 2006. Available at http://www.cdc.gov/nip/recs/provisional_recs/tdap-preg.pdf.
12. CDC. Diphtheria, tetanus, and pertussis: recommendations for vaccine use and other preventive measures: recommendations of the Immunization Practices Advisory Committee (ACIP). *MMWR* 1991; 40 (No. RR-10): 14.
13. CDC. Prevention of varicella: recommendations of the Advisory Committee on Immunization Practices (ACIP). *MMWR* 1996; 45 (No. RR-11): 19-20.
14. CDC. Use of anthrax vaccine in the United States: recommendations of the Advisory Committee on Immunization Practices (ACIP). *MMWR* 2000; 49 (No. RR-15): 11.
15. CDC. The role of BCG vaccine in the prevention and control of tuberculosis in the United States: a joint statement by the Advisory Council for the Elimination of Tuberculosis and the Advisory Committee on Immunization Practices. *MMWR* 1996; 45 (No. RR-4): 13.
16. CDC. Inactivated Japanese encephalitis vaccine: recommendations of the Advisory Committee on Immunization Practices (ACIP). *MMWR* 1993; 42 (No. RR-1): 12-13.
17. CDC. Human rabies prevention–United States, 1999: recommendations of the Advisory Committee on Immunization Practices (ACIP). *MMWR* 1999; 48 (No. RR-1): 17.
18. CDC. Typhoid immunization: recommendations of the Advisory Committee on Immunization Practices (ACIP). *MMWR* 1994; 43 (No. RR-14): 7.

Fig 7.8. Continued.

19. CDC. Vaccinia (smallpox) vaccine: recommendations of the Advisory Committee on Immunization Practices (ACIP). *MMWR* 2001; 50 (No. RR-10): 12 & 19.

20. CDC. Yellow fever vaccine: recommendations of the Advisory Committee on Immunization Practices (ACIP), 2002. *MMWR* 2002; 51 (No. RR-17): 7.

21. Zostavax (Package Insert). Whitehouse Station, NJ: Merck & Co. Inc.; 2006. Available at http://www.merck.com/product/usa/pi_circulars/z/zostavax/zostavax_pi.pdf.

For More Information

More detailed information about vaccination of pregnant women can be found in:

- ACIP statements for specific diseases.
- The ACIP's Update on Adult Immunization (*MMWR* Vol. 40, No. RR-12, November 15, 1991). See especially p. 9 and Appendix 5, pp. 82-88.

  Current ACIP recommendations can be found on the National Immunization Program's website at http://www.cdc.gov/nip/publications/ACIP-list.htm. Or call the National Immunization Program's Information Center at (404) 639-8226.

- The American College of Obstetricians and Gynecologists (ACOG) **Technical Bulletin Number 160**, October 1991. This publication is available from the American College of Obstetricians and Gynecologists, Attn: Resource Center, 409 12th Street SW, Washington, DC 20024-2188.
- The American College of Physicians' ***Guide for Adult Immunization***, Third Edition, pp. 25-29. Customer Service for the American College of Physicians can be contacted at (215) 351-2600 or (800) 523-1546.

Fig 7.8. Continued.

Adolesc Med 20 (2009) 637–663

8. Cardiorespiratory

Alain Joffe, MD, MPH
E-mail address: ajoffe@jhu.edu.

- **Classifying severity for patients who are not currently taking long-term control medications.**

Components of Severity		Classification of Asthma Severity (Youths ≥12 years of age and adults)			
			Persistent		
		Intermittent	Mild	Moderate	Severe
Impairment Normal FEV_1/FVC: 8–19 yr 85% 20–39 yr 80% 40–59 yr 75% 60–80 yr 70%	Symptoms	≤2 days/week	>2 days/week but not daily	Daily	Throughout the day
	Nighttime awakenings	≤2x/month	3–4x/month	>1x/week but not nightly	Often 7x/week
	Short-acting $beta_2$-agonist use for symptom control (not prevention of EIB)	≤2 days/week	>2 days/week but not >1x/day	Daily	Several times per day
	Interference with normal activity	None	Minor limitation	Some limitation	Extremely limited
	Lung function	• Normal FEV_1 between exacerbations • FEV_1 >80% predicted • FEV_1/FVC normal	• FEV_1 ≥80% predicted • FEV_1/FVC normal	• FEV_1 >60% but <80% predicted • FEV_1/FVC reduced 5%	• FEV_1 <60% predicted • FEV_1/FVC reduced >5%
Risk	Exacerbations requiring oral systemic corticosteroids	0-1/year (see note)	≥2/year (see note) →		
		← Consider severity and interval since exacerbation. Frequency and severity may fluctuate over time for patients in any severity category →			
		Relative annual risk of exacerbations may be related to FEV_1			

- Level of severity is determined by assessment of both impairment and risk. Assess impairment domain by patient's/caregiver's recall of previous 2–4 weeks and spirometry. Assign severity to the most severe category in which any feature occurs.
- At present, there are inadequate data to correspond frequencies of exacerbations with different levels of asthma severity. In general, more frequent and intense exacerbations (e.g., requiring urgent, unscheduled care, hospitalization, or ICU admission) indicate greater underlying disease severity. For treatment purposes, patients who had ≥2 exacerbations requiring oral systemic corticosteroids in the past year may be considered the same as patients who have persistent asthma, even in the absence of impairment levels consistent with persistent asthma.

- **Classifying severity in patients after asthma becomes well controlled, by lowest level of treatment required to maintain control.***

Lowest level of treatment required to maintain control (See figure 4–5 for treatment steps.)	Classification of Asthma Severity			
	Intermittent	Persistent		
		Mild	Moderate	Severe
	Step 1	Step 2	Step 3 or 4	Step 5 or 6

Key: EIB, exercise-induced bronchospasm; FEV_1, forced expiratory volume in 1 second; FVC, forced vital capacity; ICU, intensive care unit

***Notes:**

severity after control

- For population-based evaluations, clinical research, or characterization of a patient's overall asthma is achieved. For clinical management, the focus is on monitoring the level of control (See figure 3–5c.), not the level of severity, once treatment is established.
- See figure 3–5c for definition of asthma control.

Fig 8.1. Classifying asthma severity in youth ≥12 years of age and adults. (From National Heart Lung and Blood Institute. Expert panel report 3: guidelines for the diagnosis and management of asthma. Available at: www.nhlbi.nih.gov/guidelines/asthma/asthgdln.htm. Accessed April 25, 2009).

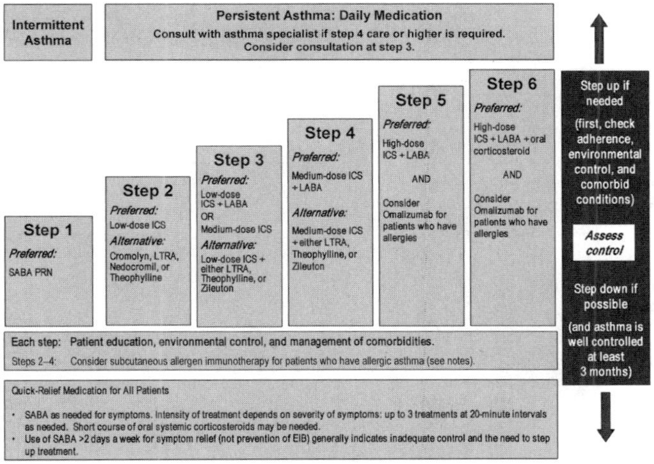

— Key: **Alphabetical order is used when more than one treatment option is listed within either preferred or alternative therapy.** EIB, exercise-induced bronchospasm; ICS, inhaled corticosteroid; LABA, long-acting inhaled beta$_2$-agonist; LTRA, leukotriene receptor antagonist; SABA, inhaled short-acting beta$_2$-agonist

Notes:

- The stepwise approach is meant to assist, not replace, the clinical decisionmaking required to meet individual patient needs.
- If alternative treatment is used and response is inadequate, discontinue it and use the preferred treatment before stepping up.
- Zileuton is a less desirable alternative due to limited studies as adjunctive therapy and the need to monitor liver function. Theophylline requires monitoring of serum concentration levels.
- In step 6, before oral systemic corticosteroids are introduced, a trial of high-dose ICS + LABA + either LTRA, theophylline, or zileuton may be considered, although this approach has not been studied in clinical trials.
- Step 1, 2, and 3 preferred therapies are based on Evidence A; step 3 alternative therapy is based on Evidence A for LTRA, Evidence B for theophylline, and Evidence D for zileuton. Step 4 preferred therapy is based on Evidence B, and alternative therapy is based on Evidence B for LTRA and theophylline and Evidence D for zileuton. Step 5 preferred therapy is based on Evidence B. Step 6 preferred therapy is based on (EPR—2 1997) and Evidence B for omalizumab.
- Immunotherapy for steps 2–4 is based on Evidence B for house-dust mites, animal danders, and pollens; evidence is weak or lacking for molds and cockroaches. Evidence is strongest for immunotherapy with single allergens. The role of allergy in asthma is greater in children than in adults.
- Clinicians who administer immunotherapy or omalizumab should be prepared and equipped to identify and treat anaphylaxis that may occur.

Fig 8.2. Stepwise approach for managing asthma in youth ≥12 years of age and adults. (From National Heart Lung and Blood Institute. Expert panel report 3: guidelines for the diagnosis and management of asthma. Available at: www.nhlbi.nih.gov/guidelines/asthma/asthgdln. htm. Accessed April 25, 2009).

Table 8.1
Predicted peak expiratory flow rates (</min) according to age, gender, and height

	Height, in																	
Age, y	42	44	46	48	50	52	54	56	57	58	60	62	64	66	68	70	72	76
Female (adolescent)																		
12	190		220		250		280		302		324		354		384		414	
14	209		239		269		298		321		343		373		403		432	
16	228		258		288		317		340		362		392		421		451	
18	247		277		306		336		358		381		411		440		470	
20	266		295		325		355		377		400		429		459		489	
Female (adult)																		
20										357	372	387	402	417	432	446		
25										350	365	379	394	409	424	439		
Male																		
12		159		206		254		301			349		398		444		491	539
14		178		226		274		321			369		416		464		511	559
16		196		246		293		341			389		436		484		531	579
18		218		266		313		361			408		456		503		551	599
20		238		286		333		381			421		476		523		571	618
22		258		306		353		401			448		496		543		591	638
24		276		326		373		421			468		516		563		611	658
25		288		336		383		431			478		526		573		621	668

Predicted peak expiratory flow rates are estimates based on age, gender, and height; value may vary depending on the type of flowmeter used. An individual's personal best may be higher or lower than the average but is usually the highest number recorded over a 2- to 3-week period. Adapted from Knudson RJ, Lebowitz MD, Holberg CJ, Burrows B. Changes in the normal maximal expiratory flow-volume curve with growth and aging. *Am Rev Respir Dis.* 1983;127(6):725–734.

C

Medication	Dosage Form	Adult Dose	Comments
Inhaled Short-Acting Beta$_2$-Agonists (SABA)			
	MDI		***Applies to all four SABAs***
Albuterol CFC	90 mcg/puff, 200 puffs/canister	■ 2 puffs 5 minutes before exercise ■ 2 puffs every 4–6 hours as needed	■ An increasing use or lack of expected effect indicates diminished control of asthma. ■ Not recommended for long-term daily treatment. Regular use exceeding 2 days/week for symptom control (not prevention of EIB) indicates the need to step up therapy. ■ Differences in potency exist, but all products are essentially comparable on a per puff basis. ■ May double usual dose for mild exacerbations. ■ Should prime the inhaler by releasing 4 actuations prior to use. ■ Periodically clean HFA activator, as drug may block/plug orifice. ■ Nonselective agents (i.e., epinephrine, isoproterenol, metaproterenol) are not recommended due to their potential for excessive cardiac stimulation, especially in high doses.
Albuterol HFA	90 mcg/puff, 200 puffs/canister		
Pirbuterol CFC	200 mcg/puff, 400 puffs/canister		
Levalbuterol HFA	45 mcg/puff, 200 puffs/canister		
	Nebulizer solution		
Albuterol	0.63 mg/3 mL 1.25 mg/3 mL 2.5 mg/3 mL 5 mg/mL (0.5%)	1.25–5 mg in 3 cc of saline q 4–8 hours as needed	■ May mix with budesonide inhalant suspension, cromolyn or ipratropium nebulizer solutions. May double dose for severe exacerbations.
Levalbuterol (R-albuterol)	0.31 mg/3 mL 0.63 mg/3 mL 1.25 mg/0.5 mL 1.25 mg/3 mL	0.63 mg–1.25 mg q 8 hours as needed	■ Compatible with budesonide inhalant suspension. The product is a sterile-filled, preservative-free, unit dose vial.

Fig 8.3. (*Continued*).

Medication	Dosage Form	Adult Dose	Comments
Anticholinergics			
	MDI		
Ipratropium HFA	17 mcg/puff, 200 puffs/canister	2–3 puffs q 6 hours	■ Evidence is lacking for anticholinergics producing added benefit to $beta_2$-agonists in long-term control asthma therapy.
	Nebulizer solution		
	0.25 mg/mL (0.025%)	0.25 mg q 6 hours	
	MDI		
Ipratropium with albuterol	18 mcg/puff of ipratropium bromide and 90 mcg/puff of albuterol	2–3 puffs q 6 hours	
	200 puffs/canister		
	Nebulizer solution		
	0.5 mg/3 mL ipratropium bromide and 2.5 mg/3 mL albuterol	3 mL q 4–6 hours	■ Contains EDTA to prevent discoloration of the solution. This additive does not induce bronchospasm.
Systemic Corticosteroids			***Applies to the first three corticosteroids***
Methylprednisolone	2, 4, 6, 8, 16, 32 mg tablets	■ Short course "burst": 40–60 mg/day as single or 2 divided doses for 3–10 days	■ Short courses or "bursts" are effective for establishing control when initiating therapy or during a period of gradual deterioration.
Prednisolone	5 mg tablets, 5 mg/5 cc, 15 mg/5 cc		■ The burst should be continued until symptoms resolve and the PEF is at least 80 percent of personal best. This usually requires 3–10 days but may require longer. There is no evidence that tapering the dose following improvement prevents relapse.
Prednisone	1, 2.5, 5, 10, 20, 50 mg tablets; 5 mg/cc, 5 mg/5 cc		
	Repository injection		
(Methylprednisolone acetate)	40 mg/mL 80 mg/mL	240 mg IM once	■ May be used in place of a short burst of oral steroids in patients who are vomiting or if adherence is a problem.

Key: CFC, chlorofluorocarbon; EIB, exercise-induced bronchospasm; HFA, hydrofluoroalkane; IM, intramuscular; MDI, metered-dose inhaler; PEF, peak expiratory flow

Fig 8.3. (*Continued*).

See insert for Figures 8.4 and 8.5.

Components of Control		Classification of Asthma Control (Youths ≥12 years of age and adults)		
		Well-Controlled	Not Well-Controlled	Very Poorly Controlled
Impairment	Symptoms	≤2 days/week	>2 days/week	Throughout the day
	Nighttime awakening	≤2x/month	1–3x/week	≥4x/week
	Interference with normal activity	None	Some limitation	Extremely limited
	Short-acting beta$_2$-agonist use for symptom control (not prevention of EIB)	≤2 days/week	>2 days/week	Several times per day
	FEV$_1$ or peak flow	>80% predicted/ personal best	60–80% predicted/ personal best	<60% predicted/ personal best
	Validated Questionnaires ATAQ ACQ ACT	 0 ≤0.75* ≥20	 1–2 ≥1.5 16–19	 3–4 N/A ≤15
Risk	Exacerbations	0–1/year	≥2/year (see note)	
		Consider severity and interval since last exacerbation		
	Progressive loss of lung function	Evaluation requires long-term followup care		
	Treatment-related adverse effects	Medication side effects can vary in intensity from none to very troublesome and worrisome. The level of intensity does not correlate to specific levels of control but should be considered in the overall assessment of risk.		

*ACQ values of 0.76–1.4 are indeterminate regarding well-controlled asthma.

Key: EIB, exercise-induced bronchospasm; FEV$_1$, forced expiratory volume in 1 second; ATAQ, Asthma Therapy Assessment Questionnaire; ACQ, Asthma Control Questionnaire; ACT, Asthma Control Test.

Notes:

- The level of control is based on the most severe impairment or risk category. Assess impairment domain by patient's recall of previous 2–4 weeks and by spirometry/or peak flow measures. Symptom assessment for longer periods should reflect a global assessment, such as inquiring whether the patient's asthma is better or worse since the last visit.
- At present, there are inadequate data to correspond frequencies of exacerbations with different levels of asthma control. In general, more frequent and intense exacerbations (e.g., requiring urgent, unscheduled care, hospitalization, or ICU admission) indicate poorer disease control. For treatment purposes, patients who had ≥2 exacerbations requiring oral systemic corticosteroids in the past year may be considered the same as patients who have not-well-controlled asthma, even in the absence of impairment levels consistent with not-well-controlled asthma.

Fig 8.6. Assessing asthma control in youth ≥12 years of age and adults. (From National Heart Lung and Blood Institute. Expert panel report 3: guidelines for the diagnosis and management of asthma. Available at: www.nhlbi.nih.gov/guidelines/asthma/asthgdln.htm. Accessed April 25, 2009).

USING THE BLOOD PRESSURE TABLES

1. Use standard height charts to determine the adolescent's height percentile for age.
2. Measure and record the adolescent's systolic (SBP) and diastolic (DBP) blood pressure (BP).
3. Use the correct gender table for SBP and DBP.
4. Locate the adolescent's age on the left-hand side of the table. Follow the age row horizontally across the table until it intersects with the vertical column for the adolescent's height percentile. Do this separately for SBP and DBP.
5. Within each height-percentile column (SBP and DBP), the numbers correlate with the 50th, 90th, 95th, and 99th BP percentiles for that age.

Example: for an 11-year-old boy at the 75th percentile for height, an SBP of 105 mm Hg represents the 50th percentile, SBPs between 106 and 119 mm Hg represent values between the 50th and 90th percentiles, an SBP of 123 mm Hg is at the 95th percentile, and a value of 130 mm Hg is at the 99th percentile.

Example: for a 15-year-old girl at the 10th percentile for height, the 90th percentile for SBP and DBP would be 121 and 78 mm Hg, respectively.

See Table 8.2 for classification of BP values, follow-up measurement frequency, and therapy.

Adapted from National High Blood Pressure Education Program Working Group on High Blood Pressure in Children and Adolescents. The fourth report on the diagnosis, evaluation, and treatment of high blood pressure in children and adolescents. *Pediatrics*. 2004;114(2 suppl 4th report):555–576.

Table 8.2
Classification of hypertension in children and adolescents, with measurement frequency and therapy recommendations

	SBP or DBP Percentile[a]	Frequency of BP Measurement	Therapeutic Lifestyle Changes	Pharmacologic Therapy
Normal	<90th	Recheck at next scheduled physical examination	Encourage healthy diet, sleep, and physical activity	—
Prehypertension	90th to <95th or if BP exceeds 120/80 mm Hg even if <90th percentile up to <95th percentile[b]	Recheck in 6 mo	Weight-management counseling if overweight; introduce physical activity and diet management[c]	None unless compelling indications such as chronic kidney disease, diabetes mellitus, heart failure, or left ventricular hypertrophy exist
Stage 1 hypertension	95th to 99th percentile plus 5 mm Hg	Recheck in 1–2 wk or sooner if the patient is symptomatic; if persistently elevated on 2 additional occasions, evaluate or refer to source of care within1 mo	Weight-management counseling if overweight; introduce physical activity and diet management[c]	Initiate therapy if compelling indications (as shown above) exist
Stage 2 hypertension	>99th percentile plus 5 mm Hg	Evaluate or refer to source of care within 1 wk or immediately if the patient is symptomatic	Weight-management counseling if overweight; introduce physical activity and diet management[c]	Initiate therapy[d]

[a] For gender, age, and height measured on at least 3 separate occasions; if systolic and diastolic categories are different, categorize according to the higher value.
[b] This occurs typically at 12 years of age for SBP and at 16 years of age for DBP.
[c] Parents and children trying to modify the eating plan to the Dietary Approaches to Stop Hypertension Study eating plan could benefit from consultation with a registered or licensed nutritionist to get them started.
[d] More than 1 drug may be required.
Adapted from National High Blood Pressure Education Program Working Group on High Blood Pressure in Children and Adolescents. The fourth report on the diagnosis, evaluation, and treatment of high blood pressure in children and adolescents. *Pediatrics*. 2004;114(2 suppl 4th report):555–576.

Table 8.3
BP levels for girls according to age and height percentile

Age, y	BP Percentile	SBP, mm Hg, According to Percentile of Height							DBP, mm Hg, According to Percentile of Height						
		5th	10th	25th	50th	75th	90th	95th	5th	10th	25th	50th	75th	90th	95th
11	50th	100	101	102	103	105	106	107	60	60	60	61	62	63	63
	90th	114	114	116	117	118	119	120	74	74	74	75	76	77	77
	95th	118	118	119	121	122	123	124	78	78	78	79	80	81	81
	99th	125	125	126	128	129	130	131	85	85	86	87	87	88	89
12	50th	102	103	104	105	107	108	109	61	61	61	62	63	64	64
	90th	116	116	117	119	120	121	122	75	75	75	76	77	78	78
	95th	119	120	121	123	124	125	126	79	79	79	80	81	82	82
	99th	127	127	128	130	131	132	133	86	86	87	88	88	89	90
13	50th	104	105	106	107	109	110	110	62	62	62	63	64	65	65
	90th	117	118	119	121	122	123	124	76	76	76	77	78	79	79
	95th	121	122	123	124	126	127	128	80	80	80	81	82	83	83
	99th	128	129	130	132	133	134	135	87	87	88	89	89	90	91
14	50th	106	106	107	109	110	111	112	63	63	63	64	65	66	66
	90th	119	120	121	122	124	125	125	77	77	77	78	79	80	80
	95th	123	123	125	126	127	129	129	81	81	81	82	83	84	84
	99th	130	131	132	133	135	136	136	88	88	89	90	90	91	92
15	50th	107	108	109	110	111	113	113	64	64	64	65	66	67	67
	90th	120	121	122	123	125	126	127	78	78	78	79	80	81	81
	95th	124	125	126	127	129	130	131	82	82	82	83	84	85	85
	99th	131	132	133	134	136	137	138	89	89	90	91	91	92	93
16	50th	108	108	110	111	112	114	114	64	64	65	66	66	67	68
	90th	121	122	123	124	126	127	128	78	78	79	80	81	81	82
	95th	125	126	127	128	130	131	132	82	82	83	84	85	85	86
	99th	132	133	134	135	137	138	139	90	90	90	91	92	93	93
17	50th	108	109	110	111	113	114	115	64	65	65	66	67	67	68
	90th	122	122	123	125	126	127	128	78	79	79	80	81	81	82
	95th	125	126	127	129	130	131	132	82	83	83	84	85	85	86
	99th	133	133	134	136	137	138	139	90	90	91	91	92	93	93

Adapted from National High Blood Pressure Education Program Working Group on High Blood Pressure in Children and Adolescents. The fourth report on the diagnosis, evaluation, and treatment of high blood pressure in children and adolescents. *Pediatrics.* 2004;114(2 suppl 4th report):555–576.

Table 8.4
BP levels for boys according to age and height percentile

Age, y	BP Percentile	SBP, mm Hg, According to Percentile of Height							DBP, mm Hg, According to Percentile of Height						
		5th	10th	25th	50th	75th	90th	95th	5th	10th	25th	50th	75th	90th	95th
11	50th	99	100	102	104	105	107	107	59	59	60	61	62	63	63
	90th	113	114	115	117	119	120	121	74	74	75	76	77	78	78
	95th	117	118	119	121	123	124	125	78	78	79	80	81	82	82
	99th	124	125	127	129	130	132	132	86	86	87	88	89	90	90
12	50th	101	102	104	106	108	109	110	59	60	61	62	63	63	64
	90th	115	116	118	120	121	123	123	74	75	75	76	77	78	79
	95th	119	120	122	123	125	127	127	78	79	80	81	82	82	83
	99th	126	127	129	131	133	134	135	86	87	88	89	90	90	91
13	50th	104	105	106	108	110	111	112	60	60	61	62	63	64	64
	90th	117	118	120	122	124	125	126	75	75	76	77	78	79	79
	95th	121	122	124	126	128	129	130	79	79	80	81	82	83	83
	99th	128	130	131	133	135	136	137	87	87	88	89	90	91	91
14	50th	106	107	109	111	113	114	115	60	61	62	63	64	65	65
	90th	120	121	123	125	126	128	128	75	76	77	78	79	79	80
	95th	124	125	127	128	130	132	132	80	80	81	82	83	84	84
	99th	131	132	134	136	138	139	140	87	88	89	90	91	92	92
15	50th	109	110	112	113	115	117	117	61	62	63	64	65	66	66
	90th	122	124	125	127	129	130	131	76	77	78	79	80	80	81
	95th	126	127	129	131	133	134	135	81	81	82	83	84	85	85
	99th	134	135	136	138	140	142	142	88	89	90	91	92	93	93
16	50th	111	112	114	116	118	119	120	63	63	64	65	66	67	67
	90th	125	126	128	130	131	133	134	78	78	79	80	81	82	82
	95th	129	130	132	134	135	137	137	82	83	83	84	85	86	87
	99th	136	137	139	141	143	144	145	90	90	91	92	93	94	94
17	50th	114	115	116	118	120	121	122	65	66	66	67	68	69	70
	90th	127	128	130	132	134	135	136	80	80	81	82	83	84	84
	95th	131	132	134	136	138	139	140	84	85	86	87	87	88	89
	99th	139	140	141	143	145	146	147	92	93	93	94	95	96	97

Adapted from National High Blood Pressure Education Program Working Group on High Blood Pressure in Children and Adolescents. The fourth report on the diagnosis, evaluation, and treatment of high blood pressure in children and adolescents. *Pediatrics*. 2004;114(2 suppl 4th report):555–576.

Table 8.5
Causes of secondary hypertension in adolescents

Renal	
	Chronic renal failure
	Renovascular disease (renal artery stenosis, fibromuscular hyperplasia, arterial or venous thrombosis); external compression of renal vessels
	Polycystic kidney disease; multicystic-dysplastic kidney
	Hydronephrosis
	Obstructive lesions (ureteropelvic or ureterovesical junction)
	Glomerulonephritis (acute or chronic, including systemic lupus erythematosis)
	Reflux nephropathy
	Hemolytic-uremic syndrome
Endocrine	
	Hyperthyroidism
	Cushing syndrome
	Insulin resistance syndrome
	Diabetes
	Congenital adrenal hyperplasia
	Hyperaldosteronism
	Hyperparathyroidism
Vascular	
	Coarctation of the aorta
	Vasculitis (Takayushu, polyarteritis nodosa)
Genetic	
	Turner syndrome
	Williams syndrome
	Liddle syndrome
	Neurocutaneous syndrome (neurofibromatosis, tuberous sclerosis)
Neoplasms	
	Pheochromocytoma
	Neuroblastoma
	Renal (renal cell carcinoma, Wilms tumor)
Drugs (includes prescription, nonprescription, and herbal medications)	

Adapted from National High Blood Pressure Education Program Working Group on High Blood Pressure in Children and Adolescents. The fourth report on the diagnosis, evaluation, and treatment of high blood pressure in children and adolescents. *Pediatrics*. 2004;114(2 suppl 4th report):555–576; and Flynn JT. Hypertension. In: Fisher M, Alderman E, Kreipe R, Rosenfield W, eds. *American Academy of Pediatrics Textbook of Adolescent Health Care*. Elk Grove Village, IL: American Academy of Pediatrics; In press.

Table 8.6
Clinical evaluation of confirmed hypertension

Study or Procedure	Purpose	Target Population
Evaluation for identifiable causes		
History, including sleep history, family history, risk factors, diet, and habits such as smoking and drinking alcohol; physical examination	History and physical examination help focus subsequent evaluation	All children with persistent BP ≥95th percentile
Serum urea nitrogen, creatinine, electrolytes, urinalysis, and urine culture	Rule out renal disease and chronic pyelonephritis	All children with persistent BP ≥95th percentile
Complete blood count	Rule out anemia, consistent with chronic renal disease	All children with persistent BP ≥95th percentile
Renal ultrasound	Rule out renal scar, congenital anomaly, or disparate renal size	All children with persistent BP ≥95th percentile
Evaluation for comorbidity		
Fasting lipid panel, fasting glucose	Identify hyperlipidemia, identify metabolic abnormalities	Overweight patients with BP at 90th–94th percentile; all patients with BP >95th percentile; family history of hypertension or CVD; child with chronic renal disease
Drug screen	Identify substances that might cause hypertension	History suggestive of possible contribution by substances or drugs
Polysomnography	Identify sleep disorder in association with hypertension	History of loud, frequent snoring
Evaluation for target-organ damage		
Echocardiogram	Identify left ventricular hypertrophy and other indications of cardiac involvement	Patients with comorbid risk factors[a] and BP at 90th–94th percentile; all patients with BP ≥95th percentile
Retinal examination	Identify retinal vascular changes	Patients with comorbid risk factors and BP at 90th–94th percentile; all patients with BP ≥95th percentile

(Continued)

Table 8.6
(Continued)

Study or Procedure	Purpose	Target Population
Additional evaluation as indicated		
American Board of Preventive Medicine	Identify white-coat hypertension, abnormal diurnal BP pattern, BP load	Patients in whom white-coat hypertension is suspected, and when other information on BP pattern is needed
Plasma renin determination	Identify low renin, suggesting mineralocorticoid-related disease	Young children with stage 1 hypertension and any child or adolescent with stage 2 hypertension; positive family history of severe hypertension
Renovascular imaging	Identify renovascular disease	Young children with stage 1 hypertension and any child or adolescent with stage 2 hypertension
Isotopic scintigraphy (renal scan)		
Magnetic resonance angiography		
Duplex Doppler flow studies		
3-Dimensional computed tomography		
Arteriography: digital subtraction angiography or classic		
Plasma and urine steroid levels	Identify steroid-mediated hypertension	Young children with stage 1 hypertension and any child or adolescent with stage 2 hypertension
Plasma and urine catecholamines	Identify catecholamine-mediated hypertension	Young children with stage 1 hypertension and any child or adolescent with stage 2 hypertension

[a] Comorbid risk factors also include diabetes mellitus and kidney disease.

Adapted from National High Blood Pressure Education Program Working Group on High Blood Pressure in Children and Adolescents. The fourth report on the diagnosis, evaluation, and treatment of high blood pressure in children and adolescents. *Pediatrics*. 2004;114(2 suppl 4th report):555–576.

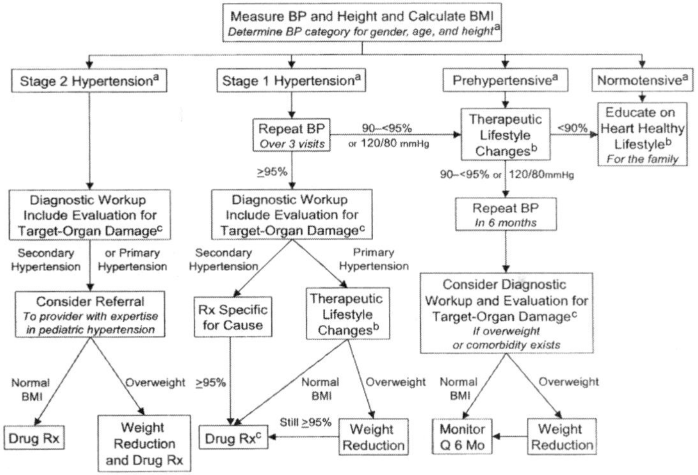

Fig 8.7. Management of elevated blood pressure in adolescents. Rx indicates prescription; Q, every. [a] See Tables 8.2 through 8.4 for definitions and blood pressure values. [b] Diet modification and physical activity. [c] Especially if younger, very high BP, little or no family history, diabetic, or other risk factors. (Reproduced from National High Blood Pressure Education Program Working Group on High Blood Pressure in Children and Adolescents. The fourth report on the diagnosis, evaluation, and treatment of high blood pressure in children and adolescents. *Pediatrics*. 2004;114(2 suppl 4th report):555–576).

See insert for Figure 8.8.

LIPID SCREENING FOR ADOLESCENTS

The following is a summary of the 2008 clinical report "Lipid Screening and Cardiovascular Health in Childhood" as it pertains to adolescents.

Screening

- The approach to screening with a fasting lipid profile remains a targeted one (see below).
- Overweight children belong to a special risk category and need cholesterol screening regardless of family history or other risk factors.

Cholesterol Concentrations

- Age-specific values for total mean cholesterol concentration peak at 9 to 11 years of age, decrease during pubertal development, and increase thereafter.
- Lipid concentrations are age, gender, and maturation dependent; they also vary according to race/ethnicity.

(text continues on p. 657)

Table 8.7
Cut points for total cholesterol and LDL concentrations in children and adolescents

Category	Percentile	Total Cholesterol, mg/dL	LDL, mg/dL
Acceptable	<75th	<170	<110
Borderline	75th–95th	170–199	110–129
Elevated	>95th	>200	>130

Adapted from Daniels SR, Greer FR; American Academy of Pediatrics, Committee on Nutrition. Lipid screening and cardiovascular health in childhood. *Pediatrics*. 2008;122(1):198–207.

Table 8.8
Lipid and lipoprotein distributions in subjects aged 5 to 19 years

	Boys			Girls		
	5–9 y	10–14 y	15–19 y	5–9 y	10–14 y	15–19 y
Total cholesterol, mg/dL						
50th percentile	153	161	152	164	159	157
75th percentile	168	173	168	177	171	176
90th percentile	183	191	183	189	191	198
95th percentile	186	201	191	197	205	208
Triglycerides, mg/dL						
50th percentile	48	58	68	57	68	64
75th percentile	58	74	88	74	85	85
90th percentile	70	94	125	103	104	112
95th percentile	85	111	143	120	120	126
LDL, mg/dL						
50th percentile	90	94	93	98	94	93
75th percentile	103	109	109	115	110	110
90th percentile	117	123	123	125	126	129
95th percentile	129	133	130	140	136	137
HDL, mg/dL						
5th percentile	38	37	30	36	37	35
10th percentile	43	40	34	38	40	38
25th percentile	49	46	39	48	45	43
50th percentile	55	55	46	52	52	51

Adapted from Daniels SR, Greer FR; American Academy of Pediatrics, Committee on Nutrition. Lipid screening and cardiovascular health in childhood. *Pediatrics*. 2008;122(1):198–207.

- In the Muscatine study, 75% of school-aged children who had total cholesterol concentrations at >90th percentile at baseline had total cholesterol concentrations of >200 mg/dL in their early 20s.
- In the Bogalusa heart study, ~70% of the children with elevated cholesterol levels had elevated levels in young adulthood.

Clinical Evaluation

- The ideal approach for screening adolescents remains controversial. Research that has focused on optimizing screening of children and adolescents has not led to a consensus. Some have advocated for screening on the basis of a positive family history, some maintain that there is insufficient evidence to recommend for or against routine screening for lipid disorders in children, and some have recommended universal screening comparable to that for adults.

Abnormal Cholesterol Concentrations

- Table 8.7 indicates cut points for total cholesterol and low-density lipoprotein (LDL) concentrations in children and adolescents. These values come from the National Cholesterol Education Program (NCEP) pediatric report. After age 18 years, values presented in the NCEP report for adults would be used.
- Data show that the sensitivity of these cut points for predicting adult lipid levels is lowest at ages 14 to 16 years and highest at ages 5 to 10 and 17 to 19 years.
- Given concerns about using the same values for all ages (2–18 years), one approach is to use percentiles: >95th percentile for LDL concentrations and <5th percentile for high-density lipoprotein (HDL) concentrations would be considered abnormal (especially if results persisted over several visits. LDL concentrations between the 90th and 95th percentiles (for LDL) and 5th to 10th percentiles would be considered borderline. Table 8.8 displays lipid and lipoprotein distributions in subjects aged 5 to 19 years (at 50th, 75th, 90th, and 95th percentiles).

Treatment of Abnormalities in Lipid and Lipoprotein Concentrations

Population Approach

- Nutrition and physical activity levels that are appropriate for all adolescents are recommended.
- Table 8.9 summarizes dietary recommendations by the American Heart Association that are based on Department of Agriculture dietary guidelines for children (>2 years old) and adolescents.
- These guidelines recommend that intake of trans fatty acids be limited to <1% of total calories.

Table 8.9
Daily estimated calories and recommended servings for grains, fruits, vegetables, and milk/dairy according to age and gender

	Age				
	1 y	2–3 y	4–8 y	9–13 y	14–18 y
Energy, kcal[a]	900	1000	—	—	—
Girls	—	—	1200	1600	1800
Boys	—	—	1400	1800	2200
Fat, % kcal	30–40	30–35	25–35	25–35	25–35
Milk/dairy, cups[b]	2[c]	2	2	3	3
Lean meat/beans, oz	2	2	—	5	—
Girls	—	—	3	—	5
Boys	—	—	4	—	6
Fruits, cups[d]	1	1	2	2	—
Girls	—	—	—	—	2-Nov
Boys	—	—	—	—	2
Vegetables, cups[d]	4	1	—	—	—
Girls	—	—	1	2	$2^{1/2}$
Boys	—	—	2	2	3
Grains, oz[e]	2	3	—	—	—
Girls	—	—	4	5	6
Boys	—	—	5	6	7

Calorie estimates are based on sedentary lifestyle. Increased physical activity will require additional calories (0–200 kcal/day if moderately physically active and 200–400 kcal/day if very physically active [1 kcal = 4.2 kJ]). — indicates data not applicable.
[a] For youth aged ≥2 years; adapted from Table 2, Table 3, and Appendix A-2 of the 2005 *Dietary Guidelines for Americans* (available at: www.healthierus.gov/dietaryguidelines; Accessed August 4, 2009). Nutrient and energy contributions from each group are calculated according to the nutrient-dense forms of food in each group (eg, lean meats and fat-free milk).
[b] Milk listed is fat free (except for children <2 years old). If 1%, 2%, or whole-fat milk is substituted, this will use, for each cup respectively, 19, 39, or 63 kcal of discretionary calories and add 2.6, 5.1, or 9.0 g of total fat, of which 1.3, 2.6, or 4.6 g are saturated fat.
[c] For 1-year-old children, 2% fat milk is included. If 2 cups of whole milk are substituted, 48 kcal of discretionary calories will be used.
[d] Serving sizes are cup for 1 year of age, cup for 2 to 3 years of age, and cup for ≥4 years of age. A variety of vegetables should be selected from each subgroup over the week.
[e] Half of all grains should be whole grains.
Adapted from American Heart Association. Table: dietary recommendations for children. Available at: www.americanheart.org/presenter.jhtml?identifier=3033999. Accessed August 4, 2009.

Individual Approach

- Focus on adolescents at high risk (adolescents who have high total cholesterol or LDL concentrations or other significant cardiovascular risk factors or who have a family history of cardiovascular disease [CVD] or high cholesterol levels).

- The initial intervention is focused on changing their diet, but if this approach does not reduce LDL levels to acceptable levels, these adolescents may be candidates for pharmacologic interventions.
- The nutritional approach for these adolescents at high risk is to limit saturated fat to 7% of total calories and dietary cholesterol to 300 mg/day.
- Adjuncts to a nutritional approach include increasing intake of soluble fiber (age plus 5 g/day up to 20 g/day at age 15 years); plant stanols and sterols (although there is concern these products reduce absorption of fat-soluble vitamins and beta carotene); and increased physical activity.

Pharmacologic Intervention

- Table 8.10 displays the LDL concentrations at which pharmacologic therapy is recommended for children ≥10 years of age.
- Adolescents with diabetes or renal, congenital heart, or collagen vascular disease, and those who are cancer survivors, require more aggressive treatment of high LDL concentrations.
- Table 8.11 lists the classes of drugs available for treatment and their adverse effects.

Report Summary

- The population approach to a healthful diet should be recommended for all adolescents according to dietary guidelines for Americans.
- The individual approach for adolescents at higher risk for CVD and with a high concentration of LDL includes changes in diet with nutritional counseling and other lifestyle interventions (physical activity).
- The most current recommendation is to screen adolescents with a positive family history of dyslipidemia or premature CVD (≤55 years for men or ≤65 years for women) with a fasting lipid profile.
- Adolescents for whom family history is unknown or who have other CVD risk factors (BMI ≥85th percentile, BP ≥95th percentile, cigarette smoking, or diabetes mellitus) should also be screened with a fasting lipid profile.
- A fasting lipid profile is recommended and should occur within the context of well-adolescent/health maintenance visits. If values are within the reference range, adolescents should be retested in 3 to 5 years.
- Adolescents who are overweight or obese and who have high triglyceride or low HDL levels should first be treated with weight management (improvement of diet with nutritional advice) and increased physical activity.
- For patients ≥8 years of age with LDL ≥190 mg/dL; LDL ≥160 mg/dL with a family history of early heart disease or ≥2 additional risk factors; or LDL ≥130 mg/dL if diabetes mellitus is present, pharmacologic intervention should be considered. The initial goal is to lower LDL concentration to <160 mg/dL. Targets as low as 130 or even 110 mg/dL may be warranted when there is a strong family history of CVD,

especially with other risk factors such as obesity, diabetes mellitus, metabolic syndrome, and other higher-risk situations.

Adapted from Daniels SR, Greer FR; American Academy of Pediatrics, Committee on Nutrition. Lipid screening and cardiovascular health in childhood. *Pediatrics*. 2008;122(1):198–207.

Table 8.10
Recommended LDL concentrations for pharmacologic treatment of children and adolescents aged ≥10 years

Patient Characteristics	Recommended Cut Points
No other risk factors for CVD	LDL concentration is persistently >190 mg/dL despite diet therapy
Other risk factors present, including obesity, hypertension, or cigarette smoking or positive family history of premature CVD	LDL concentration is persistently >160 mg/dL despite diet therapy
Children with diabetes mellitus	Pharmacologic treatment should be considered when LDL concentration is ≥130 mg/dL

Adapted from Daniels SR, Greer FR; American Academy of Pediatrics, Committee on Nutrition. Lipid screening and cardiovascular health in childhood. *Pediatrics*. 2008;122(1):198–207.

Table 8.11
Pharmacotherapeutic agents used in hyperlipidemia

Drug Class	Examples	Action	Contraindications and Adverse Effects
Statin	Atorvastatin; fluvastatin[a]; lovastatin; pravastatin; rosuvastatin[a]; simvastatin	Inhibits hepatic cholesterol synthesis	Myalgia, myositis, raised AST and ALT
Niacin	Extended-release niacin[a]	Lowers very low-density lipoprotein synthesis	Flushing, raised AST and ALT
Fibrate	Gemfibrozil[a]; fenofibrate[a]	Lowers very low density lipoprotein synthesis	Dyspepsia, constipation, myositis, anemia
Bile acid sequestrant	Cholestyramine; colesevelam[a]	Binds intestinal bile acids, interrupts enterohepatic recirculation	Gas, bloating, constipation, cramps
Cholesterol absorption inhibitor	Ezetimibe[a]	Inhibits cholesterol absorption from small intestine	Gas, bloating, constipation

AST indicates aspartate aminotransferase; ALT, alanine aminotransferase.
[a] Not approved by the US Food and Drug Administration for patients under the age of 18 years.
Jacobson MS. Atherosclerosis prevention and cholesterol management in adolescents. *Adolesc Health Update* 2007;19(3):7.

Clinical Management of High Cholesterol in Young Adults ≥20 Years of Age

Table 8.12
Recommendations for modifications to footnote the Adult Treatment Panel III treatment algorithm for LDL cholesterol

TLCs remain an essential modality in clinical management; they have the potential to reduce cardiovascular risk through several mechanisms beyond LDL lowering
In persons at high risk, the recommended LDL cholesterol goal is <100 mg/dL
An LDL cholesterol goal of <70 mg/dL is a therapeutic option based on available clinical trial evidence, especially for patients at very high risk
If LDL cholesterol is ≥100 mg/dL, an LDL-lowering drug is indicated simultaneously with lifestyle changes
If baseline LDL cholesterol is <100 mg/dL, institution of an LDL-lowering drug to achieve an LDL cholesterol level of <70 mg/dL is a therapeutic option based on available clinical trial evidence
If a person at high risk has high a triglyceride or low HDL cholesterol level, consideration can be given to combining a fibrate or nicotinic acid with an LDL-lowering drug; when triglyceride levels are ≥200 mg/dL, non-HDL cholesterol is a secondary target of therapy, with a goal 30 mg/dL higher than the identified LDL cholesterol goal
For persons at moderately high risk (≥2 risk factors and 10-year risk of 10%–20%), the recommended LDL cholesterol goal is <130 mg/dL; an LDL cholesterol goal of <100 mg/dL is a therapeutic option based on available clinical trial evidence; when LDL cholesterol level is 100–129 mg/dL, at baseline or on lifestyle therapy, initiation of an LDL-lowering drug to achieve an LDL cholesterol level of <100 mg/dL is a therapeutic option based on available clinical trial evidence
Any person at high risk or moderately high risk who has lifestyle-related risk factors (eg, obesity, physical inactivity, elevated triglyceride level, low HDL cholesterol level, or metabolic syndrome) is a candidate for TLCs to modify these risk factors regardless of LDL cholesterol level
When LDL-lowering drug therapy is used for persons at high or moderately high risk, it is advised that intensity of therapy be sufficient to achieve at least a 30%–40% reduction in LDL cholesterol levels
For people in lower-risk categories, recent clinical trials do not modify the goals and cut points of therapy

TLC indicates therapeutic lifestyle change.
Adapted from Grundy SM, Cleeman JI, Bairey CN, et al. Implications of recent clinical trials for the National Cholesterol Education Program Adult Treatment Panel III guidelines [published correction appears in *Circulation*. 2004;110(6):763]. *Circulation*. 2004;110(2):227–239. Reprinted with permission © 2004. American Heart Association.

Table 8.13
Adult Treatment Panel III LDL cholesterol goals and cut points for therapeutic lifestyle change and drug therapy in different risk categories and proposed modifications based on recent clinical trial evidence

Risk Category	LDL Cholesterol Goal, mg/dL	Initiate TLC, mg/dL	Consider Drug Therapy, mg/dL[a]
High risk: CHD[b] or CHD risk equivalents[c] (10-y risk >20%)	<100 (optional goal: <70)[d]	≥100[e]	≥100[f] (<100: consider drug options)[a]
Moderately high risk: ≥2 risk factors[g] (10-y risk 10%–20%)[h]	<130[i]	≥130[e]	≥130 (100–129; consider drug options)[j]
Moderate risk: ≥2 risk factors[g] (10-y risk <10%)[h]	<130	≥130	≥160
Lower risk: 0–1 risk factor[k]	<160	≥160	≥190 (160–189: LDL-lowering drug optional)

TLC indicates therapeutic lifestyle change; CHD, coronary heart disease.

[a] When LDL-lowering drug therapy is used, it is advised that intensity of therapy be sufficient to achieve at least a 30% to 40% reduction in LDL cholesterol levels.

[b] CHD includes history of myocardial infarction, unstable angina, stable angina, coronary artery procedures (angioplasty or bypass surgery), or evidence of clinically significant myocardial ischemia.

[c] CHD risk equivalents include clinical manifestations of noncoronary forms of atherosclerotic disease (peripheral arterial disease, abdominal aortic aneurysm, and carotid artery disease [transient ischemic attacks or stroke of carotid origin or >50% obstruction of a carotid artery]), diabetes, and ≥2 risk factors with a 10-year risk for hard CHD of >20%.

[d] Very high risk favors the optional LDL cholesterol goal of <70 mg/dL, and for patients with high triglycerides, non-HDL cholesterol of <100 mg/dL.

[e] Any person at high or moderately high risk who has lifestyle-related risk factors (eg, obesity, physical inactivity, elevated triglyceride level, low HDL cholesterol level, or metabolic syndrome) is a candidate for TLCs to modify these risk factors regardless of LDL cholesterol level.

[f] Baseline LDL cholesterol is <100 mg/dL, institution of an LDL-lowering drug is a therapeutic option based on available clinical trial results. If a person at high risk has a high triglyceride or low HDL cholesterol level, combining a fibrate or nicotinic acid with an LDL-lowering drug can be considered.

[g] Risk factors include cigarette smoking, hypertension (BP ≥140/90 mm Hg or on antihypertensive medication), low HDL cholesterol level (<40 mg/dL), family history of premature CHD (CHD in male first-degree relative <55 years of age; CHD in female first-degree relative <65 years of age), and age (men ≥45 years; women ≥55 years).

[h] Electronic 10-year risk calculators are available at www.nhlbi.nih.gov/guidelines/cholesterol.

[i] An optional LDL cholesterol goal is <100 mg/dL.

[j] For persons at moderately high risk, when LDL cholesterol level is 100 to 129 mg/dL, at baseline or on lifestyle therapy, initiation of an LDL-lowering drug to achieve an LDL cholesterol level of <100 mg/dL is a therapeutic option based on available clinical trial results.

[k] Almost all people with 0 or 1 risk factor have a 10-year risk of <10%; thus, 10-year risk assessment in people with 0 or 1 risk factor is not necessary.

Adapted from Grundy SM, Cleeman JI, Bairey CN, et al. Implications of recent clinical trials for the National Cholesterol Education Program Adult Treatment Panel III guidelines [published correction appears in *Circulation*. 2004;110(6):763]. *Circulation*. 2004;110(2):227–239. Reprinted with permission © 2004. American Heart Association.

Adolesc Med 20 (2009) 664–676

9. Genitourinary

Table 9.1
Disorders causing proteinuria

Type of Proteinemia	Disorder
Mild proteinuria: In most of these disorders, proteinuria is asymptomatic and usuallyother clinical and laboratory findings help point to the specific diagnosis	Postural proteinuria
	Physiologic or nonrenal causes of transient proteinuria
	"Benign" persistent proteinuria
	Severe obesity
	Acute or chronic pyelonephritis/reflux nephropathy
	Renal tubular disorders (eg, Fanconi syndrome, cystinosis, Dent disease)
	Congenial dysplastic lesions
	Chronic interstitial nephritis/analgesic abuse
	Hypokalemic, hypercalcemic, and uric acid nephropathy
	Early diabetes nephropathy
	Early hypertensive nephropathy
	Early hereditary nephritis (Alport syndrome)
Moderate proteinuria: Many disorders included in this category have associatedhematuria, which helps in the differential diagnosis	Acute poststreptococcal glomerulonephritis
	Membranoproliferative glomerulonephritis
	Lupus and Henoch-Schonlein purpura nephritis
	Hereditary nephritis (Alport syndrome)
	Chronic (atrophic) pyelonephritis and reflux nephropathy
	Chronic interstitial nephritis/analgesic abuse
	Diabetic nephropathy
	Hypertensive nephropathy

(Continued)

Alain Joffe, MD, MPH
E-mail address: ajoffe@jhu.edu.

 ISSN 1934-4287

Table 9.1
(Continued)

Type of Proteinemia	Disorder
Severe proteinuria (nephrotic syndrome): For all patients with severe proteinuria, appropriate workup should be performed to determine the cause	Congenital or infantile nephrotic syndrome
	Idiopathic (primary) nephrotic syndrome
	Minimal change
	Focal glomerulosclerosis
	Mesangial proliferation
	Membranoproliferative glomerulonephritis
	Membranous nephropathy
	Secondary nephrotic syndrome
	Infection: secondary syphilis, quartan malaria, hepatitis B or C, HIV
	Metabolic: diabetes mellitus
	Collagen vascular disease: lupus, Henoch-Schonlein purpura
	Malignancy: lymphoma, Hodgkin's disease, and other malignancies
	Drugs: nonsteroidal antiinflammatory drugs, gold

Adapted from Anand SK. Approach to the child with proteinuria. In: Osborn LM, DeWitt TG, First LR, Zenel JA, eds. *Pediatrics*. Philadelphia, PA: Elsevier Mosby; 2005:722, with permission from Elsevier.

Table 9.2
Available methods for testing for proteinuria

Method	Indications	Normal Range	Comments
Dipstick testing	Routine screening for proteinuria performed in the office	Negative or trace in a concentrated urine specimen (specific gravity $\geq$1.020)	False-positive test can occur if urine is very alkaline (pH >8.0) or very concentrated (specific gravity >1.025)
24-h urine for protein and creatinine excretion	Quantitation of proteinuria (as well as creatinine clearances)	<100 mg/m^2 per 24 h in a documented 24-h collection	More accurate than spot urine analysis; inconvenient for patient; limited use in pediatric practice
Spot urine for protein/creatinine ratio, preferably on first morning urine specimen	Semiquantitative assessment of proteinuria	<0.2 mg protein/mg creatinine in children aged >2 y; <0.5 mg protein/mg creatinine in those aged 6–24 mo	Simplest method to quantitate proteinuria; less accurate than measuring 24-h proteinuria
Microalbuminuria	Assess risk of progressive glomerulopathy in patients with diabetes mellitus	<30 mg urine albumin/g creatinine on first morning urine	Therapy should be intensified in diabetic patients with microalbuminuria

Note that in a 24-hour urine specimen, the creatinine content should be measured to determine whether the specimen is truly a 24-hour collection. The amount of creatinine in a 24-hour specimen can be estimated as follows: females, 15 to 20 mg/kg ideal body weight; males, 20 to 25 mg/kg ideal body weight.

Adapted from Hogg RJ, Portman RJ, Milliner D, Lemley KV, Eddy A, Ingelfinger J. Evaluation and management of proteinuria and nephrotic syndrome in children: recommendations from a pediatric nephrology panel established at the National Kidney Foundation conference on proteinuria, albuminuria, risk, assessment, detection, and elimination (PARADE). *Pediatrics*. 2000;105(6):1242–1249.

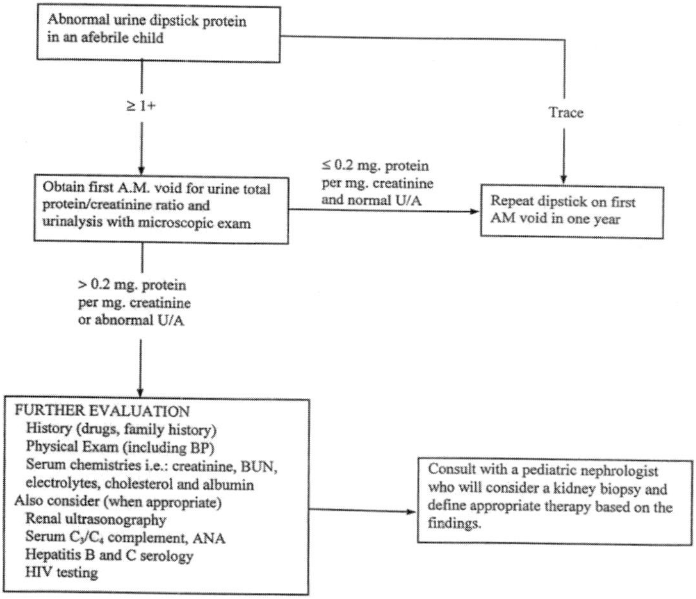

Fig 9.1. Evaluation of persistent proteinuria in children/adolescents. U/A indicates urinalysis; BP, blood pressure; BUN, serum urea nitrogen; ANA, antinuclear antibody. (From Hogg RJ, Portman RJ, Milliner D, Lemley KV, Eddy A, Ingelfinger J. Evaluation and management of proteinuria and nephrotic syndrome in children: recommendations from a pediatric nephrology panel established at the National Kidney Foundation conference on proteinuria, albuminuria, risk, assessment, detection, and elimination (PARADE). *Pediatrics*. 2000;105(6):1242–1249.)

Table 9.3
Microscopic hematuria

Transient
Thin basement membrane disease
Idiopathic hypercalciuria
Immunoglobulin A nephropathy or Alport syndrome
Sickle cell anemia or traits
Trauma or exercise
Postinfectious glomerulonephritis
Nephrolithiasis
Other glomerular disease or glomerulonephritis (focal and segmental glomerulosclerosis, Henoch-Schonlein purpura syndrome, systemic lupus erythematosis, membranoproliferative glomerulonephritis, membranous glomerulonephritis)
Congenital abnormality (ureteropelvic junction or cystic disease)
Pyelonephritis or infection
Vascular malformation
Drugs or toxins

Adapted from Reidy KJ, Del Rio M. Hematuria. In: McInerny TK, Adam HM, Campbell DE, Kamat DM, Kelleher KJ, eds. *American Academy of Pediatrics Textbook of Pediatric Care*. Elk Grove Village, IL: American Academy of Pediatrics; 2009:1566–1570.

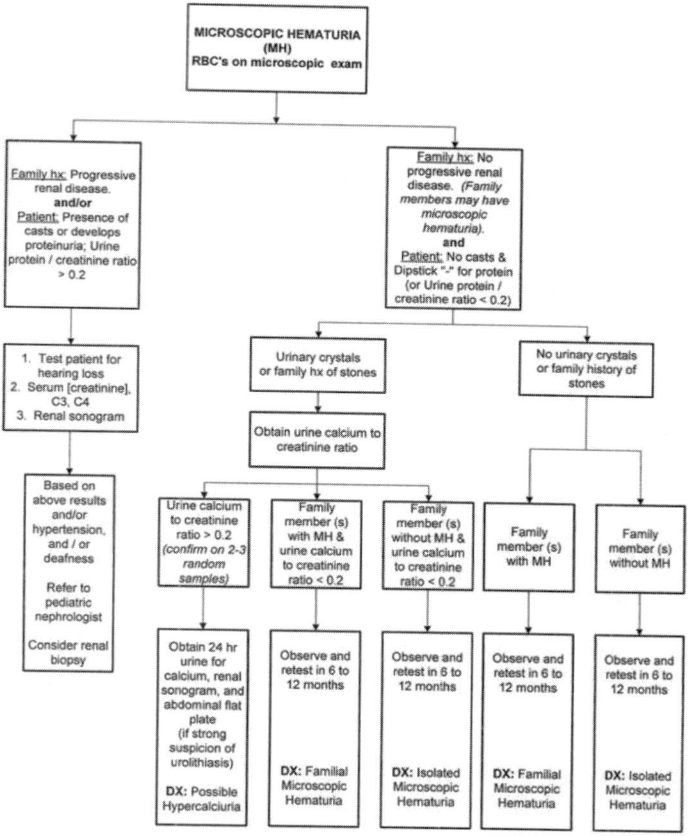

Fig 9.2. Evaluation of microscopic hematuria in children. RBCs indicates red blood cells; hx, history; DX, diagnosis. (From Feld LG, Meyers KE, Kaplan BS, Stapleton BS. Limited evaluation of microscopic hematuria in pediatrics. *Pediatrics*. 1998;102(4):e42. Available at: www.pediatrics.org/cgi/content/full/102/4/e42.)

Table 9.4
Causes of scrotal swelling

Acute, painful scrotal swelling
Torsion of spermatic cord
Torsion of appendix, testis, epididymis
Acute epididymitis, orchitis
Mumps orchitis
Henoch-Schonlein purpura
Trauma
Insect bite
Thrombosis of spermatic vein
Fat necrosis
Hernia
Folliculitis
Dermatitis, acute
Painless scrotal swelling
Tumor
Idiopathic scrotal edema
Hydrocele
Henoch-Schonlein purpura
Hernia
Chronic scrotal swelling
Hydrocele
Hernia
Varicocele
Spermatocele
Sebaceous cyst
Tumor

Adapted from Palmer LS. Scrotal swelling and pain. In: McInerny TK, Adam HM, Campbell DE, Kamat DM, Kelleher KJ, eds. *American Academy of Pediatrics Textbook of Pediatric Care*. Elk Grove Village, IL: American Academy of Pediatrics; 2009:1718.

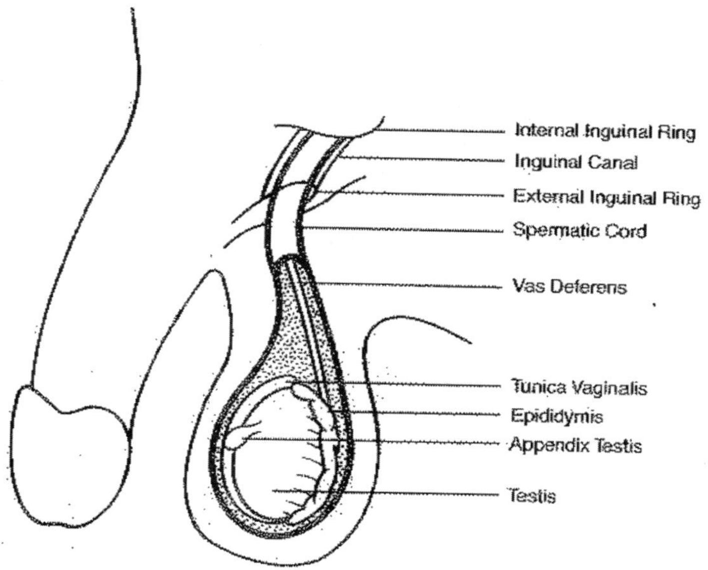

Fig 9.3. Normal scrotal anatomy. (From Kapphahn C, Schlossberger N. Male reproductive health: part 1. Painful scrotal masses. *Adolesc Health Update*. 1992;4(3):4.)

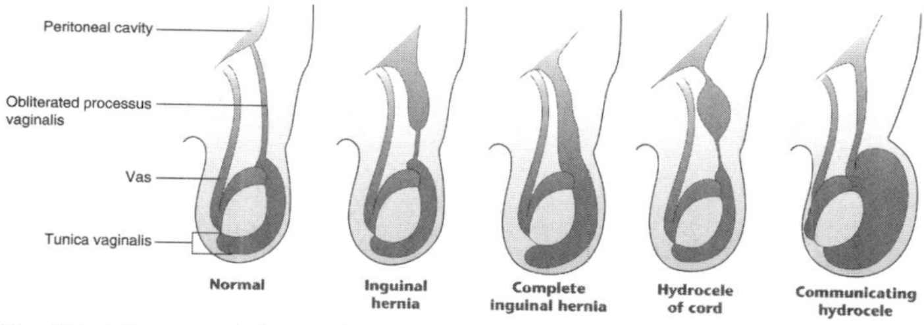

Fig 9.4. Diagram of the continuum of hernia and hydrocele. (From Palmer LS. Scrotal swelling and pain. In: McInerny TK, Adam HM, Campbell DE, Kamat DM, Kelleher KJ, eds. *American Academy of Pediatrics Textbook of Pediatric Care*. Elk Grove Village, IL: American Academy of Pediatrics; 2009:1721.)

Table 9.5
Painless and painful scrotal masses: distinguishing characteristics

Lesion	History	Physical Examination	Comments
Hydrocele (Figs 9.4 and 9.5)	May be asymptomatic; if large enough, may produce sensation of "heaviness" or "dragging" in the scrotum; may be associated with dull ache, especially if adolescent stands for long period of time or after exercise	Ill-defined soft mass without clear borders; may extend into cord; usually will transilluminate	If hydrocele is acute or of unknown duration, must rule out testicular mass, epididymitis, orchitis; consider ultrasound, especially if unable to adequately examine scrotal contents
Spermatocele/epididymal cyst (Fig 9.5D)	May be asymptomatic; if large enough, may produce sensation of "heaviness" or "dragging" in the scrotum; may be associated with dull ache, especially if adolescent stands for long period of time or after exercise; if large enough, adolescent may be concerned about "third testicle"	Firm mass with distinct borders; usually will be located in head of epididymis superior to the testicle; size varies; may or may not transilluminate	Important to determine if mass is separate from testicle
Testicular tumor (Fig 9.5A)	Usually none; may complain of scrotal swelling or "heavy" feeling; if tumor hemorrhages, may present as acute painful scrotum	Mass arising from within testicle and cannot be palpated separately from it; will feel firmer than surrounding normal testes; does not transilluminate	May be bilateral; ultrasound both testicles during evaluation

(*Continued*)

Table 9.5
(Continued)

Lesion	History	Physical Examination	Comments
Miscellaneous scrotal appendages (appendix testis, vas aberrans, appendix epididymis, organ of Giraldes)	Usually no symptoms; acute onset of pain with torsion	Incidental finding on physical examination; typical location: appendix testis—upper pole of testis or in groove between testis and epididymis; appendix epididymis—at head of epididymis (above testis); others—variable; usually small (pea-sized); do not transilluminate; with torsion, "blue-dot" appearance through scrotal sac	
Hernia (Figs 9.4 and 9.5B)	May be asymptomatic; if large enough, may produce sensation of "heaviness" or "dragging" in the scrotum; may be associated with dull ache, especially if adolescent stands for long period of time or after exercise	Soft, fluctuant; Valsalva maneuver will cause increase in size; bowel sounds may be present; should be able to follow hernia into inguinal canal	

(Continued)

Table 9.5
(Continued)

Lesion	History	Physical Examination	Comments
Varicocele (Fig 9.5E)	May be asymptomatic; if large enough, may produce sensation of "heaviness" or "dragging" in the scrotum. May be associated with dull ache especially if adolescent stands for long period of time or after exercise	Feels like "bag of worms" or "spaghetti"; does not transilluminate; usually left-sided; should decrease in size if patient lies down; will increase in size with Valsalva maneuver	Important to assess size of testicle on same side as varicocele
Testicular torsion (Fig 9.5F)	May have history of previous episodes of pain that resolved spontaneously; typically younger teenager; onset of pain is sudden; no symptoms of urethritis	Testicle may ride higher in scrotum with a more horizontal lie; epididymis may be anterior or obscured; no relief with elevation of testis (negative Prehn sign); cremasteric reflex typically absent	First-catch urine or urethral Gram-stain negative for white blood cells
Epididymitis (Fig 9.5G)	Older teenager; usually no previous episodes of pain; onset of symptoms more indolent (hours to days); may have previous symptoms of urethritis (discharge, dysuria, itching at the distal urethra	Epididymis is posterior to testicle; early on, epididymis alone will be tender, testicle will feel normal; later, entire scrotal contents may be swollen and tender; elevation of testis decreases pain (positive Prehn sign); cremasteric reflex usually present	First-catch urine or urethral Gram-stain positive for white blood cells

Data sources: Joffe A, Blythe M. Genitourinary. *Adolesc Med*. 2003;14(2):391–393; Adelman WP, Joffe A. The adolescent with a painful scrotum. *Contemp Pediatr*. 2000;17(3):111–127; and Palmer LS. Scrotal swelling and pain. In: McInerny TK, Adam HM, Campbell DE, Kamat DM, Kelleher KJ, eds. *American Academy of Pediatrics Textbook of Pediatric Care*. Elk Grove Village, IL: American Academy of Pediatrics; 2009:1717–1724.

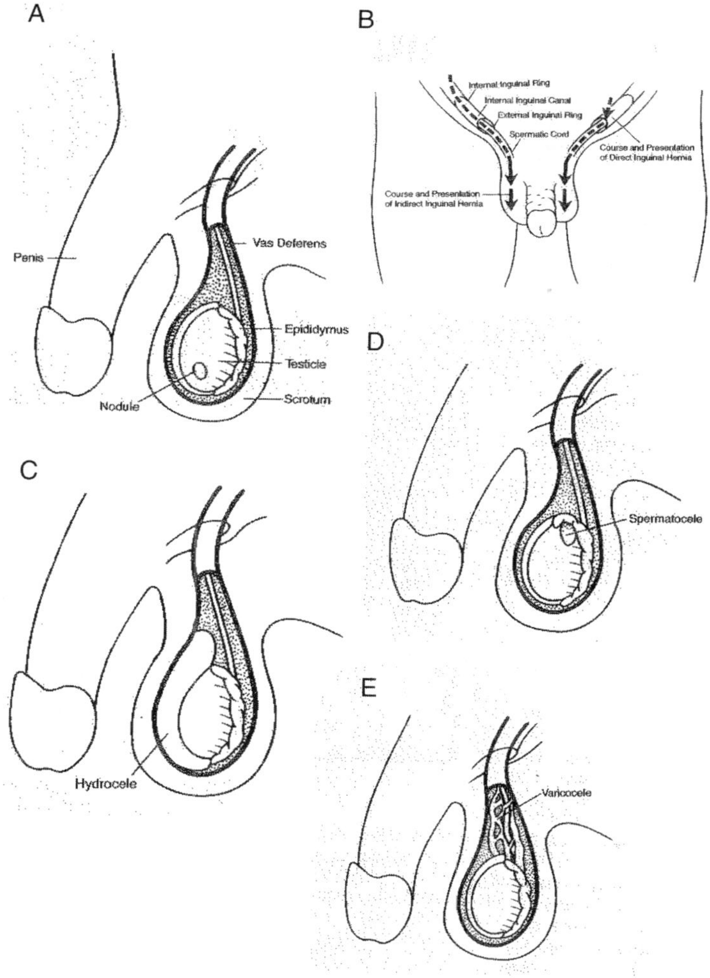

Fig 9.5. Painless and painful scrotal masses. Painless: testis tumor (A), hernia in the groin (B), hydrocele (C), spermatocele (D), and varicocele (E); painful: torsion (F) and epididymitis (G). (From Kapphahn C, Schlossberger N. Male reproductive health: part 1. Painful scrotal masses. *Adolesc Health Update.* 1992;4[3]:4 and Kapphahn C, Schlossberger N. Male reproductive health: part 2. Painless scrotal masses. *Adolesc Health Update*. 1992;5(1):4, 7.)

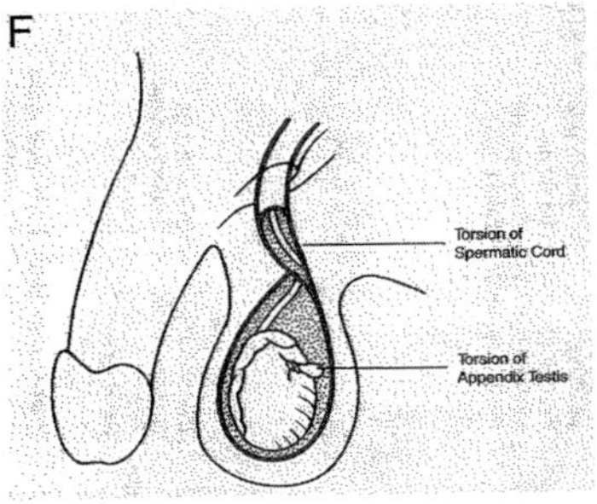

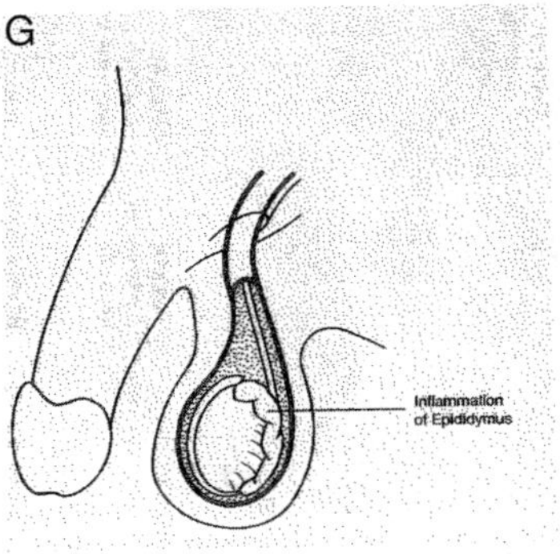

Fig 9.5. (*Continued*).

Adolesc Med 20 (2009) 677–694

10. Dermatology

ACNE

Definition

Disorder of pilosebaceous unit composed of follicle/pore, sebaceous gland, and hair on back, face, and chest.

Etiology

- Rising levels of dehydroepiandrosterone sulfate before puberty cause the sebaceous glands to enlarge and produce more sebum.
- Androgens from both the adrenal gland and gonads are important in the development of acne, because there is a positive correlation between the severity of acne and the increasing stages of puberty.

Four Primary Factors

1. Abnormal keratinization: the pilosebaceous unit is lined with squamous epithelial cells that tend to be altered and described as cohesive and not shedding, resulting in collection of cells/sebum

2. Sebum: increased by androgens

3. Bacteria: colonization of unit with *Propionibacterium acnes*, anaerobic, Gram-positive diptheroids

4. Inflammation: bacteria cause an inflammatory response and hydrolyze triglycerides in sebum to the free fatty acids

See color insert for Figure 10.1, detailing the pathogenesis of acne.

Other Factors

- Genetics
- Environmental exposures: topical/oral steroids, oils/cosmetics, physical friction

---

Margaret J. Blythe, MD
E-mail address: mblythe@iupui.edu

 ISSN 1934-4287

Summary

Pilosebaceous follicle fills with a mixture of bacteria, sebum, and keratin.

Description

- Comedonal (obstructive, noninflammatory)
  - Blackheads: dilated hair follicle with open orifice to skin; oxidation of melanin, compacted epithelial cells and/or presence of lipids may contribute
  - Whiteheads: dilated hair follicle filled with keratin, sebum, and bacteria with obstructed opening to the skin

- Papulopustular (inflammatory): papules (<5 mm) are bumps, and pustules (<5 mm) are purulent bumps; after inflammatory process, hyperpigmented or erythematous macules may persist for as long as 12 months
- Nodular/cystic (inflammatory): nodules (>5 mm) are inflammatory bumps and often involve >1 follicle
- Scars: appear like pits on face

Treatment Objectives and Agents Used

- Comedolytic agents: decrease, eliminate, or prevent follicular keratinocyte proliferation and retention—topical retinoids, benzoyl peroxides, isotretinoin, salicylic acids
- Antibacterial agents: reduce bacterial colonization and local inflammation—benzoyl peroxides, topical and oral antibiotics, salicylic acids, isotretinoin
- Antisebum: reduce sebum production—isotretinoin, hormonal contraceptives

Use of and Possible Adverse Effects of Acne Medications

Table 10.1
Acne agents: classification, use, and adverse effects

Class	Agent	How to Use	Comments
Comedolytic agents	Tretinoin 0.025%, 0.04%, 0.05%, 0.1% (cream, lotion, gel microsphere)	Apply pea-sized amount 20 min after washing face; begin with lower concentrations and increase as clinically indicated	Use sunscreen; avoid in pregnant and breastfeeding women; adverse effects are dryness, erythema, and peeling; acne may worsen during first few weeks of therapy
	Adapalene 0.1% (cream, gel)	Apply pea-sized amount nightly after gently washing face with mild soap	Use sunscreen; adverse effects are erythema, dryness, scaling, pruritus, and burning; acne may worsen during first few weeks of therapy
	Azelaic acid 15%, 20% (cream, gel)	May be used any time of day	Use sunscreen; adverse effects are dryness, erythema, and scaling; available without prescription
	Tazarotene 0.05%, 0.1% (cream, gel)		Use sunscreen; adverse effects are dryness, erythema, and scaling
Topical antibacterial agents	Benzoyl peroxide (eg, 2.5%–10% gel, liquid, face wash)	May be used morning or evening; begin with lower concentrations, especially in fair-skinned patients; back and chest acne may respond better to higher strengths	Use sunscreen; adverse effects are erythema, peeling, and possible allergic contact sensitization; may bleach clothing
Topical antibiotics	Choice of vehicle depends on type of skin (eg, clindamycin 1%, erythromycin 2% gel, solution, lotion, solution)	May be used once or twice daily	Adverse effects are dryness, tenderness, pruritus, peeling, erythema, burning, itching, and oiliness; bacteria increasingly resistant, but less with clindamycin; rare reports of pseudomembranous enterocolitis with clindamycin; may be used with comedolytic
Topical combinations	eg, 3% erythromycin/5% benzoyl peroxide, 1% clindamycin/5% benzoyl peroxide, 1.2% clindamycin phosphate-tretinoin 0.025% gel, 0.1% adapalene- 2.5%-benzoyl peroxide	May be used twice daily; may be used with comedolytic agent	Adverse effects are dryness, tenderness, pruritus; must be refrigerated; combination seems to protect against resistance of bacteria
Azelaic acid	15%, 20%	May be used once or twice daily; used with comedolytic	Adverse effects are pruritus, burning, stinging, tingling, erythema, dryness, irritation, small depigmented spots; may be beneficial in patients with postinflammatory hyperpigmentation

(*Continued*)

Table 10.1
(Continued)

Class	Agent	How to Use	Comments
Oral antibiotics	Tetracycline	600–2000 mg daily divided in 1–3 daily doses	Take on empty stomach, 1 h before or 2 h after eating, and do not take with dairy products; adverse effects are gastrointestinal discomfort, vaginal candidiasis, photosensitivity, and dental staining; use sunscreen
	Minocycline	50–100 mg once or twice daily	Can cause increased intracranial pressure, blue-black discoloration in scars, photosensitivity, and rarely hepatitis or a lupus-like syndrome; use sunscreen; better absorbed than tetracycline
	Doxycycline	50–100 mg once or twice daily	May be taken with food; photosensitivity more likely than with other tetracycline
	Erythromycin	250 mg 2–4 times daily	Bacteria increasingly resistant; adverse effects are gastrointestinal upset and interactions with certain antihistamines
Oral retinoid	Isotretinoin (Accutane)	0.5–2 mg/kg daily for 15–20 wk	Absolutely contraindicated in pregnancy; must monitor laboratory results monthly; adverse effects include drying of skin, mucous, reduced night vision, hair loss, muscle aches, joint pains, and headaches; use sunscreen
Other	Combination hormones (pill, patch, ring)		Increase SHBG, reduce free testosterone; blocks 5-α-reductase at hair-follicle level
	Spironolactone	50–150 mg daily divided	Requires 3 mo to see effect; antiandrogen at hair-follicle level; mild diuretic

SHBG, sex hormone binding globulin.
Adapted from Kristal L, Silverberg N. *Contemp Pediatr*. 1998;15(suppl):8–9.

Table 10.2
Available formulations of topical retinoids

Retinoid	Formulation	Strength, %
Tretinoin	Cream	0.025, 0.05, 0.1
	Gel	0.01, 0.025
	Liquid	0.05
	Microsphere gel (Retin-A Micro)	0.04, 0.1
	Polymerized cream (Avita)	0.025
	Polymerized gel (Avita)	0.025
Adapalene (Differin)	Cream	0.1
	Gel	0.1
	Solution	0.1
Tazarotene (Tazorac)	Cream	0.05[a], 0.1
	Gel	0.05[a], 0.1

[a] Indicated for psoriasis.
From Zaenglein AL, Thiboutot DM. Expert committee recommendations for acne management. *Pediatrics.* 2006;118(3):1192.

Table 10.3
Assessment of severity

Mild	Few to several inflammatory lesions, and comedones, no nodules, 25% of face involved
Moderate	Several to many inflammatory lesions, and comedones, few to several nodules, 50% of face involved
Severe	Numerous large inflammatory lesions, and comedones, many nodules, scars, ≥75% of face involved

Krowchuk DP. Verbal communication, 2007, Savannah, GA.

Table 10.4
Acne treatment algorithm

	Mild		Moderate		Severe, Nodular
	Comedonal	Papular/Pustular	Papular/Pustular	Nodular	
First-line therapy	Topical retinoid	Topical retinoid + BPO or BPO/AB	Topical retinoid + oral antibiotic + BPO or BPO/AB	Topical retinoid + oral antibiotic ± BPO or BPO/AB	Oral isotretinoin
Alternatives	Salicylic acid		Oral isotretinoin		Oral antibiotic + topical retinoid + BPO or BPO/AB
Alternatives for female patients			Hormonal therapy + topical retinoid ± BPO or BPO/AB	Hormonal therapy + topical retinoid ± BPO or BPO/AB	Hormonal therapy + oral antibiotic + topical retinoid ± BPO or BPO/AB
Maintenance therapy	Topical retinoid ± BPO or BPO/AB		Topical retinoid ± BPO or BPO/AB		Topical retinoid ± BPO or BPO/AB

BPO indicates benzoyl peroxide; AB, topical antibiotic.
Adapted from Gollnick H, Cunliffe W, et al. Management of Acne: a report from a global alliance to improve outcomes in acne. *J Am Acad Dermatol*. 2003;49:S1–S38.

FUNGAL INFECTIONS

Acquired from infected humans or animals or indirectly from exposure to contaminated soil or fomites.

Diagnosis

- Use of potassium hydroxide preparation of skin scales or subungual debris and heated; look for hyphae
- Culture infected hair or sample from affected area by using a cotton swab moistened with tap water

Infections

Pityriasis (Tinea) Versicolor

Etiology: yeast *Pityrosporum ovale*

- Referred to as pityrosporum versicolor to differentiate from dermatophyte infections; not true tinea
- Filamentous form of *Malassezia furfur* (*Pityrosporum orbiculare* is the yeast form)
- Interference with normal pigmentation by inhibiting tyrosinase, an enzyme that is essential in production of melanin

Clinical findings

- Multiple oval, hypopigmented or hyperpigmented, macular lesions with very fine scales usually appear on upper trunk, neck, and proximal arms
- Usually asymptomatic, chronic, and more prominent when sun-exposed areas fail to tan
- Rash can be pruritic, especially with sweating or warm weather

Diagnosis: appearance, examination with Wood's light in dark room may reveal yellow-orange fluorescence; use potassium hydroxide preparation to reveal short hyphae and spores.

Differential: pityriasis versicolor, vitiligo, pityriasis rosea, secondary syphilis.

Table 10.5
Treatment options for tinea versicolor

Topical	Selenium sulfide 2.5%; apply 10 min/d for 14 d; or single 8- to 12-h application twice, 2 weeks apart
	Ketoconazole shampoo 2%; apply 5 min/day for 1–3 d
Systemic	Ketoconazole 400 mg once day 1, 8, 15 or 200 mg ×5 d or fluconazole 400 mg once

Adapted from Trulong A, Friedlander SF. Superficial fungal infections in adolescents. In: Krowchuk DP, Lucky AW, eds. *Adol Med.* 2001;12(2):213–217.

Tinea Pedis

Etiology: fungus—*Trichophyton rubrum, Trichophyton mentagrophytes*, and *Epidermophyton floccosum* most common.

Clinical findings

- Web-space maceration, but also may have a moccasin distribution, affecting the soles and lateral feet with hyperkeratotic scale; presents with itching, redness, and scaling between toes
- Maceration, oozing, and fissuring may represent secondary infection

Differential: bacterial infection, dyshidrosis, psoriasis, foot eczema, and contact or atopic dermatitis.

Treatment: treatment options for tinea corporis/pedis/cruris (see Table 10.6 for topical treatment).

Widespread without nail involvement: Griseofulvin.

Widespread with nail involvement, refer to Table 10.7.

References: Shy R. Tinea corporis and tinea capitis. *Pediatr Rev*. 2007;28(5):167–174; Lange DS. Ketoconazole 2% shampoo in the treatment of tinea versicolor: a multicenter, randomized, double-blind, placebo-controlled trial. *J Am Acad Dermatol*. 1998;39(6):944–950.

Table 10.6
Common topical antifungal therapies

Drug Class	Drug Name	Dose (2 to 4 wk)
Tolnaftate	Tolnaftate	BID
Imidazoles	Clotrimazole	BID
	Miconazole	BID
	Econazole	QD
	Ketoconazole	QD
	Oxiconazole	QD to BID
	Sulconazole	QD
Ciclopirox[a]	Ciclopirox	BID
Benzylamine	Butenafine (eg, Lotrimin)	QD to BID
Allylamine	Terbinafine (eg, Lamisil)	BID
	Naftifine (eg, Naftin)	QD, BID

BID indicates twice daily; QD, once daily.
[a] Nail Lacquer is available.
Adapted from Shy R. Tinea corporis and tinea capitis. Pediatr Rev. 2007;28(5):164–174.

Table 10.7
Treatment options for tinea unguium

Itraconazole (Sporanox) (100 mg per capsule)	Fingernails	200 mg twice daily for 1 wk; repeat in 3 wk
	Toenails	200 mg twice daily for 1 wk/month for 3–4 mo
Terbinafine (Lamisil) (250 mg per tablet)	Fingernails	250 mg once daily for 6 wk
	Toenails	250 mg once daily for 12 wk or 500 mg orally every day for first week of month for 3–4 mo
Fluconazole	Toenails	150 mg once weekly for 3–6 mo

Adapted from Andrews M, Burns M. Common tinea infections in children. *Am Fam Physician.* 2008;77(10):1415; Trulong A, Friedlander SF. Superficial fungal infections in adolescents. In: Krowchuk DP, Lucky AW, eds. *Adol Med.* 2001;12(2):213–217.

Tinea Corporis

Etiology: fungus

- All species of *Trichophyton*, *Microsporum*, and *Epidermophyton*; most common in United States: *T rubrum*, *Trichophyton tonsurans*, *T mentagrophytes*, *Microsporum canis*, and *E floccosum*
- Animals may host specific dermatophytes: *T rubrum*, *Trichophyton tonsurans*, *T mentagrophytes*, *M canis*

Clinical findings

- Red, scaly papule spreading outward, with a coalescence of papules into plaques that become scaly
- Lesion becomes an annular, pruritic plaque on glabrous (smooth and bare) skin, with a scaly, slightly raised edge at the advancing border
- Center clears, leaving a hypopigmented or hyperpigmented postinflammatory area as the lesion advances

Differential: cutaneous lupus, drug eruption, erythema multiforme, nummular eczema, psoriasis, impetigo, granuloma annulare lesions (nonpruritic, no scale) and herald patch of pityriasis rosea, secondary syphilis.

Treatment: treatment options for tinea corporis/pedis/cruris (see Table 10.6).

References: Shy R. Tinea corporis and tinea capitis. *Pediatr Rev.* 2007;28(5):164–174.

Tinea Cruris

Etiology: fungus—*T rubrum, E flocullosum, T mentagrophytes.*

Clinical findings

- Demarcated, pruritic lesion with raised erythematous margin
- Thin, dry epidermal scaling that tends to spare the penis, scrotum, vulva, and perianal area (in contrast to candidiasis)
- Rash spreads from the groin down the inner thigh

Differential: candidal infections (more uniformly red with no central clearing), erythrasma (superficial *Corynebacterium* sp. bacterial skin infection more uniformly brown with slight scale and no border), intertrigo, psoriasis.

Treatment: treatment options for tinea corporis/pedis/cruris (see Table 10.6).

References: Shy R. Tinea corporis and tinea capitis. *Pediatr Rev*. 2007;28(5):164–174; Gupta AK, Ryder JE, Johnson AM. Cumulative meta-analysis of systemic antifungal agents for the treatment of onychomycosis. *Br J Dermatol*. 2004;150: 537–544; Finch JJ, Warshaw EM. Toenail onychomycosis: current and future treatment options. *Dermatol Ther*. 2007;20:31–46.

Tinea Unguium (Fungal Nail Infection)

Etiology: dermatophytes such as *T rubrum, E floccosum*, molds, yeast.

Clinical findings

- Local factors such as nail abnormalities-psoriasis, trauma, hyperhidrosis, water contact
- Immunocompromised

Differential: trauma, chronic paronychia, chronic skin diseases (eg, psoriasis), congenital syndromes (eg, nail-patella syndrome).

Treatment: see treatment options in Table 10.7.

HYPERSENSITIVITY SYNDROMES

- Urticaria—capillaritis
- Angioedema—Schamberg pigmented purpura
- Serum sickness–like reactions—vasculitis
- Drug reactions—erythema multiforme
- Annular erythemas (erythema migrans)—Henoch-Schonlein purpura
- Panniculitis—erythema nodosum

Urticaria

Description: cutaneous hypersensitivity reaction; lesions last few hours (<24 hours); papules, rings, and wheals and associated with angioedema (occurs in 50% of patients with urticaria, manifested as swelling of hands, feet, periorbital areas).

Etiology: infection (bacteria, viruses, parasites), bites and stings, drugs, foods (nuts, shellfish, eggs, strawberries, tomatoes), blood products.

Treatment

- Initial: nonsedating antihistamine; avoid nonsteroidal antiinflammatory drugs (NSAIDs); use lotion with menthol
- Second-line: prednisone for short courses; montelukast for longer-lasting lesions

Erythema Multiforme

Description: cutaneous hypersensitivity reaction; lesions last ≥7 days; target lesions commonly associated with prodromal symptoms; oral ulcers may be present in 25% to 50% of patients; overlaps with toxic epidermal necrolysis (TEN) with Stevens Johnson syndrome <10% body, overlap 10% to 30% of body, TEN >30% of body.

Etiology: hypersensitivity to viruses (eg herpes simplex virus); drugs such as NSAIDs, antibiotics, and antiepileptic drugs and infections.

Initial treatment: hospitalization and intravenous or oral steroids.

Erythema Nodosum

Description: tender, erythematous to violaceous nodules located over the shins.

Etiology: inflammation of fat triggered by infections such as bacteria, viruses, fungi.

Initial treatment: lesions resolve on their own; use with NSAIDs.

Warts

Etiology: human papillomavirus (>100 types).

Clinical findings

- Common warts: types 1, 2, 4, and 26 through 29
- Plantar warts: types 1 and 4 most common
- Flat warts on face, arms, legs, and hands: types 2, 3, 10, 26 through 29, and 41
- *Condyloma acuminatum*: types 6 and 11; other low-risk types are 40 and 42 through 44

Treatment: options for treating warts in adolescents

- Initial: salicylic acid, cryotherapy, podophyllin, imiquimod, tretinoin
- Aggressive: laser, electrodesiccation and curettage, topical 5-fluorouracil, intralesional interferon

Table 10.8
Conditions that are treatable with topical steroids

High-potency steroids (groups I–III)
Alopecia areata
Atopic dermatitis (resistant)
Discoid lupus
Hyperkeratotic eczema
Lichen planus
Lichen sclerosus (skin)
Lichen simplex chronicus
Nummular eczema
Poison ivy (severe)
Psoriasis
Severe hand eczema
Medium-potency steroids (groups IV and V)
Anal inflammation (severe)
Asteatotic eczema
Atopic dermatitis
Lichen sclerosus (vulva)
Nummular eczema
Scabies (after scabicide)
Seborrheic dermatitis
Severe dermatitis
Severe intertrigo (short-term)
Stasis dermatitis
Low-potency steroids (groups VI and VII)
Dermatitis (diaper)
Dermatitis (eyelids)
Dermatitis (face)
Intertrigo
Perianal inflammation

Adapted with permission from Ference JD et al. Choosing topical steroids. *Am Fam Physician.* 2009;79(2):135.

Table 10.9
Potency ratings of corticosteroids

Potency (group)	Generic Medication	Brand Medication	Dosage Vehicle	Available Sizes
Ultra high (I)	Augmented betamethasone dipropionate 0.05%	Diprolene[a]	G,[b] O	15, 45, 50 g
	Clobetasol propionate 0.05%	Clobex	L, Sh	59, 118 mL(L); 118 mL(Sh)
		Olux[a]	F	50, 100 g
		Temovate[a]	C, G, O	15, 30, 45 g (C, O); 15, 30, 60 g (G)
		Temovate E[a]	C	15, 30, 60 g
	Diflorasone diacetate 0.05%	Apexicon[a]	O	15, 30, 60 g
	Fluocinonide 0.1%	Vanos	C	30, 60 g
	Flurandrenolide 4 mcg per m^2	Cordran	T	24" × 3" rolls; 80" × 3" rolls
	Halobetasol propionate 0.05%	Ultravate[a]	C, O	15, 50 g
High (II)	Amcinonide 0.1%	NA	O	15, 30, 60 g
	Augmented betamethasone dipropionate 0.05%	Diprolene[a]	L	30, 60 mL
		Diprolene[a] AF	C	15, 50 g
	Betamethasone dipropionate 0.05%	Diprosone[a,c]	O	15, 45 g
	Desoximetasone	Topicort 0.25%[a]	C, O	15, 60 g
		Topicort 0.05%[a]	G, O	15, 60 g
	Diflorasone diacetate 0.05%	Apexicon E[a]	C	15, 30, 60 g
	Fluocinonide 0.05%	Lidex[a]	C,[b] G,[b] O	15, 30, 60 g
	Halcinonide 0.1%	Halog	C, O, So	15, 30, 60, 240 g (C, O); 30, 60 mL (So)

(*Continued*)

Table 10.9
(Continued)

Potency (group)	Generic Medication	Brand Medication	Dosage Vehicle	Available Sizes
Medium to high (III)	Amcinonide 0.1%	Cyclocort[c]	C	4, 15, 30, 60 g
	Betamethasone dipropionate 0.05%	Betanate[a]	C	15, 45 g
	Fluticasone propionate 0.005%	Cutivate[a]	O	15, 30, 60 g
	Triamcinolone acetonide 0.5%	Cinalog[a,c]	C, O	15 g
Medium (IV and V)	Betamethasone valerate	Beta-Val 0.1%[a]	C, L	14, 45 g(C); 60 mL(L)
		Luxiq 0.12%	F	100 g
	Desoximetasone 0.05%	Topicort LP[a]	C	15, 60 g
	Fluocinolone acetonide 0.025%	Synalar[a,c]	C, O	15, 60 g
	Fluticasone propionate 0.05%	Cutivate[a]	C	15, 30, 60 g
	Hydrocortisone butyrate 0.1%	Locoid[a]	O	5, 10, 15, 30, 45 g
	Hydrocortisone probutate 0.1%	Pandel	C	15, 45, 80 g
	Hydrocortisone valerate 0.2%	Westcort[a]	C, O	14, 45, 60 g(C, O); 30, 60 mL(L)
	Mometasone furoate 0.1%	Elocon[a]	C, L, O	15, 45 g (C, O); 30, 60 mL(L)
	Triamcinolone acetonide 0.025%	Kenalog[a,c]	C, L, O	15, 80, 454 g (C, O); 60 mL(L)
	Triamcinolone acetonide 0.1%	Triderm[a]	C, L,[b] O[b]	15, 80, 454 g (C, O); 15, 60 mL(L)

(Continued)

Table 10.9
(Continued)

Potency (group)	Generic Medication	Brand Medication	Dosage Vehicle	Available Sizes
Low (VI)	Alclometasone dipropionate 0.05%	Aclovate[a]	C, O	15, 45, 60 g
	Desonide 0.05%	Desonate	G	15, 30, 60 g
		Desowen[a]	C, O	15, 60 g
		Lokara	L	60, 120 mL
		Verdeso	F	100 g
	Fluocinolone 0.01%	NA	C	15, 60 g
	Hydrocortisone butyrate 0.1%	Locoid[a]	C	5, 10, 15, 30, 45 g
Least potent (VII)	Hydrocortisone 1%, 2.5%	NA	C, L, O	20, 30, 120 g (C, O); 60, 120 mL (L)

C, cream; F, foam; G, gel; L, lotion; O, ointment; Sh, shampoo; So, solution; T, tape. [a]Generic is not available; [b]Brand is not available in this formulation; [c]Brand is no longer available in the United States.

Adapted with permission from Ference JD et al. Choosing topical steroids. *Am Fam Physician.* 2009;79(2): 137–138.

Molluscum Contagiosum

Etiology: molluscum contagiosum virus types 1 and 2.

Clinical findings

- Incubation time from days to a few weeks
- Resolution in an immunocompetent person: 2 to 6 weeks; may take 6 to 9 months for resolution

Differential: verrucae vulgaris, condyloma acuminatum, trichoepithelioma.

Treatment: options for treating warts in adolescents

- Initial: salicylic acid, cryotherapy, podophyllin, imiquimod, tretinoin
- Aggressive: laser, electrodesiccation and curettage, topical 5-fluorouracil, intralesional interferon

Keratosis Pilaris: Follicular Hyperkeratosis

Etiology

- Inherited disorder
- Follicular plugging with excess keratin in follicular orifices
- Entrapment of hair

Clinical findings

- Exterior aspects of upper arms, upper legs, and buttocks

Differential: lichen spinulosus, pityriasis rubra, phrynoderma.

Treatment

- Keratolytic agents: lactic acid, salicylic acid, and urea cream (eg, 2% salicylic acid in 20% urea cream)
- Inflammatory: triamcinolone acetonide 0.1%, desonide 0.05% for 7 days

Etiology of Acquired Hair Loss

- Circumscribed: nonscarring tinea capitis, traction alopecia, trichotillomania, friction alopecia, alopecia areata
- Scarring: after infection (kerion), after inflammation (lupus), after injury (trauma, chemical, burns)
- Diffuse: telogen effluvium, endocrine (hypothyroid, hypopituitarism, hypoparthyroidism, diabetes mellitus type 1), androgenetic alopecia, nutritional (zinc, marasmus, hypervitaminosis A, chemical (thallium, heparin, coumarin, antimetabolites)

Tattoos/Body Piercing

See Immunization Action Coalition. Tattooing and body piercing information. Available at: www.immunize.org/tattoos/. Accessed July 20, 2009.

Pigmented Lesions and Photoprotection

ABCD signs of melanoma

- Asymmetry: shape of one half does not match the other (Fig 10.2 see insert)
- Border: edges are often ragged, notched, blurred, or irregular in outline; the pigment may spread into the surrounding skin (Fig 10.3 see insert)
- Color: color is uneven; shades of black, brown, and tan may be present; areas of white, gray, red, pink, or blue also may be seen (Fig 10.4 see insert)
- Diameter: there is a change in size, usually an increase; melanomas are usually larger than the eraser of a pencil (¼ in or 5 mm) (Fig 10.5 see insert)

Melanomas can vary greatly in how they look; many show all of the ABCD features or only 2 or 3 of them. Melanomas in an early stage may be found when an existing mole changes slightly (eg, new black area; newly formed fine scales and itching; texture such as hard and lumpy; itch, ooze, or bleed) (see www.cancer.gov/cancertopics/types/melanoma).

Atypical moles are larger >5 mm; are flat or flat with a raised center; are darkly or irregularly pigmented (brown, pink); have irregular or indistinct borders.

Sunscreen Facts

- How do sunscreens work? Sunscreens absorb and block ultraviolet light radiation; those that block both UV-A and UV-B light are the best.
- What is SPF (sun protection factor)? It is defined as the ratio of the minimum erythema dose required to redden unprotected skin; it refers to the UV-B protection, not UV-A.
- When and how often should sunscreens be applied? For best protection screens with SPF should be applied 30 to 45 minutes before actual sun exposure, then every 2 hours with at least 1 oz every application.
- What SPF is recommended? Sunscreens with an SPF of at least 15 are recommended, with higher ones not necessarily providing that much more protection (eg, a sunscreen with an SPF of 16 gives 93.8% protection from UV-B, whereas an SPF of 32 gives 96.9% protection).
- What are other situations in which sunscreens need to be used? Sunscreens need to be used on cloudy days, because clouds let 80% of rays penetrate; beach umbrellas offer only 50% protection, because rays reflect off sand; higher altitudes increase radiation exposure.
- Do sunscreens interfere with vitamin D production? Approximately 10 to 15 minutes of natural sunlight 2 to 3 times a week supplies adequate

vitamin D production; even this light is not necessary for normal diets that are fortified with vitamin D.
- It is estimated that one 30-minute tanning session per week increases the risk of nonmelanoma skin cancer to 30% above baseline.

Data source: Kim HJ. Photoprotection in adolescents. *Adolesc Med.* 2001;12(2):181–193.

Other Skin Conditions

Pityriasis Rosea

Etiology: unknown.

Clinical findings

- Herald patch in 50% to 80% precedes generalized rash
- 2 to 21 days generalized eruption of erythematous, oval, macular 1- to 2-cm patches with scale in center
- Rash distributed primarily on the back, chest, upper arms, neck, in a Christmas-tree pattern; usually spares face, hands, and feet and is usually nonpruritic
- In persons of color, rash may be more papular, primarily on arms, and spare torso

Differential: tinea corporis, seborrheic dermatitis, secondary syphilis, contact dermatitis.

Treatment: topical steroids, oral antihistamines if pruritic, otherwise reassurance; often takes 6 to 8 weeks to resolve.

Psoriasis

Etiology: unknown but felt to have a genetic predisposition and immunologic component; presents before 16 years of age in 25% to 45%.

Clinical findings

- Round, well-circumscribed erythematosus plaques distributed over eyebrows, ears, scalp, umbilicus; extensor surfaces of elbows and knees most common sites; uncommon in occluded sites
- Conditions such as trauma, stress, infections, and cold weather may precipitate; called "Koebner phenomenon" when areas of injury precipitate lesions
- May be associated with arthritis presenting in childhood

Differential: seborrheic dermatitis and contact dermatitis.

Treatment: topical steroids, topical synthetic retinoids, topical keratolytic agents such as salicylic acid; may require systemic treatment.

Adolesc Med 20 (2009) 695–727

11. Musculoskeletal and Sports Medicine

Alain Joffe, MD, MPH
E-mail address: ajoffe@jhu.edu.

 ISSN 1934-4287

Table 11.1
Classification of Sports According to Contact

Contact	Limited-Contact	Noncontact
Basketball	Adventure racing[a]	Badminton
Boxing[b]	Baseball	Bodybuilding[c]
Cheerleading	Bicycling	Bowling
Diving	Canoeing or kayaking (white water)	Canoeing or kayaking (flat water)
Extreme sports[d]	Fencing	Crew or rowing
Field hockey	Field events	Curling
Football, tackle	High jump	Dance
Gymnastics	Pole vault	Field events
Ice hockey[e]	Floor hockey	Discus
Lacrosse	Football, flag or touch	Javelin
Martial arts[f]	Handball	Shot-put
Rodeo	Horseback riding	Golf
Rugby	Martial arts[f]	Orienteering[g]
Skiing, downhill	Racquetball	Power lifting[c]
Ski jumping	Skating	Race walking
Snowboarding	Ice	Riflery
Soccer	In-line	Rope jumping
Team handball	Roller	Running
Ultimate Frisbee	Skiing	Sailing
Water polo	Cross-country	Scuba diving
Wrestling	Water	Swimming
	Skateboarding	
	Softball	Tennis
	Squash	Track
	Volleyball	
	Weight lifting	
	Windsurfing or surfing	

[a]Adventure racing has been added since the previous statement was published and is defined as a combination of 2 or more disciplines, including orienteering and navigation, cross-country running, mountain biking, paddling, and climbing and rope skills.
[b]The American Academy of Pediatrics opposes participation in boxing for children, adolescents, and young adults.
[c]The American Academy of Pediatrics recommends limiting bodybuilding and power lifting until the adolescent achieves sexual maturity rating 5 (Tanner stage V).
[d]Extreme sports has been added since the previous statement was published.
[e]The American Academy of Pediatrics recommends limiting the amount of body checking allowed for hockey players 15 years and younger, to reduce injuries.
[f]Martial arts can be subclassified as judo, jujitsu, karate, kung fu, and tae kwon do; some forms are contact sports and others are limited-contact sports.
[g]Orienteering is a race (contest) in which competitors use a map and a compass to find their way through unfamiliar territory.
Adapted from American Academy of Pediatrics, Committee on Sports Medicine and Fitness. Medical conditions affecting sports participation. *Pediatrics*. 2008;121(4):841–848.

Table 11.2
Medical Conditions and Sports Participation

Condition	May Participate
Atlantoaxial instability (instability of the joint between cervical vertebrae 1 and 2)	Qualified yes
Explanation: Athlete (particularly if he or she has Down syndrome or juvenile rheumatoid arthritis with cervical involvement) needs evaluation to assess the risk of spinal cord injury during sports participation, especially when using a trampoline.	
Bleeding disorder	Qualified yes
Explanation: Athlete needs evaluation.	
Cardiovascular disease	
Carditis (inflammation of the heart)	No
Explanation: Carditis may result in sudden death with exertion.	
Hypertension (high blood pressure)	Qualified yes
Explanation: Those with hypertension >5 mm Hg above the 99th percentile for age, gender, and height should avoid heavy weightlifting and power lifting, bodybuilding, and high-static component sports. Those with sustained hypertension (>95th percentile for age, gender, and height) need evaluation. The National High Blood Pressure Education Program Working Group report defined prehypertension and stage 1 and stage 2 hypertension in children and adolescents younger than 18 years of age.	
Congenital heart disease (structural heart defects present at birth)	Qualified yes
Explanation: Consultation with a cardiologist is recommended. Those who have mild forms may participate fully in most cases; those who have moderate or severe forms or who have undergone surgery need evaluation. The 36th Bethesda Conference defined mild, moderate, and severe disease for common cardiac lesions.	
Dysrhythmia (irregular heart rhythm)	Qualified yes
Long-QT syndrome	
Malignant ventricular arrhythmias	
Symptomatic Wolff-Parkinson-White syndrome	
Advanced heart block	
Family history of sudden death or previous sudden cardiac event	

(*Continued*)

Table 11.2
(Continued)

Condition	May Participate
Implantation of a cardioverter-defibrillator	
Explanation: Consultation with a cardiologist is advised. Those with symptoms (chest pain, syncope, near-syncope, dizziness, shortness of breath, or other symptoms of possible dysrhythmia) or evidence of mitral regurgitation on physical examination need evaluation. All others may participate fully.	
Heart murmur	Qualified yes
Explanation: If the murmur is innocent (does not indicate heart disease), full participation is permitted. Otherwise, athlete needs evaluation (see structural heart disease, especially hypertrophic cardiomyopathy and mitral valve prolapse).	
Structural/acquired heart disease	
Hypertrophic cardiomyopathy	Qualified no
Coronary artery anomalies	Qualified no
Arrhythmogenic right ventricular cardiomyopathy	Qualified no
Acute rheumatic fever with carditis	Qualified no
Ehlers-Danlos syndrome, vascular form	Qualified no
Marfan syndrome	Qualified yes
Mitral valve prolapse	Qualified yes
Anthracycline use	Qualified yes
Explanation: Consultation with a cardiologist is recommended. The 36th Bethesda Conference provided detailed recommendations. Most of these conditions carry a significant risk of sudden cardiac death associated with intense physical exercise. Hypertrophic cardiomyopathy requires thorough and repeated evaluations, because disease may change manifestations during later adolescence. Marfan syndrome with an aortic aneurysm also can cause sudden death during intense physical exercise. Athlete who has ever received chemotherapy with anthracyclines may be at increased risk of cardiac problems because of the cardiotoxic effects of the medications, and resistance training in this population should be approached with caution; strength training that avoids isometric contractions may be permitted. Athlete needs evaluation.	

(*Continued*)

Table 11.2
(Continued)

Condition	May Participate
Vasculitis/vascular disease Kawasaki disease (coronary artery vasculitis) Pulmonary hypertension Explanation: Consultation with a cardiologist is recommended. Athlete needs individual evaluation to assess risk on the basis of disease activity, pathologic changes, and medical regimen.	Qualified yes
Cerebral palsy Explanation: Athlete needs evaluation to assess functional capacity to perform sports-specific activity.	Qualified yes
Diabetes mellitus Explanation: All sports can be played with proper attention and appropriate adjustments to diet (particularly carbohydrate intake), blood glucose concentrations, hydration, and insulin therapy. Blood glucose concentrations should be monitored before exercise, every 30 minutes during continuous exercise, 15 minutes after completion of exercise, and at bedtime.	Yes
Diarrhea, infectious Explanation: Unless symptoms are mild and athlete is fully hydrated, no participation is permitted, because diarrhea may increase risk of dehydration and heat illness (see fever).	Qualified no
Eating disorders Explanation: Athlete with an eating disorder needs medical and psychiatric assessment before participation.	Qualified yes
Eyes Functionally 1-eyed athlete Loss of an eye Detached retina or family history of retinal detachment at young age High myopia Connective tissue disorder, such as Marfan or Stickler syndrome	Qualified yes

(*Continued*)

Table 11.2
(Continued)

Condition	May Participate
Previous intraocular eye surgery or serious eye injury Explanation: A functionally 1-eyed athlete is defined as having best-corrected visual acuity worse than 20/40 in the poorer-seeing eye. Such an athlete would suffer significant disability if the better eye were seriously injured, as would an athlete with loss of an eye. Specifically, boxing and full-contact martial arts are not recommended for functionally 1-eyed athletes, because eye protection is impractical and/or not permitted. Some athletes who previously underwent intraocular eye surgery or had a serious eye injury may have increased risk of injury because of weakened eye tissue. Availability of eye guards approved by the American Society for Testing and Materials and other protective equipment may allow participation in most sports, but this must be judged on an individual basis.	
Conjunctivitis, infectious Explanation: Athlete with active infectious conjunctivitis should be excluded from swimming.	Qualified no
Fever Explanation: Elevated core temperature may be indicative of a pathologic medical condition (infection or disease) that is often manifest by increased resting metabolism and heart rate. Accordingly, during athlete's usual exercise regimen, the presence of fever can result in greater heat storage, decreased heat tolerance, increased risk of heat illness, increased cardiopulmonary effort, reduced maximal exercise capacity, and increased risk of hypotension because of altered vascular tone and dehydration. On rare occasions, fever may accompany myocarditis or other conditions that may make usual exercise dangerous.	No
Gastrointestinal Malabsorption syndromes (celiac disease or cystic fibrosis)	Qualified yes

(Continued)

Table 11.2
(Continued)

Condition	May Participate
Explanation: Athlete needs individual assessment for general malnutrition or specific deficits resulting in coagulation or other defects; with appropriate treatment, these deficits can be treated adequately to permit normal activities.	
Short-bowel syndrome or other disorders requiring specialized nutritional support, including parenteral or enteral nutrition	
Explanation: Athlete needs individual assessment for collision, contact, or limited-contact sports. Presence of central or peripheral, indwelling, venous catheter may require special considerations for activities and emergency preparedness for unexpected trauma to the device(s).	
Heat illness, history of	Qualified yes
Explanation: Because of the likelihood of recurrence, athlete needs individual assessment to determine the presence of predisposing conditions and behaviors and to develop a prevention strategy that includes sufficient acclimatization (to the environment and to exercise intensity and duration), conditioning, hydration, and salt intake, as well as other effective measures to improve heat tolerance and to reduce heat injury risk (such as protective equipment and uniform configurations).	
Hepatitis, infectious (primarily hepatitis C)	Yes
Explanation: All athletes should receive hepatitis B vaccination before participation. Because of the apparent minimal risk to others, all sports may be played as athlete's state of health allows. For all athletes, skin lesions should be covered properly, and athletic personnel should use universal precautions when handling blood or body fluids with visible blood.	

(Continued)

Table 11.2
(Continued)

Condition	May Participate
HIV infection	Yes
Explanation: Because of the apparent minimal risk to others, all sports may be played as athlete's state of health allows (especially if viral load is undetectable or very low). For all athletes, skin lesions should be covered properly, and athletic personnel should use universal precautions when handling blood or body fluids with visible blood. However, certain sports (such as wrestling and boxing) may create a situation that favors viral transmission (likely bleeding plus skin breaks). If viral load is detectable, then athletes should be advised to avoid such high-contact sports.	
Kidney, absence of one	Qualified yes
Explanation: Athlete needs individual assessment for contact, collision, and limited-contact sports. Protective equipment may reduce risk of injury to the remaining kidney sufficiently to allow participation in most sports, providing such equipment remains in place during activity.	
Liver, enlarged	Qualified yes
Explanation: If the liver is acutely enlarged, then participation should be avoided because of risk of rupture. If the liver is chronically enlarged, then individual assessment is needed before collision, contact, or limited-contact sports are played. Patients with chronic liver disease may have changes in liver function that affect stamina, mental status, coagulation, or nutritional status.	
Malignant neoplasm	Qualified yes
Explanation: Athlete needs individual assessment.	
Musculoskeletal disorders	Qualified yes
Explanation: Athlete needs individual assessment.	
Neurologic disorders	
History of serious head or spine trauma or abnormality, including craniotomy, epidural bleeding, subdural hematoma, intracerebral hemorrhage, second-impact syndrome, vascular malformation, and neck fracture.	Qualified yes
Explanation: Athlete needs individual assessment for collision, contact, or limited-contact sports.	

(*Continued*)

Table 11.2
(Continued)

Condition	May Participate
History of simple concussion (mild traumatic brain injury), multiple simple concussions, and/or complex concussion	Qualified yes
Explanation: Athlete needs individual assessment. Research supports a conservative approach to concussion management, including no athletic participation while symptomatic or when deficits in judgment or cognition are detected, followed by graduated return to full activity.	
Myopathies	Qualified yes
Explanation: Athlete needs individual assessment.	
Recurrent headaches	Yes
Explanation: Athlete needs individual assessment.	
Recurrent plexopathy (burner or stinger) and cervical cord neuropraxia with persistent defects	Qualified yes
Explanation: Athlete needs individual assessment for collision, contact, or limited-contact sports; regaining normal strength is important benchmark for return to play.	
Seizure disorder, well controlled	Yes
Explanation: Risk of seizure during participation is minimal.	
Seizure disorder, poorly controlled	Qualified yes
Explanation: Athlete needs individual assessment for collision, contact, or limited-contact sports. The following noncontact sports should be avoided: archery, riflery, swimming, weightlifting, power lifting, strength training, and sports involving heights. In these sports, occurrence of a seizure during activity may pose a risk to self or others.	
Obesity	Yes
Explanation: Because of the increased risk of heat illness and cardiovascular strain, obese athlete particularly needs careful acclimatization (to the environment and to exercise intensity and duration), sufficient hydration, and potential activity and recovery modifications during competition and training.	
Organ transplant recipient (and those taking immunosuppressive medications)	Qualified yes

(*Continued*)

Table 11.2
(Continued)

Condition	May Participate
Explanation: Athlete needs individual assessment for contact, collision, and limited-contact sports. In addition to potential risk of infections, some medications (eg, prednisone) may increase tendency for bruising.	
Ovary, absence of one	Yes
Explanation: Risk of severe injury to remaining ovary is minimal.	
Pregnancy/postpartum	Qualified yes
Explanation: Athlete needs individual assessment. As pregnancy progresses, modifications to usual exercise routines will become necessary. Activities with high risk of falling or abdominal trauma should be avoided. Scuba diving and activities posing risk of altitude sickness should also be avoided during pregnancy. After the birth, physiological and morphologic changes of pregnancy take 4 to 6 weeks to return to baseline.	
Respiratory conditions	
Pulmonary compromise, including cystic fibrosis	Qualified yes
Explanation: Athlete needs individual assessment but, generally, all sports may be played if oxygenation remains satisfactory during graded exercise test. Athletes with cystic fibrosis need acclimatization and good hydration to reduce risk of heat illness.	
Asthma	Yes
Explanation: With proper medication and education, only athletes with severe asthma need to modify their participation. For those using inhalers, recommend having a written action plan and using a peak flow meter daily. Athletes with asthma may encounter risks when scuba diving.	
Acute upper respiratory infection	Qualified yes
Explanation: Upper respiratory obstruction may affect pulmonary function. Athlete needs individual assessment for all except mild disease (see fever).	

(*Continued*)

Table 11.2
(Continued)

Condition	May Participate
Rheumatologic diseases	Qualified yes
Juvenile rheumatoid arthritis	
Explanation: Athletes with systemic or polyarticular juvenile rheumatoid arthritis and history of cervical spine involvement need radiographs of vertebrae C1 and C2 to assess risk of spinal cord injury. Athletes with systemic or HLA-B27 -associated arthritis require cardiovascular assessment for possible cardiac complications during exercise. For those with micrognathia (open bite and exposed teeth), mouth guards are helpful. If uveitis is present, risk of eye damage from trauma is increased; ophthalmologic assessment is recommended. If visually impaired, guidelines for functionally 1-eyed athletes should be followed.	
Juvenile dermatomyositis, idiopathic myositis	
Systemic lupus erythematosis	
Raynaud phenomenon	
Explanation: Athlete with juvenile dermatomyositis or systemic lupus erythematosis with cardiac involvement requires cardiology assessment before participation. Athletes receiving systemic corticosteroid therapy are at higher risk of osteoporotic fractures and avascular necrosis, which should be assessed before clearance; those receiving immunosuppressive medications are at higher risk of serious infection. Sports activities should be avoided when myositis is active. Rhabdomyolysis during intensive exercise may cause renal injury in athletes with idiopathic myositis and other myopathies. Because of photosensitivity with juvenile dermatomyositis and systemic lupus erythematosis, sun protection is necessary during outdoor activities. With Raynaud phenomenon, exposure to the cold presents risk to hands and feet.	

(*Continued*)

Table 11.2
(Continued)

Condition	May Participate
Sickle cell disease Explanation: Athlete needs individual assessment. In general, if illness status permits, all sports may be played; however, any sport or activity that entails overexertion, overheating, dehydration, or chilling should be avoided. Participation at high altitude, especially when not acclimatized, also poses risk of sickle cell crisis.	Qualified yes
Sickle cell trait Explanation: Athletes with sickle cell trait generally do not have increased risk of sudden death or other medical problems during athletic participation under normal environmental conditions. However, when high exertional activity is performed under extreme conditions of heat and humidity or increased altitude, such catastrophic complications have occurred rarely. Athletes with sickle cell trait, like all athletes, should be progressively acclimatized to the environment and to the intensity and duration of activities and should be sufficiently hydrated to reduce the risk of exertional heat illness and/or rhabdomyolysis. According to National Institutes of Health management guidelines, sickle cell trait is not a contraindication to participation in competitive athletics, and there is no requirement for screening before participation. More research is needed to assess fully potential risks and benefits of screening athletes for sickle cell trait.	Yes
Skin infections, including herpes simplex, molluscum contagiosum, verrucae (warts), staphylococcal and streptococcal infections (furuncles [boils], carbuncles, impetigo, methicillin-resistant *Staphylococcus aureus* [cellulitis and/or abscesses]), scabies, and tinea Explanation: During contagious periods, participation in gymnastics or cheerleading with mats, martial arts, wrestling, or other collision, contact, or limited-contact sports is not allowed.	Qualified yes

(*Continued*)

Table 11.2
(Continued)

Condition	May Participate
Spleen, enlarged Explanation: If the spleen is acutely enlarged, then participation should be avoided because of risk of rupture. If the spleen is chronically enlarged, then individual assessment is needed before collision, contact, or limited-contact sports are played.	Qualified yes
Testicle, undescended or absence of one Explanation: Certain sports may require a protective cup.	Yes

This table is designed for use by medical and nonmedical personnel. "Needs evaluation" means that a physician with appropriate knowledge and experience should assess the safety of a given sport for an athlete with the listed medical condition. Unless otherwise noted, this need for special consideration is because of variability in the severity of the disease, the risk of injury for the specific sports, or both.

Adapted from American Academy of Pediatrics, Committee on Sports Medicine and Fitness. Medical conditions affecting sports participation. *Pediatrics*. 2008;121(4):841–848.

INCREASING DYNAMIC COMPONENT →

INCREASING STATIC COMPONENT ↑

	A. Low (< 40% Max O_2)	B. Moderate (40-70% Max O_2)	C. High (> 70% Max O_2)
III. High (>50% MVC)	**IIIA (Moderate)** Bobsledding/luge[a,b] Field events (throwing) Gymnastics[a,b] Martial arts[a] Sailing Sport climbing Water skiing[a,b] Weight lifting[a,b] Windsurfing[a,b]	**IIIB (High Moderate)** Body building[a,b] Downhill skiing[a,b] Skateboarding[a,b] Snowboarding[a,b] Wrestling[a]	**IIIC (High)** Boxing[a,c] Canoeing/kayaking Cycling[a,b] Decathlon Rowing Speed-skating[a,b] Triathlon[a,b]
II. Moderate (20-50% MVC)	**IIA (Low Moderate)** Archery Auto racing[a,b] Diving[a,b] Equestrian[a,b] Motorcycling[a,b]	**IIB (Moderate)** American football[a] Field events (jumping) Figure skating[a] Rodeoing[a,b] Rugby[a] Running (sprint) Surfing[a,b] Synchronized swimming[b]	**IIC (High Moderate)** Basketball[a] Ice hockey[a] Cross-country skiing (skating technique) Lacrosse[a] Running (middle distance) Swimming Team handball
I. Low (< 20% MVC)	**IA (Low)** Billiards Bowling Cricket[d] Curling Golf Riflery	**IB (Low Moderate)** Baseball/softball[a] Fencing Table tennis Volleyball	**IC (Moderate)** Badminton Cross-country skiing (classic technique) Field hockey[a] Orienteering Race walking Racquetball/squash Running (long distance) Soccer[a] Tennis

Fig 11.1. Classification of sports according to cardiovascular demands (based on combined static and dynamic components).12 This classification is based on peak static and dynamic components achieved during competition. It should be noted, however, that the higher values may be reached during training. The increasing dynamic component is defined in terms of the estimated percentage of maximal oxygen uptake (Max O2) achieved and results in increasing cardiac output. The increasing static component is related to the estimated percentage of maximal voluntary contraction (MVC) reached and results in increasing blood pressure load. Activities with the lowest total cardiovascular demands (cardiac output and blood pressure) are shown in box IA, and those with the highest demands are shown in box IIIC. Boxes IIA and IB depict activities with low/moderate total cardiovascular demands, boxes IIIA, IIB, and IC depict activities with moderate total cardiovascular demands, and boxes IIIB and IIC depict high/moderate total cardiovascular demands. These categories progress diagonally across the graph from lower left to upper right. [a] Danger of bodily collision. [b] Increased risk if syncope occurs. [c] Participation is not recommended by the American Academy of Pediatrics. [d] The American Academy of Pediatrics classifies cricket in the IB box (low static component and moderate dynamic component). (Reproduced with permission from Mitchell JH, Haskell W, Snell P, Van Camp SP. 36th Bethesda Conference. Task force 8: classification of sports. *J Am Coll Cardiol.* 2005;45(8):1364–1367.)

See foldout for figures 11.2–11.4.

Table 11.3
Categories of sports eye-injury risk to the unprotected player

High Risk	Moderate Risk	Low Risk	Eye Safe
Small, fast projectiles	Tennis	Swimming	Track and field[a]
Air rifle	Badminton	Diving	Gymnastics
BB gun	Soccer	Skiing (snow and water)	
Paintball	Volleyball	Noncontact martial arts	
Hard projectiles, "sticks," close contact	Water polo	Wrestling	
Basketball	Football	Bicycling	
Baseball/softball	Fishing		
Cricket	Golf		
Lacrosse (men's and women's)			
Hockey (field and ice)			
Squash			
Racquetball			
Fencing			
Intentional injury			
Boxing			
Full-contact martial arts			

[a] Javelin and discus have a small but definite potential for injury. However, good field supervision can reduce the extremely low risk of injury to a near-negligible level.
Adapted from Vinger PF. A practical guide for sports eye protection. *Phys Sportsmed.* 2000;28(6):49–69. Reprinted by permission.

Table 11.4
Recommended eye protectors for selected sports

Sport	Minimal Eye Protector	Comment
Baseball/softball (youth batter and base runner)	ASTM standard F910	Face guard attached to helmet
Baseball/softball (fielder)	ASTM standard F803 for baseball	ASTM specifies age ranges
Basketball	ASTM standard F803 for basketball	ASTM specifies age ranges
Bicycling	Helmet plus streetwear/ fashion eyewear	
Boxing	None available; not permitted in the sport	Contraindicated for functionally 1-eyed athletes
Fencing	Protector with neck bib	
Field hockey (men and women)	ASTM standard F803 for women's lacrosse (goalie: full face mask)	Protectors that pass for women's lacrosse also pass for field hockey
Football	Polycarbonate eye shield attached to helmet-mounted wire face mask	
Full-contact martial arts	None available; not permitted in the sport	Contraindicated for functionally 1-eyed athletes
Ice hockey	ASTM standard F513 face mask on helmet (goaltenders: ASTM standard F1587)	HECC- or CSA-certified full-face shield
Lacrosse (men)	Face mask attached to lacrosse helmet	Should have option to wear helmet
Lacrosse (women)	ASTM standard F803 for women's lacrosse	
Paintball	ASTM standard F1776 for paintball	
Racquet sports (badminton, tennis, paddle tennis, handball, squash, and racquetball)	ASTM standard F803 for selected sport	
Soccer	ASTM standard F803 for selected sport	
Street hockey	ASTM standard 513 face mask on helmet	Must be HECC or CSA certified

(*Continued*)

Table 11.4
(Continued)

Sport	Minimal Eye Protector	Comment
Track and field	Streetwear with polycarbonate lenses/ fashion eyewear[a]	
Water polo/swimming	Swim goggles with polycarbonate lenses	
Wrestling	No standard available	Custom protective eyewear can be made

ASTM indicates American Society for Testing and Materials; HECC, Hockey Equipment Certification Council; CSA, Canadian Standards Association

[a] Eyewear that passes American Society for Testing and Materials standard F803 is safer than streetwear eyewear for all sports activities with impact potential.

Adapted from American Academy of Pediatrics, Committee on Sports Medicine and Fitness. Protective eyewear for young athletes. *Pediatrics*. 2004;113(3 pt 1):619–622.

Returning to Play After a Sport-Related Concussion

Background

- Definition of concussion: "A trauma-induced alteration in mental status that may or may not involve loss of consciousness" (Meehan WP 3rd, Bachur RG. Sport-related concussion. *Pediatrics*. 2009;123[1]:114–123).
- Loss of consciousness is not a reliable predictor of the extent of the injury or of the time to recovery. Signs and symptoms of concussion are listed in Table 11.5.
- The current classification scheme for concussions is as follows
  - Simple concussions are ones in which the injury resolves in 7 to 10 days.
  - Complex concussions are characterized by persistence of symptoms, multiple concussions, or prolonged cognitive impairment, or the athlete suffers sequelae such as convulsions or loss of consciousness lasting >1 minute.
- Signs and symptoms of concussion can evolve over days; hence, determining whether a concussion is simple or complex cannot be made in an acute setting.
- After a first concussion, an athlete's risk for a repeat concussion is increased.
- An athlete who experiences loss of consciousness is 6 times more likely to sustain another concussion than one who never had loss of consciousness.

Return to Play

- There is no uniformly accepted gold standard for returning an athlete to play after a concussion.
- The American Academy of Pediatrics recommends conservative management of concussions (see Table 11.2–Neurologic disorders). It is recommended that the return to play for an athlete who has sustained a complex concussion be managed by individuals with expertise in the management of sport-related concussion.
- An athlete cannot return to play until:
  - no signs or symptoms of any kind are present at rest or during exercise;
  - the neurologic examination is normal; and
  - if performed, results of neuroimaging studies are normal.
- The generally preferred approach to returning an athlete to play is outlined in Table 11.6. Return to play for young athletes may warrant an even more conservative approach. Such an approach might be to remove a young athlete sustaining a concussion from competition for the rest of the day and not allowing him or her to return to play until medically cleared, rather than allowing him or her to return if symptoms have resolved within 20 minutes.

Adapted from: Kirkwood MW, Yeates KO, Wilson PE. Pediatric sport-related concussion: a review of the clinical management of an oft-neglected population. *Pediatrics*. 2006;117(4):1359–1371; and Meehan WP 3rd, Bachur RG. Sport-related concussion. *Pediatrics*. 2009;123(1):114–123.

Table 11.5
List of symptoms reported in athletes after sustaining a sport-related concussion

Signs of Concussion	Symptoms of Concussion
Loss of consciousness	Headache
Amnesia, retrograde or antegrade	Dizziness
Disorientation	Nausea or vomiting
Appearing dazed	Difficulty balancing
Acting confused	Vision changes
Forgetting game rules or play assignments	Photophobia
Inability to recall score or opponent	Phonophobia
Inappropriate emotionality	Feeling "out of it"
Poor physical coordination	Difficulty concentrating
Imbalance	Tinnitus
Seizure	Drowsiness
Slow verbal responses	Sadness
Personality changes	Hallucinations

Adapted from Meehan WP 3rd, Bachur RG. Sport-related concussion. *Pediatrics*. 2009; 123(1);114–123.

Table 11.6
Return-to-play protocol recommended by the Second International Conference on Concussion in Sport[a]

Step	Level of Activity
1	No activity, complete rest; proceed to level 2 once symptoms resolve
2	Light aerobic exercise (eg, walking, stationary cycling)
3	Sport-specific exercise (eg, skating in hockey, running in soccer); addition of light resistance training
4	Noncontact training drills; progressively increased resistance training
5	Full-contact training after medical clearance
6	Game play

[a] McCrory P, Johnson K, Meeuwisse W, et al. Summary and agreement statement of the 2nd International Conference on Concussion in Sport, Prague 2004. *Br J Sports Med*. 2005;39(4):196–204.

Reprinted from Meehan WP 3rd, Bachur RG. Sport-related concussion. *Pediatrics*. 2009;123(1):117.

Return to Sports Participation After Infectious Mononucleosis

Background

- Concerns about resumption of athletic activity after acute infectious mononucleosis center on 2 issues:
  - the athlete's readiness to resume activity; and
  - potential rupture of the spleen, especially in contact sports.
- Splenic rupture almost always occurs between days 3 and 21 of the illness; rupture can, on occasion, occur later (4–7 weeks after symptom onset). Up to 50% of cases of ruptured spleen are not associated with trauma.
- Compared to baseline, an athlete's exercise capacity ($\dot{V}O_{2\,max}$) declines during a viral illness.
- Studies in the military did not demonstrate differences in aerobic capacity between athletes who resumed light activity as soon as they became afebrile compared with those held out for 2 weeks. No detrimental effect of light activity (no abdominal or chest trauma and no significant exertion or Valsalva activity) on afebrile athletes was observed.
- Recent studies suggest that use of ultrasound is not a reliable method for determining whether splenomegaly is present because assessments are usually based on a single measurement, and spleen size in healthy athletes is quite variable.

Recommendations

- Athletes should not resume exercise or sports activity until they are afebrile, have a good energy level, and do not have any significant associated abnormalities. This generally occurs ~3 weeks after onset of illness.
- Return to contact sports is more controversial, and there are no uniformly accepted guidelines; return to play must be individualized.
- Use of imaging studies (generally ultrasound) to guide the decision is controversial. It is generally assumed (on the basis of observations that risk of splenic rupture is greatest during the first 3–4 weeks of the illness) that the spleen is most susceptible to rupture as it enlarges. Hence, documentation by ultrasound of a reduction in splenic size would suggest a lower risk for rupture. However, there have been no data to support such an approach.

References: Hosey RG, Mattacola CG, Kriss V, Armsey T, Quarles JD, Jagger J. Ultrasound assessment of spleen size in collegiate athletes. *Br J Sports Med.* 2006;40(3):251–254; Hosey RG, Kriss V, Uhl TL, DiFiori J, Hecht S, Wen DY. Ultrasonographic evaluation of splenic enlargement in athletes with acute infectious mononucleosis. *Br J Sports Med.* 2008;42(12):974–977; Putukian M, O'Connor FG, Stricker PR, et al. Mononucleosis and athletic participation: an evidence-based subject review. *Clin J Sport Med.* 2008;18(4): 309–315; and Welch MJ, Wheeler L. Aerobic capacity after contracting infectious mononucleosis. *J Orthop Sports Phys Ther.* 1986;8:199–202.

RESOURCES FOR MUSCULOSKELETAL PROBLEMS AND SPORT-RELATED INJURIES

Table 11.7
Common sports and sites of pain associated with stress fractures

Sport	Sites of Pain
Baseball	Tibia
	Humerus, shaft
	Proximal humeral growth plate
Basketball	Anterior cortex of the tibia
	Tarsal navicular
Football	Lumbar spine: pars interarticularis
Gymnastics	Lumbar spine: pars interarticularis
	Distal radial growth plate
	Tibia
	Fibula
Ice skating	Distal fibula
Running	Proximal tibial metaphysis
	Distal tibial metaphysis
	Fibula
	Tarsal navicular
	Midshaft of femur
	Distal femur
	Femoral neck
	Sacrum
Soccer	Patella
Swimming	Proximal tibia
Tennis	Nondominant ulna (from 2-handed backhand stroke)
	Dominant side metacarpal
Volleyball	Ulna
	Tibia

Adapted from Yngve DA. Stress Fractures. In: Sullivan JA, Anderson SJ, eds. *Care of the Young Athlete*. Rosemont, IL: American Academy of Orthopaedic Surgeons and American Academy of Pediatrics; 2000: 283.

See the foldout for Table 11.8.

Table 11.9
Key Palpation Landmarks

Site of Tenderness	Possible Injury
Tibial tubercle	Fracture Osgood-Schlatter disease
Patellar tendon	Patellar tendinitis
Patella	Fracture Bipartite patella
Inferior pole	Sinding-Larsen-Johansson disease
Superior pole	Quadriceps tendinitis
Medial joint line	Medial meniscal tear Pes anserinus bursitis
Lateral joint line	Lateral meniscal tear
Medial epicondyle	Medial collateral ligament tear Physeal injury
Lateral epicondyle	Lateral collateral ligament tear
Physeal injury	Physeal injury Iliotibial band syndrome
Fibular head	Lateral collateral ligament tear Biceps femoris tendinitis
Medial retinaculum	Patellar subluxation and/or dislocation Medial plica

Adapted from Pasque CB, McGinns DW. Knee. In: Sullivan JA, Anderson SJ, eds. *Care of the Young Athlete*. Rosemont, IL: American Academy of Orthopaedic Surgeons and American Academy of Pediatrics; 2000:382.

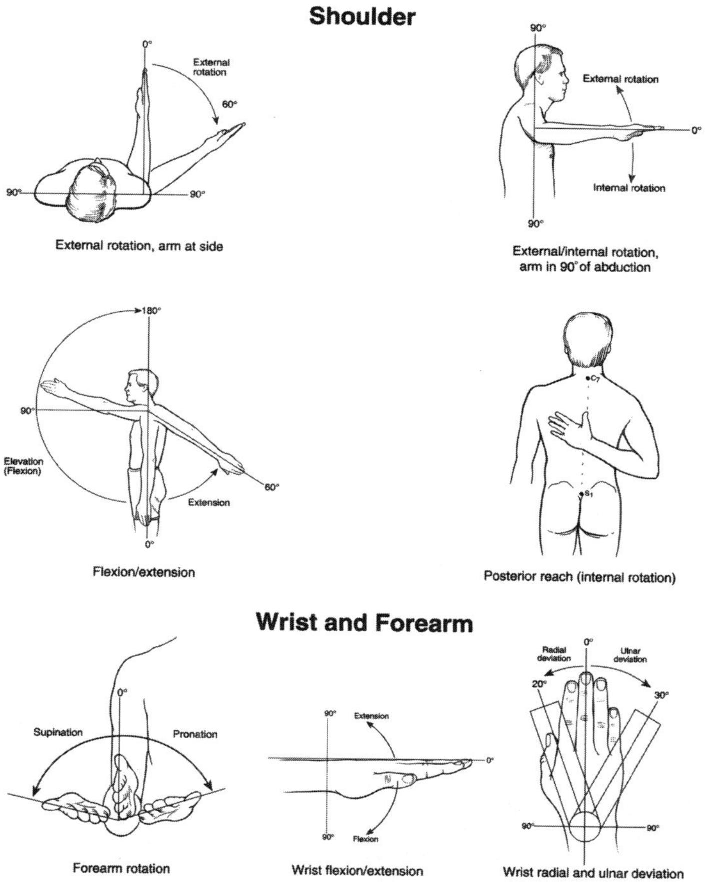

Fig 11.5. Measuring joint motion in the upper extremity. (Reprinted with permission from *The Clinical Measurement of Joint Motion*. Rosemont, IL: American Academy of Orthopaedic Surgeons; 1993.)

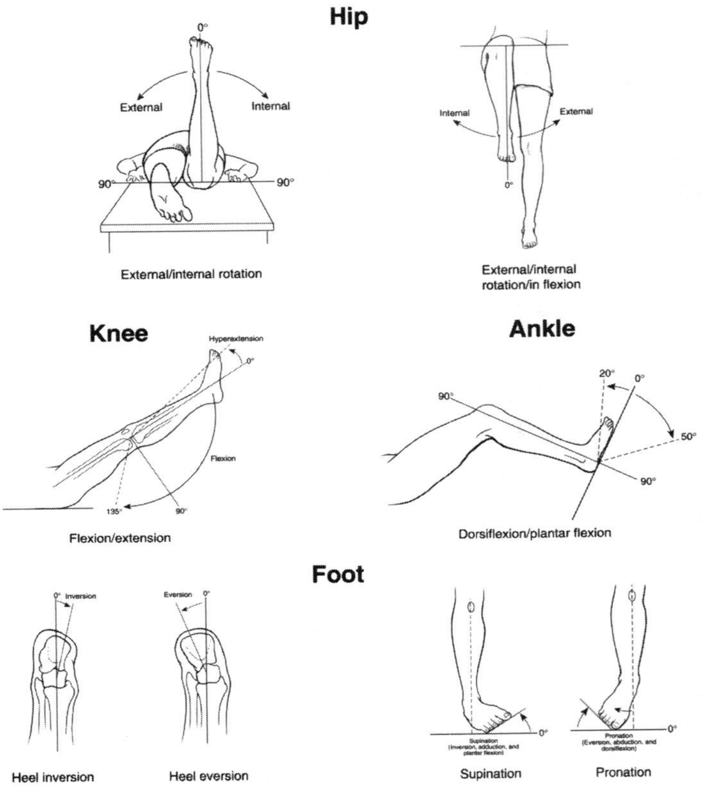

Fig 11.6. Measuring joint motion in the lower extremity. (Reprinted with permission from *The Clinical Measurement of Joint Motion*. Rosemont, IL; American Academy of Orthopaedic Surgeons; 1993.)

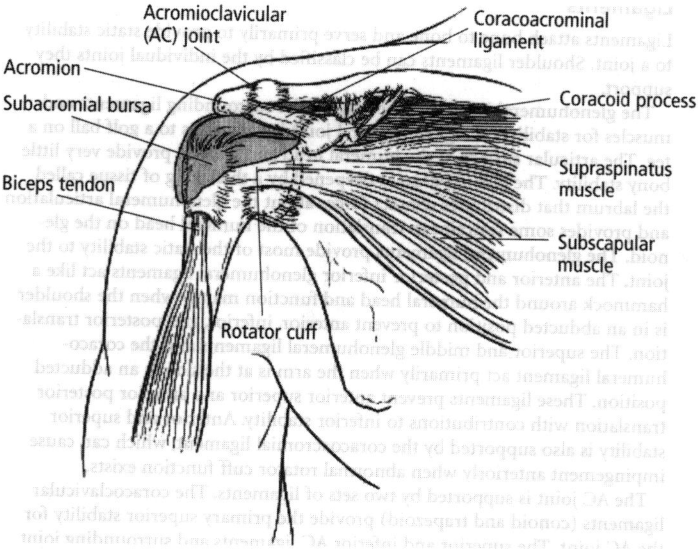

Fig 11.7. Anatomy of the shoulder (anterior view). (Reproduced from Pasque CB, McGinnis DW, Yurko-Griffin L. Shoulder. In: Sullivan JA, Anderson SJ, eds. *Care of the Young Athlete*. Rosemont, IL: American Academy of Orthopaedic Surgeons and American Academy of Pediatrics; 2000:326).

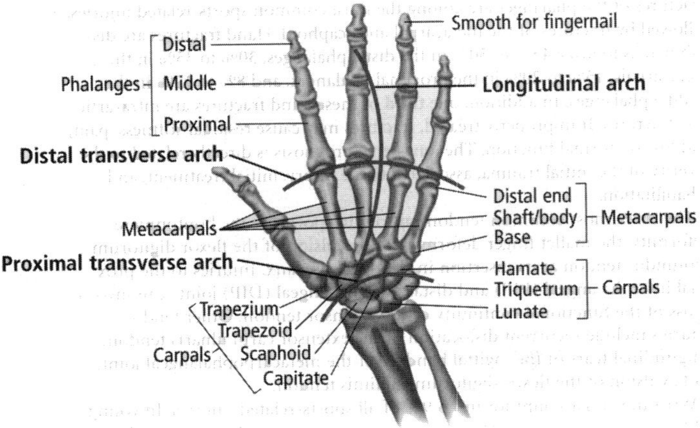

Fig 11.8. Bony anatomy of the hand and wrist. (Reproduced from Garcia-Moral CA, Green NE, Fox JA. Hand and wrist. In: Sullivan JA, Anderson SJ, eds. *Care of the Young Athlete*. Rosemont, IL: American Academy of Orthopaedic Surgeons and American Academy of Pediatrics; 2000:350).

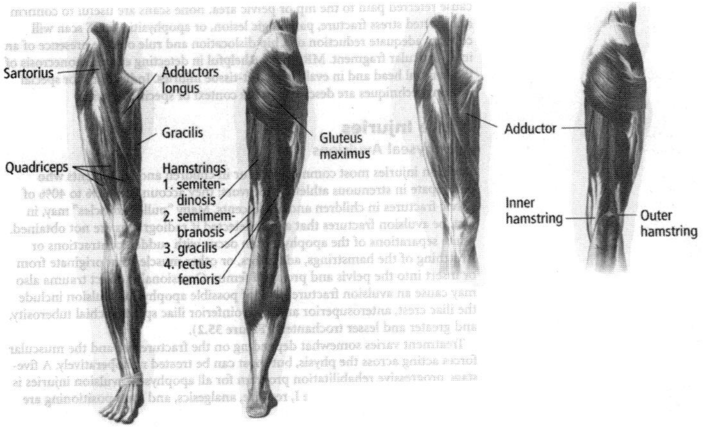

Fig 11.9. Muscles around the femur. (Reproduced from Beatty JH, Hip, pelvis, and thigh. In: Sullivan JA, Anderson SJ, eds. *Care of the Young Athlete*. Rosemont, IL: American Academy of Orthopaedic Surgeons and American Academy of Pediatrics; 2000:367).

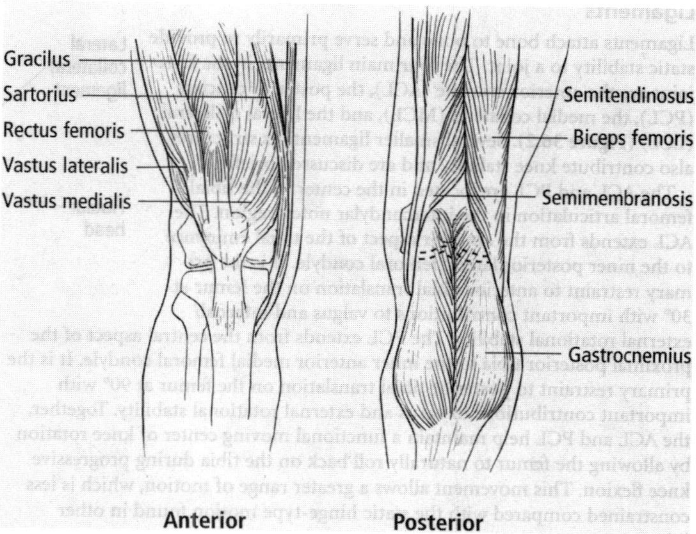

Fig 11.10. Musculature of the knee. (Reproduced from Pasque CB, McGinnis DW. Knee. In: Sullivan JA, Anderson SJ, eds. *Care of the Young Athlete*. Rosemont, IL: American Academy of Orthopaedic Surgeons and American Academy of Pediatrics; 2000:380).

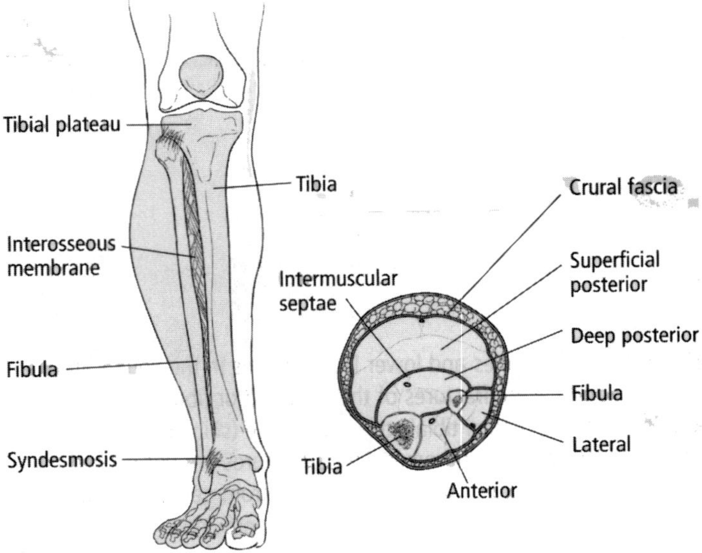

Fig 11.11. Compartments of the lower extremity. (Reproduced from Gruel CR. Lower leg. In: Sullivan JA, Anderson SJ, eds. *Care of the Young Athlete*. Rosemont, IL: American Academy of Orthopaedic Surgeons and American Academy of Pediatrics; 2000:406).

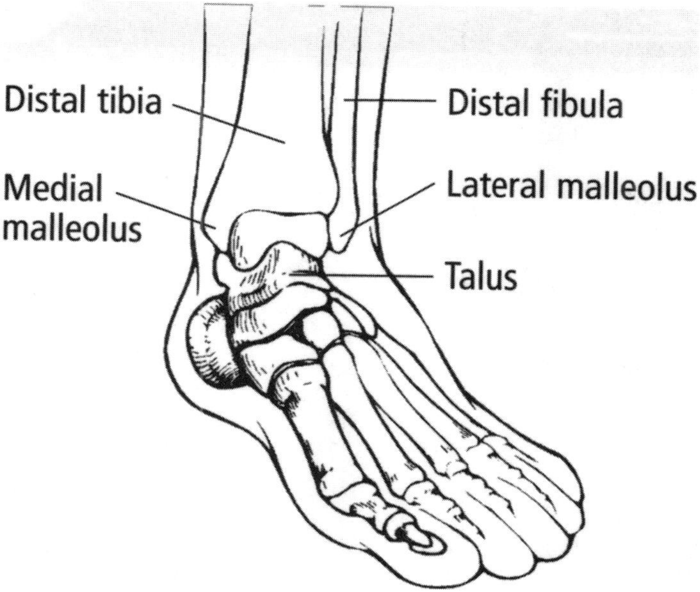

Fig 11.12. Bony anatomy of the ankle. (Reproduced from Anderson SJ, Sullivan JA. Ankle. In: Sullivan JA, Anderson SJ, eds. *Care of the Young Athlete*. Rosemont, IL: American Academy of Orthopaedic Surgeons and American Academy of Pediatrics; 2000:414).

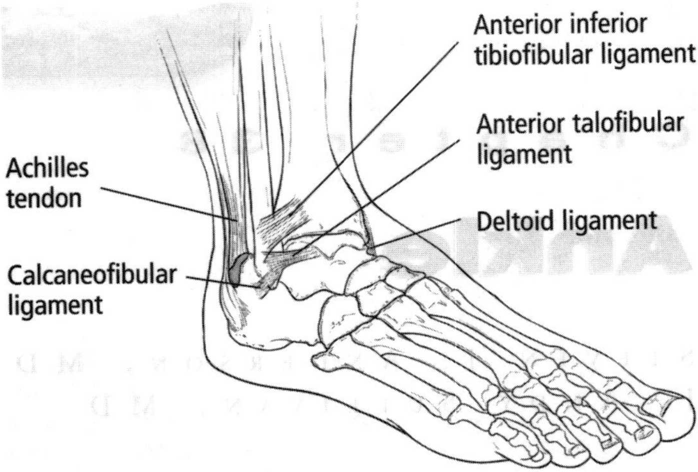

Fig 11.13. Major ligaments of the ankle and the Achilles tendon. (Reproduced from Anderson SJ, Sullivan JA. Ankle. In: Sullivan JA, Anderson SJ, eds. *Care of the Young Athlete*. Rosemont, IL: American Academy of Orthopaedic Surgeons and American Academy of Pediatrics; 2000:414).

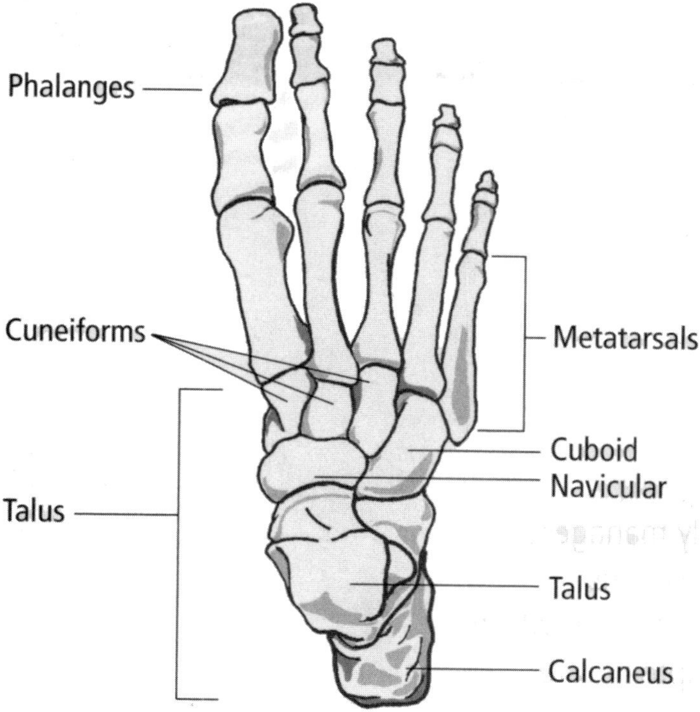

Fig 11.14. Bony anatomy of the foot. (Reproduced from Sullivan JA. Foot. In: Sullivan JA, Anderson SJ, eds. *Care of the Young Athlete*. Rosemont, IL: American Academy of Orthopaedic Surgeons and American Academy of Pediatrics; 2000:426).

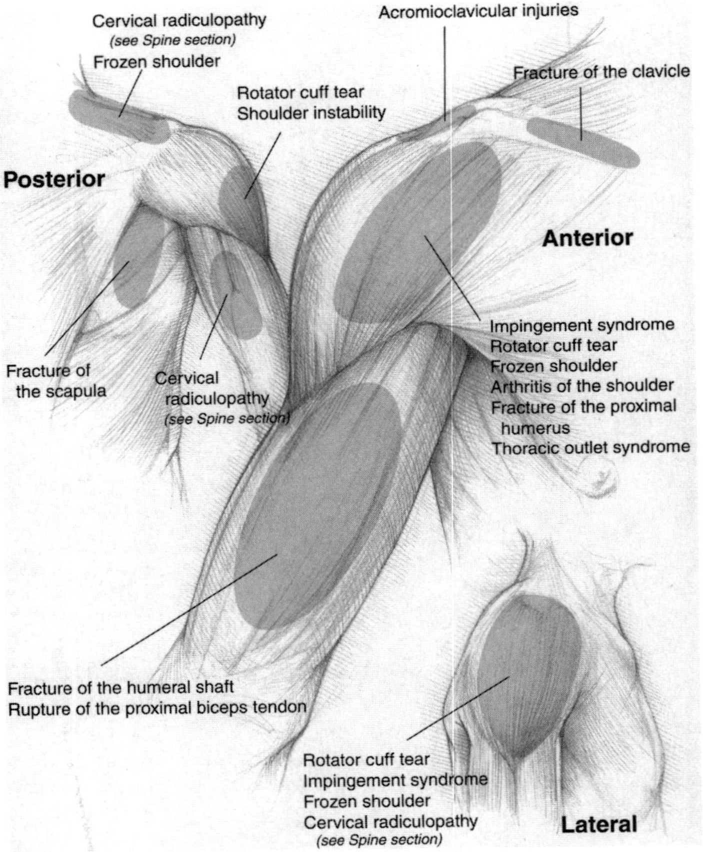

Fig 11.15. Pain diagram: shoulder. (Reproduced from Griffin LY, ed. *Essentials of Musculoskeletal Care*. 3rd ed. Rosemont, IL: American Academy of Orthopaedic Surgeons; 2005:144).

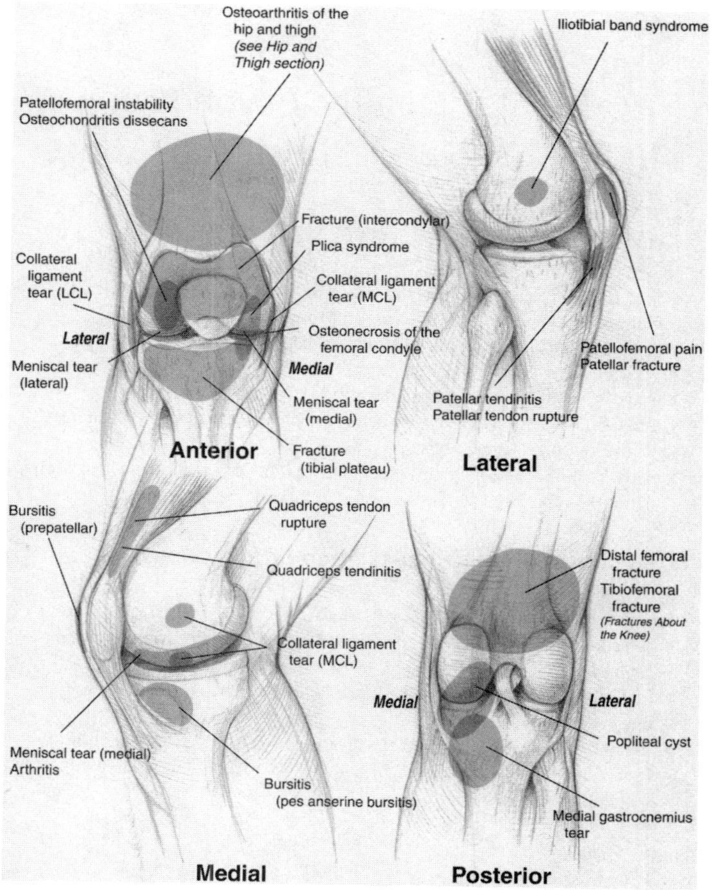

Fig 11.16. Pain diagram: knee and lower leg. (Reproduced from Griffin LY, ed. *Essentials of Musculoskeletal Care*. 3rd ed. Rosemont, IL: American Academy of Orthopaedic Surgeons; 2005:468).

Adolesc Med 20 (2009) 728–787

12. Mental Health, Psychotropic Medications, and Substance Abuse

COMMON MENTAL HEALTH DIAGNOSES

Five axes to help plan treatment and describe general medical conditions, psychosocial and environmental problems, and functioning.

- Axis I: clinical psychiatric disorder or diagnosis (eg, anxiety)
- Axis II: personality disorder, mental retardation
- Axis III: general medical condition (eg, cystic fibrosis)
- Axis IV: psychosocial/environmental problems (eg, divorce of parents, victim of child sexual abuse)
- Axis V: global assessment of functioning (eg, 35) (scale from 1 to 100 with 100 superior, 1 to 10 in danger of hurting self or others)

Core Symptoms and Manifestation of Symptoms

Inattentiveness: distractibility, task persistence, memory organization.

- Avoiding tasks that require sustained attention; daydreaming, poor concentration
- Inability to shift attention from 1 task to another; forgetfulness, losing or misplacing things
- Inability to complete tasks at hand; disorganization, easy distractibility
- Procrastination
- Inattentive errors in driving

Impulse control.

- Poor frustration tolerance
- Losing temper easily
- Being impatient
- Getting easily bored
- Making irresponsible choices

Hyperactivity.

- Avoiding situation in which one is expected to sit still for prolonged periods of time

---

Margaret J. Blythe, MD
E-mail address: mblythe@iupui.edu.

Table 12.1
Diagnostic criteria for attention-deficit/hyperactivity disorder

A. Either (1) or (2)
   1. Six (or more) symptoms of inattention, persisting for at least 6 mo
      Inattention
      a. Fails to give close attention to details, makes careless mistakes in schoolwork, work, or other activities
      b. Difficulty sustaining attention in tasks: school or work
      c. Does not seem to listen when spoken to directly
      d. Does not follow through on instructions (eg, fails to finish schoolwork, chores, or assignments in the workplace)
      e. Difficulty with organizational skills
      f. Difficulty engaging in tasks that require "sustained" mental effort (eg, schoolwork, homework)
      g. Often loses things necessary for tasks or activities (eg, school assignments, pencils, books, or tools)
      h. Easily distracted by extraneous stimuli
      i. Often forgetful
   2. Six (or more) symptoms of hyperactivity or impulsivity persisted for at least 6 mo
      Hyperactivity
      a. Fidgets, unable to stay still
      b. Leaves seat in classroom or in other situations in which remaining seated is expected
      c. Runs about, climbs excessively in situations where inappropriate; described as feelings of restlessness in adolescents or adults
      d. Difficulty playing or engaging in activities quietly
      e. Often "on the go" or often acts as if "driven by a motor"
      f. Often talks excessively
      Impulsivity
      a. Blurts out answers before questions are completed
      b. Difficulty waiting turn
      c. Interrupts or intrudes on others

B. Hyperactive-impulsive or inattentive symptoms causing impairment present before 7 y old

C. Some impairment from symptoms present in ≥2 settings (eg, school, work, home)

D. Clear evidence of significant impairment in social, academic, or occupational functioning

E. Symptoms not occurring exclusively during the course of pervasive developmental disorder, schizophrenia, or other psychotic disorder and are not better accounted for by another mental disorder (eg, mood disorder, anxiety disorder, dissociative disorder, or a personality disorder)

- Choosing roles with high levels of constant physical activity
- Reporting subjective feeling of restlessness

References: Robin A, Schubiner H, Coleman WL. Adolescent attention-deficit/hyperactivity disorder and learning disorders: preface. *Adolesc Med State Art Rev*. 2008;19(2):xiii–xv.

Scales

- Connors/Wells Adolescent Self-report of Symptoms (CASS): 27 or 87 items (www.pearsonassessments.com/crsr.aspx. Accessed August 4, 2009)
- Teacher's Report Form (TRF) for ages 6 to 18 years and Youth Self-report Form for ages 1 to 18 years (www.aseba.org/products/forms.html. Accessed August 4, 2009)
- National Resource Center on ADHD (www.help4adhd.org/en/treatment/scales. Accessed August 4, 2009)

Comorbid Conditions Presenting by Middle Adolescence

- Conduct/oppositional disorder: 30% to 50%; language disorders: 30% to 35%; learning disabilities (dyslexia, dysgraphia, dyscalculia): 15% to 45%; depression: 30% to 45%; anxiety: 15% to 30%; bipolar: 23%; smoking: 20%; substance abuse: 15%; tic disorders: 50%

Epidemiology

- 6% to 10% of school-aged children, with 70% to 85% persisting into adolescence
- Childhood: 5 boys:1 girl
- Adolescence: 2 boys:1 girl
- Parents with attention-deficit/hyperactivity disorder (ADHD): ≥50% chance of having children with ADHD; 25% of teenagers with ADHD have a parent with ADHD
- Evaluate for symptoms: inattention, impulsivity, hyperactivity, academic underachievement, mood lability, irritability and hot temper, impaired stress intolerance, disorganization (organization, forgetfulness, careless work, procrastination, trouble paying attention, struggling to complete work, not turning in work), behavior problems (truancy, substance abuse, oppositional behavior, fighting, family conflict, risky sexual behavior)

Medications

- Methylphenidate: Concerta (12 hours); Metadate CD (methylphenidate) (8 hours); Ritalin LA (methylphenidate) (8 hours); Ritalin SR (8

Table 12.2
Criteria for major depressive episode

A. Five (or more) symptoms present during the same 2-wk period; represent a change from previous functioning
B. One of the 2 symptoms depressed mood or loss of interest or pleasure are present
   1. Depressed mood most of the day: self-report (eg, feels sad or empty) or observation made by others (eg, appears tearful) or described as irritable
   2. Diminished interest or pleasure in all, or almost all, activities
   3. Significant appetite and/or weight change; loss or weight gain of >5% when not attempting to lose weight
   4. Insomnia or hypersomnia
   5. Agitation or retardation noticed by others as well
   6. Fatigue or loss of energy
   7. Feelings of worthlessness or excessive/inappropriate guilt that may be unwarranted
   8. Diminished ability to think or concentrate, or indecisiveness, nearly every day (either by subjective account or as observed by others)
   9. Recurrent thoughts of death/suicidal ideation without or with a specific plan or suicide attempt
C. The symptoms do not meet criteria for a mixed episode
D. Symptoms cause significant distress/impairment in social, occupational, or other important areas of functioning
E. Symptoms not caused by physiological effects of a substance (eg, a drug of abuse, a medication) or a general medical condition (eg, hypothyroidism)
F. Symptoms not better accounted for by bereavement (ie, after the loss of a loved one) unless symptoms last >2 mo

hours); Methylin ER (8 hours); Daytrana transdermal patch* (worn 12–15 hours)

- Dexmethylphenidate: Focalin XR (8 hours); Focalin (dexmethylphenidate) (4–5 hours)
- Dextroamphetamine and mixed amphetamine salts: Dexedrine (4–5 hours); Dexedrine Spansule (8 hours); Adderall (4–5 hours); Adderall XR (8–9 hours); and Vyvanse (12 hours); doses increase every 3 days, usually with maximum of 1 to 2 mg/kg for methylphenidate and 1 to 1.5 mg/kg for mixed amphetamine salts
- Atomoxetine: Strattera; start with 18 to 25 mg and advance every 3 days; maximum of 100 mg/day or 1.8 mg/kg; may be used to lower dose of stimulant; selective norepinephrine uptake inhibitor
- Bupropion (Wellbutrin), venlafaxine (Effexor): work at norepinephrine receptors

Table 12.3
Diagnostic criteria for dysthymic disorder

A. Depressed mood or irritability (self-report or by others) for at least previous year or longer
B. Depression accompanied by ≥2 symptoms
   1. Significant appetite change
   2. Insomnia or hypersomnia
   3. Low energy or fatigue
   4. Low self-esteem
   5. Poor concentration or difficulty making decisions
   6. Feelings of hopelessness
C. No resolution of symptoms of depression and/or irritability for >2 mo at a time
D. Major depressive episode could have occurred in past but is not part of the current clinical picture
E. Clinical criteria for other clinical disorders such as manic episode, a mixed episode, or a hypomanic episode or cyclothymic disorder not met
F. Mood disturbance not part of a chronic psychotic disorder, such as schizophrenia or delusional disorder
G. Symptoms not caused by physiological effects of a substance (eg, a drug of abuse, a medication) or a general medical condition (eg, hypothyroidism)
H. Symptoms cause significant distress or impairment in social, occupational, or other areas of functioning

- Clonidine: α_2-adrenergic–blocking agent that can decrease overactivity and impulsiveness and promote sleep; dose: 0.1, 0.2, or 0.3 mg at night before bed; other medications for sleep include trazodone, melatonin 3 to 6 mg, and mirtazapine (Remeron)

- Adverse effects: appetite suppression, weight loss, abdominal pain, irritability, insomnia, nausea, vomiting, tics, agitation

*Patch is 10, 15, 20, and 30 mg, equivalent to 27, 36, 54, and 72 mg of methylphenidate, respectively; adverse effects: headache, stomachache, jittery, overfocused, agitated).

SIGECAPS Mnemonic for Depression

- Sleep
- Interest
- Guilt

- Energy
- Concentration
- Appetite changes
- Psychomotor agitation or retardation
- Suicidality

Resources

National Adolescent Health Information Center. The mental health of adolescents: a national profile, 2008. Available at: http://nahic.ucsf.edu/index.php/nahic/article/the_mental_health_of_adolescents_a_national_profile_2008. Accessed August 4, 2009.

Shain BN; American Academy of Pediatrics, Committee on Adolescence. Suicide and suicide attempts in adolescents. *Pediatrics*. 2007;120(3):669–676.

TeensHealth From Nemours. Your mind. Available at: http://kidshealth.org/teen/your_mind. Accessed August 4, 2009.

American Academy of Pediatrics. Children's mental health in primary care. Available at: www.aap.org/mentalhealth/mh8mL.html. Accessed August 4, 2009.

American Academy of Pediatrics. Feelings need check ups too. Available at: www.aap.org/disasters/pdf/Feelings% 20Need%20Check%20ups%20Toolkit_0823.pdf. Accessed August 4, 2009.

Zuckerbrot RA, Cheung AH, Jensen PS, Stein RE, Laraque D; GLAD-PC Steering Group. Guidelines for Adolescent Depression in Primary Care (GLAD-PC): I. Identification, assessment, and initial management. *Pediatrics*. 2007; 120(5). Available at: www.pediatrics.org/cgi/content/full/120/5/e1299.

Cheung AH, Zuckerbrot RA, Jensen PS, Ghalib K, Laraque D, Stein RE; GLAD-PC Steering Group. Guidelines for Adolescent Depression in Primary Care (GLAD-PC): II. Treatment and ongoing management [published correction appears in *Pediatrics*. 2008;121(1):227]. *Pediatrics*. 2007;120(5). Available at: www.pediatrics.org/cgi/content/full/120/5/e1313.

The REACH Institute. Guidelines for Adolescent Depression in Primary Care (GLAD-PC). Available at: www. glad-pc.org. Accessed August 4, 2009.

Risk factors: history, family history, other psychiatric disorders (ADHD, anxiety), substance abuse, trauma (history of physical or sexual abuse), psychosocial adversity (divorce, death of family member).

Behaviors: irritability, physical complaints such as stomachaches and headaches, fights with family members or friends, skipping school, grades dropping, or substance use.

Other diagnoses: thyroid disease, anemia, sleep disorder, infection such as mononucleosis, or medications such as steroids, asthma treatment, acne treatment.

Consider bipolar diagnosis with following symptoms: rapid onset of depression, psychotic symptoms, family history, previous symptoms of mania on depression medications such as hyperactivity, rapid speech, decreased need for sleep.

National Center for Mental Health Checkups, TeenScreen. Start a primary care program. Available at: www.teenscreen.org/start-a-primary-care-program. Accessed August 4, 2009.

Self-report check lists available with permission: Kutcher Adolescent Depression Scale. www.cprf.ca/education/Openmind2006/KADS11.pdf. Accessed August 4, 2009.

US Preventive Services Task Force: Major Depressive Disorder in Children and Adolescents—Summary of Recommendations

- Recommends screening of adolescents (12–18 years of age) for major depressive disorder when systems are in place to ensure accurate diagnosis, psychotherapy (cognitive-behavioral or interpersonal), and follow-up
- Concludes that the current evidence is insufficient to assess the balance of benefits and harms of screening children (7–11 years of age)

Reference: US Department of Health and Human Services, Agency for Healthcare Research and Quality, US Preventive Services Task Force. Major depressive disorder in children and adolescents. Available at: www.ahrq.gov/clinic/uspstf/uspschdepr.htm. Accessed August 4, 2009.

US Preventive Services Task Force screening questions for depression in adult primary care patients when positive response requires further evaluation

- Over the past 2 weeks, have you ever felt down, depressed, or hopeless?
- Over the past 2 weeks, have you felt little interest or pleasure in doing things?

Reference: US Department of Health and Human Services, Agency for Healthcare Research and Quality. Screening for depression. Available at: www.ahrq.gov/clinic/3rduspstf/depression/depressrr.htm. Accessed August 4, 2009.

Describe Bipolar

Manic

During this time, you must have had ≥3 symptoms of mania: needing less sleep, being more talkative, behaving wildly or irresponsibly in activities that could have serious outcomes, or feeling as if your thoughts are racing.

In a manic episode, you may feel very happy, energetic, or on edge. You may feel like you need very little sleep. You may feel overly self-confident. Some people spend a lot of money or get involved in dangerous activities when they are manic.

In bipolar 2, the manic episode may be less severe and shorter.

Depression

This describes mood going in the opposite direction: feelings of sadness, depression, and hopelessness; trouble thinking and making decisions; memory problems. Loss of interest in things enjoyed in the past with even thoughts about killing yourself.

Onset usually at 15 to 24 years of age.

Table 12.4
Bipolar I disorder

Criteria for manic episode

A. Distinct period of abnormally and persistently elevated expansive or irritable mood, lasting at least 1 wk
B. Three or more of symptoms persisted and present
   1. Inflated self-esteem or grandiosity
   2. Decreased need for sleep
   3. More talkative
   4. Flight of ideas
   5. Distractibility
   6. Increase in goal-directed activity (work, school, sex)
   7. Excessive involvement in "pleasurable" activities with potential for unwanted consequences (eg, buying, sex, foolish investments)
C. Do not meet criteria for mixed
D. Severe enough to cause marked impairment
E. Symptoms not caused by the direct physiological effects of a substance (eg, a drug of abuse, a medication) or a general medical condition (eg, hypothyroidism)

Occurrence of $\geq$1 manic episode or mixed episode. Multiple mood episodes are often described: manic, depressed (Table 12.2), mixed, hypomanic (Table 12.5). Untreated, an average of 4 cycles per year is described with full functionality in between episodes.

Reprinted with permission from the *Diagnostic and Statistical Manual of Mental Disorders*. Text Revision. Fourth Edition. (Copyright 2000). American Psychiatric Association.

Table 12.5
Bipolar II disorder

Criteria for hypomania

A. Distinct period of elevated, expansive or irritable mood lasting at least 4 days
B. Three or more symptoms persisted or present
   1. Inflated self-esteem or grandiosity
   2. Decreased need for sleep
   3. More talkative
   4. Flight of ideas
   5. Distractibility
   6. Increase in goal-directed activity (work, school, sex)
   7. Excessive involvement in "pleasurable" activities with potential for unwanted consequences (eg, buying, sex, foolish investments)
C. Change in functioning
D. Disturbance and change in function noticed by those around
E. Not severe enough to cause marked impairment
F. Symptoms not caused by the direct physiological effects of a substance (eg, a drug of abuse, a medication) or a general medical condition (eg, hypothyroidism)

Occurrence of recurrent major depression episodes with hypomania. Depressed patients with "agitated depression" or depressed patients with irritability, anger, hostility.
Reprinted with permission from the *Diagnostic and Statistical Manual of Mental Disorders*. Text Revision. Fourth Edition. (Copyright 2000). American Psychiatric Association.

Table 12.6
Mixed episode

Criteria for mixed episode

A. Criteria met for both manic (Table 12.4) and major depression (Table 12.2) over at least a 1-wk period
B. Severe enough to cause impairment in function
C. Symptoms not caused by the direct physiological effects of a substance (eg, a drug of abuse, a medication) or a general medical condition (eg, hypothyroidism)

Reprinted with permission from the *Diagnostic and Statistical Manual of Mental Disorders*. Text Revision. Fourth Edition. American Psychiatric Association.

Table 12.7
Distinguishing bipolar from unipolar depression

Symptom	Bipolar	Unipolar
Substance abuse	Very high	Moderate
Family history	Almost uniform	Sometimes
Seasonality	Common	Occasional
First episode <25 y	Very common	Sometimes
Psychotic features <35 y	Highly predictive	Uncommon
Rapid turn-on/off pattern	Typical	Unusual
>3 recurrent major depressive episodes	Common	Unusual
Antidepressant-induced mania/hypomania	Predictive	Uncommon
Mixed depression with hypomania	Predictive	Rare

Adapted with permission from Kaye NS. Is your depressed patient bipolar? *J Am Board Fam Pract.* 2005;18(4):271–281.

Table 12.8
Diagnostic criteria for obsessive compulsive disorder

A. Either obsessions or compulsions
   Obsessions defined by
   1. Recurrent, persistent thoughts, impulses, images (described as intrusive, inappropriate); causes marked anxiety or distress
   2. Not simply excessive worries about real-life events
   3. Attempts to ignore or suppress such thoughts, impulses, or images
   4. Recognizes thoughts, impulses, or images are a result of his or her own mind

   Compulsions defined by (1) and (2)
   1. Repetitive behaviors (eg, hand-washing, ordering, checking) or mental acts (eg, praying, counting, repeating words silently)
   2. Behaviors or mental acts performed to prevent or reduce distress or some dreaded event or situation → not realistic connection

B. Person recognizes obsessions or compulsions as excessive or unreasonable
C. The obsessions or compulsions cause marked distress → time consuming → significantly interfere with normal routine (occupational, academic, or usual social activities or relationships)
D. If another Axis I disorder is present, content of the obsessions or compulsions not restricted to disorder (eg, preoccupation with food in the presence of an eating disorder)
E. Disturbance not caused by the direct physiological effects of a substance (eg, a drug of abuse, a medication) or a general medical condition

Reprinted with permission from the *Diagnostic and Statistical Manual of Mental Disorders*. Text Revision. Fourth Edition. (Copyright 2000). American Psychiatric Association.

Table 12.9
Diagnostic criteria for posttraumatic stress disorder

A. Person exposed to a traumatic event in which both of the following were present
   1. Experienced, witnessed, or confronted with an event or events involving actual or threatened death or serious injury or threat/risk of physical injury to self or others
   2. Response involved intense fear, helplessness, or horror
B. Traumatic event persistently reexperienced in 1 (or more) ways
   1. Recurrent, intrusive distressing recollections of the event: images, thoughts, or perceptions
   2. Recurrent distressing dreams of the event
   3. Acting or feeling as if the traumatic event were recurring (eg, sense of reliving experience, illusions, hallucinations, dissociative flashback episodes)
   4. Intense psychological distress with any reminders of traumatic event
   5. Physiological response to reminders of traumatic event
C. Avoidance of any reminders associated with trauma; attempts to eliminate in 3 (or more) of the following ways
   1. Avoid thoughts, feelings, or conversations associated with the trauma
   2. Avoid activities, places, or people that arouse recollections of the trauma
   3. Inability to recall an important aspect of the trauma
   4. Diminished interest or participation in significant activities
   5. Feeling detached or estranged from others
   6. Restricted range of affect (eg, unable to have loving feelings)
   7. Sense of a foreshortened future (eg, does not expect to have a career, marriage, children, or a normal life span)
D. Persistent symptoms/problems not present before the trauma indicated by 2 (or more) of the following
   1. Difficulty falling or staying asleep
   2. Irritability or outbursts of anger
   3. Difficulty concentrating
   4. Hypervigilance
   5. Exaggerated startle response
E. Duration of the symptoms >1 mo
F. Disturbance causes clinical and significant distress with impairment in social, occupational, or other important areas

Specify if
   Acute: if duration of symptoms is <3 mo
   Chronic: if duration of symptoms is ≥3 mo

Specify if
   With delayed onset: if onset of symptoms is at least 6 mo after the stressor

Reprinted with permission from the *Diagnostic and Statistical Manual of Mental Disorders*. Text Revision. Fourth Edition. (Copyright 2000). American Psychiatric Association.

Table 12.10
Diagnostic criteria for generalized anxiety disorder

A. Excessive anxiety and worry on more days than not for at least 6 mo (eg, work or school performance)
B. Difficult to control the worry
C. Associated with ≥3 of 6 symptoms
   1. Restlessness or feeling keyed up or on edge
   2. Being easily fatigued
   3. Difficulty concentrating or mind going blank
   4. Irritability
   5. Muscle tension
   6. Sleep disturbance
D. Focus of the anxiety and worry not confined to features of an Axis I disorder (eg, anxiety or worry is not about having a panic attack [as in panic disorder])
E. Anxiety, worry, or physical symptoms cause clinically significant distress or impairment in social, occupational, or other important areas
F. Disturbance not caused by the direct physiological effects of a substance (eg, a drug of abuse, a medication) or a general medical condition (eg, hyperthyroidism) and does not occur exclusively during a mood disorder, a psychotic disorder, or a pervasive developmental disorder

Reprinted with permission from the *Diagnostic and Statistical Manual of Mental Disorders*. Text Revision. Fourth Edition. (Copyright 2000). American Psychiatric Association.

Table 12.11
Symptoms of panic attack (period of intense fear or discomfort; may experience a number of symptoms listed; symptoms develop suddenly, peaking within 10 min)

System	Examples
Cardiovascular	Palpitations, sensation of heart pounding, tachycardia
	Chest discomfort or chest pain
	Dizziness, lightheadedness, feeling unsteady or faint as if one were going to fall or pass out
Neurologic	Numbness or tingling
	Trembling or shaking
Respiratory	Feeling short of breath
	Feeling like one were smothering
	Choking sensation
Gastrointestinal	Nausea or abdominal discomfort
Autonomic	Sweating
	Chills
Psychiatric	Feeling hot and flushed
	Feelings of unreality
	Feeling detached from oneself
	Fear of dying
	Fear of losing control
	Fear of going crazy

Reprinted with permission from the *Diagnostic and Statistical Manual of Mental Disorders*. Text Revision. Fourth Edition. (Copyright 2000). American Psychiatric Association.

Table 12.12
Screening/diagnostic questions to assess for presence of common mental health illnesses

Major depressive disorder and dysthymic disorder
- Have you been feeling sad, down, or depressed or in a bad mood?
- Have you lost interest in the things that you used to enjoy doing, or are you getting less pleasure from the things you used to enjoy?
- Some people tell me that they are "bored all the time" or that they are just "going through the motions." Does that describe you at all?
- Do little things seem to irritate you more than they used to? Does it seem like pretty much anything can put you in a bad mood?
- Has there been any change in your appetite or weight?
- How have you been sleeping?
  - Are you having problems falling asleep? Staying asleep? Waking up too early in the morning? Sleeping too much?
- Have you been feeling fidgety or restless or had trouble sitting still?
- Some people feel slowed down or like they are moving in slow motion. Do you?
- How is your energy level?
- Are you feeling guilty or blaming yourself for things?
- Have you had problems thinking, concentrating, remembering, or making decisions?
- Have you been having any thoughts about dying?
  - Sometimes when people feel really bad, they think about hurting or killing themselves. Have you had thoughts like that?
  - Have you thought about ways that you might hurt/kill yourself?
  - Have you made any plans to hurt/kill yourself?
  - Have you already tried to hurt/kill yourself?
  - Is there a gun in your home or do you know of anyone who has a gun?
- What problems have you had because of the way you have been feeling?
  - Have you had problems at home? At school? At work? With friends? Getting things done? In your social life?

Mania/hypomania
- Have there ever been days at a time when you've been in an especially good mood, almost high, in a way that was definitely different than your normal self?
  - Can you think of anything that caused your good mood?
  - Did you feel hyper or like you were taking drugs even though you weren't?
  - During this time, did you feel more self-confident than usual, that you had special talents or powers, or that you would do something great or become famous?
  - During this time, how was your sleep? Did you need less sleep than usual?
  - During this time, were you more talkative than usual? Did you talk faster than usual? Did you feel like you couldn't stop talking? Did people have a hard time getting you to stop talking?

(*Continued*)

Table 12.12
(Continued)

During this time, did you feel like you got more done than usual? Did you do more schoolwork? Did you do more around the house? Were you more fidgety, restless, or edgy than usual, or did you feel like you were always moving?
During this time, did you do anything that might have gotten you into trouble? Shopping sprees? Sexually?
Generalized anxiety disorder
Have you been overly worried or anxious about things in your everyday life?
Do you or do other people think you worry about things too much, even little things?
Do you worry that something really bad is going to happen to you or someone else?
How often/how much do you worry about these things?
Is it hard for you to stop or control your worrying?
When you're anxious or worried, do you feel restless, fidgety, or jittery? Feel tired all the time? Have muscle pain or soreness? Have problems concentrating or keeping your mind on things? Feel irritable or "on edge"? Have sleeping problems, especially problems falling asleep?
What problems have you had because of the way you have been feeling?
Have you had problems at home? At school? At work? With friends? Getting things done? In your social life?
Posttraumatic stress disorder
Have you ever seen or been part of a traumatic event during which you or someone else was in danger?
At the time, how did you feel (terrified/helpless/out of control)?
Does what happened still bother you?
Do you still think about it or remember it?
Do you have dreams or nightmares about it?
Do you ever have flashbacks or feel like it is happening all over again?
Are there things that remind you of what happened and get you upset?
Do you ever have physical symptoms when you remember what happened?
Do you try to forget what happened by trying to block out thoughts of it? By trying to avoid situations/places/activities that remind you of it?
Have you felt different since it happened?
Loss of interest in activities? Feeling distant or like you don't fit in anymore? No longer able to experience certain emotions? Feel like your future has changed or been affected?
Has your behavior changed since it happened?
Trouble sleeping? More irritable or lose your temper more often? Difficulty concentrating? More vigilant and always looking out for trouble?
What problems have you had because of the way you have been feeling?
Do you often feel upset because of it?
Have you had problems at home? At school? At work? With friends? Getting things done? In your social life?

(*Continued*)

Table 12.12
(Continued)

Panic attacks/panic disorder
- A panic attack is a sudden attack of fear, anxiety, or panic that comes unexpectedly and for no obvious reason. Have you ever had anything like that?
  - Have these attacks included: racing, pounding, fluttering, or irregular heartbeat?
  - Chest pain or pressure? Sweating? Shaking? Shortness of breath or trouble breathing? Choking sensation? Nausea or belly pain? Dizziness, lightheadedness, or the feeling you might faint? Numbness or tingling? Hot flashes or chills? Fear you were going crazy, losing control, or not yourself? Fear you might die?
  - How long does it take for the attack to come on? How long before it goes away?
- Do you worry about having more of these attacks?
- Do you worry that something really bad is happening when you have these attacks?

Obsessive-compulsive disorder
- Some people have repetitive thoughts that don't seem to make sense but that they can't seem to get out of their head. Do you have any thoughts like that?
  - Do you try to ignore or get rid of the thoughts, or do you try to think of other things to try to get the thoughts out of your head?
- Some people have to do things over and over without really wanting to, and without being able to stop themselves. For example, they wash their hands, or they have to check things, or they have to count things over and over. Do you do anything like that?
  - Do you get really tense or anxious if you don't _, or do you think something bad would happen if you don't _?
- Do you feel that your thoughts/behaviors are out of control and don't make much sense? Do you still feel like you have to do it?
- Does it bother you that you have these thoughts/behaviors?
- What problems have you had because of the way you have been feeling?
  - Have you had problems at home? At school? At work? With friends? Getting things done? In your social life?

Adapted from Rosen D. Management of mental illness in primary care practice: part 1. *Adolesc Health Update*. 2005;17(3):5.

Table 12.13
Initial treatment choices for managing mental illness in primary care

Condition[a]	Medication	Psychotherapy
Major depressive disorder	Medication indicated for moderate-severe depression; best evidence to support use of fluoxetine as drug of first choice; consider alternative SSRIs if fluoxetine is not effective; Bupropion is another alternative for some patients (see text); seek consultation if augmentation strategies are indicated	Good evidence for effectiveness of CBT in management of acute symptoms and prevention of relapse; CBT reduces risk of suicidality; CBT shown to protect against increased risk of suicidality associated with medications
Dysthymic disorder	Limited evidence in adolescents; antidepressant medication often used to manage symptoms and to reduce risk of progression to major depressive disorder	CBT is treatment of choice
Anxiety disorders	SSRIs are effective in managing symptoms and are often effective in low doses; both short-term and long-term benefit established; benzodiazepines are sometimes appropriate for short-term use while SSRIs are being titrated	CBT is the psychotherapy treatment of choice; specialized strategies are useful in social anxiety , separation anxiety, and in the management of phobias
Obsessive-compulsive disorder	SSRIs are effective in managing symptoms, and several SSRIs are approved for treatment of child and adolescent obsessive-compulsive disorder	Psychotherapy helps patients to extinguish specific symptoms; focused techniques (eg, exposure and response prevention) are often useful
Post-traumatic stress disorder	Medications (SSRIs) are helpful in reducing symptom burden	Trauma-focused CBT is the treatment of choice; debriefing strategies to prevent posttraumatic stress disorder have not been well validated

SSRI indicates selective serotonin reuptake inhibitor; CBT, cognitive behavioral therapy.

[a] For detailed definitions, please see American Psychiatric Association. *Diagnostic and Statistical Manual of Mental Disorders*. 4th ed, Text Revision. American Psychiatric Association: Washington, DC; 2000.

Adapted from Rosen D. Management of mental illness in primary care practice: part 2. *Adolesc Health Update*. 2005;18(1):3.

Table 12.14
Psychotherapeutic modalities

Cognitive behavioral therapy	An interactive, problem-oriented form of psychotherapy that has been shown to be helpful in the mood and anxiety disorders. Its goal is to identify and change maladaptive beliefs, attitudes, and behaviors. A variety of general strategies may be used, including correcting cognitive distortions, challenging dysfunctional attitudes and beliefs, reframing negative expectations, improving problem solving, enhancing social skills, and increasing participation in social and other activities. Special techniques such as reinforced practice (anxiety disorders) or exposure and response prevention (phobias and obsessive-compulsive disorder) may be used to treat specific disorders.
Interpersonal therapy	Focuses specifically on addressing relationship issues (eg, interpersonal conflict, role transitions, or grief) that may contribute to the development or maintenance of mental illness or symptoms. It has been used mainly in the treatment of depression but has also been shown to be useful for bulimia nervosa, posttraumatic stress disorder, and other conditions.
Behavioral therapies	Have been shown to be useful in the disruptive behavior disorders such as ADHD. Behavioral classroom interventions and behavioral parent training both aim to define specific target behaviors, precipitating circumstances, and alternative productive or prosocial behaviors. Parents and teachers learn effective use of consequences to reward positive behavior and to avoid rewarding unwanted behavior. Limit setting and problem solving are components of this intervention.
Dialectical behavioral therapy	A specific treatment approach for managing patients with borderline personality disorder with or without associated self-harm behaviors. Its focus is on emotional regulation, interpersonal effectiveness, tolerating distress, and development of more adaptive coping strategies. There is an increasing body of evidence supporting the use of dialectical behavioral therapy, which has also been adapted for treatment of patients with eating disorders, substance abuse, and other health-risk behaviors.
Psychodynamic therapy	Based on the idea that current symptoms are related to past events and to feelings and thoughts that are part of the subconscious mind. By revealing these unconscious influences, therapy allows for greater self-awareness, change, and recovery. Although it is one of the oldest psychotherapeutic modalities, the effectiveness of psychodynamic therapy has not been well studied.

Adapted from Rosen D. Management of mental illness in primary care practice: part 2. *Adolesc Health Update*. 2005;18 (1):6.

OTHER PSYCHIATRIC DISORDERS

I. Personality Disorders
   A. Persistent pattern of behavior and experience deviating from that expected
   B. Pattern of behavior described as
      1. Pervasive, inflexible in both personal and social situations
      2. Significant distress or impairment
      3. Long duration beginning in adolescent or early adulthood
   C. Not a result of another mental disorder, effects of substance abuse, or general medical condition
   D. Group A (described as odd-eccentric)
      1. Paranoid personality disorder
         a. "Pattern of distrust and suspiciousness such that others' motives are interpreted as malevolent"
         b. Distrust and suspicion of others without justification in 4 or more of the following:
            i. Suspects that others are exploiting, harming, or deceiving him or her
            ii. Doubts the loyalty or trustworthiness of friends or associates
            iii. Reluctant to confide in others for fear the information will be used against him or her
            iv. Reads hidden negative meanings into benign remarks or events
            v. Harbors grudges
            vi. Feels character attacked even when not apparent to others
            vii. Recurrent suspicions of fidelity of spouse or sexual partner
      2. Schizoid personality disorder
         a. "Pattern of detachment from social relationships and restricted range of emotional expression"
         b. Detachment from social relationships, limited range of expression of emotions in 4 or more of the following:
            i. Does not desire close relationships
            ii. Prefers solitary activities
            iii. Experiences little interest in sexual relationships
            iv. Takes pleasure in no or few activities
            v. Lacks close friends except perhaps relatives
            vi. Indifferent to praise or criticism
            vii. Displays emotional detachment, emotional coldness
         c. Not within the context of a psychotic illness or mood disorder
      3. Schizotypal personality disorder
         a. "Pattern of acute discomfort in close relationships, cognitive or perceptual distortions, and eccentricities of behavior"
         b. Social and interpersonal deficits with acute distortions indicated by 5 or more of the following:
            i. Ideas of reference
            ii. Odd beliefs or magical thinking that influences behavior
            iii. Unusual perceptual experiences
            iv. Odd thinking and speech
            v. Suspiciousness or paranoid ideation
            vi. Inappropriate or constricted affect

vii. Odd, eccentric, or peculiar behavior or appearance
viii. Lack of close friends other than first-degree relatives
ix. Excessive social anxiety

E. Group B (described as dramatic-emotional)
1. Antisocial disorder
a. "Pattern of disregard for and violation of the rights of others"
b. Disregard for and violation of the rights of others as indicated by 3 or more of the following:
i. Lack of respect for law; repeatedly performing behaviors or acts that are grounds for arrest
ii. Deceitful, often repeatedly lying, using aliases, or conning others
iii. Impulsivity
iv. Irritable and aggressive, with repeated physical fights or assaults
v. Disregard for safety
vi. Consistently irresponsible with inability to maintain job
vii. Lacking remorse
c. At least 18 years of age
d. Conduct disorder with onset before 15 years of age
e. Behavior not associated with schizophrenia or manic episode
2. Borderline personality disorder
a. "Pattern of instability in interpersonal relationships, self-image, and affects and marked impulsivity"
b. Instable interpersonal relationships, self-image, and affect with marked impulsivity indicated by 5 or more of the following:
i. Displays effort to avoid real or imagined abandonment
ii. Pattern of unstable and intense interpersonal relationships
iii. Identity disturbance-unstable sense of self
iv. Impulsivity
v. Recurrent suicidal behaviors, gestures, or self-mutilating behavior
vi. Instability of affect with marked reactivity of mood
vii. Chronic feelings of emptiness
viii. Inappropriate intense anger or difficulty controlling anger
ix. Stress-related paranoid ideation or severe dissociation symptoms
3. Histrionic personality disorder
a. "Pattern of excessive emotionality and attention seeking"
b. Excessive emotionality and attention seeking, presenting in a variety of contexts in 5 or more of the following:
i. Uncomfortable when not the center of attention
ii. Often displays inappropriately sexually seductive or provocative behavior
iii. Displays rapidly shifting and shallow expression of emotion
iv. Uses physical appearance to get attention
v. Uses style of speech that is excessively impressionistic and lacking in detail
vi. Shows self-dramatization, theatrical and exaggerated expression
vii. Easily influenced by others
viii. Considers relationships more intimate than usually are

4. Narcissistic personality
   a. "Pattern of grandiosity, need for admiration, and lack of empathy"
   b. Grandiosity, need for admiration, and lack of empathy as indicated by 5 or more of the following:
      i. Grandiose sense of self
      ii. Preoccupied with fantasies such as unlimited success and power
      iii. Believes unique and should associate with others of special or high status
      iv. Requires excessive admiration
      v. Sense of entitlement
      vi. Exploitative taking advantage of others to achieve his or her own goals
      vii. Lacks empathy
      viii. Often envious of others or believes others are envious of him or her
      ix. Shows arrogant, haughty behaviors or attitudes

A. Group C (described as anxious-fearful)
   1. Avoidant personality disorder
      a. "Pattern of social inhibition, feelings of inadequacy and hypersensitivity"
      b. Social inhibition, feelings of inadequacy, and hypersensitivity to negative evaluation as indicated by 4 or more of the following:
         i. Avoids occupational activities that involve interpersonal contact for fear of criticism, disapproval, or rejection
         ii. Unwilling to get involved with people unless certain of being liked
         iii. Restraint within intimate relationships for fear of being shamed or ridiculed
         iv. Preoccupied with being criticized or rejected in social situations
         v. Inhibited in new interpersonal situations because of feelings of inadequacies
         vi. View self as socially inept
         vii. Unusually reluctant to take personal risks or to engage in any new activities
   2. Dependent personality
      a. "Pattern of submissive and clinging behavior related to an excessive need to be taken care of"
      b. Excessive need to be taken care of leading to submissive and clinging behavior and fears of separation indicated by 5 or more of following:
         i. Difficulty making everyday decisions
         ii. Needs others to assume responsibility for most major areas of life
         iii. Difficulty expressing disagreement with others for fear of loss of support or approval
         iv. Lack of self-confidence in judgment or abilities
         v. Needs to obtain support from others
         vi. Feels uncomfortable or helpless when alone

vii. Seeks another relationship as source of care and support when a close relationship ends
viii. Unrealistically preoccupied with fears of being left to take care of himself or herself
3. Obsessive-compulsive personality disorder
a. "Pattern of preoccupation with orderliness, perfectionism, and control"
b. Preoccupation with orderliness, perfectionism, and mental and interpersonal control as indicated by 4 or more of the following:
i. Preoccupied with details, rules, lists, order, organization
ii. Shows perfectionism that interferes with task completion
iii. Excessively devoted to work and productivity to the exclusion of leisure activities and friendships
iv. Overly conscientious, scrupulous, and inflexible about matters of morality, ethics, or values
v. Unable to discard worn-out or worthless objects
vi. Reluctant to delegate tasks or to work with others
vii. Adopts a miserly spending style toward both self and others
viii. Shows rigidity and stubbornness
4. Personality disorder not otherwise specified
a. "Category for disorders of personality functioning that does not meet criteria for any specific personality disorder . . . but causes clinically significant distress or impairment in one or more areas of functioning"

II. Conduct Disorder
A. Repetitive and persistent pattern of behavior in which the basic rights of others or societal norms or rules are violated, manifested by the presence of 3 or more of the following criteria:
1. Aggression to people and animals
2. Destruction of property
3. Deceitfulness or theft
4. Serious violations of rules
B. Disturbance in behavior causes clinically significant impairment in social, academic, or occupational functioning
C. Criteria are not met for antisocial personality disorder
D. Types
1. Childhood-onset type: onset of at least 1 criterion characteristic of conduct disorder
2. Adolescent-onset type: absence of any criteria characteristic of conduct disorder before 10 years of age

III. Oppositional Defiant Disorder
A. Pattern of negative, hostile, and defiant behavior lasting at least 6 months during which 4 or more of the following are present:
1. Often loses temper
2. Often argues with adults
3. Often actively defies or refuses to comply with adults' requests or rules

4. Often deliberately annoys people
5. Often blame others for his/her mistakes for misbehavior
6. Is often touchy or easily annoyed by others
7. Often angry and resentful
8. Often spiteful or vindictive

B. Disturbance in behavior causes clinically significant impairment in social, academic, or occupational functioning
C. Behaviors do not occur exclusively during the course of psychotic or mood disorder
D. Criteria are not met for conduct disorder, and if the individual is 18 years old or older, criteria are not met for antisocial personality disorder

References American Psychiatric Association. *Diagnostic and Statistical Manual of Mental Disorders*. Text Revision. Fourth Edition. Washington, DC: American Psychiatric Association; 2000:685–729; Frances A, First MD, Pincus HA. *The Essential Companion to the Diagnostic and Statistical Manual of Mental Disorders*, 4th ed. Washington, DC: American Psychiatric Association; 1995:357–380; and American Academy of Pediatrics. *The Classification of Child and Adolescent Mental Diagnoses in Primary Care: Diagnostic and Statistical Manual for Primary Care (DSM-PC)*. Elk Grove Village, IL: American Academy of Pediatrics; 1996

EATING DISORDERS

Table 12.15
Diagnostic criteria for anorexia nervosa

A. Refusal to maintain body weight at or above a minimally normal weight for age and height (eg, weight loss or failure to make expected weight gain during period of growth to <85% of expected weight)
B. Intense fear of gaining weight or becoming fat, even though underweight
C. Disturbance in view of body image, weight, or shape with denial of the seriousness of the current low body weight
D. In postmenarcheal females, amenorrhea (ie, the absence of at least 3 consecutive menstrual cycles without hormone supplementation)
E. Specify type
   Restricting type
   Binge-eating/purging type

Reprinted with permission from the *Diagnostic and Statistical Manual of Mental Disorders*. Text Revision. Fourth Edition. (Copyright 2000). American Psychiatric Association.

Table 12.16
Diagnostic criteria for bulimia nervosa

A. Recurrent episodes of binge eating
   1. Eating in a limited amount of time (eg, within any 2-h period) an amount of food that is definitely larger than most people
   2. A sense of lack of control (eg, cannot stop eating or control what or how much)
B. Recurrent inappropriate compensatory behavior to prevent weight gain (eg, self-induced vomiting; misuse of laxatives, diuretics, enemas, or other medications; fasting; or excessive exercise)
C. Inappropriate eating and behaviors both occur, on average, at least twice per week for 3 mo
D. Self-evaluation is unduly influenced by body shape and weight
E. The disturbance does not occur exclusively during episodes of anorexia nervosa

Specify type
   Purging type: self-induced vomiting or the misuse of laxatives, diuretics, or enemas
   Nonpurging type: other inappropriate compensatory behaviors such as fasting or excessive exercise

Table 12.17
Diagnostic criteria for eating disorder not otherwise specified

Category for disorders of eating that do not meet the criteria for specific eating disorder; examples include
   1. For females, all criteria for anorexia nervosa met except individual still has regular menses
   2. All criteria for anorexia nervosa met except despite significant weight loss, current weight is in normal range
   3. All criteria for bulimia nervosa met except that binge-eating and inappropriate compensatory behaviors occur less than twice per week or for a duration of <3 mo
   4. Regular use of inappropriate compensatory behaviors by an individual of normal body weight but after eating small amounts of food (eg, self-induced vomiting after eating 2 cookies)
   5. Repeatedly chewing and spitting out, but not swallowing, large amounts of food
   6. Binge-eating disorder: recurrent episodes of binge eating in the absence of the regular use of inappropriate compensatory behaviors characteristic of bulimia nervosa

Table 12.18
Research criteria for binge-eating disorder

A. Recurrent episodes of binge eating
   1. Eating an amount of food definitely larger than most eat in a similar period of time under similar circumstances
   2. Sense of lack of control over eating
B. Episodes associated with 3 (or more) of the following
   1. Eating much more rapidly than normal
   2. Eating until feeling uncomfortably full
   3. Eating large amounts of food when not feeling physically hungry
   4. Eating alone because of being embarrassed by how much one is eating
   5. Feeling disgusted with oneself, depressed, or very guilty after overeating
C. Marked distress regarding binge eating present
D. Occurs, on average, at least 2 d/wk for 6 mo
E. Not associated with the regular use of inappropriate compensatory behaviors

Table 12.19
Specific questions to screen for weight-control measures

General questions
- "How do you feel about your weight?"
- "Have you had a recent change in your weight?"
- "What have you done to change your weight or body shape?"
- "Are you afraid of gaining weight or being overweight?"
- "Have you had a menstrual period?" If yes, "When was your last menstrual period?"

Fasting
- "Have you ever tried to go for a long period of time without eating anything?"
- "For how long would you do that?"
- "When was the last time you did this?"
- "How typical has that been for you over the past week/month?"
- "Do you have any thoughts about what causes you to do this?"

Binging
- "Do you ever eat an amount of food that is larger than what other young people your age would eat?"
- "Do you ever feel that your eating is out of control or that you are powerless to stop eating?"
- "Are there times when you can't stop eating even when you are full?"
- "Are there certain things that "set you off" like being stressed, upset, or angry that causes you to binge?"

(Continued)

Table 12.19
(Continued)

Self-induced vomiting
"Do you ever vomit to keep yourself from gaining weight?"
"How often in the last month?"
"Are there certain things that &lquote;set you off,' such as being stressed, upset, or angry, that cause you to vomit?
"How do you make yourself vomit (fingers, spoon, automatic, etc)?"
"Have you ever vomited blood?"
Medication and substance use
"Do you ever use laxatives, diuretics, ipecac, diet pills, other medications, complementary or alternative medications, or other supplements to keep yourself from gaining weight?"
"How often do you take them?"
"How many at one time?"
"Have you ever experienced a side effect or unpleasant consequence from taking these things?"
Excessive exercise
"What kind do you do?"
"How long at one time?"
"How many times per day? Per week?"
"Do you exercise alone or with others?"
"Do you ever force yourself to exercise, even if you don't want to or when you are injured?"
"Do you ever get upset if you miss a workout or can't exercise?"
"Do you primarily exercise to influence your weight and body shape?"

Adapted with permission from Steinegger C, Katzman DK. Interviewing the adolescent with an eating disorder. *Adolesc Med.* 2008;19(1):28.

Table 12.20
Scoff questions to screen for eating disorders

Do you make yourself sick (induce vomiting) because you feel uncomfortably full?
Do you worry that you have lost control over how much you eat?
Have you recently lost more than 1 stone or 14 lb in a 3-mo period?
Do you think you are too fat although others say you are too thin?
Would you say that food dominated your life?

Score 1 point for every yes answer; a score of ≥2 indicates a likely eating disorder.
Adapted from Morgan JF, Reid F, Lacey JH. The SCOFF questionnaire: assessment of a new screening tool for eating disorders. *BMJ.* 1999;319(7223):1467–1468 with permission from BMJ Publishing Group, Ltd.

Table 12.21
Possible findings on physical examination in adolescents with eating disorders

Anorexia Nervosa	Bulimia Nervosa
Bradycardia	Sinus bradycardia
Orthostatic by pulse or blood pressure	Orthostatic by pulse or blood pressure
Hypothermia	Hypothermia
Cardiac murmur (one third with mitral valve prolapse)	Cardiac murmur (mitral valve prolapse)
Dull, thinning scalp hair	Hair without shine
Sunken cheeks, sallow skin	Dry skin
Lanugo	Parotitis
Atrophic breasts (postpubertal)	Russell's sign (callous on knuckles from self-induced emesis)
Atrophic vaginitis (postpubertal)	Mouth sores
Pitting edema of extremities	Palatal scratches
Emaciated, may wear oversized clothes	Dental enamel erosions
Flat affect	May look entirely normal
Cold extremities, acrocyanosis	Other cardiac arrhythmias

Adapted from American Academy of Pediatrics, Committee on Adolescence. Identifying and treating eating disorders. *Pediatrics*. 2003;111(1):206.

Table 12.22
Medical complications resulting from eating disorders

Medical complications resulting from purging

1. Fluid and electrolyte imbalance; hypokalemia; hyponatremia; hypochloremic alkalosis
2. Use of ipecac: irreversible myocardial damage and a diffuse myositis
3. Chronic vomiting: esophagitis; dental erosions; Mallory-Weiss tears; rare esophageal or gastric rupture; rare aspiration pneumonia
4. Use of laxatives: depletion of potassium bicarbonate, causing metabolic acidosis; increased serum urea nitrogen concentration and predisposition to renal stones from dehydration; hyperuricemia; hypocalcemia; hypomagnesemia; chronic dehydration; with laxative withdrawal, may get fluid retention (may gain up to 10 lb in 24 h)
5. Amenorrhea (can be seen in normal or overweight individuals with bulimia nervosa), menstrual irregularities, osteopenia

Medical complications from caloric restriction

1. Cardiovascular electrocardiographic abnormalities: low voltage; sinus bradycardia (from malnutrition); T wave inversions; ST segment depression (from electrolyte imbalances). Prolonged corrected QT interval is uncommon but may predispose patient to sudden death; dysrhythmias include supraventricular beats and ventricular tachycardia, with or without exercise; pericardial effusions can occur in those who are severely malnourished; all cardiac abnormalities except those secondary to emetine (ipecac) toxicity are completely reversible with weight gain
2. Gastrointestinal system: delayed gastric emptying; slowed gastrointestinal motility; constipation; bloating; fullness; hypercholesterolemia (from abnormal lipoprotein metabolism); abnormal liver function test results (probably from fatty infiltration of the liver); all are reversible with weight gain
3. Renal: increased serum urea nitrogen concentration (from dehydration, decreased glomerular filtration rate) with increased risk of renal stones; polyuria (from abnormal vasopressin secretion, rare partial diabetes insipidus); total body sodium and potassium depletion caused by starvation; with refeeding, 25% can get peripheral edema attributable to increased renal sensitivity to aldosterone and increased insulin secretion (affects renal tubules)
4. Hematologic: leukopenia; anemia; iron deficiency; thrombocytopenia
5. Endocrine: euthyroid sick syndrome; amenorrhea; osteopenia
6. Neurologic: cortical atrophy; seizures

Adapted from American Academy of Pediatrics, Committee on Adolescence. Identifying and treating eating disorders. *Pediatrics*. 2003;111(1):207.

Table 12.23
Criteria for hospital admission for children, adolescents, and young adults with eating disorders

Anorexia nervosa
<75% ideal body weight or ongoing weight loss despite intensive management
Refusal to eat
Body fat <10%
Heart rate <50 beats per min daytime; <45 beats per min nighttime
Systolic pressure <90 mm Hg
Orthostatic changes in pulse (>20 beats per min) or blood pressure (>10 mm Hg)
Temperature <96°F
Arrhythmia
Bulimia nervosa
Syncope
Serum potassium concentration <3.2 mmol/L
Serum chloride concentration <88 mmol/L
Esophageal tears
Cardiac arrhythmias including prolonged QTc
Hypothermia
Suicide risk
Intractable vomiting
Hematemesis
Failure to respond to outpatient treatment

Adapted from American Academy of Pediatrics, Committee on Adolescence. Identifying and treating eating disorders. *Pediatrics*. 2003;111(1):208.

Resources

US Department of Health and Human Services. Body image: loving yourself inside and out. Available at: www. womenshealth.gov/bodyimage/eatingdisorders. Accessed August 4, 2009.

National Eating Disorders Association. Home page. Available at: www. nationaleatingdisorders.org. Accessed August 4, 2009.

US Department of Health and Human Services. Women's health. Available at: www.hrsa.gov/womenshealth. Accessed August 4, 2009.

Substance Abuse

Table 12.24
Drugs of abuse to consider according to specific clinical effect

System	Possible Drug of Abuse
Eyes/pupils	
Mydriasis	Amphetamines/stimulants, cocaine, glutethimide, jimsonweed, LSD; withdrawal from alcohol, opiates
Miosis	Alcohol, barbiturates, benzodiazepines, opiates, PCP
Nystagmus	Alcohol, barbiturates, benzodiazepines, inhalants, PCP
Conjunctival injection	LSD, marijuana
Lacrimation	Inhalants, LSD; withdrawal from opiates
Cardiovascular	
Tachycardia	Amphetamines/stimulants, cocaine, LSD, marijuana, PCP; withdrawal from alcohol, barbiturates, benzodiazepines
Hypertension	Amphetamines/stimulants, cocaine, LSD, marijuana, PCP; withdrawal from alcohol, barbiturates, benzodiazepines
Hypotension	Barbiturates, opiates; orthostatic: marijuana; withdrawal from depressants
Arrhythmias	Amphetamines/stimulants, cocaine, inhalants, opiates, PCP
Core body temperature	
Elevated	Amphetamines/stimulants, cocaine, PCP; withdrawal from alcohol, barbiturates, benzodiazepines, opiates
Decreased	Alcohol, barbiturates, benzodiazepines, opiates
Peripheral nervous system response	
Hyperreflexia	Amphetamines/stimulants, cocaine, LSD, marijuana, methaqualone, PCP; withdrawal from alcohol, barbiturates, benzodiazepines
Hyporeflexia	Alcohol, barbiturates, benzodiazepines, inhalants, opiates
Tremor	Amphetamines/stimulants, cocaine, LSD; withdrawal from alcohol, barbiturates, benzodiazepines, cocaine
Ataxia	Alcohol, amphetamines/stimulants, barbiturates, benzodiazepines, inhalants, LSD, PCP

(*Continued*)

Table 12.24
(Continued)

System	Possible Drug of Abuse
Central nervous system response	
Hyperalertness	Amphetamines/stimulants, cocaine
Sedation/somnolence	Alcohol, barbiturates, benzodiazepines, inhalants, marijuana, opiates
Seizure	Alcohol, amphetamines/stimulants, cocaine, inhalants, methaqualone, opiates (particularly meperidine, propoxyphene); withdrawal from alcohol, barbiturates, benzodiazepines
Hallucinations	Amphetamines/stimulants, cocaine, inhalants, LSD, marijuana, PCP; withdrawal from alcohol, barbiturates, benzodiazepines
Gastrointestinal	
Nausea/vomiting	Alcohol, amphetamines/stimulants, cocaine, inhalants, LSD, opiates, peyote; withdrawal from alcohol, barbiturates, benzodiazepines, cocaine, opiates

LSD indicates D -lysergic acid diethylamide; PCP, phencyclidine.
Adapted from Schwartz B, Alderman EM. Substances of abuse. Pediatr Rev. 1997;18:204–215.

Table 12.25
Select pharmacology, effects, and treatment of specific drugs of abuse with select additional information

Pharmacology	Intoxication Effects	Intoxication Treatment	Withdrawal Effects	Withdrawal Treatment	Comments
Alcohol (ethanol)					
Mechanism of action: CNS depression; increases fluidity of neuronal cell membranes	Mild (blood level <0.1 g/dL): disinhibition, euphoria, mild impaired coordination, mild sedation	Mild intoxication:	Mild ("hangover"): headache, mild tremulousness, nausea/ vomiting	Mild: bed rest and hydration	• Most commonly abused drug
Dose: ~10 g per drink (1 drink = 12 oz beer, 4 oz wine, 1.5 oz 80-proof liquor); each drink increases blood concentration ~0.025 g/dL (varies by weight)	Moderate (0.1–0.2 g/dL): increased sedation, impaired mentation and judgment, mood swings, slurred speech, ataxia	• Observation (can be at home for adolescents who have stable home environment)	Severe:	Severe:	• Use in high school seniors[a]: 80% ever, 74% past year, 51% past month, 3% daily
Onset: 10 min (rapidly absorbed)	Severe (>0.3 g/dL): confusion, stupor; (>0.4 g/dL): coma, respiratory depression, death	Overdose (stupor, coma):	• Prevalence: extremely rare in adolescents; only seen with chronic use	Benzodiazepine taper:	• Major health risk: motor vehicle accidents, violence, other injuries secondary to intoxication
Peak: 40–60 min	Other effects:	• Airway protection, respiratory support	• Onset: several hours after last drink	• Chlordiazepoxide 25–50 mg q 4–6 h or diazepam 10 mg q 4–6 h	• Significantly increased risk of toxicity when used with other sedatives
Elimination rate: 7–10 g/h	• Skin: flushed	• Gastric lavage and charcoal (avoid ipecac because of aspiration risk)	• Temperature: elevated; sweating	• Decrease by 20% qd × 3–5 d	• Diagnostic test: blood alcohol level; breath test used in law enforcement

(Continued)

Table 12.25
(Continued)

Pharmacology	Intoxication Effects	Intoxication Treatment	Withdrawal Effects	Withdrawal Treatment	Comments
Legal intoxication level: 0.05–0.10 g/dL (varies by state)	• Eyes: pupils normal size and sluggish, nystagmus	• Thiamine 100 mg IV	• Eyes: dilated pupils	Consider antipsychotics for psychosis (but will lower seizure threshold)	• Tolerance develops with prolonged use
	• Neurologic: decreased reflexes	• Follow finger-stick glucose; administer IV fluid with glucose as necessary	• Neurologic: tremulousness, hyperactive reflexes, seizures • Cardiovascular: tachycardia, hypertension		Acute complications (occur with large, single doses):
	• GI: nausea/vomiting				• Gastritis, pancreatitis
	• Metabolic: hypoglycemia		• GI: nausea/vomiting		Chronic complications (extremely rare in adolescent):
	Blackouts: anterograde amnesia while intoxicated (with heavy use)		• Psychiatric: anxiety, agitation, insomnia, confusion, hallucinations		• Liver disease
	Idiosyncratic intoxication: sudden onset, marked behavior change (eg, impulsive, aggressive, depressed) with consumption of a small amount; lasts a few hours; most common in young males		Delirium tremens:		• Cardiomyopathy, hypertension, hyperlipidemia

(Continued)

Table 12.25
(Continued)

Pharmacology	Intoxication Effects	Intoxication Treatment	Withdrawal Effects	Withdrawal Treatment	Comments
			• Chronic users only; extremely rare in adolescents		• Wernicke encephalopathy: delirium, eye-muscle paralysis, ataxia
			• Mortality: 20% in adults		• Korsakoff syndrome: dementia with marked anterograde amnesia
			• Onset: 3–5 d after last drink • Autonomic hyperactivity, disorientation/clouding of consciousness, perceptual disturbances/hallucinations • Fluids and electrolytes important to manage		
Marijuana (cannabis)					
Active agent: THC	Low dose: euphoria, laughter, relaxation, time distortion, auditory and visual enhancement; impaired concentration, thinking, memory	For severe anxiety or agitation:	• Relatively mild and occur with chronic use only	No specific treatment	• Most commonly used illicit drug
Derived from leaves and stems of *Cannabis sativa*	High dose: mood fluctuations, depersonalization, hallucinations	• Benzodiazepine	• Psychiatric: irritability, sleep disturbances		• Use in high school seniors[a]: 42% ever, 35% past year, 21% past month, 4.6% daily

(Continued)

Table 12.25
(Continued)

Pharmacology	Intoxication Effects	Intoxication Treatment	Withdrawal Effects	Withdrawal Treatment	Comments
Hashish/hash is a high-potency resin derived from flower of female plant	Toxic reaction: anxiety, panic, delusions, hallucinations, paranoia, psychosis	• Calm environment	• Neurologic: tremor, nystagmus		• Potentiates other drugs of abuse
Potency: 4%–6% THC typical; 20%–30% for hashish	Other effects:	Otherwise, no specific treatment	• GI: anorexia, nausea/vomiting, diarrhea		• May be adulterated by other drugs (eg, PCP) without user's knowledge • Virtually no lethal potential other than from accident or injury secondary to intoxication
Routes of administration: smoking (greater bioavailability), ingestion	• GI: increased appetite, dry mouth, decreased nausea				
Onset: 5–10 min smoked; 30–60 min ingested	• Eyes: injected conjunctiva, normal to dilated pupils				• Detectability in urine: 5 d for single dose, 10 d for casual use, 14–30 d for daily use
Peak: 20 min smoked; 3–4 h ingested	• Cardiovascular: increased heart rate, orthostatic hypotension (sometimes elevated blood pressure)				Complications of chronic use:
Duration: 3 h smoked; 6–8 h ingested	• Neurologic: normal to increased reflexes, drowsiness; impaired coordination, tracking, reaction times				• Pulmonary (cough, bronchitis, decreased diffusion capacity, and FEV_1)

(Continued)

Table 12.25
(Continued)

Pharmacology	Intoxication Effects	Intoxication Treatment	Withdrawal Effects	Withdrawal Treatment	Comments
Common street names: pot, weed, grass, reefer, joints (cigarettes), blunts (cigars)	• Respiratory: bronchodilation (acutely)				• Gynecomastia
	May precipitate seizures, psychosis, or emotional disorder in persons who have those underlying disorders				• Decreased sperm count and motility
					• "Amotivational syndrome" (controversial): apathy, loss of ambition, withdrawal from work and recreational activities
Heroin and other opiates					
Derived from opium poppy, *Papaver somniferum*, or synthesized	General: euphoria followed by sedation ("nod"), somnolence, analgesia	Overdose:	Seen with >3 wk of regular use; not seen with intermittent use	Primarily supportive (almost never fatal)	• Heroin is most widely abused of the opiates

(Continued)

Table 12.25
(Continued)

Pharmacology	Intoxication Effects	Intoxication Treatment	Withdrawal Effects	Withdrawal Treatment	Comments
Examples: heroin, morphine, meperidine, oxycodone, opium, codeine, methadone, hydromorphone, propoxyphene, fentanyl	Neurologic: slowed comprehension, impaired mentation, decreased reflexes	• Respiratory and circulatory support	Onset (varies by drug): 6–8 h after last dose of heroin; 24–48 h after methadone	Severe withdrawal: detoxification with methadone (20–40 mg qd tapered by 5 mg/d) and/or clonidine (0.2 mg tid to qid for 7–10 d, then tapered over 2–3 d)	• Use of heroin in high school seniors[a]: 1.6% ever, 1.1% past year, 0.6% past month, 0.1% daily; for other opiates: 7.2% ever, 4.7% past year, 1.8% past month, 0.1% daily (underestimates actual use by adolescents because of higher use in high school dropouts)
Mechanism of action: binds to opioid receptors in the CNS, causing CNS depression	Eyes: constricted/pinpoint pupils	• Treat any arrhythmias	Duration: 7–10 d		• Potentially fatal interaction between meperidine and monamine oxidase inhibitors
Heroin:	Cardiovascular: decreased blood pressure, arrhythmias	• Gastric lavage and charcoal may be useful if drugs taken PO	General: drug craving, rhinorrhea, lacrimation, muscle aches, yawning		• Detectability in urine: 24 h for heroin, 3 d for methadone; synthetic opiates such as fentanyl will not be detected

(Continued)

Table 12.25
(Continued)

Pharmacology	Intoxication Effects	Intoxication Treatment	Withdrawal Effects	Withdrawal Treatment	Comments
• Dose: 1–25 mg; concentration usually ~5%, but varies considerably (1%–20%)	Temperature: decreased	• Naloxone 2.0 mg (0.1 mg/kg in children) IV q 3 min until response or maximum of 10 mg; may need to readminister in 2–3 h or use IV drip (of total initial dose per hour) because half-life is shorter than that of many opiates	Temperature: elevated; chills, hot and cold flashes, sweating, piloerection		Complications of IV administration: "track marks," endocarditis, cellulitis, phlebitis; pulmonary emboli (septic and talc); hepatitis and HIV infection (with shared needles)
• Routes of administration: snorting (most common in adolescents), intravenous ("shooting up, mainlining"), subcutaneous ("skin popping"), ingestion, smoking	Respiratory: respiratory depression, cough suppression	• Monitor for 24 h (72 h for methadone and long-acting agents)	Respiratory: increased respiration rate		
• Onset: IV, immediate; snorted, 30 min; subcutaneous, 15 min	GI: nausea/vomiting, constipation		GI: nausea/vomiting, abdominal cramps, diarrhea		
• Duration: 3–6 h (IV)	Urologic: urinary retention		Psychiatric: restlessness, anxiety, sleep disturbance		
• Common street names: junk, smack, dope	Overdose:		Cardiovascular: hypertension, tachycardia		
Methadone:	• Hypotension, bradycardia, circulatory collapse		Eyes: dilated pupils		

(Continued)

Table 12.25
(Continued)

Pharmacology	Intoxication Effects	Intoxication Treatment	Withdrawal Effects	Withdrawal Treatment	Comments
• Onset: 30 min PO	• Severe respiratory depression, pulmonary edema		Neurologic: tremor		
• Duration: >24 h	• Stupor, coma, death • Seizures (especially with meperidine and propoxyphene)				
Cocaine					
Derived from leaves of cocoa bush, *Erythroxylon coca*	General: hyperalertness, increased energy, confidence, restlessness, stimulation and enhancement of mood, elation, euphoria	• Benzodiazepine for agitation, anxiety, seizures; helpful for hypertension	"Crash": the immediate appearance of unpleasant effects; also a withdrawal syndrome that appears later	Consider antidepressant for depression	• Use in high school seniors[a]: 6% ever, 4% past year, 1.8% past month, 0.2% daily; for crack: 3% ever, 2.1% past year, 1% past month, 0.1% daily (underestimates actual use by adolescents because of higher use in high school dropouts)
Mechanism of action: Increased release and decreased reuptake of biogenic amines, causing:	Psychiatric: insomnia, labile affect, agitation, anxiety, paranoia, delirium, hallucinations, psychosis	• For severe hypertension: nitroprusside, labetalol, or phentolamine	• Craving for cocaine		• Detectability in urine: 4–6 d (also detectable in blood)
CNS and peripheral nervous system stimulation	Eyes: dilated pupils	• Cardiac monitor; treat arrhythmias (avoid lidocaine: can cause seizures)	• Depression, dysphoria, anhedonia, irritability		• Addicts use in binges with escalating doses and frequency

(*Continued*)

Table 12.25
(Continued)

Pharmacology	Intoxication Effects	Intoxication Treatment	Withdrawal Effects	Withdrawal Treatment	Comments
Local anesthesia	Neurologic: dizziness, paresthesias, hyperreflexia, tremor, local anesthesia, seizures	• Treat ischemic chest pain with nitrates, heparin, aspirin, calcium channel blockers (β-blocker use is controversial because of possible unopposed α-agonist activity)	• Lethargy, fatigue, weakness		• Crack has higher addiction potential because of more intense, shorter high and lower cost per dose
Vasoconstriction	Cardiovascular: hypertension, tachycardia, arrhythmia	• Haloperidol for psychosis	• Tremor		• With concomitant ethanol use: prolonged effects caused by formation of ethyl cocaine
Routes of administration: snorting, smoking (freebase form, "crack"), IV	GI: nausea, dry mouth, anorexia	• Cooling blanket for hyperthermia	• Nausea, hunger		• "Speedball": cocaine and heroin used together IV
Onset: very rapid	Temperature: elevated; sweating				• Sometimes smuggled in ingested packets
Peak: smoked, <1 min; snorted, 2–30 min; IV, 0.5–2 min	Overdose: coma, toxic psychosis, chest pain/angina, myocardial infarction, hyperthermia, rhabdomyolysis, stroke, seizures				Complications of administration:
Duration: smoked, 4–15 min; snorted, 30–60 min; IV, 12–30 min					• Nasal septum ulceration, epistaxis with snorting

(Continued)

Table 12.25
(Continued)

Pharmacology	Intoxication Effects	Intoxication Treatment	Withdrawal Effects	Withdrawal Treatment	Comments
Common street names: coke, nose candy, snow; crack, rock (freebase)					• Same IV complications as with IV heroin • Lung damage from smoking
Amphetamines and other stimulants					
Examples: dextroamphetamine sulfate, methamphetamine (also available in a crystal form), amphetamine sulfate, benzphetamine, methylphenidate	General: euphoria, reduced fatigue, alertness, restlessness, hyperactivity	• Gastric lavage and charcoal for drugs taken PO	"Crash" is the immediate appearance of withdrawal symptoms (similar to cocaine)	Consider antidepressant for depression	• Effects, treatment, and use patterns similar to those of cocaine
Mechanism of action: CNS stimulation; sympathomimetic through:	Psychiatric: insomnia, irritability, impulsivity, anxiety, panic, hallucinations (especially visual, tactile, olfactory) possible psychosis	• Treat hypertension and arrhythmias	Withdrawal usually appears in 2–4 d after last use		• Use in high school seniors[a]: 15% ever, 9% past year, 4% past month, 0.3% daily; for crystal methamphetamine: 3.9% ever, 2.4% past year, 1.1% past month, 0.1% daily
Release of presynaptic neurotransmitters	Temperature: elevated; flushing, sweating	• Benzodiazepine for agitation, hypertension	• Lethargy, fatigue		• Detectability in urine: 48 h (amphetamine and methamphetamine)

(Continued)

Table 12.25
(Continued)

Pharmacology	Intoxication Effects	Intoxication Treatment	Withdrawal Effects	Withdrawal Treatment	Comments
Direct stimulation of postsynaptic catecholamine receptors	Eyes: dilated pupils	• Cooling blanket for hyperthermia	• Depression, anxiety, nightmares		• Sometimes used in "runs" (ie, frequent, repeated doses)
Prevention of reuptake of neurotransmitters	Neurologic: tremor, ataxia, headache, hyperreflexia, possible seizures	• Haloperidol for psychosis (avoid phenothiazines)	• Sweating, muscle cramps		
Mild inhibition of monamine oxidase	GI: decreased appetite, dry mouth, nausea/vomiting	• Although acidification of urine increases clearance, it's not recommended	• Abdominal cramps, hunger		
Routes of administration: PO (most common), smoking (crystal methamphetamine), snorting, and IV (possible, but much less common)	Cardiovascular: palpitations, tachycardia, elevated blood pressure, possible arrhythmia	• Hemodialysis may be helpful in overdose			
Onset: PO, 30 min; IV, immediate	Overdose: coma, circulatory collapse, hypertensive crisis, hyperthermia, seizures (rarely), arrhythmias, cerebral hemorrhage				
Common street names: uppers, speed, meth; ice, crystal (crystal methamphetamine)					

(Continued)

Table 12.25
(Continued)

Pharmacology	Intoxication Effects	Intoxication Treatment	Withdrawal Effects	Withdrawal Treatment	Comments
LSD and other hallucinogens					
Active agent: LSD	General: perceptual alterations, illusions, synesthesias (1 sense is perceived as another), loss of time sense, body-image changes, euphoria, depersonalization, derealization, hallucinations	• Peaceful, calm environment	No specific syndrome	No treatment necessary	• Use in high school seniors[a]: 12% ever, 8% past year, 4% past month, 0.1% daily
Derived from an alkaloid in rye fungus	Psychiatric: labile affect, anxiety, restlessness, paranoia, sleep disturbances	• Help restore contact with reality: talk about familiar things and reassure patient ("talking down")			• Detectability: not detected in standard urine screens
Mechanism of action: inhibits release of serotonin	Eyes: dilated pupils, conjunctival injection, lacrimation	• Benzodiazepine, if needed for sedation			• No deaths have been reported from direct effect of drug
Route of administration: PO	Neurologic: dizziness, paresthesias, hyperreflexia, tremor, ataxia	• Avoid phenothiazines because of possible synergistic anticholinergic and CNS depressant effects			• Flashback: occurrence of effects after drug has worn off; selective serotonin reuptake inhibitor may induce or worsen
Available as tablets, gelatin squares, or applied to pieces of paper ("blotters")	GI: dry mouth, anorexia, nausea	• Treat hypertension, hyperthermia, seizures as necessary			

(Continued)

Table 12.25
(Continued)

Pharmacology	Intoxication Effects	Intoxication Treatment	Withdrawal Effects	Withdrawal Treatment	Comments
Dose: usually 25–100 μg; >250 μg especially dangerous	Temperature: elevated; flushing, piloerection				
Onset: 30 min	Cardiovascular: elevated blood pressure, tachycardia				
Peak: 2–4 h	Overdose: coma				
Duration: 6–12 h	"Bad trip": extremely negative response causing terror, panic, "feeling of going crazy"				
Tolerance: rapid and short-lived					
Common street name: acid					
PCP					
Mechanism of action: dissociative anesthetic with analgesic, stimulant, depressant, and hallucinogenic properties	Low dose (<5 mg):	• Reduce stimulation	No specific syndrome	No specific treatment	• Use in high school seniors[a]: 2.7% ever, 1.8% past year, 0.6% past month, 0.3% daily

(Continued)

Table 12.25
(Continued)

Pharmacology	Intoxication Effects	Intoxication Treatment	Withdrawal Effects	Withdrawal Treatment	Comments
Routes of administration: PO, IV, intramuscular, snorting, smoking	• Psychiatric: illusions, hallucinations, disordered thought, distortion of body image, amnesia, euphoria, dysphoria, anxiety, psychosis, catatonia, paranoia, agitation, combative/violent behavior	• Do not try to "talk down" as for other hallucinogens			• Fat-soluble and may remain in body for prolonged periods
Available forms: liquid, powder, tablet, rock crystal, mixed with leaves (eg, marijuana)	• Eyes: vertical and horizontal nystagmus, miosis, blank stare	• Benzodiazepine for sedation, if necessary			• Flashbacks occur; more common than with LSD
Dose: 3 mg smoked, 5 mg PO and snorted, 10 mg IV, on average	• Neurologic: analgesia, ataxia, dysarthria, hyperreflexia, reduced proprioception and sensation, impaired coordination	• Respiratory and cardiovascular support			• Recovery usually within 24 h, but coma can last 5 d with high dose
Onset: IV, seconds; smoked and snorted, 2–5 min; PO, 30 min	• Cardiovascular: tachycardia, elevated blood pressure	• Treat seizures			• Use caution in treating patients; behavior can be violent and unpredictable
Peak: smoked and snorted, 15–30 min; PO, 2–5 h	• Skin: diaphoresis, flushing	• Cooling blanket for hyperthermia			• Detectability in urine: 1–2 wk

(*Continued*)

Table 12.25
(Continued)

Pharmacology	Intoxication Effects	Intoxication Treatment	Withdrawal Effects	Withdrawal Treatment	Comments
Duration: up to 12 h	Moderate dose (5–10 mg): see above plus hyperthermia, hypersalivation, myoclonus	• Treat hypertension with nitroprusside, labetalol, or phentolamine			
Common street names: angel dust, dust, hog	High dose (>10 mg): see above plus unresponsiveness, muscle rigidity, eyes-open coma, hypoventilation, extensor posturing, seizures, arrhythmias, death, rhabdomyolysis, and renal failure	• Haloperidol if needed for psychosis/very severe agitation (avoid phenothiazines)			
Ketamine (common street name: "special K") is a short-acting anesthetic that has psychoactive properties similar to PCP		• Gastric lavage and charcoal; continuous nasogastric suction hastens removal			
		• Acidifying urine increases excretion, but not recommended • Diuresis is controversial			
Depressants (sedatives, hypnotics, tranquilizers)					

(Continued)

Table 12.25
(Continued)

Pharmacology	Intoxication Effects	Intoxication Treatment	Withdrawal Effects	Withdrawal Treatment	Comments
Examples:	Depend on previous exposure because of tolerance	Overdose:	Requires more than several weeks of regular use	For barbiturates and similar agents: detoxification with slow phenobarbital taper	• Barbiturate use in high school seniors[a]: 7.4% ever, 4.7% past year, 2.2% past month, 0.1% daily
Barbiturates:	General: sedation, drowsiness, fatigue, lethargy, yawning, euphoria	• Respiratory and circulatory support	More severe and appears earlier with shorter-acting drugs	• Starting dose: administer until mild toxicity (ataxia, nystagmus, dysarthria)	• Benzodiazepine abuse mostly seen in adults; rare in adolescents
• Very short acting (duration: 3–4 h): thiopental	Eyes: pupils normal to constricted, lateral nystagmus	• Gastric lavage	Withdrawal syndrome can be fatal	• Taper: by 120 mg/d	• Barbiturates are second most common cause of fatal accidental overdose in children
• Short acting (duration: 4–8 h): secobarbital, pentobarbital	Neurologic: ataxia, diplopia, dizziness, dysmetria, slurred speech, hypotonia, diminished reflexes, impaired mentation and memory	• Charcoal: repeated doses (q 2–4 h) for long-acting barbiturates may hasten removal	Psychiatric: agitation, restlessness, anxiety, insomnia, irritability, delirium, hallucinations, psychosis	For benzodiazepines: detoxification with slow taper of long-acting benzodiazepine (eg, chlordiazepoxide)	• Benzodiazepines significantly less lethal than barbiturates; overdose is rare
• Intermediate acting (duration: 8–10 h): amobarbital	Psychiatric: anxiety, delirium, depression, irritability, psychosis	For barbiturates:	Neurologic: headache, weakness, tremulousness, hyperreflexia, seizures		• Especially dangerous in combination with alcohol
• Long acting (duration: 12–24 h): phenobarbital	Temperature: decreased	• Hemodialysis or hemoperfusion may be helpful in removal of all barbiturates	Temperature: elevated; flushing, sweating		• Causes tolerance and physical dependence

(Continued)

Table 12.25
(Continued)

Pharmacology	Intoxication Effects	Intoxication Treatment	Withdrawal Effects	Withdrawal Treatment	Comments
Nonbarbiturates that have similar properties: meprobamate, glutethimide, methaqualone	Cardiovascular: decreased blood pressure	• Hemoperfusion particularly helpful in removal of short-acting barbiturates	GI: abdominal cramps, nausea/ vomiting		• Detectability in urine:
Benzodiazepines: diazepam, chlordiazepoxide, flurazepam	Respiratory: respiratory depression	• Alkalinization of urine hastens removal of long-acting barbiturates (eg, phenobarbital); forced diuresis is no longer recommended	Cardiovascular: tachycardia, hypertension or orthostatic hypotension		• Barbiturates: short acting, 1 d; intermediate acting, 2–3 d; long acting, >7 d
Mechanism of action: CNS depression; benzodiazepines bind to a specific receptor that potentiates GABA	Overdose: stupor, coma, severe hypotension, cardiac arrest, respiratory arrest, pulmonary edema, hypothermia, death	For benzodiazepines:			• Benzodiazepines: ~3 d; very high rate of false-negative screens
Routes of administration: usually PO, but certain agents can be used IV	With methaqualone: seizures, hyperreflexia, muscle hypertonicity and spasm	• Flumazenil: 0.2 mg IV followed in 30 s by 0.3 mg followed q 1 min by 0.5 mg until response or total of 3–5 mg given (all doses administered over 30 s)			• Barbiturates and benzodiazepines also detectable in blood
Common street name: downers	With glutethimide: dilated pupils	• May need to retreat or start IV drip with long-acting benzodiazepines			

(Continued)

Table 12.25
(Continued)

Pharmacology	Intoxication Effects	Intoxication Treatment	Withdrawal Effects	Withdrawal Treatment	Comments
	With benzodiazepines: little respiratory depression or hypotension; antianxiety	• Contraindicated in mixed overdose with tricyclic antidepressants or stimulants (can cause seizures) or in cases of long-term physical addiction (can precipitate withdrawal)			
Inhalants					
Active agents: volatile solvents—toluene, benzene, other hydrocarbons, fluorocarbons	General: euphoria, giddiness, drowsiness, impaired judgment	• Respiratory and circulatory support	No withdrawal syndrome	No withdrawal treatment	• Use highest among young male adolescents, often as a group activity
Examples: model airplane glue, rubber cement, correction fluid, paint thinner, spray paint, shoe polish, gasoline, propane, butane, aerosol propellants	Psychiatric: hallucinations, psychosis	• Treat arrhythmias			• Use in 8th-graders[a]: 22% ever, 13% past year, 6% past month, 0.2% daily
Mechanism of action: CNS stimulation and excitement, progressing to depression	Eyes: nystagmus, lacrimation	• Avoid use of epinephrine or other proarrhythmic drugs, if possible			• Use in high school seniors[a]: 17% ever, 8% past year, 3% past month, 0.1% daily

(Continued)

Table 12.25
(Continued)

Pharmacology	Intoxication Effects	Intoxication Treatment	Withdrawal Effects	Withdrawal Treatment	Comments
Route of administration: inhaled from a bag or cloth ("huffing") saturated with substance	Neurologic: dizziness, headache, ataxia, slurred speech, diplopia, diminished reflexes	• Check complete blood count, PT/PTT, liver tests, and renal function tests			• May have rash on face, odor on breath, or irritation of eyes
Onset: immediate	Respiratory: rhinorrhea, mucosal irritation				• Can cause permanent hepatic, renal, cardiac, CNS, and peripheral nerve damage • Not detectable in blood or urine
Duration: 5–15 min	GI: anorexia, nausea/vomiting, salivation Overdose: respiratory depression, arrhythmia, cardiac arrest, seizure, delirium, stupor, coma Sudden sniffing death syndrome: sudden death, probably caused by cardiac arrhythmias				

CNS indicates central nervous system; q, every; qd, every day; IV, intravenously; GI, gastrointestinal; THC, δ-9-tetrahydrocannabinol; PCP, phencyclidine; FEV_1, forced expiratory volume in 1 second; PO, by mouth; tid, 3 times per day; qid, 4 times per day; LSD, D -lysergic acid diethylamide tartrate; GABA, γ-aminobutyric acid; PT, prothrombin time; PTT, partial thromboplastin time.

(*Continued*)

Table 12.25
(Continued)

Other important stimulants:

- "Designer drug" amphetamines: eg, methylenedioxymethamphetamine (MDMA, "ecstasy," "X"), methylenedioxymethamphetamine (MDEA); similar to amphetamines with mild euphorigenic and hallucinogenic properties; overdoses treated same as those with amphetamines.
- Khat leaves (*Catha edulis*) contain methcathinone; chewed, smoked, or made into a tea.
- Amphetamine "look-alikes": eg, ephedrine, pseudoephedrine, phenylpropanolamine, caffeine; sold in various combinations as amphetamines or as legal substitutes ("herbal ecstasy," "ma huang").

Other important hallucinogens:

- Peyote: cactus in southwest United States and Mexico; tops contain hallucinogenic alkaloids, including mescaline.
- Mescaline (3,4,5-trimethoxyphenethylamine): effects similar to those of LSD but much less potent; fewer "bad trips"; dose: usually 100 to 500 μg; onset: 30 to 120 minutes; duration: 6 to 12 hours; frequently accompanied by nausea/vomiting; drugs sold as mescaline are often LSD and/or PCP.
- Psychedelic mushrooms (psilocybin, psilocin): effects similar to those of LSD but much less potent; dose: 4 to 10 mg psilocybin; route: oral; onset: 15 minutes; peak: 90 minutes; duration: 5 to 6 hours; common street names: mushrooms, shrooms.
- Morning glory seeds (*Rivea corymbosa* and *Ipomoea* sp): effects similar to LSD but less potent; often causes nausea, dizziness, diarrhea.
- Dimethyltryptamine (DMT): found in seeds from several plants in West Indies and South America; tobacco, marijuana, or parsley is soaked in the liquid and smoked; duration: 1 to 3 hours.
- Nutmeg: contains lysergide and other hallucinatory alkaloids.

- Jimsonweed (*Datura stramonium*): grows wild in the southwest United States; contains atropine and scopolamine; hallucinogenic and anticholinergic properties; may have anticholinergic syndrome (delirium, flushing, dry mucous membranes, dilated pupils); gastric lavage recommended; consider physostigmine in severe cases.

(*Continued*)

Table 12.25
(Continued)

Other important inhalants:

- Nitrites (amyl nitrite ["poppers"], butyl nitrite, isobutyl nitrite): cause vasodilatation and smooth muscle relaxation; common effects: lightheadedness ("rush"), giddiness, headache, dizziness, orthostatic hypotension, tachycardia, flushing; often abused for purpose of enhancing sexual pleasure; use can cause methemoglobinemia.
- Nitrous oxide ("laughing gas"): available as whipped cream propellant; usually inhaled from balloon; deaths have occurred with 100% N_2O.

[a] *Johnson LD, O'Malley PM, Bachman JG. Monitoring the Future Study*. Ann Arbor, MI: News and Information Services of the University of Michigan; 1995.

Adapted from Joffe A, Blythe MJ, eds. Handbook of adolescent medicine. *Adolesc Med*. 2003;14(2):455.

Table 12.26
Alcohol impairment chart: women

No. of Drinks	Approximate Blood Alcohol Percentage by Body Weight, lb									Comment
	90	100	120	140	160	180	200	220	240	
0	.00	.00	.00	.00	.00	.00	.00	.00	.00	Only safe driving limit
1	.05	.05	.04	.03	.03	.03	.02	.02	.02	Impairment begins
2	.10	.09	.08	.07	.06	.05	.05	.04	.04	Driving skills affected
3	.15	.14	.11	.10	.09	.08	.07	.06	.06	Possible criminal penalties
4	.20	.18	.15	.13	.11	.10	.09	.08	.08	
5	.25	.23	.19	.16	.14	.13	.11	.10	.09	
6	.30	.27	.23	.19	.17	.15	.14	.12	.11	Legally intoxicated
7	.35	.32	.27	.23	.20	.18	.16	.14	.13	—
8	.40	.36	.30	.26	.23	.20	.18	.17	.15	Criminal penalties
9	.45	.41	.34	.29	.26	.23	.20	.19	.17	
10	.51	.45	.38	.32	.28	.25	.23	.21	.19	

Your body can get rid of 1 drink per hour. Each 1 oz. of 80-proof liquor, 12 oz of beer, or 5 oz of table wine = 1 drink.

Adapted from Pennsylvania Liquor Control Board, Bureau of Alcohol Education. Alcohol impairment chart: females. Available at: www.lcb.state.pa.us/edu/cwp/view.asp?a=1346&q=555677. Accessed April 13, 2009.

Table 12.27
Alcohol impairment chart: men

No. of Drinks	Approximate Blood Alcohol Percentage by Body Weight, lb								Comment
	100	120	140	160	180	200	220	240	
0	.00	.00	.00	.00	.00	.00	.00	.00	Only safe driving limit
1	.04	.03	.03	.02	.02	.02	.02	.02	Impairment begins
2	.08	.06	.05	.05	.04	.04	.03	.03	
3	.11	.09	.08	.07	.06	.06	.05	.05	Driving skills affected
4	.15	.12	.11	.09	.08	.08	.07	.06	Possible criminal penalties
5	.19	.16	.13	.12	.11	.09	.09	.08	
6	.23	.19	.16	.14	.13	.11	.10	.09	
7	.26	.22	.19	.16	.15	.13	.12	.11	Legally intoxicated
8	.30	.25	.21	.19	.17	.15	.14	.13	Criminal penalties
9	.34	.28	.24	.21	.19	.17	.15	.14	
10	.38	.31	.27	.23	.21	.19	.17	.16	

Your body can get rid of 1 drink per hour. Each 1 oz. of 80-proof liquor, 12 oz of beer, or 5 oz of table wine = 1 drink.

Adapted from Pennsylvania Liquor Control Board, Bureau of Alcohol Education. Alcohol impairment chart: males. Available at: www.lcb.state.pa.us/edu/cwp/view.asp?a=1346&q=555684. Accessed April 13, 2009.

Table 12.28
Opening questions about drug and alcohol use and the CRAFFT questions

Initial questions
"Have you ever drank alcohol (more than a few sips)?"
"Have you ever used marijuana or hashish?"
"Have you ever used any other drug to get high? By other 'drug' we mean illicit drugs (such as ecstasy or heroin), prescription drugs such as OxyContin or Klonopin that were not prescribed by your doctor or taken the way the doctor said to, over-the-counter medications such as dextromethorphan), and inhalants such as glue or nitrous from spray cans."
CRAFFT questions: during the past 12 mo
"Have you ever ridden in a car driven by someone (including yourself) who was 'high' or had been using alcohol or drugs?"
"Do you ever use alcohol or drugs to relax, feel better about yourself, or fit in?"
"Do you ever use alcohol or drugs while you are by yourself, alone?"
"Do you ever forget things you did while using alcohol or drugs?"
"Do your family or friends ever tell you that you should cut down on your drinking or drug use?"
"Have you ever gotten into trouble while you were using alcohol or drugs?"

Adapted with permission from Levy S, Knight JR. *Adolesc Med.* 2008;19(1):84.

Resources

US Department of Health and Human Services and SAMSHA National Clearing House for Alcohol and Drug Information: Available at: http://ncadi.samhsa.gov.

Top 50 Publications. Available at: http://ncadistore.samhsa. gov/catalog/top.aspx.

Table 12.29
Sample brief advice

Health effects of substance use
"Drugs and alcohol affect your brain and can damage it for life."
"Alcohol can hurt your liver."
"Smoked drugs, including marijuana, can hurt your lungs."
"Smoking marijuana increases your risk of developing depression and schizophrenia (psychosis)."
"Alcohol and drugs, including marijuana, impair driving ability and can cause accidents."
"Drug and alcohol use puts teens at higher risk of sexual assault, sexually transmitted infections, and unwanted pregnancy."
"If a girl becomes pregnant, drug and alcohol use can hurt the baby."
Driving/riding while intoxicated:
"Drug- and alcohol-related car crashes are a leading cause of death for young people."
"Don't ever drive a car after using drugs or drinking, even if you don't feel 'high' or drunk."
"Make arrangements ahead of time for safe transportation."
"Please talk to your parents about the 'contrast for life.' I'd like you to come back in a week and let me know how that conversation went."

Adapted with permission from Levy S, Knight JR. *Adolesc Med.* 2008;19(1):84.

Table 12.30
Stages of use

Stage	Description
Abstinence	The time before a teenager has ever tried drugs or more than a few sips of alcohol
Experimentation	The first 1 or 2 times that a substance is used; experimentation is generally of shorter duration; an adolescent who is experimenting is curious to know what it feels like to be intoxicated
Regular (nonproblematic) use	Drug use together with ≥1 friend for recreational purposes in relatively low-risk situations and without related problems; regular use typically occurs at predictable times such as on weekends
Problematic use	Drug use in a high-risk situation (such as in a car or when baby-sitting), associated with a problem (such as a fight while intoxicated, a school suspension or arrest), or for purposes other than recreation (such as to relieve stress or depression)

(*Continued*)

Table 12.30
(Continued)

Stage	Description
Substance abuse	Continued substance use despite a significant negative impact on functioning as defined in the DSM-IV A maladaptive pattern of substance use that leads to clinically significant impairment or distress as manifested by ≥1 of the following, occurring within a 12-mo period Recurrent substance use that results in a failure to fulfill major role obligations at work, school, or home Recurrent substance use in situations in which it is physically hazardous Recurrent substance-related legal problems Continued use despite having persistent or recurrent social or interpersonal problems caused or exacerbated by the effects of the substance
Substance dependence	Loss of control over use of a substance, or compulsion to use a substance, as defined in the DSM-IV A maladaptive pattern of substance use that leads to clinically significant impairment or distress, as manifested by ≥3 of the following, occurring any time in the same 12-mo period Tolerance Withdrawal The substance is often taken in larger amounts or over a longer period than intended There is a persistent desire or unsuccessful efforts to cut down or control substance use A great deal of time is spent in activities necessary to obtain the substance, use the substance, or recover from its effects Important social, occupational, or recreational activities are given up or reduced because of substance use The substance use is continued despite knowledge of having a persistent physical or psychological problem that is likely to have been caused or exacerbated by the substance

DSM-IV indicates *Diagnostic and Statistical Manual of Mental Disorders*, 4th edition.
Adapted with permission from Levy S, Knight JR. *Adolesc Med*. 2008;19(1):86.

Table 12.31
Stages of change

Stage	Description
Precontemplation	The adolescent does not believe that his or her substance use has or will cause problems and has not begun to consider a change.
Contemplation	The adolescent begins to consider the negative impact of substance use and weighs the reasons to continue against the reasons to stop.
Determination	The adolescent has decided to make a change, but no action has occurred yet. This stage may involve setting a quit date or agreeing to see a counselor.
Action	The adolescent has made a behavioral change.
Maintenance	The behavior change has been well established. The adolescent may continue to develop new strategies to avoid substance use in a variety of settings.
Relapse	A recurrence of substance use after achieving abstinence. A single use or use over a brief period of time with a quick return to commitment to abstinence is often referred to as a "slip." This is in distinction to a loss of commitment to change, which is referred to as a relapse.

Adapted with permission from Levy S, Knight JR. *Adolesc Med.* 2008;19(1):87.

Table 12.32
Strategies appropriate for various stages of use and stages of change

Stage of Use	Stage of Change	Intervention Strategy	Intervention Goal
Abstinence	NA	Praise and encouragement.	Indicate to the adolescent an openness to discussing drug and alcohol use in the future.
Experimentation or regular use	Precontemplation	Ask open-ended questions about the risks associated with drug use.	Raise concern regarding continued drug use.
	Contemplation	Ask about the reasons for considering a behavior change.	Draw out and further explore reasons for quitting.
		Provide valid medical information.	
Problem use or abuse	Precontemplation	Have the patient describe the problem associated with use. Listen reflectively by repeating the problem and any associated negative affect.	Consider the personal negative effects of drug use.
		Listen reflectively by repeating the problem and any associated negative affect.	
	Contemplation	Ask about problems associated with drug use and personal goals, and explore the discrepancy between those goals and current behavior.	Agree to a trial of abstinence.
		Weigh the pros and cons of continued use, and the pros and cons of behavioral change.	
	Action	Ask about confidence in ability to sustain the change and previous motivations to use drugs.	Maintain abstinence.
		Develop strategies for avoiding drug use.	
	Maintenance	Ask about risky situations and how drug use was avoided.	Promote continued motivation to maintain abstinence.
		Devise new strategies for avoiding use.	
		Ask about pros and cons of abstinence.	
	Relapse	Ask about the context of repeat drug use.	Return to abstinence.
		Determine strength of commitment to abstinence.	
		Develop new strategies for use in high-risk situations.	
		Identify additional supports.	

(Continued)

Table 12.32
(Continued)

Stage of Use	Stage of Change	Intervention Strategy	Intervention Goal
Dependence	Contemplation	Determine the importance of change and confidence in ability to make a change.	Agree to work toward change.
		Support self-efficacy.	Accept a referral to treatment.
	Action	Ask about barriers to change.	Identify appropriate level of services.
	Maintenance	Ask about the treatment, progress, and personal goals for the future.	Maintain therapeutic alliance.
	Relapse	Support self-efficacy.	Assist in getting back into treatment.
		Reaffirm goals.	
		Discuss the medical model of drug dependence and need for ongoing treatment.	

NA indicates not applicable.
Adapted with permission from Levy S, Knight JR. *Adolesc Med.* 2008;19(1):89.

Adolesc Med 20 (2009) 788–793

13. Nutrition

Alain Joffe, MD, MPH
E-mail address: ajoffe@jhu.edu.

 ISSN 1934-4287

Table 13.1
Food sources of calcium

Nondairy		Dairy	
Food	Calcium, mg	Food	Calcium, mg
Fortified cereals, various (1 oz)	236–1043	Plain, nonfat yogurt, 8 oz	452
Soy beverage, calcium fortified, 1 cup	368	Romano cheese, 1.5 oz	452
Rhubarb, 1 cup	348	Pasteurized process, Swiss cheese, 2 oz	438
Sardines, Atlantic, in oil, drained, 3 oz	325	Plain yogurt, low-fat, 8 oz	415
Tofu, firm, with nigari,[a] 1 cup	253	Fruit yogurt, low-fat, 8 oz	345
Broccoli, 1 cup	188	Swiss cheese, 1.5 oz	336
Pink salmon, canned, with bone, 3 oz	181	Ricotta cheese, part-skim, cup	335
Collards, cooked from frozen, cup	178		
Molasses, blackstrap, 1 tbsp	172	Pasteurized process American cheese food, 2 oz	323
Beet greens, 1 cup	165	Provolone cheese, 1.5 oz	321
Spinach, cooked from frozen, cup	146	Mozzarella cheese, part-skim, 1.5 oz	311
Soybeans, green, cooked, cup	130	Cheddar cheese, 1.5 oz	307
Turnip greens, cooked from frozen, cup	124	Fat-free (skim) milk, 1 cup	306
Ocean perch, Atlantic, cooked, 3 oz	116	Muenster cheese, 1.5 oz	305
Oatmeal, instant, fortified, 1 packet	99–110	1% low-fat milk, 1 cup	290
White beans, canned, cup	96	Low-fat (1%) chocolate milk, 1 cup	288
Kale, cooked from frozen, cup	90	2% reduced-fat milk	285
Okra, cooked from frozen, cup	88	Buttermilk, low-fat, 1 cup	284
Soybeans, mature, cooked, cup	88	Chocolate milk, 1 cup	280
Blue crab, canned, 3 oz	86	Whole milk, 1 cup	276
Beet greens, cooked from fresh, 1/2 cup	82	Yogurt, plain, whole milk, 1 cup	275
Pak-choi, Chinese cabbage, cooked from fresh, cup	79	Ricotta cheese, whole milk, 1 cup	255
Clams, canned, 3 oz	78	Mozzarella cheese, whole milk, 1.5 oz	215
Dandelion greens, cooked from fresh, cup	74	Feta cheese, 1.5 oz	210
Rainbow trout, farmed, cooked, 3 oz	73		

[a] Calcium sulfate and magnesium chloride.

Data sources: US Department of Health and Human Services. Dietary guidelines for Americans, 2005: appendix B-5. Available at: www.health.gov/dietaryguidelines/dga2005/document/html/AppendixB.htm. Accessed May 5, 2009; and University of Michigan Health System. Calcium and vitamin D: patient education handout associated with UMHS clinical care guideline. Available at: www.med.umich.edu/1libr/guides/calcium.htm. Accessed May 17, 2009.

Table 13.2
Calcium and vitamin D supplements

Preparation	Elemental Calcium per Tablet, mg	Vitamin D per Tablet, IU	Relative Cost (per Tablet), $[a]
Calcium carbonate			
Caltrate 600-D	600	400	0.12
Viactiv soft chews	500	200	0.13
Nature's Bounty calcium 600 plus vitamin D	600	125	0.08
Rite Aid calcium soft chews, 500 mg, plus vitamins D and K	500	100	0.09
Nature Made calcium 600	600	200	0.10
Os-Cal + D	500	200	0.14
Tums Ultra 1000	1000	—	0.06
CVS calcium 500 tablets with vitamin D	500	200	0.07
Calcium citrate			
Rite Aid calcium citrate plus vitamin D	315	200	0.06
Citracal calcium citrate caplets plus D	315	200	0.10
Calcium complex (carbonate, lactate, gluconate)	150	100	0.08
Calcium phosphate			
Posture-D	600	125	0.18

[a] Relative cost per tablet was calculated from search of multiple internet pharmacy websites (eg, www.drugstore.com, www.cvs.com, and www.riteaid.com).

Table 13.3
Dietary sources of iron

Source	Serving Size	Total Iron per Serving, mg[a]
Meats		
Liver, giblets, organ meats	3 oz	5.2–9.9
Beef	3 oz	2.0–3.1
Pork (excluding loin chop)	3 oz	1.2–1.3
Lamb	3 oz	1.8–2.3
Poultry/fowl		
Chicken	3 oz	0.9–1.1
Turkey	3 oz	1.3–2.2
Duck	3 oz	2.3
Fish		
Shrimp	3 oz	2.3–2.6
Tuna, light meat, canned	3 oz	1.3
Clams, canned	3 oz	23.8
Oysters, wild, cooked	3 oz	10.2
Oysters, raw	6 oysters	4.8
Sardines, canned, in oil	3 oz	2.5
Cereals		
Corn flakes, dry	1 cup	8.7
Raisin bran, dry	1 cup	5.0
Oatmeal, instant, fortified	1 cup	4.2
Fruits/fruit juices		
Apricots, dried	7 halves	1.2
Prune juice	¾ cup	2.3
Vegetables/beans/legumes		
Potato, baked, with skin	1 medium	2.8
Peas, cooked	½ cup	1.3
Spinach, cooked from fresh	½ cup	3.2
Spinach, raw	1 cup	1.6
Soybeans, mature, cooked	½ cup	4.4
Soybeans, green, cooked	½ cup	2.2
White beans, canned	½ cup	3.9
Lentils, cooked	½ cup	3.3
Kidney beans		
Canned	½ cup	1.6
Cooked	½ cup	2.6
Chickpeas		
Canned	½ cup	1.6
Cooked	½ cup	2.4
Lima beans, cooked	½ cup	2.2
Navy beans, cooked	½ cup	2.1
Refried beans	½ cup	2.1
Tomato paste	¼ cup	2.0
Tomato puree	½ cup	2.2

(*Continued*)

Table 13.3
(Continued)

Source	Serving Size	Total Iron per Serving, mg[a]
Miscellaneous foods		
Blackstrap molasses	1 tbsp	3.5
Pumpkin or squash seed kernels, roasted	1 oz	4.2
Tofu, raw, regular	2.5 × 2.75 × 1 in	6.4

Only food sources with ≥1.0 mg of iron per serving are listed.
[a] Available iron will be less.
Data sources: US Department of Health and Human Services. Dietary guidelines for Americans, 2005: appendix B-3. Available at: www.health.gov/dietaryguidelines/dga2005/document/html/AppendixB.htm. Accessed May 4, 2009; and USDA Nutrient Database for Standard Reference, Release 11-1, 1997.

See color insert for figures 13.1–13.2, food pyramids.

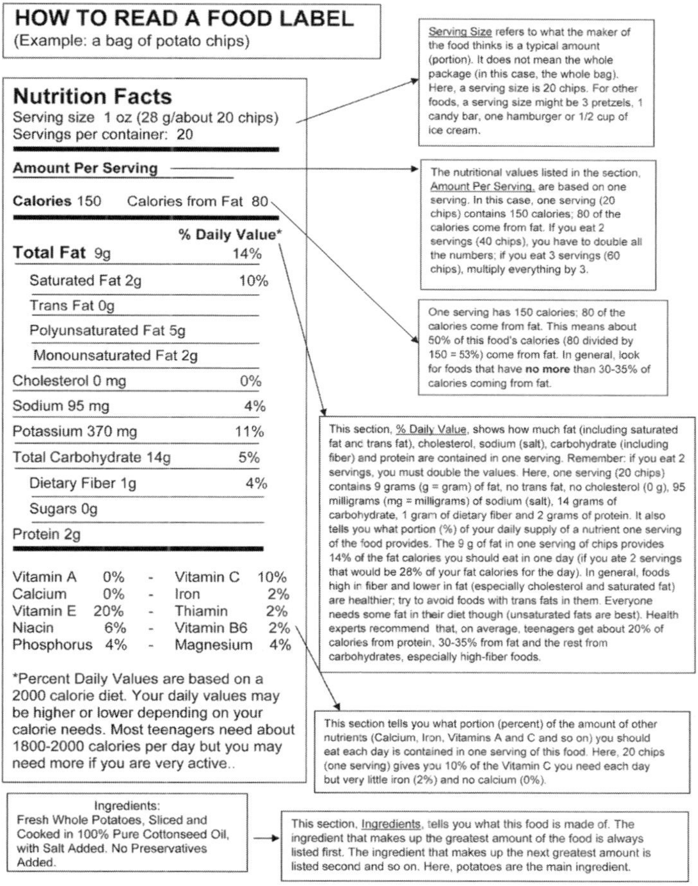

Fig 13.3. How to read a food label.

Adolesc Med 20 (2009) 794–822

14. Rheumatology and Miscellaneous Clinical Conditions

I. CAUSES OF MUSCULOSKELETAL COMPLAINTS IN ADOLESCENTS

Table 14.1
Causes of musculoskeletal complaints in adolescents

Category	Selected Conditions
Rheumatic diseases	Chronic juvenile arthritis
	Systemic arthritis
	Juvenile ankylosing spondylitis
	Psoriatic arthritis
	Juvenile dermatomyositis
	Scleroderma
Chronic pain syndromes	Fibromyalgia
	Hypermobility syndrome
	Complex regional pain syndrome
Vasculitis	Henoch-Schonlein purpura
	Kawasaki disease
Infections	Disseminated gonococcal infection and arthritis
	Lyme arthritis
	Postinfectious reactive arthritis
	Viral synovitis and arthritis
	Bacterial osteomyelitis
Overuse syndromes	Stress injury of the distal physis of radius
	Stress injury of proximal physis of the humerus
	Juvenile osteochondritis dissecans
	Osgood-Schlatter disease
	Stress fractures
	Tendonitis
	Bursitis
	Lateral epicondylitis
	Idiopathic anterior knee pain

(Continued)

Margaret J. Blythe, MD
E-mail address: mblythe@iupui.edu

 ISSN 1934-4287

Table 14.1
(Continued)

Category	Selected Conditions
Orthopedic conditions	Legg-Calve-Perthes disease
	Slipped capital femoral epiphysis
	Scheuermann disease
Systemic disease	Rickets
	Osteoporosis
	Sickle cell disease
	Hemophilia
	Diabetes mellitus
	Sphingolipidoses
Neoplasms of bone	
Benign	Osteoid osteoma
	Osteoblastoma
Malignant	Osteosarcoma
	Chondrosarcoma
	Ewing's sarcoma
Psychosomatic	Various somatic complaints and psychosomatic disorders
Peripheral neuropathy	Median nerve (carpal tunnel syndrome) compressive neuropathy
Muscle disease	Muscular dystrophies
	Myopathies
Acute trauma	Soft tissue injuries
	Bone fractures
	Ligament sprains
	Intraarticular cartilage injuries

From Patel DR. Musculoskeletal diagnosis. *Adolesc Med.* 2007;18(1):8.

II. ACUTE RHEUMATIC FEVER

- "Exaggerated" autoimmune response to infection with group A streptococcus in a susceptible host
- Repeated infection is necessary to prime the immune response before the first episode of acute rheumatic fever (ARF) occurs
- Structural and immunologic similarities between streptococcal M protein and myosin (both α-helical, coiled-coil molecules) seem essential to the development of rheumatic carditis
- Major clinical and public health effects derive from the long-term damage to heart valves (ie, rheumatic heart disease [RHD])
- ARF and RHD are largely restricted to developing countries and some poor, mainly indigenous populations of wealthy countries

- Most recent ARF incidence data for industrialized country came from the nonindigenous population of New Zealand (incidence: <10 in 100 000)
- More than half of the patients who have no evidence of carditis during episodes of Sydenham chorea subsequently develop RHD
- If clinical diagnosis of carditis had been relied on, ~90% of echocardiographically detected cases would have been missed
- Recommend that either carbamazepine or valproic acid be used for Sydenham chorea
- Intravenous immunoglobulin seems to have no effect on cardiac outcome in ARF
- Course of antibiotics started within 9 days of the onset of a sore throat caused by group A streptococcus prevents most cases of ARF
- Differential for polyarthritis and fever: septic arthritis, connective tissue and other autoimmune disease, viral arthropathy, reactive arthropathy, Lyme disease, sickle cell anemia infective endocarditis, leukemia, gout
- Differential for carditis: innocent murmur, mitral valve prolapse, congenital heart disease, infective endocarditis, hypertrophic cardiomyopathy, myocarditis, pericarditis

Reference: Carapetis JR, McDonald M, Wilson NJ. Acute rheumatic fever. *Lancet*. 2005;366(9480): 155–168.

Jones Criteria

- 2 major or 1 major and 2 minor manifestations must be present, plus evidence of antecedent group A streptococcus infection
- Chorea and indolent carditis do not require evidence of antecedent group A streptococcus infection
- Recurrent episode requires only 1 major or several minor manifestations, plus evidence of antecedent group A streptococcus infection

Major Manifestations

- Carditis (mitral valve involvement most common)
- Polyarthritis
- Chorea
- Erythema marginatum
- Subcutaneous nodules

Minor Manifestations

- Arthralgia
- Fever
- Raised erythrocyte sedimentation rate (ESR) or C-reactive protein (CRP) concentrations
- Prolonged PR interval on electrocardiogram

Evidence of Antecedent Group A Streptococcus Infection

- Positive throat culture or rapid antigen test for group A streptococcus.
- Raised or rising streptococcal antibody titer.

Reference: Special Writing Group of the Committee on Rheumatic Fever, Endocarditis, and Kawasaki Disease of the Council on Cardiovascular Disease in the Young of the American Heart Association. Guidelines for the diagnosis of rheumatic fever. Jones Criteria, 1992 update [published correction appears in *JAMA*. 1993;269(4):476]. *JAMA*. 1992;268(15):2069–2073.

World Health Organization Criteria (2002–2003)

Chorea and indolent carditis do not require evidence of antecedent group A streptococcus infection.

First Episode

- As per Jones criteria

Recurrent Episode

- In a patient without established RHD: as per first episode
- In a patient with established RHD: requires 2 minor manifestations, plus evidence of antecedent group A streptococcus infection
- Evidence of antecedent group A streptococcus infection as per Jones criteria, but with addition of recent scarlet fever

Reference: World Health Organization. *Rheumatic Fever and Rheumatic Heart Disease: Report of a WHO Expert Consultation*. Geneva, Switzerland: World Health Organization; 2004. WHO technical report series 923. Available at: www.who.int/cardiovascular_diseases/resources/en/cvd_trs923.pdf. Accessed June 26, 2009.

Table 14.2
Recommended antibiotic regimens for primary and secondary prophylaxis of ARF

	Dose	Frequency	Duration
Primary prophylaxis (treatment of group A streptococcal pharyngitis)			
Benzathine penicillin G	1.2 million units intramuscularly (600 000 units if body weight is <27 kg)	Single dose	Single dose
Phenoxymethylpenicillin (penicillin V) or amoxicillin	Children: 250 mg orally; adolescents and adults: 500 mg orally	2–3 times daily	10 d
First-generation cephalosporins or erythromycin (only if allergic to penicillin[a])	Orally: dose varies with drug and formulation	Varies with agent and formulation	10 d
Secondary prophylaxis (long-term preventive therapy for patients with a history of ARF or RHD)			
Benzathine penicillin G	1.2 million units intramuscularly (600 000 units if body weight is <20 kg)	Every 3–4 wk	5 y since last episode or age 18 y (whichever is longer), 10 y since last episode or age 25 y (whichever is longer) if mild or healed carditis; lifelong if more severe carditis or valve surgery[b]
Phenoxymethylpenicillin (penicillin V) Erythromycin	250 mg orally	Twice daily	

[a] Small portions of patients allergic to penicillin, allergic to cephalosporins.
[b] World Health Organization. Rheumatic fever and rheumatic disease: report of WHO Expert Consultation, Geneva, 29 October–1 November 2001. Geneva: Who; 2001.
Adapted from Carapetis JR, McDonald M, Wilson NJ. Acute rheumatic fever. *Lancet.* 2005;366(9480):155–168, with permission from Elsevier.

III. LABORATORY TESTS FOR CONNECTIVE TISSUE DISEASE

Estimated Sedimentation Rate (ESR)

- Measures distance that anticoagulated red blood cells (RBCs) settle in a sedimentation tube for 1 hour
- Measures (mm/hour) the distance from the top of the blood column to the top of the RBC layer as gravity causes RBCs to settle

- Upward displacement of plasma counterbalances the downward force
- Plasma proteins directly proportional to the protein's molecular weight and degree of asymmetry have greatest effect on RBC aggregation
- As fibrinogen increases, as in various inflammatory states, the ESR increases concomitantly; for this reason, ESR is considered an indirect measure of fibrinogen
- ESR tends to rise slowly after the onset of inflammation and can stay elevated for days to weeks after resolution of the inflammation
- Noninflammatory conditions with abnormal RBCs and anemia have less of a tendency to form rouleaux, thereby producing lower ESRs

C-Reactive Protein (CRP)

- Acute-phase reactant synthesized in the liver primarily in response to cytokines interleukin 1-β, interleukin 6, and tumor necrosis factor α
- CRP functions by binding directly to microorganisms as an opsonin for complement, activating neutrophils and inhibiting platelet aggregation
- Concentration of CRP may increase several hundred–fold within 4 to 6 hours of onset of inflammation and peaks between 36 and 50 hours
- Concentrations decline rapidly because of its short 4- to 7-hour half-life; in general, CRP both rises and normalizes faster than does the ESR

Because CRP is a directly measured plasma protein, it is unaffected by the external conditions that alter ESR values.

Reference: Batlivala SP. Focus on diagnosis: the erythrocyte sedimentation rate and the C-reactive protein test. *Pediatr Rev*. 2009;30(2):72–74.

Selected Conditions Other Than Autoimmune Disease in Which Antinuclear Antibodies May Be Positive

Infections

- Epstein-Barr virus
- Tuberculosis
- Subacute bacterial endocarditis
- Malaria
- Hepatitis C

Drugs

- Anticonvulsants
- Procainamide
- Hydralazine
- Isoniazid
- Minocycline
- Oral contraceptives
- Penicillamine

- Quinidine
- Chlorpromazine
- Methyldopa

Reference: Wagner-Weiner L. Laboratory evaluation of children with rheumatic disease. *Pediatr Ann.* 2002;31(6):366. Reprinted by permission of Slack, Inc.

IV. JUVENILE IDIOPATHIC ARTHRITIS

Classification Criteria for Juvenile Idiopathic Arthritis (JIA)

- Objective arthritis in ≥1 joint for ≥2 weeks (arthritis: swelling of a joint or limitation of motion with heat, pain, or tenderness)
- Onset before the age of 17 years
- Male/female ratio 1:1
- Exclusion of other causes of joint inflammation

Classification Criteria for JIA

- Systemic
- Oligoarthritis: persistent or extended
- Polyarthritis (rheumatoid factor [RF]-negative)
- Polyarthritis (RF-positive)
- Psoriatic arthritis
- Enthesitis-related arthritis
- Undifferentiated arthritis: fits no other category or fits >1 category

Adapted from Siegel DM. Chronic arthritis in adolescence. *Adolesc Med.* 2007;18(1):48.

Differential in Adolescents

- Infections: bacterial arthritis (gonococcal infection), osteomyelitis, chronic infections of drug abusers, Lyme disease, postinfectious response from viruses (Epstein-Barr, parvovirus B19, HIV, hepatitis B, hepatitis C), bacteria (eg, salmonella, *Campylobacter*, streptococci)
- Malignancies, localized as well as systemic
- Noninflammatory and orthopedic conditions: trauma, hypermobility, spondylolisthesis, slipped capital femoral epiphysis, patellofemoral syndrome
- Pain syndromes: fibromyalgia, reflex sympathetic dystrophy, psychogenic pain syndrome
- Systemic inflammatory conditions: inflammatory bowel disease, erythema nodosum, drug reactions, Behçet disease, sarcoidosis
- Immunodeficiencies: HIV infection
- Other rheumatic disease: all rheumatic diseases present with polyarteritis nodosa, rheumatoid arthritis, Raynaud phenomenon rare in JIA or spondyloarthropathies

- Laboratory studies: joint fluid, elevated ESR and CRP, RF, antinuclear antibody (ANA)

Three Types of JIA

Systemic

May begin at any age with equal distribution between males and females and joint destruction; presents as 10% of the arthritis in children.

- Fevers
- Rheumatoid rash, salmon colored
- Polyserositis: pericarditis, pleuritis, peritonitis
- Lymphadenopathy and hepatosplenomegaly
- Arthritis
- Laboratory test results: anemia, elevated white cell counts, elevated ESR and CRP, negative RF, and negative ANA

Polyarticular

≥5 joints in the absence of systemic signs and divided into RF-negative and RF-positive disease; presents as 30% of cases of arthritis.

RF-Negative (Type 1)

- Arthritis for >6 weeks; usually ≥5 joints in first 6 months; less symmetric and erosive
- Younger children usually under the age of 6 years, with girls more than boys (3:1)
- Most joints can be involved, including small joints in the hands and feet
- Less often associated with iridocyclitis or uveitis (insidious onset, diagnosed only by slit-lamp examination) (5%)
- Laboratory test results: elevated ESR and CRP, usually negative RF (~10%), positive ANA in 40% to 50%

RF-Positive (Type 2)

- Arthritis for >6 weeks; usually ≥5 joints in first 6 months; symmetric and erosive
- Usually begins in older children as adolescents, affecting girls more than boys
- Adult disease beginning in childhood/adolescence
- Associated with rheumatoid nodules in 50%, vasculitis, lung disease, Felty syndrome
- Deformities similar as adults including ulnar deviations of metacarpophalangeal joints, laxity of ligaments
- Laboratory test results: elevated ESR and CRP, positive RF, 50% positive ANA

Pauciarticular

Oligoarthritis affects <5 joints in the absence of systemic signs; presents as 60% of cases.

Type 1

- Affects young children at a mean of 2 years of age and by 5 years of age and predominantly females (5:1 ratio)
- Knees and ankles are the predominant joints involved, although wrists, elbows, cervical spine, and occasionally finger joints can be involved; 1 to 4 joints in first 6 months
- Associated with flexion contractures and limb-length discrepancy
- Associated with iridocyclitis, uveitis in 5% to 15% (correlates with positive ANA), must treat to avoid cataracts
- Laboratory test results: elevated ESR and CRP, negative RF, positive ANA in 60% to 90%

Type 2

- Predominantly affects older children, usually older than 8 years
- Affected joints predominantly lower extremity, including hips, knees, ankle, and tarsal joints
- Enthesitis: inflammation of tendons is common (eg, Achilles, patellar, and plantar fasciitis); often involves attachments of ligaments as well as the spine; more often have joint pain without obvious swelling and may complain of back pain and stiffness
- Laboratory test results: associated with being HLA-B27–positive, elevated ESR and CRP, RF negative, ANA negative

References: American College of Rheumatology. Arthritis in children. Available at: www.rheumatology.org/public/factsheets/diseases_and_conditions/juvenilearthritis.asp?aud=pat. Accessed June 4, 2009; Cassidy JT. Rheumatic diseases of childhood: section XIII—connective tissue diseases. In: McMillian JA, Feigin RD, DeAngelis CD, Jones MD, eds. *Oski's Pediatrics*. 4th ed. Philadelphia, PA: Lippincott, Williams & Wilkins; 2006:2537–2557; and American College of Rheumatology. Patient education: diseases and conditions. Available at: www.rheumatology.org/public/factsheets/diseases_and_conditions/index.asp. Accessed June 4, 2009.

V. SPONDYLOARTHROPATHIES

Shared features: inflammation of joints of axial skeleton, enthesitis, high frequency of HLA-27 in patient and family; HLA-27 not found in JIA, nor is enthesitis; onset primarily in adolescence.

Classic Juvenile Ankylosing Spondylitis

Description and Epidemiology

- Most common in teenaged and young adult males with symptoms of lower back pain and stiffness, limitation of lumbosacral mobility

- Physical signs include sacroiliac joint and lower lumber back tenderness and may progress up the spine
- Joint pain may occur with swelling and stiffness but more often affects axial skeleton, sites at which tendons and muscles attach to bone (enthuses), and sacroiliac joints
- 20% develop iritis (acute onset of erythema, pain, photophobia)
- Other sites: eyes (iritis), aorta valve (aortic valve insufficiency), aorta (aortitis)
- Laboratory test results: associated with being HLA-B27–positive, elevated ESR and CRP, RF negative, and ANA negative
- Radiologic results: sacroiliitis (erosions, pseudowidening, and sclerosis)

Reactive Arthritis (Reiter Syndrome)

Description

- Reactive asymmetric monoarthritis or oligoarthritis of often lower extremities
- Other possible involvements: conjunctivitis (most common 30%), urethritis, skin rash (balanitis circinata [20%–40%], keratodermal blennorrhagica [5%–10%]); musculoskeletal, cardiovascular (aortitis [1%–2%])
- Manifests as a postinfection reactive arthritis from a variety of organisms
  - Genitourinary (*Chlamydia trachomatis, Chlamydia psittaci, Chlamydia pneumoniae, Mycoplasma genitalium, Mycoplasma fermentans, Ureaplasma urealyticum*)
  - Gastrointestinal (*Campylobacter jejuni, Campylobacter fetus, Clostridia difficile, Escherichia coli, Giardia, Entamoeba histolytica, Salmonella enteriditis, Salmonella heidelberg, Salmonella paratyphi, Salmonella typhimurium, Shigella flexneri, Yersinia enterocolitica, Yersinia pseudotuberculosis*)
  - Other (*Cryptosporidium, Streptococcus pyogenes*)
- Laboratory test results: associated with being HLA-B27–positive, elevated ESR and CRP, RF negative, and ANA negative.

Enteropathic Arthritis

Description

- Associated with large joint involvement such as hip, knee, and wrists in 10% to 20%
- Laboratory test results: associated with being HLA-B27–positive, elevated ESR and CRP, RF negative, and ANA negative; associated with anti–*Saccharomyces cerevisiae* mannan antibodies test and perinuclear staining antineutrophil cytoplasmic antibody

Psoriatic Arthritis

Description

- Inflammatory, asymmetric oligoarthritis with involvement of distal joints
- Other sites: nails, skin
- Laboratory test results: associated with negative RF

Reference: Kim PS, Klausmeier TL, Orr DP. Reactive arthritis: a review. *J Adolesc Health*. 2009;44(4):309–315. American College of Rheumatology. Reactive arthritis. Available at: www.rheumatology.org/public/factsheets/diseases·and·conditions/reactivearthritis.asp?aud·pat. Accessed June 8, 2009.

VI. SYSTEMIC LUPUS ERYTHEMATOSUS (SEE TABLE 14.3)

Pathogenesis, Epidemiology, and Presentation

- Unknown but genetic susceptibility and environmental factors lead to disease
- Immune-complex vasculitis with fibrinoid necrosis such as basic inflammatory lesion
- May occur at any age but after 5 years of age, more common in adolescence, female/male ratio of 8:1
- Diagnosis usually made within 6 months
- Unpredictable clinical presentation with multisystem autoimmune disease, which may include rash, joint complaints, renal abnormalities, hematologic abnormalities, or central nervous system problems

References: American College of Rheumatology. The 1982 revised criteria for classification of systemic lupus erythematosus. Available at: www.rheumatology.org/publications/classification/SLE/sle.asp?aud=mem. Accessed June 4, 2009; and American College of Rheumatology. Systemic lupus erythematosus (lupus). Available at: www.rheumatology.org/public/factsheets/diseases_and_conditions/lupus.asp?aud=pat. Accessed June 4, 2009.

VII. DERMATOMYOSITIS/POLYMYOSITIS

Description

- Patients with dermatomyositis have a skin rash preceding or accompanying a progressive, symmetrical weakness of the proximal limbs and anterior flexor muscles. In some cases distal muscles, such as those in the forearms and around the ankles and wrists, become affected as the disease progresses.
- Patients with polymyositis have the weakness and no rash

Diagnostic Criteria

- Characteristic dermatitis of eyelids, metacarpophalangeal, and proximal interphalangeal joints, elbows, knees, and medial malleoli
- Symmetrical proximal muscle weakness

Table 14.3
1982 revised criteria for the classification of systemic lupus erythematosus

Criterion	Definition
Malar rash	Flat or raised erythremic rash sparing nasolabial folds
Discoid rash	Erythematous raised patches with scaling/follicular plugging
Photosensitivity	Skin rash caused by unusual reaction to sunlight
Oral ulcers	Painless oral/nasopharyngeal ulcerations
Arthritis	Nonerosive arthritis involving ≥2 peripheral joints; characterized by tenderness, swelling, or effusion
Serositis	Pleuritis: history of pleuritic pain and/or rubbing heard by provider and/or evidence of pleural effusion; or
	Pericarditis, documented by electrocardiogram and/or rub and/or evidence of pericardial effusion
Renal disorder	Persistent proteinuria: >0.5 g/d or >3 if quantitation not performed; or
	Cellular casts: may be red cell, hemoglobin, granular, tubular, or mixed
Neurologic disorder	Seizures, in the absence of other diagnoses; or
	Psychosis, in the absence of other diagnoses
Hematologic disorder	Cytopenia
Immunologic disorder	Antibodies to native DNA; or
	Antibodies to Sm nuclear antigen;
	Biological false-positive test for syphilis
Antinuclear antibody	Abnormal titer in the absence of drugs known to be associated with "drug-induced lupus" syndrome

Four or more of the 11 criteria provide a sensitivity of 96% and a specificity of 96% for systemic lupus erythematosus.

Data sources: Tan EM, Cohen AS, Fries JF, et al. The 1982 revised criteria for the classification of systemic lupus erythematosus. *Arthritis Rheum.* 1982;25(11):1271–1277; Hochberg MC. Updating the American College of Rheumatology revised criteria for the classification of systemic lupus erythematosus. *Arthritis Rheum.* 1997;40(9):1725; and Cassidy JT. Rheumatic disease of childhood. In: McMillian JA, Feigin RD, DeAngelis, Jones MD, eds. *Oski's Pediatrics.* 4th ed. Philadelphia, PA: Lippincott, Williams & Wilkins; 2006:2537–2557.

Adapted from American College of Rheumatology. The 1982 revised criteria for classification of systemic lupus erythematosus. Available at: www.rheumatology.org/publications/classification/SLE/sle.asp?aud=mem. Accessed June 4, 2009.

- Elevated muscle-derived enzyme levels
- Muscle histology on biopsy confirming inflammatory myositis
- Electromyographic evidence of myopathy and denervation

Clinical Features

Two modes of muscle presentation.

Mode 1

- Onset of fatigue, weakness, and rash
- Arthralgias, myalgias, muscle weakness

Mode 2

- Acute onset with fever, muscle tenderness, and weakness
- Proximal muscles commonly affected, with shoulder and hip girdle weakness; weakness of neck flexors not uncommon
- Oropharyngeal muscle weakness with nasal voice, dysphagia, and difficulty swallowing
- Characteristic rash
    - Heliotrope sign: violaceous suffusion of eyelid
    - Gottron sign: erythematous scaly papules associated with an atrophic, hyperkeratotic rash over the dorsa of the interphalangeal joints, elbows, knees
    - Shawl sign: erythema over the sun-exposed areas of the back and chest
    - Nail-bed capillary changes
- Other findings: calcinosis on pressure points, gastrointestinal complications secondary to small vessel disease, myocarditis, and conduction defects
- Laboratory test results: abnormal muscle-derived enzymes (creatinine phosphokinase, aminotransferases, aldolase; ANAs are positive in up to 60%; electromyography reveals characteristic pattern of muscle irritability; muscle histopathology reveals characteristic inflammatory changes; myositis-specific antibodies

References: Hom C, Ilowite NT. Other rheumatic diseases in adolescence: dermatomyositis, scleroderma, overlap syndromes, systemic vasculitis, and panniculitis. *Adolesc Med.* 1998;9(1):69–83, vi; Bohan A, Peter JB. Polymyositis and dermatomyositis (first of two parts). *N Engl J Med.* 1975;292(7):344–347; and Cassidy JT. Rheumatic diseases of childhood: section XIII—connective tissue diseases. In: McMillian JA, Feigin RD, DeAngelis CD, Jones MD, eds. *Oski's Pediatrics.* 4th ed. Philadelphia, PA: Lippincott, Williams & Wilkins; 2006:2537–2557.

VIII. SCLERODERMA

Diagnosis

Progressive thickening and fibrosis of skin in localized disease of skin and involvement of vessels and organs in the systemic form of scleroderma.

Clinical Presentations

Localized Scleroderma

- Confined to skin, self-limited, resolves in 3 to 4 years
- Skin lesions take the form of morphea, linear scleroderma, or en coup de sabre (scleroderma of scalp or face)
  - Morphea: erythematous lesions on trunk, legs; lesions become firm, waxy with atrophy of skin; may result in joint contractures with disfigurement
  - Linear scleroderma: asymptomatic linear area of erythema on single extremity; induration and thickening of skin; binding underlying tissues may result in joint contracture and asymmetrical growth of limb
  - En coup de saber: scleroderma of scalp or face

Systemic Scleroderma (SS)

- Single major criterion for SS: sclerodermatous skin change proximal to the metacarpophalangeal joints
- Minor criteria: sclerodactyly, digital pitting scars, and even loss of digits with bibasilar pulmonary fibrosis
- CREST syndrome: limited cutaneous SS
  - Involvement of hands and lower forearms; edema, thickening, and loss of skin elasticity, proximal to the elbow
  - Tightening of skin results in tapered fingers, pinched nose, smoother facies
  - Contractures occur with thickening of skin, generalized hyperpigmentation with vitiligo, telangiectasia, and calcium deposition
  - Multisystem involvement (gastrointestinal, pulmonary, cardiac, and renal) because of local fibrosis and vascular involvement
  - 90% of patients with SS have Raynaud phenomena

References: American College of Rheumatology. 1980 criteria for the classification of systemic sclerosis. Available at: www.rheumatology.org/publications/classification/systsclr.asp?aud=mem. Accessed June 8, 2009; Hom C, Ilowite NT. Other rheumatic diseases in adolescence: dermatomyositis, scleroderma, overlap syndromes, systemic vasculitis, and panniculitis. *Adolesc Med.* 1998;9(1):69–83, vi; and American College of Rheumatology. Scleroderma (systemic sclerosis). Available at: www.rheumatology.org/public/factsheets/diseases_and_conditions/scleroderma.asp?aud=pat. Accessed June 8, 2009.

IX. VASCULITIS SYNDROMES

Henoch-Schonlein Vasculitis: Polyarteritis

- Necrotizing arteritis of small and medium-sized muscular arteries affecting multiple organ systems
- Diagnosis confirmed by demonstration of typical angiographic appearance/histology
- Of the 10 criteria proposed by the American College of Rheumatology in 1990, $\geq$3 are required for diagnosis and include:
  - Weight loss >4 lb
  - Livedo reticularis

- Testicular pain or tenderness
- Myalgias, weakness, or leg tenderness
- Mononeuropathy or polyneuropathy
- Diastolic blood pressure >90 mm Hg
- Elevated serum urea nitrogen
- Hepatitis B infection
- Arteriographic abnormality
- Biopsy of a small or medium-sized artery demonstrating polymorphonuclear cell infiltrate

- Diagnostic test results: elevated acute-phase reactants
- Etiology: evidence of immune complex deposition against surface endothelial antigens

Adapted from Lightfoot RW Jr, Michel BA, Bloch DA, et al. The American College of Rheumatology 1990 criteria for the classification of polyarteritis nodosa. *Arthritis Rheum.* 1990;33(8):1088–1093. Other references: American College of Rheumatology. Vasculitis. Available at: www.rheumatology.org/public/fact sheets/diseases_and_conditions/vasculitis.asp?aud=pat. Accessed June 8, 2009; and Hom C, Ilowite NT. Other rheumatic diseases in adolescence: dermatomyositis, scleroderma, overlap syndromes, systemic vasculitis, and panniculitis. *Adolesc Med.* 1998;9(1):69–83.

Kawasaki Disease

Description

- Inflammatory arthritis of large vessels
- Symptoms: headache, shortness of breath, fevers, arthralgias, and myalgias; night sweats, anorexia, and weight loss; vessel pain and tenderness; ischemic symptoms may be absent in younger patients with only the prominent systemic symptoms; different patterns of vessel involvement have been described
- Diagnostic test results: elevation of acute phase reactants, normocytic anemia, but unusual to have elevated ANA; use MRI and/or ultrasound of vessels to diagnose

Panniculitis: Erythema Nodosum

Etiology

- Inflammatory disease of the subcutaneous fat tissue associated with systemic inflammation
- Associated with β-hemolytic streptococcal infection, tuberculosis, histoplasmosis, coccidioidomycosis, and leprosy
- Associated with use of sulfonamides and oral contraceptives
- Associated with sarcoid and inflammatory bowel disease

Clinical Appearance

- Erythematous, indurated, tender, and heal without scarring
- Lesions may be associated with malaise, fatigue, and fever

Reference: Hom C, Ilowite NT. Other rheumatic diseases in adolescence: dermatomyositis, scleroderma, overlap syndromes, systemic vasculitis, and panniculitis. *Adolesc Med.* 1998;9(1):69–83.

X. CHRONIC PAIN SYNDROMES

Fibromyalgia

- Etiology: unknown
- Epidemiology: 80% to 90% female and white; peak age at diagnosis: adolescence to midadulthood
- Description
  - Widespread musculoskeletal pain not associated with arthritis
  - Fatigue
  - Specific areas of soft tissue point tenderness on physical examination
  - Symptoms present for at least 3 months
- Pathophysiology: disturbed sleep or nonrestorative sleep
- Diagnosis: history of widespread pain, including
  - Left side of body
  - Right side of body
  - Above the waist
  - Below the waist
  - Axial skeletal pain (eg, cervical, anterior chest, thoracic spine, or low back)
  - Pain in 11 of 18 tender point sites on digital palpation (See figures 14.1 and 14.2)

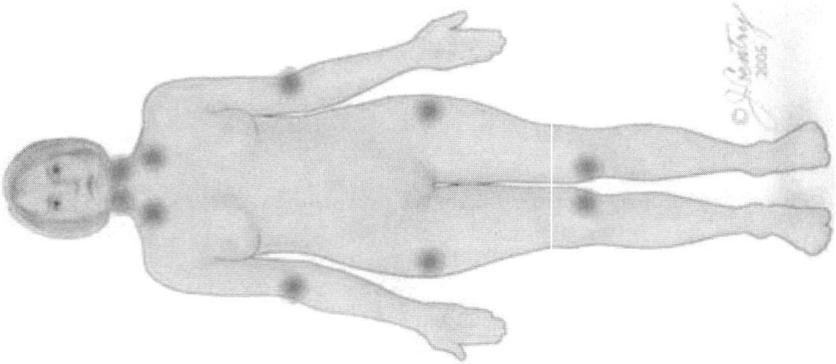

Fig 14.1. Point sites of tenderness for fibromyalgia–anterior. (Reproduced with permission from American College of Rheumatology. Fibromyalgia. Available at: www.rheumatology.org/public/factsheets/diseases_and_conditions/fibromyalgia.asp?aud=pat. Accessed June 8, 2009).

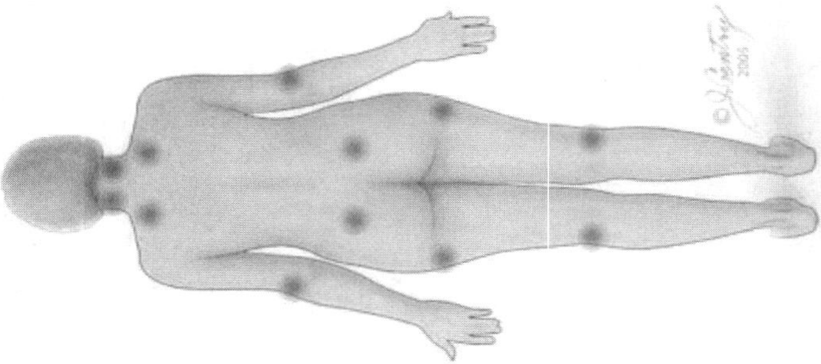

Fig 14.2. Point sites of tenderness for fibromyalgia–posterior. (Reproduced with permission from American College of Rheumatology. Fibromyalgia. Available at: www.rheumatology.org/public/factsheets/diseases_and_conditions/fibromyalgia.asp?aud_pat. Accessed June 8, 2009).

Clinical Presentation

Table 14.4
Prevalence of symptoms and signs in adolescents with fibromyalgia syndrome

Symptom/Sign	Percentage of Patients at Initial Presentation	Percentage of Patients Over Time
Sleep disturbance	96	94
Diffuse pain	93	94
Headache	71	82
Fatigue	62	97
Morning stiffness	53	88
Morning fatigue	49	82
Depression	43	61
Subjective swelling[a]	40	59
Irritable bowel	38	46
Dysmenorrhea	36	42
Paresthesias	24	36
Anxiety	22	58
Raynaud phenomenon	13	30

[a] Swelling reported by the patient (typically in the hands and fingers) but not confirmed by physician on physical examination (eg, "My rings are tighter than they used to be"). From Siegel DM. Fibromyalgia syndrome. *Adolesc Health Update*. 2003;15 (2):1–8.

Laboratory Tests

All laboratory test results are normal, including ESR, CRP, negative RF, and negative ANA.

References: Siegel DM. Fibromyalgia syndrome. *Adolesc Health Update*. 2003;15(2):1–8; and American College of Rheumatology. Fibromyalgia. Available at: www.rheumatology.org/public/factsheets/diseases_and_conditions/fibromyalgia.asp?aud=pat. Accessed June 8, 2009.

Chronic Fatigue Syndrome

- Etiology: unknown; consider infectious agents, immune dysfunction, stress, nutritional deficiency, neurally mediated hypotension
- Epidemiology: predominantly white females with average age of 30 years but has presented in teenagers no younger than 12 years
- Description/diagnosis: severe chronic fatigue of ≥6 months' duration with other known medical conditions excluded by conical diagnosis
- Symptoms, which generally predate the fatigue and persist or recur during 6 more consecutive months of illness, include
  - Impairment of short-term memory or concentration
  - Sore throat
  - Tender cervical or axillary lymph nodes
  - Muscle pain

Differential

Table 14.5
Features of fibromyalgia syndrome that help exclude other diagnoses

Diagnosis	Clinical Features Not Seen in FS	Laboratory Results Not Seen in FS
Infectious mononucleosis	Fever	Epstein-Barr viral titers consistent with acute infection
	Enlarged tonsils	
	Adenopathy	
	Hepatosplenomegaly	Elevated LFTs
Chronic Lyme disease	History of tick bite with typical cutaneous eruption (erythema migrans)	Positive Lyme antibody with confirmatory test
	Erythema migrans	
Juvenile arthritis (systemic or polyarticular)	Fever	Elevated ESR
	Rash	Elevated WBC
	Swollen, red, warm joints	Anemia
	Hepatosplenomegaly	
Systemic lupus erythematosus	Fever	Positive ANA
	Rash	Positive anti-dsDNA
	Oral lesions	Positive anti-Smith
	Alopecia	Leukopenia
	Serositis	Anemia
	Renal disease	Thrombocytopenia
Obstructive sleep apnea	Snoring	Diagnostic sleep study
	Apnea	

FS indicates fibromyalgia syndrome; LFTs, liver function tests; WBC, white blood cell count; dsDNA, double-stranded DNA.
From Siegel DM. Fibromyalgia syndrome. *Adolesc Health Update*. 2003;15(2):1–8.

Chronic Fatigue Syndrome (continued)

- Multijoint pain without swelling or redness
- Headaches of a new type, pattern, or severity
- Unrefreshing sleep
- Postexertional malaise lasting for >24 hours

- Other symptoms: irritable bowel; abdominal pain; nausea; diarrhea or bloating; chills and night sweats; brain fog; chest pain; shortness of breath; chronic cough; visual disturbances (blurring, sensitivity to light, eye pain, or dry eyes); allergies or sensitivities to foods, alcohol, odors, chemicals, medications, or noise; difficulty maintaining upright position (orthostatic instability, irregular heartbeat, dizziness, balance problems, or fainting); psychological problems (depression, irritability, mood swings, anxiety, panic attacks); jaw pain; weight loss or gain

- Pathophysiology: disturbed sleep or nonrestorative sleep
- Differential: fibromyalgia, myalgic encephalitis, neurasthenia, multiple chemical sensitivities, chronic mononucleosis; other: hypothyroidism, sleep apnea, narcolepsy, major depressive disorder, bipolar affective disorder, eating disorder, cancer, autoimmune disease, hormonal disorder
- Laboratory tests to consider: alanine aminotransferase, albumin, alkaline phosphatase, serum urea nitrogen, calcium, complete blood count, creatinine, electrolytes, ESR, globulin, glucose, phosphorus, thyrotropin, total protein, transferrin saturation, and urinalysis
- All laboratory test results normal, including ESR, CRP, negative RF, and negative ANA
- Diagnosis: an empirical definition—3 questionnaires are available: Medical Outcomes Study: 36-item Short Form Survey Instrument, Multidimensional Fatigue Inventory, and the Centers for Disease Control and Prevention Symptom Inventory; this approach can be useful in identifying and monitoring response to treatment

References: Centers for Disease Control and Prevention. Chronic fatigue syndrome: healthcare professionals. Available at: www.cdc.gov/cfs/healthcareprofessionals.htm. Accessed June 8, 2009; and Centers for Disease Control and Prevention. Chronic fatigue syndrome: diagnosis. Available at: www.cdc.gov/cfs/cfsdiagnosis HCP.htm. Accessed June 8, 2009.

Reflex Sympathetic Dystrophy

- Etiology: unknown
- Epidemiology: more girls than boys
- Description/diagnosis
  - History of constant pain and increasing disability in a distal extremity exacerbated with even mild use
  - No specific history of injury or trauma
  - Increasing pain with decreasing use results in vicious cycle of limitation
- Pathophysiology: Disturbed sleep or nonrestorative sleep
- Differential: injury, trauma
- Clinical presentation
  - Exquisite and deep pain in extremity exacerbated with any movement
  - Extremity held in bizarre posture with refusal to move it
  - Extremity characteristically tender, swollen, cool, and even mottled (blue/purple discoloration of skin) and even with increased sweating, suggesting autonomic dysfunction
  - Even light touch or passive movement causes extreme pain, often described as burning
  - Inappropriate affect of happiness except when limb is touched or manipulated

- Laboratory test results: radiographs unremarkable; bone scans unremarkable or may show decrease or increase in uptake; Doppler studies may show changes in blood flow; acute phase reactants are all normal

Reference: Cassidy JT. Progress in diagnosis and understanding chronic pain syndromes in children and adolescents. *Adolesc Med*. 1998;9(1):101–114.

OTHER CLINICAL CONDITIONS

Headaches in Adolescence

Table 14.6
Types of headaches most commonly seen in adolescents

Episodic tension-type headache
$<$15 d/mo
Less severe pain compared to migraine
Band-like sensation
No nausea or vomiting
Chronic tension-type headache
Frequent ($\geq$15 d/mo) or daily, sometimes continuous
Less severe pain compared to migraine
Band-like sensation
No nausea or vomiting
Rebound (medication-overuse headache)
Chronic tension-type headache caused by medication overuse ($\geq$3 doses weekly for weeks on end)
Migraine headache
May or may not be preceded by aura
Often a family history of migraine
Variable frequency and severity
Sometimes associated with menses
Severe, pounding or throbbing pain
Intermittent (2–4 times per month, not daily)
Often characterized by pallor
Often accompanied by nausea and/or vomiting
Often causes sensitivity to light and noise
Attacks are typically followed by sleep

Four types of headache are frequently seen in adolescents. Some patients experience $>$1 type of headache, and others will experience combined or mixed headaches. None of these headaches have associated neurologic symptoms or signs. Life-threatening headaches are rare in adolescents.

Adapted from Rothner AD. Headache in adolescence. *Adolesc Health Update*. 2006; 18(2):2.

Table 14.7
Differential diagnosis of headache types most commonly seen in adolescents

Acute generalized	
	Fever
	Systemic infection
	Central nervous system infection
	Toxins (carbon monoxide, amphetamines)
	Trauma
Acute localized	
	Trauma
	Sinusitis with fever
	Otitis
	Pharyngitis
	Temporomandibular joint disorder
Acute recurrent	
	Migraine
	Chronic progressive
	Hydrocephalus
	Neoplasm
	Benign intracranial hypertension (formerly pseudotumor cerebri)
	Trauma
Chronic nonprogressive	
	Episodic tension-type
	Chronic tension-type
	Medication overuse (rebound)
Mixed	
	Combined migraine and tension headaches

Adapted from Rothner AD. Headache in adolescence. *Adolesc Health Update*. 2006;18(2):3.

Table 14.8
Diagnostic criteria for pediatric migraine

Migraine without aura
- A. At least 5 attacks fulfilling criteria B–D (below)
- B. Headache attacks lasting 1–72 h
- C. Headache having at least 2 of the following characteristics
  1. Unilateral location, may be bilateral, frontotemporal (not occipital)
  2. Pulsing quality
  3. Moderate or severe pain intensity
  4. Aggravation by or causing avoidance of routine physical activity (eg, walking, climbing stairs)
- D. During the headache, at least 1 of the following
  1. Nausea or vomiting
  2. Photophobia and phonophobia, which may be inferred from behavior
- E. Not attributed to another disorder

Migraine with aura
- A. At least 2 attacks fulfilling criteria B–D (below)
- B. Aura consisting of at least 1 of the following, but no motor weakness
  1. Fully reversible visual symptoms, including positive features or negative features (eg, flickering lights, spots, or lines)
  2. Fully reversible sensory symptoms, including positive features (ie, pins and needles) or negative features (ie, numbness)
  3. Fully reversible dysphasic speech disturbances
- C. At least 2 of the following
  1. Homonymous visual symptoms or unilateral sensory symptoms
  2. At least 1 aura symptom develops gradually over ≥5 min or different aura symptoms occur in succession over ≥5 min
  3. Each symptom lasts ≥5 min but ≤60 min
- D. Not attributable to another disorder

Headache Classification Subcommittee of the International Headache Society. The International classification of headache disorders. *Cephalal.* 2004;24(suppl 1):1–160. Reprinted with permission from John Wiley and Sons, Ltd.

Table 14.9
A quick checklist for headache history

1. When did your headache(s) start?
2. How often do your headaches occur?
3. Are your headaches occurring more often?
4. Are your headaches becoming more severe?
5. Does anything special bring them on?
6. Can you tell 15 to 30 min before that a headache is coming? How?
7. Where is your pain and what does the pain feel like?
8. Do you have other symptoms with the headache? Nausea or vomiting?
9. Does anything make your headache worse? Better?
10. Do you take anything for your headache? How often?
11. How long does your headache last?
12. Does anyone else in the family have headaches?
13. Are you taking any medications regularly, including over-the-counter medications?
14. How do you feel between your headaches?
15. How many days of school have you missed because of your headaches?
16. What do you think is causing your headaches?

Along with the headache-specific history, the pediatrician should observe the patient along with patient/parent interaction. It is important to ask about depression and anxiety and take into account any mental health problems that might be present.
Adapted from Rothner AD. Evaluation of headaches. In: Winner P, Rothner AD. Headache in Children and Adolescents. Hamilton, Ontario; BC Decker; 2001:7, 21–23 with permission from PMPH-USA, Ltd.

Indications for Additional Testing

From the History

- No family history
- First and worst headache ever
- Onset of new type of headache (<1 months' duration)
- Changes in headache pattern
- Consistently localized or occipital pain
- Pain that awakens the patient
- Pain caused by straining and exertion (eg, sports, bowel movement)
- Pain unrelieved by initial treatments
- Pain with neurologic symptoms or signs
- Vomiting, especially in the morning
- Seizures

From the Physical Examination

- Patient critically ill
- Signs of trauma

Table 14.10
Examples of medications used to treat migraine headaches in adolescents

Therapeutic Purpose	Medication Class	Example	Adolescent Starting Dose
Acute symptomatic	Analgesic	Acetaminophen[a]	325 mg PO Q 4 h
	Analgesic	Ibuprofen[a]	400 mg PO Q 6 h
Abortive	Triptan	Sumatriptan[a]	5 mg nasal spray[b]; 25 mg PO[b,c]
	Triptan	Almotriptan[d]	6.25 mg PO[b,c]
	Triptan	Rizatriptan[d]	5 mg PO[b,c]
	Triptan	Eletriptan[d]	20 mg PO[b,c]
	Triptan	Zolmitriptan[d]	5 mg nasal spray[b]; 2.5 mg PO[b,c]
	Long-acting triptan	Frovatriptan[d]	2.5 mg PO[c,e]
	Long-acting triptan	Naratriptan[d]	1 mg PO[c,e]
	Ergot compound	Dihydroergotamine mesylate[d]	1 spray in each nostril; may repeat once(20–60 min later)
Preventive[f]	Antidepressant	Amitriptyline[g]	5–10 mg PO nightly, titrating up to 20–30 mg nightly
	Anticonvulsant	Divalproex sodium[g]	125 mg PO per d
	Anticonvulsant	Topiramate[g]	25 mg PO per d

- Nuchal rigidity
- Presence of cranial bruits or macrocephaly
- Skin lesions suggesting neurocutaneous syndromes
- Localized tenderness of scalp of skull indicating injury

From the Neurologic Examination

- Abnormal funduscopic findings (eg, retinal hemorrhages, papilledema)
- Abnormal eye movements (eg, nystagmus, sixth-nerve palsy, double vision)
- Decreased or asymmetric muscle strength, tone, bulk
- Gait abnormalities or balance difficulties (ataxia, dysmetria)
- Altered affect or level of consciousness

Need an MRI

- Are the headaches of recent onset (in last month?)
- Are there any neurologic symptoms or signs in additions to the headaches (eg, gait disturbance, seizures)?
- Are these symptoms getting worse over time? Slowly? Quickly?
- Is there an absence of family history of migraine?
- Are there any red flags on the examination? Abnormal vital signs such as blood pressure? Tachycardia? Fever? Significant skin lesions? Neurologic deficits?

Adapted from Rothner AD. Headache in adolescence. *Adolesc Health Update*. 2006;18(2):5–6.

Table 14.10
(Continued)

Usual Dose	Adverse Effects	Comments
650 mg Q 4 h		Maximum: 4 g/d; 15 mg/kg
600 mg Q 6 h	Gastric irritation	Maximum: 3.2 g/d; 10 mg/kg
20 mg nasal spray[b]; 50–100 mg[b,c]	Tingling, hot sensation; feeling of tightness in chest and neck	No more than 2 doses per day and no more than 2 d/wk
12.5 mg[b,c]	As above	As above
10 mg[b,c]	As above	As above
40 mg[b,c]	As above	As above
5 mg nasal spray[b]; 5 mg[b,c]	As above	As above
2.5 mg PO[c,e]	As above	As above
2.5 mg PO[c,e]	As above	As above
1 spray in each nostril; may repeat once (20–60 min later)	Nausea, bad taste, rhinitis	As above
Depending on response and with careful monitoring, up to 1 mg/kg per d	Sedation, weight gain	Not more than 100 mg/d; consider electrocardiogram (see text)
500 mg/d	Tremor, sedation	Not more than 1000 mg/d
100 mg/d	Paresthesia	Not more than 200 mg/d

These are suggested doses; all dosages should be checked with additional sources before prescribing. PO indicates orally; Q, every.

[a] See the American Academy of Neurology practice parameter on effectiveness of ibuprofen, acetaminophen, and nasal sumatriptan for treatment of migraine.

[b] If headache persists or recurs, may repeat dose once 2 hours later.

[c] See American Academy of Neurology practice parameter on lack of data either supporting or refuting use of oral triptan preparations.

[d] No specific recommendation about the use of this drug in American Academy of Neurology practice parameter on treatment.

[e] If headache persists or recurs, may repeat dose once 4 to 6 hours later.

[f] Preventive medications often take 6 to 8 weeks to become effective.

[g] American Academy of Neurology practice parameter on treatment finds insufficient evidence to make any recommendations concerning the use of this drug.

Adapted from Rothner AD. Headache in adolescence. *Adolesc Health Update*. 2006;18(2):7.

Syncope

Differential Diagnosis

Evaluation

- Was there loss of consciousness completely (true syncope or near syncope?)
- Did anything trigger the event?
- What was the duration of loss of consciousness? After regaining consciousness, how long until there was a complete recovery?
- In what position was the patient when he or she lost consciousness?
- Was there a prodrome?
- Did the patient have clonic or tonic/clonic movements? Loss of bowel or bladder control and/or an audible cry before the episode?
- Is there a family history of early sudden death, heart muscle problem, epilepsy migraines, or sleep disorder?

Adapted from Franklin WH. Syncope. *Adolesc Health Update*. 2006;18(3):5.

Table 14.11
Differential diagnosis: syncope

Neurocardiogenic causes
True syncope
Neurocardiogenic syncope
Vasovagal, neurally mediated vasodepressor, micturition, cough, sneeze, trumpet players, weight lifters, defecation, swallow (deglutition), hair-grooming and church syncope (also known as the simple faint or the benign faint), carotid sinus hypersensitivity
Near syncope
Postural orthostatic tachycardia syndrome
Primary cardiac causes
Arrhythmias
Tachyarrhythmias
Ventricular fibrillation
Long QT syndrome
Wolff-Parkinson-White syndrome
Brugada syndrome
Ventricular tachycardia
Catecholaminergic polymorphic ventricular tachycardia
Torsades de pointes (long QT syndrome)
Operated congenital heart disease
Supraventricular tachycardia (Rare in adolescents with a structurally normal heart)
Bradyarrhythmias
Heart block
Congenital complete heart block
Kearns-Sayre syndrome
NKX2.5 gene defect
Long QT syndrome
Sinus node dysfunction/sinus bradycardia/junctional bradycardia
Postoperative congenital heart disease
Rare types of congenital long QT syndrome
Structural causes
Cardiomyopathy/myocarditis
Dilated
Hypertrophic (also known as idiopathic hypertrophic subaortic stenosis and asymmetric septal hypertrophy)
Arrhythmogenic right ventricular dysplasia/cardiomyopathy
Aortic stenosis
Coronary artery anomaly
Primary pulmonary hypertension

(*Continued*)

Table 14.11
(Continued)

Primary neurologic causes
Epilepsy
Migraine (atypical)
Sleep disorders
Cataplexy
Narcolepsy
Other causes of syncope and conditions confused with syncope
Psychiatric
Conversion disorder (hysteric faint)
Factitious disorders (malingering and Munchausen syndrome)
Panic disorder (hyperventilation)
Eating disorders
Drugs
Illicit drugs/club drugs (cocaine, methamphetamine)
Prescription medications (diuretics, antihypertensive agents)
Medications that prolong the QT
Hypoglycemia

Adapted from Franklin WH. Syncope. *Adolesc Health Update.* 2006;18(3):2.

Table 14.12
Red flags in the history and reasons for a cardiology consultation

Syncope during activity, particularly swimming
Syncope when cardiopulmonary resuscitation was performed
Patient's history of documented congenital heart disease (operated or unoperated)
Medications that prolong the QT interval
Family history of sudden depth before the age of 35 y
Family history of drowning before the age of 35 y
Family history of a motor vehicle crash/death, particularly a single-car accident, before the age of 35 y and unexplained by alcohol, drugs, or sleep deprivation
Family history of long QT syndrome, Brugada syndrome, or catecholaminergic polymorphic ventricular tachycardia
Family history of a person under the age of 35 y with a pacemaker or implantable defibrillator
Family history of heart muscle problem (heart too big, heart muscle too thick), hypertrophic cardiomyopathy, hypertrophic obstructive cardiomyopathy, asymmetric septal hypertrophy, idiopathic hypertrophic subaortic stenosis, or dilated cardiomyopathy

Adapted from Franklin WH. Syncope. *Adolesc Health Update.* 2006;18(3):6.

Adolesc Med 20 (2009) 823–859

Table 1

Adolescent Drug Formulary

This table lists a broad range of medications likely to be used by adolescent medicine clinicians. Wherever possible, both brand and generic names are listed. Brand names listed are not an indication that a particular product is preferred; rather brand names likely to be familiar to clinicians are included to help identify a particular medication. Dosages and formulations are also listed.

This formulary is not meant to be a comprehensive prescribing guide. Clinicians should also consult the product label for complete prescribing information, especially concerning serious side-effects, laboratory and symptom monitoring, and whether dosages should be adjusted in patients with renal or hepatic disease. Clinicians should also obtain a complete medication history (including use of complementary and alternative medicines) and consider possible drug-drug interactions when prescribing any medication. Many of the drugs listed in the table have not been approved for use in patients under 18 years of age.

 ISSN 1934-4287

Table 1
Adolescent Drug Formulary

Drug	Available as	Dosage	Comments
Acetaminophen (Tylenol)	325, 500, 650 mg tabs, gelcaps, caps	≥12 years: 500 mg-1 g q 4–6 hours; max dose 4 g/24 hr	Pregnancy category A
Acetaminophen + codeine (Tylenol with codeine No. 3)	300 mg acetaminophen + 30 mg codeine tabs	1–2 tabs q 4 hours as needed	Sedating; high abuse potential. Avoid use with acute or severe asthma. Codeine is pregnancy category C/D. Schedule II
Abilify	*See* Aripiprazole		
Acyclovir (Zovirax)	200 mg caps; 400, 800 mg tabs; 5% cream (2 g) or ointment (15 g)	*See* chapter on infectious diseases for dosing in genital herpes. Varicella: 800 mg qid for 5 days for pts. >40 kg	Pregnancy category C
Adapalene (Differin)	0.1% cream (15 g, 45 g), gel (15 g, 45 g), solution (30 mL), pledgets (#60)	Apply small amount to clean, dry skin once daily at bedtime	Reduce dosing frequency if irritation develops. Avoid sunlight or use sunscreen. Pregnancy category C
Adderall, Adderall XR	*See* Amphetamine/dextroamphetamine in formulary Table 2–ADHD medications		
Albuterol (several)	0.63 mg/3 mL NS, 1.25 mg/3 mL NS, 2.5 mg/3 mL NS solution for inhalation; 90 mcg/inhalation MDI	2.5–5 mg/dose over 5–15 minutes or 1–2 inhalations q 4–6 hours as needed. 2 inhalations 15 minutes before exercise for exercise-induced symptoms	Pregnancy category C
Alprazolam (Xanax)	0.25, 0.5, 1, 2 mg tabs	Initial: 0.25–0.5 mg tid; may increase at 3–4 day intervals to max 4 mg/d	Benzodiazepines may be habit-forming. Monitor blood count and hepatic function. Pregnancy category D. Schedule IV
Aluminum chloride hexahydrate (Drysol)	20% solution (35 mL)	Initial: apply once daily at bedtime; wash next morning. Maintenance: apply once-twice weekly	
Ambien	*See* Zolpidem		
Amitriptyline (Elavil)	10 , 25, 50, 75, 100, 150 mg tabs	Initial: 25–50 mg once daily at bedtime; may increase gradually to max 200 mg/24 hr. Migraine prophylaxis: 10–25 mg once daily at bedtime; may increase q 2–4 weeks to 100 mg daily if needed	High toxicity in overdose. Monitor levels, EKG, liver enzymes. Note black box warning regarding suicidality. Pregnancy category D

(*Continued*)

Table 1
(Continued)

Drug	Available as	Dosage	Comments
Amlodipine (Norvasc)	2.5, 5, 10 mg tabs	2.5–5 mg daily. May increase to 10 mg/24 hr.	Pregnancy category C
Amoxicillin (several)	250, 500 mg caps; 500 mg, 875 mg tabs; 125, 200, 250, 400 mg chewable tabs	Mild-moderate ENT, skin, GU infections: 500 mg q 12 hours or 250 mg q 8 hours. Lower respiratory, severe ENT, skin, GU infections: 875 mg q 12 hours or 500 mg q 8 hours	Dosing/duration of therapy varies depending on condition being treated. Recommended for treatment of chlamydial infection during pregnancy: 500 mg tid for 7 days. Adjust dose in renal failure. Pregnancy category B
Amoxicillin plus clavulanate potassium (Augmentin)	Tabs consisting of 125 mg clavulanate potassium plus either 250, 500, or 875 mg amoxicillin	Usual dose of amoxicillin: 250 mg tid or 500 mg bid; for more severe infections 875 mg bid or 500 mg tid	Take with meals. Dosing/duration of therapy varies depending on condition being treated. Pregnancy category B
Amphetamine/dextroamphetamine mixed salts (Adderall, Adderall XR)	*See* formulary Table 2 -- ADHD medications		Pregnancy category C. Schedule II
Ampicillin (several)	250, 500 mg caps	250–500 mg qid	Dosage and duration of therapy varies depending on condition being treated. Pregnancy category B
Aripiprazole (Abilify)	5, 10, 15, 20, 30 mg tabs; 10, 15 mg orally disintegrating tabs	2 mg qd for 2 days, then 5 mg qd for 2 days to target dose 10 mg qd; max dose 30 mg/24 hr. Adult: 10–15 mg qd to max dose of 30 mg/24 hr	Note black box warning regarding suicidality. Doses are for monotherapy only. Pregnancy category C
Atarax	*See* Hydroxizine		
Atenolol (Tenormin)	25, 50, 100 mg tabs	25–100 mg/dose qd	Use with caution in asthma. Pregnancy category D
Ativan	*See* Lorazepam		
Atomoxetine (Strattera)	10, 18, 25, 40, 60, 80, 100 mg caps	≤70 kg: start at 0.5 mg/kg/d; increase after intervals of 3 days or more to dose of 1.2 mg/kg/d. Max dose 1.4 mg/kg/d or 100 mg, whichever is less. >70 kg: Initial – 40 mg/24 hr; may increase after intervals of 3 days or more to 80 mg, then after 2–4 weeks may increase to max of 100 mg/24 hr as single dose or divided bid	Monitor hepatic function. Pregnancy category C

(*Continued*)

Table 1
(Continued)

Drug	Available as	Dosage	Comments
Atorvastatin (Lipitor)	10, 20, 40, 80 mg tabs	≤17 years: 10 mg qd titrated up to max 20 mg qd. Adult: 10–20 mg qd; max 80 mg/24 hr	Monitor lipid levels to titrate dose. Pregnancy category X
Aventyl	*See* Nortriptyline		
Azelaic acid (Azelex)	20% cream (30, 50 g)	Apply small amounts to clean, dry skin bid	Pregnancy category B
Azelastine (Astelin, Optivar)	1% nasal spray (137 mcg/spray, #200, 30 mL); Ophthalmic drops (0.05%, 0.5 mg/mL, 6 mL)	2 sprays each nostril bid 1 drop into each affected eye bid	Pregnancy category C
Azithromycin (Zithromax)	250, 500, 600 mg tabs; 1 g sachet.	500 mg on day 1, then 250 mg days 2–4 (Z-Pack); 500 mg qd for 3 days (Tri-Pak)	*See* chapter on infectious diseases for treatment of chlamydial or gonococcal infections
Baclofen	10, 20 mg tabs	10–15 mg/d divided bid-tid. Max 60–80 mg/d	Pregnancy category C
Beclomethasone dipropionate (Qvar, Beconase AQ)	40 or 80 mcg per inhalation (#100, 7.3 g) 42 mcg/spray (#200, 25 g)	Initial: 40–80 mcg bid. Max 320 mcg bid. 1–2 sprays each nostril bid	Rinse mouth after use. Pregnancy category C *See* Cardiorespiratory chapter for more information on asthma drugs.
Benadryl	*See* Diphenhydramine		
Benzoyl peroxide (several)	Many preparations (liquid or liquid cream wash, bar, lotion, cleanser, cream, gel). Strengths include 2.5, 3, 3.5, 4, 4.5, 5, 5.5, 6, 7, 8, 8.5, 9, 10%.	Cleanser, liquid wash, bar: wet affected areas, apply and wash qd-bid. Rinse and dry. Lotion, cream or gel: Apply small amount to clean, dry skin daily-bid depending on other medications used	May start with reduced dosing frequency to avoid skin irritation; reduce dosing frequency if irritation develops. May bleach hair or fabrics. Pregnancy category C
Benzoyl peroxide with erythromycin (Benzamycin) or clindamycin (Benzaclin, Duac)	30 mg erythromycin/50 mg BP per g (0.8, 23.3, 46 g); 10 mg clindamycin/ 50 mg BP per g (25, 45 g)	Apply bid to affected areas after washing and drying skin. Apply Duac qhs	Pregnancy category C

(Continued)

Table 1
(Continued)

Drug	Available as	Dosage	Comments
Budesonide inhaled (Pulmicort Turbuhaler, Flexhaler)	Turbuhaler: 200 mcg/inhalation (#200, 104 mg); Flexhaler: 90 mcg (#60, 165 mg), 180 mcg (#120, 225 mg) per metered dose	Turbuhaler: 1–2 inhalations bid; max 4 inhalations bid; Flexhaler: 180–360 mcg bid. Max 1440 mcg/24 hours.	*See* Cardiorespiratory chapter for more information on asthma drugs. Rinse mouth after using. Pregnancy category C
Budesonide nasal spray (Rhinocort aqua)	32 mcg/spray (#120 sprays, 8.6 g)	1–4 sprays to each nostril qd; max 8 sprays/24 hr.	Direct spray laterally, away from nasal septum. Use regularly for maximum effect. Consider initiating use 1 week prior to exposure to known allergens or 2–4 weeks prior to anticipated start of pollen season. Pregnancy Category C
Budesonide and formoterol (Symbicort)	80 mcg budesonide plus 4.5 mcg formoterol (#60, 6.9 g; #120, 10.2 g); 160 mcg budesonide plus 4.5 mcg formoterol (#60, 6.9 g; #120, 10.2 g)	160 mcg budesonide bid. Max dose 320 mcg budesonide bid	*See* Cardiorespiratory chapter for more information on asthma drugs. Pregnancy category C
Bupropion HCl (Wellbutrin, Welbutrin SR, Wellbutrin XL, Zyban)	75, 100 mg tabs (Wellbutrin); 100, 150 mg sustained release (SR) tabs, 150 mg, 300 mg extended-release (XL) tabs	>18 years: SR: initial dose 150 mg once daily in am for 3 days; if tolerated increase to 150 mg bid. XL: initial 150 mg once daily in am for 3 days; if tolerated increase to 300 mg once daily. Smoking cessation: 150 mg QAM for 3 days, then increase to 150 mg bid	Note black box warning regarding suicidality; contraindicated in bulimia; seizures associated with doses >300 mg/24 hr or >150 mg/dose. Pregnancy category C
Buspirone HCl (BuSpar)	5, 10, 15, 30 mg tabs	Initial: 7.5 mg bid; may increase every 2–3 days by 5 mg/d up to 60 mg/24 hr divided bid or tid	Pregnancy Category B
Captopril (Capoten)	12.5, 25, 50, 100 mg tabs	Initial: 12.5–25 mg bid-tid; increase weekly if needed by 25 mg/dose to max 450 mg/d	Take 1 hour before or 2 hours after meals; may add diuretic before increasing to max dose. Pregnancy category C/D

(*Continued*)

Table 1
(Continued)

Drug	Available as	Dosage	Comments
Carbamazepine (Tegretol, Tegretol –XR, Carbatrol, Aretol, Epitol)	100 mg chewable tabs; 200 mg tabs; 200, 300 mg extended–release caps; 100, 200, 400 mg extended-release tabs	>12 years: 200 mg bid; increase as needed by 200 mg/24 hr at 7 day intervals (divided bid or qid). Max dose (12–15 years): 1000 mg/24 hr; >15 years: 1200 mg/24 hr; adult: 1.6–2.4 g/24 hr	Monitor levels; hepatic, ophthalmic, renal function; may reduce hormonal contraceptive effectiveness via increased estrogen metabolism. Pregnancy category D
Catapres	*See* Clonidine		
Cefaclor (Ceclor)	250, 500 mg tabs; 375, 500 mg extended-release tabs	250–500 mg bid-tid; 375–500 mg extended-release bid	Dosing/duration of therapy varies depending on condition being treated. Pregnancy category B
Cefadroxil (Duricef)	500 mg caps	1–2 g/24 hr daily or bid	Dosing/duration of therapy varies depending on condition being treated. Pregnancy catgeory B
Cefdinir (Omnicef)	300 mg caps	300 mg q 12 hours or 600 mg q 24 hr	Dosing/duration of therapy varies depending on condition being treated. Pregnancy category B
Cefixime	400 mg tablet	*See* chapter on infectious diseases for dosage in treating gonococcal infections	Pregnancy category B.
Cefoxitin sodium (Mefoxin)	1, 2, 10 g injection powder for solution	*See* chapter on infectious diseases for dosing in PID or epididymitis	Pregnancy category B
Cefpodoxime proxetil (Vantin)	100, 200 mg tabs	100–400 mg q 12 hours; *see* chapter on infectious diseases for use in gonococcal infections	Pregnancy category B
Cefprozil (Cefzil)	250, 500 mg tabs	250–500 mg q 12 hours or 500–1000 mg once daily	Dosing/duration of therapy varies depending on condition being treated. Pregnancy category B
Ceftibuten HCl (Cedax)	400 mg caps	400 mg daily	Dosing/duration of therapy varies depending on condition being treated. Pregnancy category B
Ceftriaxone sodium (Rocephin)	250, 500 mg, 1, 2, 10 g powder for reconstitution and injection	*See* chapter on infectious diseases for use in gonococcal infections	Pregnancy category B
Cefuroxime axetil (Ceftin)	250, 500 mg tabs	250–500 mg bid. *See* chapter on infectious diseases for use in gonococcal infections	Pregnancy category B
Celexa	*See* Citalopram		

(*Continued*)

Table 1
(Continued)

Drug	Available as	Dosage	Comments
Cephalexin (Keflex)	250, 500 mg caps or tabs	250 mg q 6 hours or 500 mg mg q 12 hours; max 1 g qid	Dosing/duration of therapy varies depending on condition being treated. Pregnancy category B
Cetirizine HCl (Zyrtec, Zyrtec –D)	5, 10 mg tabs; extended release tabs (5 mg) with 120 mg pseudoephedrine (Zyrtec-D)	5–10 mg/24 hr; Zyrtec-D: 1 tab bid	Pregnancy category B
Chlorpheniramine maleate (Chlor-Trimeton)	4 mg tabs; 8 mg caps; 8, 12 mg sustained-release tabs	>12 years: 4 mg q 4–6 hours (max: 24 mg/24 hr); sustained release 8–12 mg bid	Pregnancy category B
Chlorpromazine (Thorazine)	10, 25, 50, 100, 200 mg tabs; 30, 75, 150 mg extended-release caps; 25 mg/mL injection	Nausea: 10–25 mg q 4–6 hours; 25 mg IM (if blood pressure normal, may repeat q 3–4 hours) until able to convert to oral meds	Pregnancy category C
Cholestyramine (Questran, Questran Light)	4 g anhydrous resin per 9 g powder (9, 378 g); Light versions (all with aspartame): 4 g anhydrous resin per 5.5 g powder (Prevalite–5.5, 231 g); 4 g anhydrous resin per 5.7 g powder (Cholestyramine Light - 5.7, 210, 231, 239 g); 4 g anhydrous resin per 6.4 g powder (Questran Light - 6.4, 268 g)	240 mg/kg/ 24 hr divided tid. Adult: 4 g qd-bid; maintenance 8–16 g bid-qid	Pregnancy category C
Ciclopirox (Loprox)	0.77% cream (15, 30, 90 g), gel (30, 45, 60, 90, 100g); 1% shampoo (120 mL); 8% solution (6.6 mL)	Apply bid up to 4 weeks. Shampoo (>16 y): apply 5 mL to wet hair, leave on 3 minutes, rinse. Repeat twice weekly with 3 or more days between applications	Dosing/duration of therapy varies depending on condition being treated. Pregnancy category B
Cimetidine (Tagamet, Tagamet HB)	100, 200 (OTC), 300, 400, 800 mg tabs	300 mg qid or 400 mg bid or 800 mg qhs	Dosing/duration of therapy varies depending on condition being treated. Pregnancy category B

(*Continued*)

Table 1
(Continued)

Drug	Available as	Dosage	Comments
Ciprofloxacin (Cipro, Cipro XR, Ciloxan, Ciprodex)	100, 250, 500, 750 mg tabs; 500, 1000 mg extended-release tabs; 3.5 mg/mL (2.5, 5, 10 mL) ophthalmic solution	UTI: 250–500 mg bid. Ophthalmic soln: 1–2 drops q 2 hr while awake ×2 days, then 1–2 drops q 4 hr while awake ×5 days	Dosing/duration of therapy varies depending on condition being treated. *See* black box warning regarding tendon injuries. Not approved <18. No longer recommended for treatment of gonococcal infections unless organism is proven sensitive. Pregnancy category C
Ciprofloxacin + hydrocortisone (Cipro HC Otic)	Ciprofloxacin 2 mg/mL plus 10 mg/mL hydrocortisone otic susp (10 mL)	3 drops in affected ear(s) bid for 7 days	Do not use with perforated tympanic membrane(s). Pregnancy category C
Citalopram hydrobromide (Celexa)	10, 20, 40 mg tabs	Initial: 10–20 mg once daily; after 7 days may increase by 20 mg to 40 mg daily; max 60 mg/24 hr	Note black box warning regarding suicidality. Pregnancy category C
Clarithromycin (Biaxin, Biaxin XL)	250, 500 mg tabs; 500 mg extended-release tabs (XL)	250–500 mg bid; XL: 1 g once daily	Dosing/duration of therapy varies depending on condition being treated. Pregnancy category C
Clindamycin (Cleocin, Cleocin-T, Benzaclin, Duac)	75, 150, 300 mg caps. Topical: 1% soln (1, 30, 60 mL); pledgets (#60); 1% gel (7.5, 30, 42, 60, 77 g); 1% lotion (60 mL); 1% foam (50 g); 1% gel with 5% benzoyl peroxide (25, 50 g pump). Vaginal cream 2% (40 g); ovules 100 mg (#3)	150–450 mg q6–8 hours. Acne: Apply small amount to clean, dry skin daily or bid. Bacterial vaginosis: 300 mg orally bid for 7 days OR 100 mg ovule intravaginally qhs for 3 days or 1 applicatorful cream for 3 or 7 days qhs	Dosing/duration of therapy varies depending on condition being treated. Pregnancy category B Reduce dosing frequency if irritation develops. Pregnancy category (with benzoyl peroxide) C

(*Continued*)

Table 1
(Continued)

Drug	Available as	Dosage	Comments
Clonazepam (Klonopin)	0.5, 1, 2 mg tabs; 0.125, 0.25, 0.5, 1, 2 mg disintegrating oral tabs	0.25 – 0.5 mg bid-tid; may increase by 0.5–1 mg /24 hr every 3 days to max dose of 4 mg/24 hr divided bid-tid	Benzodiazepines may be habit-forming; monitor blood count and hepatic function. Pregnancy category C. Schedule IV
Clonidine (Catapres, Catapres TTS)	0.1, 0.2, 0.3 mg tabs; 0.1, 0.2, 0.3 mg/24 hr transdermal patch (TTS)–patch lasts 7 days	0.1 mg bid; may increase in 0.05–0.1 mg increments every 7 days. Max dose 0.9–2.4 mg/24 hr depending on age/wgt. TTS: younger adolescent–convert to patch after establishing dose closest to oral maintenance dose. Older adolescent: initial 0.1 mg/24 hr patch for 7 days; may increase by 0.1 mg/24 hr at 1–2 week intervals. No benefit to doses >0.6 mg/24 hr	Pregnancy category C
Clotrimazole (Lotrimin AF, Gyne-Lotrimin)	1% cream, soln, lotion; 100 mg vaginal tablet; 1%, 2% vaginal cream	Apply bid up to 4 weeks for skin infection Vulvovaginal candidiasis: *see* chapter on infectious diseases	Pregnancy category C
Concerta	*See* Methylphenidate		
Cromolyn sodium (Intal, Nasalcrom, Opticrom)	800 mcg/inhalation MDI (#112, 8.1 g; #200, 14.2 g); 4% nasal spray (5.2 mg/spray −13, 26 mL); 4% ophthalmic soln (2.5, 5, 10 mL)	Asthma: 2–4 inhalations tid-qid; 2–4 inhalations 10–60 minutes before exercise. Rhinitis: 1 spray to each nostril tid-qid; 1–2 gtts each eye 4–6 times/24 hr	Use regularly for maximum effect. Consider initiating use 1 week prior to exposure to known allergens or 2–4 weeks prior to anticipated start of pollen season. Pregnancy category B
Cyclobenzaprine HCl (Flexeril)	5, 7.5, 10 mg tabs; 15, 30 mg extended-release tabs	5 mg tid; may increase to 10 mg tid. Extended-release: 15–30 mg daily; max duration of use (either form) 2–3 weeks	Sedating. Not approved for <15. Pregnancy category B
Cyproheptadine (Periactin)	4 mg tabs	Younger teen: 4 mg bid-tid; max 16 mg/24 hr. Older teen/adult: 4 mg bid-qid; may titrate up to max 32 mg/24 hr (migraine prophylaxis)	Dosing depends on condition being treated and age of patient. Stimulates appetite. Pregnancy category B
Depakote; Depakote ER	*See* Divalproex (valproic acid)		

(*Continued*)

Table 1
(Continued)

Drug	Available as	Dosage	Comments
Desloratidine (Clarinex)	5 mg tabs; 2.5, 5 mg orally disintegrating tabs. Extended release tabs with pseudoephedrine: 2.5 mg desloratadine/120 mg pseudoephedrine (Clarinex-D 12 hr); 5/240 (Clarinex-D 24 hour)	5 mg daily. Clarinex-D 12 hr: 1 tab bid; Clarinex-D 24 hr: 1 tab daily	Pregnancy category C
Desmopressin acetate (DDAVP)	0.1, 0.2 mg tabs.	Nocturnal enuresis: Initial: 0.2 mg at bedtime; max 0.6 mg oral	Pregnancy category B
Desyrel	*See* Trazodone		
Dexedrine	*See* Dextroamphetamine		
Dexmethyphenidate (Focalin)	2.5, 5, 10 mg tabs	For dosage, see formulary Table 2–ADHD medications	When switching from racemic methylphenidate, use half the dose. Pregnancy category C. Schedule II
Dextroamphetamine sulfate (Dexedrine, Dexedrine spansules)	5, 10 mg tabs; 5, 10, 15 mg sustained release caps (spansules)	For dosage, see formulary Table 2–ADHD medications	High abuse potential. Pregnancy category C. Schedule II
Diazepam (Valium)	2, 5, 10 mg tabs	1–10 mg bid-qid as needed depending on symptom severity	Sedating. Potentially addictive. Avoid abrupt cessation. Prolonged use not recommended. Pregnancy category D. Schedule IV
Dicyclomine HCl (Bentyl)	10 mg caps, 20 mg tabs	Initial: 20 mg qid; increase to 40 mg qid if tolerated	Anticholinergic. Discontinue if not effective in 2 weeks or not tolerated. Antacids may inhibit absorption. Pregnancy category B
Dihydroergotamine mesylate with caffeine (Migranal)	4 mg/mL nasal spray; 0.5 mg/spray (3 mL)	One spray to each nostril; may repeat in 15 minutes; max 3 mg/24 hr	Not for use in persons <18. Avoid simultaneous use of macrolides. Pregnancy category X

(*Continued*)

Table 1
(Continued)

Drug	Availale as	Dosage	Comments
Diltiazem (Cardiazem, Cardiazem XR, Dilacor XR)	30, 60, 90, 120 mg tabs; 120, 180, 240, 300, 360, 420 mg extended-release tabs; 60, 90, 120, 180, 240, 300, 360, 420 mg extended-release caps	30–120 mg/dose tid-qid immediate release; 120–300 mg/24 hr (divided bid with Cardiazem XR; qd with other extended-release forms). Max: 540 mg/24 hr	Pregnancy category C
Dimenhydrinate (Dramamine)	50 mg	>40 kg: 50–100 mg/dose 30 minutes prior to travel for motion sickness; max 400 mg/24 hr	Pregnancy category B
Diphenhydramine (Benadryl)	25, 50 mg tabs	25–50 mg q 4–6 hours; max 300 mg/24 hr	Pregnancy category B
Divalproex sodium (Depakote, Depakote ER)	125, 250, 500 mg delayed-release tabs; 250, 500 mg extended-release (ER) tabs	Initial: 500–750 mg daily divided qd-tid; max 60 mg/kg/24 hr. Migraine prophylaxis: 250 mg bid-tid; ER: 500 mg qd; after 7 days may increase to 1000 mg qd	Extended-release dose generally 8%–20% higher than delayed-release dose. Monitor levels, hepatic function, platelet count. Pregnancy category D
Docosonal (Abreva)	10% cream (2 g)	Apply 5 times daily until healed	Begin treatment at earliest indication of outbreak. Avoid eyes/mucous membranes. Pregnancy category: fetal risk cannot be ruled out
Docusate sodium (Colace)	50, 100, 250 mg caps	50–400 mg daily divided qd-qid	Pregnancy category C
Doxycycline (several)	50, 75, 100 mg caps, tabs	100–200 mg/24 hr divided qd-bid. Max dose 300 mg/24 hr	*See* chapter on infectious diseases for treatment of STIs. Dosing/duration of therapy varies depending on condition being treated. Take with fluids. Avoid sun/UV light. Monitor blood, renal and hepatic function with long-term use. Pregnancy category D
Econazole nitrate (Spectazole)	1% cream (15, 30, 85 g)	*Tinea cruris*, *t versicolor*, *t corporis*: apply daily for 2 weeks. *T pedis*: apply daily for 4 weeks. Cutaneous candidiasis: apply bid for 2 weeks	Pregnancy category C

(*Continued*)

Table 1
(Continued)

Drug	Available as	Dosage	Comments
Effexor, Effexor XR	*See* Venlafaxine		
Eflornithine HCl (Vaniqua)	13.9% cream (30 g)	Apply bid at least 8 hours apart; do not wash area for at least 4 hours	Pregnancy category C
Elavil	*See* Amitriptyline		
Enalapril maleate (Vasotec)	2.5, 5, 10, 20 mg tabs	Initial: 2.5–5 mg daily; titrate up to 10–40 mg/24 hr divided qd-bid as needed	Pregnancy category D
Epinastine HCl (Elestat)	0.05% soln (5 mL)	1 drop in each eye bid	Remove contact lenses before applying; may reinsert after 10 minutes if eye not red. Pregnancy category C
Erythromycin (several)	Base: 250, 500 mg tabs; 250, 333, 500 mg extended release tabs; 250 mg delayed release capsules. Ethyl succinate: 400 mg tabs; stearate: 250 mg tabs	250 mg q 6 hours; 333 mg q 8 hours; 500 mg q 12 hours. Max 4 g/24 hr	Dosing/duration of therapy varies depending on condition being treated. Pregnancy category B
Erythromycin topical	2% saturated swab (#60); 1.5, 2% soln (60 mL); 2% gel (30, 60 g); 3% with 5% benzoyl peroxide gel (46.6 g)	Apply small amount to clean, dry skin bid (gel apply qd-bid)	Topical antibiotics should not be used as single therapy for acne (rapid emergence of resistant organisms). Reduce dosing frequency or strength if irritation develops. Benzoyl peroxide may bleach hair or fabrics. Pregnancy category (with benzoyl peroxide) C
Escitalopram oxalate (Lexapro)	5, 10, 20 mg tabs	Initial: 10 mg daily; may increase to 20 mg daily after 1–3 weeks (longer interval for younger adolescents)	Note black box warning regarding suicidality. Pregnancy category C

(Continued)

Table 1
(Continued)

Drug	Available as	Dosage	Comments
Eskalith, Eskalith SR	*See* Lithium		
Esomeprazole (Nexium)	20, 40 mg caps	20–40 mg daily	Dosing/duration of therapy varies depending on condition being treated. Pregnancy category B
Famciclovir (Famvir)	125, 250, 500 mg tabs	*See* chapter on infectious diseases for use in genital herpes	Pregnancy category B
Famotidine (Pepcid)	10, 20 (OTC), 40 mg tabs	20–40 mg bid or 40 mg qhs	Dosing/duration of therapy varies depending on condition being treated. Pregnancy category B
Fexofenadine HCL (Allegra, Allegra-D)	30, 60, 180 mg tabs (Allegra); 60 mg fexofenadine with 120 mg pseudoephedrine (Allegra D 12 hr); 180 mg fexofendadine with 240 mg pseudoephedrine (Allegra-D 24 hr)	60 mg bid or 180 mg daily; Allegra-D 12 hr: 1 tab bid; Allegra-D 24 hr: 1 tab qd	Do not take D-12 hr or D-24 hr with food. Pregnancy category C
Fluconazole	50, 100, 150, 200 mg tabs	Vulvovaginal candidiasis: 150 mg as single dose	Other: dosing/duration of therapy varies depending on condition being treated. Pregnancy category C
Flunisolide (Aerobid, Aerospan, Nasarel)	80 mcg/dose inhaler (Aerospan: #60, 5.1 g; #120, 8.9 g); 250 mcg/dose inhaler (Aerobid: #100, 7 g); nasal soln (25 mcg/spray (#200, 25 mL))	Aerobid: Two inhalations bid; max dose 4 inhalations/24 hr if <16 years and 8 inhalations/24 hr if ≥16 years. Aerospan (>12 years): 2 inhalations bid; max 8 inhalations/24 hr; Nasal soln: 2 sprays per nostril bid; max (>14 years): 4 sprays per nostril/24 hr	*See* Cardiorespiratory chapter for more information on asthma drugs. Rinse mouth after use. Pregnancy category C
Fluoxetine (Prozac)	10, 20, 40 mg caps; 10, 20 mg tabs; 90 mg delayed-release caps	Initial: 10–20 mg daily; may increase by 10–20 mg after 1–2 weeks; max 80 mg/24 hr (adults). Bulimia: 60 mg QAM; titrate up to this dose over several days. Premenstrual dysphoric disorder (PMDD): initiate at 20 mg qd; max dose 80 mg/24 hr	Note black box warning regarding suicidality. Doses >20 mg/24 hr should be given bid. For PMDD, can give continuously or start 14 days before menses through 1st full day of menses. Pregnancy category C

(Continued)

Table 1
(Continued)

Drug	Available as	Dosage	Comments
Fluticasone propionate inhaled (Flovent HFA, Flovent Diskus)	MDI: 44, 110, 220 mcg/inhalation (#60, 7.9 g; #120, 13 g). Dry powder inhaler (DPI): 50, 100, 150 mcg/dose (#60-15 Rotadisks, 4 doses per disk)	MDI: Initiate with 2 inhalations (44 mcg) bid; max 880 mcg/24 hr. DPI: Initiate with 2 inhalations (50 mcg) bid; max 1000 mcg/24 hr	*See* Cardiorespiratory chapter for more information on asthma drugs. Use higher doses at start if previous use of steroids. Pregnancy category C
Fluticasone propionate nasal spray (Flonase)	50 mcg/spray (#120, 16g)	Initial: 1–2 sprays to each nostril daily or 1 spray to each nostril bid; may reduce to 1 spray each nostril for maintenance	Direct spray laterally away from nasal septum. Consider initiating use 1 week prior to exposure to known allergens or 2–4 weeks prior to anticipated start of pollen season. Pregnancy category C
Fluticasone propionate plus salmeterol (Advair Diskus-dry powder inhaler; Advair HFA-aerosol inhaler)	Diskus: 100, 250, 500 mcg fluticasone each combined with 50 mcg salmeterol per inhalation. HFA: 45, 115, 230 mcg fluticasone each combined with 21 mcg salmtererol per inhalation	No prior steroid use: Diskus: One inhalation bid, starting with 100 mcg/dose; increase as needed every 2 weeks; max dose 1 inhalation bid of 500 mcg fluticasone. HFA: 2 inhalations of 45 or 115 mcg bid; max dose two 230 mcg inhalations bid. Prior steroid use: *see* Cardiorespiratory chapter	Do not initiate in significantly worsening or acutely deteriorating asthma. *See* Cardiorespiratory chapter for more information on asthma drugs. Pregnancy category C
Fluvoxamine (Luvox)	25, 50, 100 mg tabs	≤17 years: start at 25 mg qhs. May increase by 25 mg/d every 4–7 days. Daily doses >50 mg should be divided bid. ≥18 years: start at 50 mg; dose may be increased by 50 mg/24 hr every 4–7 days. Max dose 300 mg/24 hr. Daily doses >100 mg should be divided bid	Females may require lower doses than males. Note black box warning regarding suicidality. Pregnancy category C
Focalin	*See* Dexmethylphenidate		

(*Continued*)

Table 1
(Continued)

Drug	Available as	Dosage	Comments
Formoterol fumarate (Foradil)	12 mcg dry powder capsules for inhalation with inhaler device (#12, #60 blister pack)	One inhalation q 12 hours. One inhalation at least 15 minutes before exercise	Should not be used as single therapy for asthma. Long-acting β-2 agonists may increase risk of asthma deaths. Do not initiate in significantly worsening or acutely deteriorating asthma. Pregnancy category C
Gabapentin (Neuronton, Gabarone)	100, 300, 400 mg caps; 100, 300, 400, 600, 800 mg tabs	300 mg tid; may increase to 1800 mg/24 hr divided tid. Migraine prophylaxis: 300 mg tid; may increase up to 800 mg tid	Do not stop medication abruptly. Pregnancy category C
Griseofulvin (several)	500 mg microcrystalline tabs; 125, 250, 330 mg ultramicrocrystalline tabs	Micro: 500–1000 mg/24 hr divided daily-bid; ultramicrosize: 330–750 mg/24 hr divided daily or bid	250 mg ultramicrocrystalline = 500 mg microcrystalline. Dosing/duration of therapy depends on condition being treated. Monitor blood, liver and renal parameters with prolonged therapy. Pregnancy category C
Guanfacine HCl (Tenex)	1, 2 mg tabs	1–4 mg/24 hr divided bid	Pregnancy category B
Haloperidol (generic)	0.5, 1, 2, 5, 10, 20 mg tabs	0.5–2.0 mg bid-tid (moderate symptoms) or 3–5 mg bid-tid (severe symptoms)	Pregnancy category C
Hydrochlorothiazide (Hydrodiuril, Microzide)	12.5, 25, 50 mg tabs	Initial: 12.5–25 mg daily; may increase up to max dose of 100 mg divided qd or bid	Doses >50 mg/24 hr may result in hypokalemia. Pregnancy category B/D
Hydrocodone plus acetaminophen (Vicodin)	5 mg hydrocodone/500 mg acetaminophen cap; 5, 7.5, 10 mg hydrocodone in combination with 325 mg acetaminophen (tabs); 2.5, 5, 7.5, 10 mg hydrocodone in combination with 500 mg acetaminophen (tabs)	>14 years: 7.5 mg hydrocodone q4–6 hours for mod-severe pain; max 6 doses/24 hr. Adults: max 60 mg hydrocodone/4 g acetaminophen/24 hr	Sedating. High abuse potential. Avoid with severe or acute asthma. Pregnancy category C. Schedule III

(Continued)

Table 1
(Continued)

Drug	Available as	Dosage	Comments
Hydrocodone bitartrate plus homatropine methyl bromide (Hycodan)	5 mg hydrocodone/1.5 mg homatropine per tab or per 5 mL syrup	1 tab or 5 mL q 4–6 hours prn; max 6 doses/24 hr	Sedating. High abuse potential. Avoid with severe or acute asthma. Pregnancy category C. Schedule III
Hydromorphone (Dilaudid)	2, 4, 8 mg tabs	1–4 mg q 4–6 hours as needed	Sedating. High abuse potential. Pregnancy category C/D depending on timing and duration of use. Schedule II
Hydroxyzine HCl (Atarax)	10, 25, 50 mg tabs; 25, 50, 100 mg caps	25 mg tid-qid; max 600 mg/24 hr	Pregnancy category C
Ibuprofen	100, 200 mg tabs/caps/caplets (OTC); 400, 600, 800 mg tabs	400–800 mg q 6–8 hours prn	Pregnancy category C/D
Imipramine (Tofranil, Tofranil PM)	10, 25, 50 mg tabs; 75, 100, 125, 150 mg caps	Initial: 25–50 mg/24 hr divided qd-tid; max 200 mg/24 hr. Adult 75–100 mg/24 hr divided qd-tid; max 200 mg/24 hr. Enuresis: 25 mg qhs; may increase in 25 mg increments to max 75 mg/24 hr	Note black box warning regarding suicidality. Pregnancy category D
Imiquimod (Aldara)	5% cream (12 single-use packets with applicators)	Apply only to lesions and rub in at bedtime 3 days per week (eg, M-W-F); wash off 6–10 hours later. Use up to 16 weeks	Can skip applications if significant reddening/irritation develops. *See* chapter on infectous diseases for use in genital warts. Pregnancy category C
Ipratroprium bromide (Atrovent)	17 mcg/inhalation MDI (#200, 12.9 g)	2–3 inhalations qid; max 12 inhalations/24 hr	Pregnancy category B

(*Continued*)

Table 1
(Continued)

Drug	Available as	Dosage	Comments
Iron (Fe) preparations (many)	12% elemental Fe (mg Fe/gluconate), tabs: 27/240 (Fergon); 28/246, 34/300, 36/325 20% elemental Fe (mg Fe/sulfate), tabs: 60/300, 65/324, 65/325) 30% elemental Fe (dried, mg Fe/sulfate): 65/200; extended release 50/160 33% elemental Fe (mg Fe/fumarate), tabs: 29.5/90, 66/200, 106/324, 106/325, 115/350; chewable: 33/100; timed release: 50/150 Polysaccharide-iron complex and ferrous bis-glycinate chelate (Niferex): 60 mg (elemental Fe) cap; 150 mg (elemental Fe) cap containing 50 mg Vit C	Treatment of iron deficiency/iron deficiency anemia: 60–100 mg elemental iron bid-qid. Prophylaxis: 60–100 mg elemental iron/24 hr	Take with Vitamin C (eg, orange juice) to enhance absorption. Pregnancy category A
Isometheptene mucate + dichloralphenazone + acetaminophen (Midrin)	65 mg isometheptene/100 mg dichloralphenazone /325 mg acetaminophen caps	2 caps initially, followed by 1 cap q 1 hr until relief. Max 5 caps/12 hr period	Frequent use may lead to analgesic withdrawal headache. Dichloralphenazone may be sedating and addictive. Pregnancy category: fetal risk cannot be ruled out
Isoniazid (INH)	300 mg tabs	Tuberculosis prophylaxis: 300 mg once daily for 9 months	Some recommend monitoring liver function tests before and during therapy. Caution about alcohol use. Pregnancy category C
Itraconzaole (Sporanox)	100 mg caps	Onychomycosis: Toenail-200 mg daily for 12 weeks; Fingernail–200 mg bid for 1 week, then 3 weeks off, then 200 mg bid for an additional wk	Pregnancy category C

(Continued)

Table 1
(Continued)

Drug	Available as	Dosage	Comments
Ketoconazole (Nizoral)	2% cream (15, 30, 60 g); 200 mg tabs Shampoo: 1% (OTC), 2%	*T cruris, t versicolor, t corporis*: apply cream daily for at least 2 weeks. *T pedis*: treat for 6 weeks. Oral: Initial: 200 mg daily. Max: 400 mg/24 hours. Shampoo: Use twice weekly with at least 3 days between applications for up to 8 weeks, then pm to control symptoms	Dosing/duration of therapy varies depending on condition being treated. Pregnancy category C
Ketorolac tromethamine (Toradol)	10 mg tabs	10–20 mg (lower dose in younger teens <50 kg) followed by 10 mg q 6 hours. Max 40 mg/24 hours	Maximum use–5 days. Pregnancy category C/D
Klonopin	*See* Clonazepam		
Labetalol HCl (Trandate)	100, 200, 300 mg tabs	Initial: 100 mg bid; may increase at 2–3 day intervals in increments of 100 mg bid. Max: 2.4 g/24 hours	Pregnancy category C/D
Lactulose (Kristalose)	10, 20 g packets for reconstitution (#30); 10 g/15 mL (30, 237, 473, 960, 1893 mL)	Younger teens: 40 to 90 mL (20 g/30 mL) daily in 3 to 4 divided doses. Older teens/adults: 15 to 45 mL (20 g/30 mL) 3 to 4 times daily for 24 to 48 hours; max 40 g/24 hr	May be antagonized by nonabsorbable antacids. Pregnancy category B
Lamotrigine (Lamictal)	25, 100, 150, 200 mg tabs	Migraine prophylaxis: 50 mg daily; may titrate up to 50 mg bid	Pregnancy category C
Lansoprazole (Prevacid)	15, 30 mg delayed-release caps; 15, 30 mg disintegrating delayed-release tabs	15–30 mg daily	Dosing/duration of therapy varies depending on condition being treated. Pregnancy category B

(*Continued*)

Table 1
(Continued)

Drug	Available as	Dosage	Comments
Levofloxacin (Levaquin)	250, 500, 750 mg tabs. Ophthalmic drops 0.5% (2.5, 5 mL)	UTI (uncomplicated): 250 mg qd for 3 days; UTI (complicated)/pyelonephritis: 250 mg qd for 10 days or 750 mg qd for 5 days; Community-acquired pneumonia: 500 mg qd for 7–14 days or 750 mg qd for 5 days; Acute sinusitis: 500 mg qd for 10–14 days or 750 mg qd for 5 days. *See* chapter on infectious diseases for use in STIs. Conjunctivitis: 1–2 gtts in affected eye(s) q 2 hours (max 8 times/24 hr) while awake days 1–2, then q 4 hours while awake (max 4 times/24 hr) days 3–7	Increased risk of tendinitis and tendon rupture in all ages. Take with full glass of water. Not generally recommended for <18 years old. Pregnancy category A
Levothyroxine sodium (Levoxyl, Synthroid)	25, 50, 75, 88, 100, 112, 125, 137, 150, 175, 200, 300 mcg tabs	2–3 mcg/kg/dose once daily; titrate as needed in 12.5–25 mcg/d increments every 1–2 weeks. Start with 25% of recommended full maintenance dose	100 mcg levothyroxine = 65 mg thyroid USP. Pregnancy category A
Lexapro	*See* Citalopram		
Lindane	1% shampoo (30, 60, 473 mL); 1% lotion (30, 60, 473 mL)	Scabies: Apply thin layer of lotion to skin. Thoroughly rinse off medication after 8–12 hr. May repeat 1 time in 1 week. Pediculosis capitis: apply 15–30 mL of shampoo, lather 4–5 minutes, rinse hair, comb to remove nits. May repeat 1 time in 1 week. Pediculosis pubis: use shampoo or lotion as above	Avoid contact with face, mucous membranes, urethra or any area of damaged skin. Pregnancy category B
Lisinopril (Prinivil, Zestril)	2.5, 5, 10, 20, 30, 40 mg tabs	≤16 years: start with 0.07 mg/kg/dose daily; max starting dose 5 mg. Titrate up as needed to max dose of 0.61 mg/kg/24 hr or 40 mg/24 hr. ≥16 years: start at 10 mg qd; max dose 80 mg/24 hr	Pregnancy category C/D
Lithium (Lithobid, Eskalith)	150, 300, 600 mg caps; 300 mg tabs; 300, 450 mg extended-release tabs	600–1800 mg/24 hr divided tid-qid. Give bid if using extended-release tabs	Therapeutic level 0.6–1.5 mEq/L depending on condition being treated. Pregnancy category D

(*Continued*)

Table 1
(Continued)

Drug	Available as	Dosage	Comments
Loperamide HCl (Imodium, Imodium AD)	2 mg caps, tabs, or caplets (all OTC)	Initial: 4 mg, then 2 mg after each loose stool; max 16 mg/24 hr	Pregnancy category C
Loratidine (Alavert, Claritin) or Loratidine + pseudoephedrine sulfate (Claritin-D 12 or 24 hr)	Loratidine 10 mg or loratidine 5 mg plus 120 mg pseudoephedrine (Claritin-D 12 hr) or loratidine 10 mg plus 240 mg pseudoephedrine (Claritin-D 24 hr)	10 mg loratidine (without pseudoephedrine) qd; D-12 hr - 1 tab bid; D-24 hr-1 qd	Pregnancy category B/C
Lorazepam (Ativan)	0.5, 1, 2 mg tabs	Initial: 2–3 mg daily divided bid or tid; may titrate up to 10 mg daily divided bid or tid	Consider 0.5 mg test dose to evaluate for behavioral activation. Pregnancy category D. Schedule IV
Losartan potassium (Cozaar)	25, 50, 100 mg tabs	Initial: 0.7 mg/kg (max 50 mg) qd; may titrate up to max 100 mg/24 hr. Adult: initial dose 50 mg qd.	Pregnancy category C/D
Lovastatin (Altroprev, Mevacor)	10, 20, 40 mg tabs; 20, 40, 60 mg extended-release tabs	≤17 years: 10 mg qd; max 40 mg qd. Adults-immediate release: 20 mg qd; maintenance 10–80 mg/24 hr divided qd-bid. Extended release: 20–60 mg qhs	Manufacturer does not recommend use of extended release formulation for <18-year-olds. Pregnancy category X
Luvox	*See* Fluvoxamine		
Lysdexamfetamine (Vyvanse)	20, 30, 40, 50, 60, 70 mg capsules (sprinkle in water and drink immediately)	*See* formulary Table 2-ADHD medications - for dosage	Pregnancy category C. Schedule II
Mebendazole (Vermox)	100 mg chewable tabs	*Enterobius vermicularis*: 100 mg once; may repeat in 2 weeks if not cured. *Ascaris*: 100 mg bid for 3 days; may repeat in 3–4 weeks if not cured; alternate dose: 500 mg once	Dose/duration of treatment for other infections varies. Pregnancy category C
Meclizine HCl (Antivert)	12.5, 25, 50 mg tabs	Motion sickness: 12.5–50 mg 60 minutes prior to departure; repeat q 24 hr as needed. Vertigo: 25–100 mg/24 hr in divided doses	Pregnancy category B

(*Continued*)

Table 1
(Continued)

Drug	Available as	Dosage	Comments
Mefenamic acid (Ponstel)	250 mg caps	Dysmenorrhea (>14 years): 500 mg at start of menses, then 250 mg q 6 hr	Typical duration of use for 2–3 days after bleeding starts. Pregnancy category C
Meperidine HCl (Demerol)	50, 100 mg tabs	40–70 mg (younger teen) to 50–150 mg (older teen/adult) q 3–4 hr as needed	Sedating. High abuse potential. Contraindicated in asthma. Pregnancy category C/D. Schedule II
Metadate	*See* Methylphenidate in formulary Table 2–ADHD medications		
Metformin HCl (Glucophage, Glucophage XR)	500, 850, 1000 mg tabs; 500, 750, 1000 mg extended-release tabs	10–16 years: initial dose 500 mg bid; can increase every 7 days by 500 mg/24 hr in 2 divided doses. Max: 2000 mg/24 hr. >16 years: 500 mg bid; can increase dose every 7 days by 500 mg/24 hr in 2 divided doses up to max of 2500 mg/24 hr. At 2500 mg/24 hr, administer divided tid. 850 mg tabs: 850 mg with breakfast; increase as needed after 2 weeks to 850 mg bid; may increase after 2 additional wks to max dose 2550 mg/24 hr (divided tid). Extended-release: 500 mg qd with evening meal; increase as needed by 500 mg q 7 days to 2000 mg/24 hr max (max dose given qd or divided bid)	Administer doses with meals. Extended-release tabs not evaluated in <17 years. Pregnancy category B
Methylin	See Methylphenidate		

(Continued)

Table 1
(Continued)

Drug	Available as	Dosage	Comments
Methylphenidate (Concerta, Metadate CD, Metadate ER, Ritalin, Ritalin LA, Ritalin SR)	5, 10, 20 mg immediate release tabs; 10, 20 mg extended-release tabs (Metadate ER, Methylin ER); 18, 27, 36, 54 mg extended-release tabs (Concerta); 20 mg sustained-release tabs (Ritalin SR); 10, 20, 30, 40, 50, 60 mg extended-release caps (Metadate CD, Ritalin LA); transdermal patch (Daytrana)	*See* formulary Table 2–ADHD medications	Pregnancy category C. Schedule II
Methylprednisolone (Medrol)	2, 4, 8, 16, 32 mg tabs; Medrol Dosepak contains 21 4-mg tabs	Asthma exacerbation: 40–80 mg/24 hr divided daily-bid. Allergic disorder (adults): 4–48 mg daily depending on condition being treated	Adjust dose in asthma after peak flow reaches >70%. Pregnancy category C
Metoclopramide HCl (Reglan)	5, 10 mg tabs	0.1–0.2 mg/kg/dose with meals and qhs; max dose 32 mg/24 hr. Adult: 10–15 mg/dose with meals and qhs.	Can cause tardive dyskinesia that is often irreversible. Pregnancy category B
Metronidazole (Flagyl, Flagyl ER, MetroGel-Vaginal)	250, 500 mg tabs; 375 mg caps; 750 mg extended release tabs; 0.75% vaginal gel (#5 applicators, 70 g)	Bacterial vaginosis: 500 mg bid for 7 days or 1 applicator intravaginally daily for 5 days Trichomoniasis: 2 g as single dose; alternative regimen: 500 mg bid for 7 days	Avoid alcohol during therapy. Pregnancy category B

(*Continued*)

Table 1
(Continued)

Drug	Available as	Dosage	Comments
Miconazole nitrate (Lotrimin AF, Monistat)	2% cream (15, 30, 90 g); 2% lotion (30, 60 mL); 2% ointment (28.4 g); 2% soln (7.39, 29.57 mL); 2% gel (24 g). Spray: 2% powder (85, 90, 100 g), liquid (105 mL). 2% powder (70, 90 g). Vaginal preps: 2% cream (15, 25, 45 g); supps -100 mg (#7), 200 mg (#3), 1200 mg (#1); combination packs (supps plus cream)	Fungal skin infections: apply bid for 2–4 weeks. Vulvovaginal candidiasis–*See* chapter on infectious diseases for dosing	Pregnancy category C
Minocycline (Minocin)	50, 75, 100 mg caps; 50, 75, 100 mg tabs; 45, 90, 135 mg extended-release tabs; 50, 100 mg pellet-filled caps	Infections: 200 mg once then 100 mg q 12 hours Acne: 50–100 mg qd-bid (immediate-release) Extended-release: 45 mg qd for 45–59 kg teen; 90 mg qd for 60–90 kg teen; 135 mg qd for >90 kg teen	Dosing/duration of therapy varies on condition being treated. Swallow whole, take on an empty stomach with fluids. Monitor blood, renal, hepatic function in long-term use. Avoid sunlight or use sunscreen. Pregnancy category D
Mometasone furoate (Nasonex, Asmanex Twisthaler, Elocon)	50 mcg/spray (#120, 17 g); 220 mcg per actuation (#14, 30, 60, 120) powder for inhalation; 0.1% cream, ointment (15, 45 g); lotion/soln (30, 60 mL)	2 sprays to each nostril qd; 220 mcg qd in the evening; may increase to 440 mcg/24 hr in evening or divided bid; Apply thin film or a few drops to affected areas qd	Direct spray laterally away from septum. Use regularly for maximum effect. Consider initiating 1 week prior to exposure to known allergen or 2–4 weeks prior to anticipated start of pollen season. Safety >3 weeks not established for pediatric patients. *See* Cardiorespiratory chapter for more information on asthma drugs. Pregnancy category C
Montelukast (Singulair)	10 mg tabs; 5 mg chewable tabs	≤14 years: 5 mg qd; >14 years: 10 mg qd For exercise-induced asthma (>15 years): 10 mg >2 hrs before exercise. Do not repeat at <24 hr intervals	Pregnancy category B

(*Continued*)

Table 1
(Continued)

Drug	Available as	Dosage	Comments
Mupirocin (Bactroban)	2% ointment (15, 22, 30 g), cream (15, 30 g) or ointment for nasal use (2% (1 g)	Skin infections: Apply tid for 5–14 days Nasal: Small amount intransally bid-qid for 5–14 days	Pregnancy category B
Naphazoline HCl plus pheniramine maleate (Naphcon A)	Naphazoline HCl 0.025% plus pheniramine maleate 0.3% soln (15 mL)	1–2 drops to affected eye(s) up to qid	Remove contact lenses. Pregnancy category C
Naproxen (Naprosyn)	250, 375, 500 mg immediate-release tabs, caps, gel-caps; 375, 500 mg delayed-release tabs	250–500 mg initially, then 250 mg q 12 hr. Max dose 2 tabs in 8–12 hr, 3 tabs in 24 hr. Delayed-release (adult): 375–500 mg bid. Dysmenorrhea: 500 mg bid or 500 mg followd by 275 mg q 6–8 hours; max dose 1250 mg/24 hr	Pregnancy category C/D
Naproxen sodium (Aleve, Anaprox, Anaprox DS)	220 mg (200 mg naproxen), 275 mg (250 mg naproxen), 550 mg (500 mg naproxen) tabs; 412.5 mg (375 mg naproxen), 550 mg (500 mg naproxen) controlled-release tabs	*See* naproxen; dose based on mg naproxen.	Pregnancy category C/D
Naratriptan HCl (Amerge)	1, 2.5 mg tabs	1–2.5 mg; may repeat once in 4 hr. Max 5 mg/24 hr	Safety not established in pediatric/adolescent patients. Pregnancy category C
Nedocromil sodium (Alocril)	2% soln (5 mL)	1–2 drops to each eye bid	Remove contact lenses during use. Pregnancy category B
Neurontin	*See* Gabapentin		
Nifedipine (Adalat CC, Procardia, Procardia XL)	30, 60, 90 mg extended-release tabs	Extended-release (>40 kg): Start at 10–20 mg/24 hr divided bid-qd; max dose 120 mg/24 hr. Adult: 30–60 mg qd; may titrate up to max dose 120 mg/24 hr over 7–14 days	Pregnancy category C
Nitrofurantoin (Macrobid, Macrodantin)	25, 50, 100 mg (macrocystals) caps; 100 mg dual release caps (25 mg macrocrystals/75 mg monohydrate)	50–100 mg (macrocrystals) q 6 hours. Dual release: 100 mg bid	Dosing/duration of therapy varies depending on condition being treated. Pregnancy category B

(*Continued*)

Table 1
(Continued)

Drug	Available as	Dosage	Comments
Nizatidine (Axid)	75 mg tabs; 150, 300 mg caps	GERD: 150 mg bid up to 8 (younger teens) - 12 weeks	Pregnancy category B
Norethindrone acetate (Aygestin)	5 mg tabs	2.5–10 mg daily for 5–10 days during 2nd half of theoretical menstrual cycle (after estrogens if needed)	Pregnancy category X
Norfloxacin (Noroxin, Chibroxin)	400 mg tabs; 3 mg/mL (5 mL) ophthalmic drops	Adults and teens >55 kg: 400 mg q 12 hr for 7–10 days (uncomplicated UTI) or 10–21 days for complicated UTI. Prostatitis: 300 mg q 12 hr for 28 days. 1–2 gtts qid for up to 7 days (may give q 2 hours in 1st 24 hours if infection severe)	Limited data in <18 years. Increased risk of tendinitis and tendon rupture in all ages. Pregnancy category C
Nortriptyline HCl (Pamelor, Aventyl)	10, 25, 50, 75 mg caps	Adolescent: 1–3 mg/kg/24 hr divided tid-qid or 30–50 mg/24 hr divided tid-qid. Adult: 75–100 mg/24 hr divided tid-qid. Max dose 150 mg/24 hr. Enuresis (>11 years): 25–35 mg qhs	Note black box warning regarding suicidality. Pregnancy category D
Ofloxacin (Floxin, Floxin Otic, Ocuflox)	200, 300, 400 mg tabs; Otic soln: 0.3% (5, 10 mL); Ophthalmic soln 0.3% (1, 5, 10 mL)	Respiratory: 400 mg q 12 hours Otitis externa: 10 gtts to affected ear(s) bid for 10–14 days. Chronic suppurative otitis media: 10 gtts to affected ear(s) bid for 14 days. Acute otitis media with tubes: 5 gtts to affected ear(s) bid for 5 days; 1–2 gtts to affected eye(s) q 2–4 hr ×2 days, then qid for 5 days	Dosing/duration of therapy varies depending on condition being treated. Safety and efficacy of oral formulations in children <18 years of age have not been established. Increased risk of tendinitis and tendon rupture in all ages Take on an empty stomach with full glass of water. Pregnancy category C
Olanzapine (Zyprexa)	2.5, 5, 7.5, 10, 15, 20 mg tabs; 5, 10, 15, 20 mg oral disintegrating tab	5 mg qd; increase q 3–4 days to max dose 20 mg/24 hr	Pregnancy category C

(Continued)

Table 1
(Continued)

Drug	Available as	Dosage	Comments
Olopatadine HCL (Patanol)	0.1% (5 mL), 0.2% soln (2.5 mL)	1–2 gtts to affected eye(s) bid (0.1%); 1 drop in affected eye(s) daily (0.2%)	For allergic conjunctivitis. Remove contact lenses. Wait at least 10 minutes after instilling drops before reinserting lenses. Pregnancy category C
Omeprazole (Prilosec, Prilosec OTC)	10, 20, 40 mg sustained-release caps; 20 mg delayed-release tabs (OTC)	GERD: 20 mg qd up to 4 weeks Gastric ulcer (adults): 40 mg/24 hr divided qd-bid for 4–8 weeks	Dosing/duration of therapy varies depending on condition being treated. Take before eating; can take with antacids. Pregnancy category C
Ondansetron (Zofran)	8 mg oral disintergrating tab (ODT)	Vomiting in acute gastroenteritis: 8 mg ODT tid prn nausea	Off-label use. Pregnancy category B
Oseltamivir phosphate (Tamiflu)	75 mg	75 mg bid for 5 days	Start therapy within 48 hr of onset of influenza symptoms. Pregnancy category C
Oxycodone (Oxycontin)	5, 15, 30 mg tabs; 10, 20, 40 mg controlled-release tabs	Dose range for younger adolescent: 0.05–0.15 mg/kg/dose q 4–6 hours (max 5 mg/dose). Older adolescent: 5–10 mg regular tabs q 4–6 hr as needed. Take total daily dose and administer divided bid using controlled-release tabs	Pregnancy category B/D (if used for prolonged time or at term). Schedule II
Oxycodone HCl plus acetaminophen (Percocet)	2.5 mg oxycodone/325 mg acetaminophen; 5 mg/325 mg; 7.5 mg/325 mg; 7.5 mg/500 mg; 10 mg/325 mg; 10 mg/650 mg tabs	Dosage based on age and amount of oxycodone/acetaminophen. *See* oxycodone above. Max dose acetaminophen 4 g/24 hr	Pregnancy category B/D (D if used for prolonged time or at term). Schedule II
Pamelor	*See* Nortriptyline		
Pantoprazole (Protonix)	20, 40 mg enteric-coated tabs	>40 kg: 40 mg qd. Adult: 40–80 mg qd for 4–8 weeks	Dosing/duration of therapy varies depending on condition being treated. Pregnancy category B

(Continued)

Table 1
(Continued)

Drug	Available as	Dosage	Comments
Paroxetine (Paxil, Paxil CR)	10, 20, 30, 40 mg tabs; 12.5, 25, 37.5 mg controlled-release tabs (CR)	Obsessive-compulsive disorder or social anxiety disorder ≤17 years: 10 mg daily; titrate up as needed by 10 mg/24 hours every 7 days. Max 50 mg/24 hr. ≥18 years: Depression: 20 mg q am for 4 weeks; can titrate up by 10 mg/24 hr q 7 days to max of 50 mg/24 hr. Paxil CR: start with 25 mg q am for 4 weeks. If needed, increase by 12.5 mg/24 hr every 7 days to max dose of 62.5 mg/24 hr. Panic disorder: 10 mg daily; increase dose by 10 mg/24 hr q 7 days to max 60 mg/24 hr. Paxil CR: Start with 12.5 mg q am; can increase by 12.5 mg/24 hr q 7 days to max dose 75 mg/24 hr	Note black box warning regarding suicidality. The FDA does not recommend the use of paroxetine to treat depression in those ≤17 years of age. Pregnancy category D
Penciclovir (Denavir)	1% cream (2 g)	Apply q 2 hours while awake for 4 days	Begin treatment at earliest symptom or sign of an outbreak. Avoid eyes and mucous membranes. Pregnancy category B
Penicillin V potassium (Veetids)	250, 500 mg tabs	250–500 mg/dose q 6–8 hours. Group A streptococcal pharyngitis: 500 mg bid (if good compliance expected) - tid for 10 days	Dosing/duration of therapy varies depending on condition being treated. Take 1 hr before or 2 hours after meals. Pregnancy category B
Permethrin (Acticin, Elimite, Nix)	5% cream (60 g); 1% cream rinse with comb (OTC, 2 oz); 1% lotion (OTC, 60 mL)	Scabies: apply 5% cream from neck to soles of feet and wash off 8–14 hours later. May repeat in 7 days. Lice (head or pubic hair): Shampoo, rinse and towel-dry hair. Apply 1% cream rinse, wait 10 minutes, rinse. Remove nits with comb; may reapply in 7–10 days	Pregnancy category B

(Continued)

Table 1
(Continued)

Drug	Available as	Dosage	Comments
Phenazopyridine HCl (Pyridium, Urostat, Azo-Standard)	95, 97.2, 100 mg tabs (OTC); 100, 150, 200 mg tabs	100–200 mg tid after meals. Do not use >2 days	Turns urine orange; may stain contact lens. Pregnancy category B
Pimecrolimus (Elidel)	1% cream (15, 30, 100 g)	Apply thin layer bid	Avoid sun/UV light. May increase cancer risk. Pregnancy category C
Pirbuterol acetate (Maxair)	200 mcg/inhalation breath-actuated MDI (Autohaler); 200 mcg/inhalation MDI (inhaler)	2 inhalations q 4–6 hours as needed. Max 12 inhalations/24 hr	Pregnancy category C
Podofilox (Condylox)	0.5% topical solution (3.5 mL), gel (3.5 g)	Apply q 12 hours for 3 days, then discontinue for 4 days; may repeat up to 4 treatment cycles	Pregnancy category C
Polyethylene glycol (PEG) (Glycolax, Miralax, GoLYTELY)	PEG 3350 powder for reconstitution: 236 g (Miralax), 255, 527 g (with dosing cup; single dose packets [17 g, #12])	17 g dissolved in 4–8 oz water, juice, soda, coffee, or tea	Avoid use if bowel obstruction is a possibility. Pregnancy category C
Polymixin plus neomycin plus hydrocortisone (Cortisporin Otic)	Polymyxin B sulfate 10 000 units, neomycin sulfate 3.5 mg, hydrocortisone 10 mg/mL solution, suspension (10 mL)	3–4 gtts in affected ear(s) tid-qid for 7–10 days	Do not use with perforated tympanic membrane. Pregnancy category C
Polymyxin plus trimethoprim sulfate (Polytrim)	Polymyxin B sulfate 10 000 units, trimethoprim sulfate 1 mg/mL (10 mL) ophthalmic soln	1 drop to affected eye(s) q 3 hours (max 6 doses/24 hr) for 7–10 days	Pregnancy category C
Pravastatin (Pravachol)	10, 20, 40, 80 mg tabs	≤13: 20 mg qd; 14–18 and adults: 40 mg qd. Adult maintenance dose 40–80 mg qd	Pregnancy category X
Prochlorperazine (Compazine)	5, 10 mg tabs; 10, 15 mg slow-release caps	5–10 mg/dose immediate release bid-qid; 10 mg bid or 15 mg qd (extended-release)	Pregnancy category C

(Continued)

Table 1
(Continued)

Drug	Available as	Dosage	Comments
Promethazine HCl (Phenergan)	12.5, 25, 50 mg tabs 25, 50 mg/mL injection (1 mL)	Motion sickness: 25 mg 30–60 minutes before travel; may repeat q 8–12 hours. Nausea/vomiting: 12.5–25 mg q 4–6 hours	If giving injection, IM preferred (do not give subcutaneous or IV). Pregnancy category C
Propanalol (Inderal)	10, 20, 40, 60, 80, 90 mg tabs; 60, 80, 120, 160 mg extended-release caps	Dosing depends on weight. Hypertension (younger adolescent): 0.5–1 mg/kg/24 hr divided q6–12 hours; may increase dose q 3–5 days (max 8 mg/kg/24 hr). Older adolescent/adult: 40 mg/dose bid or 60–80 mg qd (sustained-release); may increase 10–20 mg/dose q3–5 days to max 640 mg/24 hr. Migraine prophylaxis: (≥35) kg: 20–40 mg tid; older adolescent/adult: 80 mg/24 hours divided q 6–8 hours; may increase by 20–40 mg/dose q 3–4 weeks (usual dosc rangc 160–240 mg/24 hr)	Do not give if patient has asthma. Pregnancy category C/D
Prozac	*See* Fluoxetine		
Quetiapine fumarate (Seroquel, Seroquel XR)	25, 50, 100, 200, 300, 400 mg tabs; 50, 150, 200, 300, 400 mg extended-release tabs (XR)	50 mg bid; target dose range 150–750 mg/24 hr	Note black box warning regarding suicidality. Baseline and semiannual eye exams recommended (cataract formation). Pregnancy category C
Ranitidine HCl	75, 150 mg (OTC); 300 mg tabs	75–150 mg bid depending on age; max 300 mg/24 hr	Dose/duration of therapy varies depending on condition being treated. Pregnancy category B
Rimantidine (Flumadine)	100 mg tabs	>40 kg: 100 mg bid for 5–7 days	Start within 48 hours of symptom onset. Pregnancy category C

(*Continued*)

Table 1
(Continued)

Drug	Available as	Dosage	Comments
Risperidone (Risperdal)	0.25, 0.5, 1, 2, 3, 4 mg tabs; 0.5, 1, 2, 3, 4 mg orally disintegrating tabs (ODT)	10–17 years: 0.5 mg/24 hours q am or qhs. May increase by 0.5–1.0 mg increments (at intervals at least 24 hrs apart) to recommended dose of 2.5 (bipolar mania) - 3 mg (schizophrenia)/24 hours. >17 years: Bipolar mania: 2–3 mg qd; may increase by 1 mg/24 hr to max dose 6 mg/24 hr. Schizophrenia: 1 mg bid; can increase by 1–2 mg q 7 days to max dose 16 mg/24 hours.	Pregnancy category C
Ritalin	*See* Methylphenidate		
Rizatriptan benzoate (Maxalt, Maxalt ODT)	5, 10 mg tabs; 5, 10 mg oral disintegrating tabs (ODT)	5–10 mg; may repeat q2 hours (max 30 mg/24hr)	Not recommended in patients <18 years. Interacts with propanalol. Pregnancy category C
Salmeterol (Serevent Diskus)	50 mcg/inhalation dry powder (#28, #60 inhalations)	1 inhalation q 12 hours; exercise induced bronchospasm: 1 inhalation 30–60 minutes before exercise (do not repeat <12 hours)	Long-acting β-2 agonists may increase risk of asthma deaths. Pregnancy category C
Sarafem	*See* Fluoxetine		
Selenium sulfide (Selsun)	1% lotion (OTC-210, 325, 400 mL); 2.5% lotion (120 mL)	*Tinea versicolor*: apply 2.5% lotion qd for 7 days to affected areas; leave on 30 minutes and rinse thoroughly. May repeat monthly for 3 months for prophylaxis. Seborrhea/dandruff: Apply 5–10 mL of 1% or 2.5% lotion to wet scalp, wait 2–3 minutes; rinse thoroughly. Repeat twice weekly for 2 weeks, then 1–4 times per month as needed.	Pregnancy category C
Seroquel	*See* Quetiapine		
Sertraline HCl (Zoloft)	25, 50, 100 mg	>13 y: 50 mg daily; may increase dose by 50 mg q 7 days to max 200 mg/24 hr	Note black box warning regarding suicidality. Pregnancy category C

(Continued)

Table 1
(Continued)

Drug	Available as	Dosage	Comments
Simvastatin (Zocor)	5, 10, 20, 40, 80 mg tabs	<17 years: 10 mg daily in the evening; maintenance 10–40 mg qd. Adults: 20–40 mg qd in the evening; maintenance dose range 5–80 mg/24 hr	Pregnancy category X
Sonata	*See* Zaleplon		
Spironolactone (Aldactone)	25, 50, 100 mg tabs	Hirsutism: 50–200 mg/24 hr divided qd-bid	Pregnancy category C/D
Strattera	See Atomoxetine		
Sumatriptan succinate (Imitrex)	25, 50, 100 mg tabs; 5, 20 mg/dose in 100 microliter single dose units (6 units per pack) nasal spray	25 mg as soon as headache apparent; if no relief in 2 hr may give 25–100 mg q 2 hours up to daily max of 200 mg. Nasal spray: 5–20 mg into 1 nostril or divided into each nostril at onset of headache. May repeat dose in 2 hr to max 40 mg/24 hours	Efficacy of sumatriptan in <18 y questionable–some do not recommend use. Pregnancy category C
Tacrolimus (Protopic)	0.03, 0.1% ointment (30, 60, 100 g)	Apply thin layer to affected areas bid	May increase risk for cancer. Pregnancy category C
Tazarotene (Tazorac)	0.05%, 0.1% gel (30, 60, 100 g)	Apply to clean dry skin once daily at bedtime	Avoid exposure to sun/UV light. Reduce dosing frequency if irritation develops. Pregnancy category X
Tegretol	*See* Carbamazepine		
Tenex	*See* Guanfacine		
Terbinafine (Lamisil, Lamisil AT)	1% cream, spray; 250 mg tabs	Onychomycosis (adults): 250 mg qd for 6 weeks (fingernails) or 12 weeks (toenails); *tinea capitis* (>40 kg): 250 mg qd	Dosing/duration of therapy varies depending on condition being treated. Onychomycosis: liver function tests at baseline; monitor for hepatic dysfunction during therapy. Pregnancy category B
Tetracycline HCl	250, 500 mg caps	1–2 g/24 hr divided q 6–12 hours	Avoid prolonged exposure to sunlight. Pregnancy category D
Tofranil	*See* imipramine		

(*Continued*)

Table 1
(Continued)

Drug	Available as	Dosage	Comments
Tolnaftate (Tinactin)	1% topical aerosol liquid (60, 120 mL) or powder (100, 105, 150 g); cream (15, 21, 30 g), gel (15 g); 1% powder (45, 90 g) or soln (10 mL)–all formulations OTC	Apply small amt gel, liquid, cream, powder or 1–3 drops soln bid-tid for 2–4 weeks	Pregnancy category C
Topiramate (Topamax)	15, 25 mg caps; 25, 50, 100, 200 mg tabs	Migraine prophylaxis: start at 25 mg qhs for 7 days, then increase as needed after 1 week to 25 mg bid, then if needed after 7 days, increase to 25 mg q am, 50 mg qhs, then after 7 days if needed to 50 mg bid.	May reduce effectiveness of hormonal contraceptives via increased metabolism of estrogen. Pregnancy category C
Tramadol (Ultram)	50 mg tabs; 100, 200, 300 mg extended-release tabs	50–100 mg q 4–6 hours	Safety of immediate/extended release not established <16 years and extended release <18 years. Do not give if opioids contraindicated. Pregnancy category C
Trazodone HCl (Desyrel)	50, 100, 150, 300 mg tabs	<18 years: 1.5–2 mg/kg/24 hr divided bid-tid. Can increase dose q 3–4 days to max of 6 mg/kg/24 hr divided tid. Adult: 150 mg/24 hr divided tid; may increase by 50 mg/d q3–4 days to max 400 mg/24 hr divided tid	Note black box warning regarding suicidality. Use with caution in patients taking antihypertensive meds. Pregnancy category C
Tretinoin (Retin-A, Retin-A Micro, many others)	0.02% (40 g) , 0.025% (20, 45 g), 0.05% (20, 40, 45, 60g), 0.1% (20, 45 g) cream; 0.01% (15, 45 g), 0.025% (15, 20, 45 g), 0.04% (20, 40 g) gel; Retin-A Micro gel: 0.04% (20, 45g), 0.1% (20, 45 g)	Wash face and pat dry, wait 30 minutes, then apply small amount to skin once daily.	Reduce dosing frequency or strength if irritation develops; Avoid sunlight/use sunscreen. Pregnancy category C

(Continued)

Table 1
(Continued)

Drug	Available as	Dosage	Comments
Triamcinolone acetonide (Azmacort)	75 mcg/inhalation MDI (#240, 20 g)	Two inhalations tid-qid or 4 inhalations bid. Max 16 inhalations/ 24 hr	Rinse mouth after use. Pregnancy category C/D
Triamcinolone acetonide (Nasocort AQ, Nasocort HFA)	AQ: 55 mcg/spray (#30, 6.5 g, #120,16.5 g); HFA: 55 mcg/spray (#100, 9.3 g)	AQ: 2 sprays each nostril qd; HFA: 2 sprays each nostril qd; after 4–7 days, may increase to 4 sprays/nostril/24 hr divided qd-qid	May reduce dose if symptom reduction warrants. Pregnancy category C/D
Triamcinolone acetonide (Kenalog)	Cream and ointment: 0.025%, 0.1% (15, 80, 454 g); 0.5% (15 g); lotion: 0.025%, 0.1% (60 mL); aerosol: 0.2 mg/2 second spray (23, 63 g)	Apply to affected area bid-tid	Pregnancy category C/D
Trimethoprim (TMP) plus sulfamethoxazole (SMX) (Bactrim, Septra, Co-Trimoxazole)	Single strength (SS) tabs: 80 mg TMP/ 400 mg SMX. Double strength (DS) tabs: 160 mg TMP/800 mg SMX	>40 kg: 160 mg TMP/800 mg SMX (1 DS tab) bid	Dosing/duration of therapy varies depending on condition being treated. Pregnancy category C/D
Valacyclovir (Valtrex)	500, 1000 mg tabs	Herpes labialis: 2 g/dose q12 hr for 1 day. *See* chapter on infectious diseases for dosing in genital herpes	Pregnancy category B
Valium	*See* Diazepam		
Valproic acid (Depakene)	250 mg caps; 125, 250, 500 mg delayed-release caps	Migraine prophylaxis: 250 mg delayed-release cap bid; max dose 1000 mg/24 hr	Pregnancy category D
Venlafaxine (Effexor, Effexor XR)	25, 37.5, 50, 75, 150 mg caps; 37.5, 75, 150 mg extended-release tabs, caps; 225 mg extended-release tab	Initial: 37.5–75 mg daily; may increase by 37.5–75 mg increments/d after 4 or more day intervals to maintenance range 150–300 mg/24 hr	Note black box warning regarding suicidality. Pregnancy category C
Verapamil (Calan, Calan SR, Isoptin)	40, 80, 120 mg tabs; 120, 180, 240 mg extended/sustained-release tabs; 100 120, 180, 200, 240, 300, 360 mg extended/sustained-release caps	Hypertension Under 60 kg: 4–8 mg/kg/24 hr divided tid; ≥60 kg: 240–480 mg/24 hr divided tid-qid or divided qd-bid with sustained-release tabs/caps Migraine prophylaxis: 80 mg tid-qid	Pregnancy category C

(Continued)

Table 1
(Continued)

Drug	Available as	Dosage	Comments
Vyvanse	*See* Lysdexamfetamine		
Wellbutrin, Wellbutrin SR, Wellbutrin XL	*See* Bupropion		
Xanax	*See* Alprazolam		
Zaleplon (Sonata)	5, 10 mg caps	5–10 mg qhs	Pregnancy category C. Schedule IV
Zafirlukast (Accolate)	10, 20 mg tabs	20 mg po bid	Pregnancy category B
Zolmitriptan (Zomig, Zomig ZMT)	2.5, 5 mg tabs; 2.5, 5 mg orally-disintegrating tabs, 5 mg/ 100 microliters nasal spray (6 single use units)	2.5–5 mg; may repeat once in 2 hours; max dose 10 mg/ 24 hr. Spray: 1 spray; may repeat in 2 hr. Max dose 10 mg/24 hr	Pregnancy category C
Zoloft	*See* Sertraline		
Zolpidem tartrate (Ambien)	5, 10 mg tabs; 6.25, 12.5 mg extended-release tabs	5–10 mg at bedtime or 6.25–12.5 mg extended release at bedtime	Safety and efficacy in children not established. Pregnancy category C. Schedule IV
Zyban	*See* Buproprion		
Zyprexa	*See* Olanzapine		

References

This table is based on a table that originally appeared in: Strasburger VC, Brown RT, Braverman PK, Rogers PD, Holland-Hall CM. *Adolescent Medicine: A Handbook for Primary Care*; 2005. Philadelphia, PA: Lippincott Williams & Wilkins, pp. 293–311. Reprinted with permission.

Other sources used in the preparation of this table include:

Custer JW, Rau RE, eds. *The Harriet Lane Handbook*, 18th ed; 2009. Philadelphia, PA: Mosby, Inc.

Scharf MA, Williams TP. Psychopharmacology in adolescent medicine. *Adolesc Med*;2006:165–181.

Singh MK, Pfeifer JC, Barzman DH, Kowatch RA, DelBello MP. Medical management of pediatric mood disorders. *Pediatr Ann.* 2007;36: 552–563.

Micromedex Healthcare Series. Thomson Micromedex (internet database), Updated periodically. Greeenwood Village, CO: Thomson Healthcare.

Table 2
Stimulant Medications, Dosing, and Duration of Effects

Active Ingredient	Drug Name	Dosing	Duration of Behavioral Effects
Mixed salts of amphetamine (dextroamphetamine/ levoamphetamine)	ADDERALL tablets *(scored)*: 5, 7.5, 10, 12.5, 15, 20, 30 mg	Start with 5 mg 1–2 times per day and increase by 5 mg each week until good control achieved. Maximal recommended dose: 40 mg	4–6 hr
	ADDERALL RX Extended-Release capsule *(can be sprinkled)*: 5, 10, 15, 20, 25, 30 mg extended-release capsules	Start at 5 mg in the morning and increase by 5 mg each week until good control is achieved. Maximal recommended dose: 30 mg	10–12 hr
Dextroamphetamine	DEXEDRINE tablet: 5 mg DEXTROSTAT tablet *(scored)*: 5, 10 mg	Tablet: Start with 5 mg 1–2 times per day and increase by 5 mg each week until good control achieved. Maximal recommended dose: 40 mg	4–6 hr
	DEXEDRINE SPANSULES Sustained-Release capsule *(cannot be chewed)*: 5, 10, 15 mg	Capsule: start with 5 mg one time per day and increase by 5 mg each week until good control is achieved.	6–10 hr
Methylphenidate	RITALIN tablets: 5, 10, 20 mg METHYLIN tablets (*scored*): 5, 10, 20 mg METHYLIN Chewable tablets: 5, 10, 20 mg METHYLIN Oral Solution: 5, 10 mg/5 mL	Start with 5 mg 1–2 times per day and increase by 5 mg each week until good control is achieved. May need third reduced dose in the evening. Maximal recommended dose: 60 mg	

(*Continued*)

Table 2
(Continued)

Active Ingredient	Drug Name	Dosing	Duration of Behavioral Effects
	FOCALIN tablets *(scored)*: 2.5, 5, 10 mg	Start with 2.5 mg 1–2 times per day and increase by 2.5 mg each week until good control is achieved. May need third reduced dose in the evening. Maximal recommended dose: 30 mg	4–5 hr
	RITALIN-LA capsule *(can be sprinkled)*: 10, 20, 30, 40 mg RITALIN-SR tablet: 20 mg SR METADATE ER tablet: 10, 20 mg extended release METHYLIN ER tablet: 10 mg extended release METADATE CD capsule *(can be sprinkled)*: 10, 20, 30 mg extended release	Start with 10–20 mg in the morning and increase each week until good control is achieved. Alternatively, titrate using short-acting methylphenidate and then switch over to a longer-acting form. May need second dose or regular methylphenidate dose in the evening. Maximal recommended dose: 60 mg	6–10 hr
	FOCALIN XR capsule *(can be sprinkled)*: 5, 10, 20 mg	Start with 5 mg in the morning and increase by 5 mg each week until good control is achieved. Maximal recommended dose: 30 mg	8–10 hr
	CONCERTA capsule *(noncrushable)*: 18, 27, 36, 54 mg	Start at 18 mg in the morning and increase by 18 mg each week until good control is achieved. Maximal recommended dose: 72 mg	8–12 hr

(Continued)

Table 2
(Continued)

Active Ingredient	Drug Name	Dosing	Duration of Behavioral Effects
	DAYTRANA Patch 1.1, 1.8, 2.2, 3 mg/hr	Worn daily for 9 hours. Patch is to be replaced once a day in the morning. Skin sensitization as compared with contact rash may occur rarely, causing FDA advisory board to recommend oral methylphenidate use before the patch	Approximately 12 hr
Lysdexamfetamine	VYVANSE capsule *(sprinkle in water and drink immediately)*: 30, 50, 70 mg	Start at 30 mg in the morning and increase by 20 mg each week until good control is achieved. Maximal recommended dose: 70 mg	Approximately 12 hr

FDA, US Food and Drug Administration.

From Leslie LK, Guevara JP. Attention-deficit/Hyperactivity Disorder. In: McInerny TK, Adam HM, Campbell DE, Kamat DM, Kelleher KJ, eds. *American Academy of Pediatrics Textbook of Pediatric Care*. Elk Grove Village, IL: American Academy of Pediatrics; 2009.

Adolesc Med 20 (2009) 860–872

Note: Page numbers of article titles are in **boldface** type.

A

Abortions
- for teenagers, 335
- parent/guardian involvement, 395–397

ACHES mnemonic, 407
Achilles tendon, 724
Acne
- assessment of, 681
- definition, 677
- description, 678
- etiology, 677
- scoring systems, 472
- treatment, 678, 679–680, 682

Acute rheumatic fever (ARF), 795–798
Adolescence. *See also* Specific issues
- characteristics of, 380–381
- checklist, 414
- developmental assets of, 385

Adolescents. *See also* Specific conditions; Specific issues
- contraindications for COCs, 504
- global evaluation of functioning, 401–405
- health statistics, **261–349**
- psychosocial history and, 400–401

Adrenal glands, androgen production, 350
Age
- alcohol use before 13yrs, 334
- at first marijuana use, 333
- birth rates and, 336
- BMI cut-offs, 442
- BP levels by height, 650, 651
- causes of deaths, 296–305
- *Chlamydia* infection rates, 344
- contraceptives and, 338
- deaths and death rates by, 293–295
- dieting and, 288
- experience of sexual violence and, 272
- fasting and diet aid use, 291
- feelings of sadness/hopelessness and, 273
- gonorrhea infection rates and, 346–347
- HIV/AIDS diagnosis and, 341
- induced vomiting and laxative use, 292
- lipid levels and, 656
- number of outpatient visits and, 388
- nutrition/exercise and, 290
- obese and overweight students and, 288
- peak expiratory flow rates, 640
- receipt of HIV/AIDS education, 339
- sexual intercourse among students, 337
- sexual intercourse before 13yrs, 337
- sexually-transmitted diseases and, 341–349
- smoking behaviors and, 332, 334
- suicidal ideation and, 274
- suicide attempts and, 275
- syphilis infection rates and, 348–349

Age groups, projected population, 264
Alcohol use
- 30 day prevalence of abuse, 328, 329–330
- annual prevalence of abuse, 322
- before sexual intercourse, 339
- driving and, 271
- impairment charts, 781
- intoxication and withdrawal, 760–762
- questions about, 782
- survey of, 271, 334
- survey on use of, 334
- trends in heavy drinking, 307
- trends in lifetime abuse, 312

Amenorrhea, 457
- differential diagnoses, 464

evaluation of, 478
primary, 468–469
Amphetamines
30 day prevalence of use, 327
annual prevalence of illicit use, 320
intoxication and withdrawal, 769–770
trends in lifetime use, 311
Androgens
adrenal production of, 350
insensitivity to, 476
sources in adult women, 473
Androstenedione, in puberty, 350
Ankle
bony anatomy of, 723
major ligaments of, 724
range of motion, 718
Anorexia nervosa, 751, 757
Anthrax vaccination, 632
Antinuclear antibody tests, 799–800
Antisocial disorder, 748
Anxiety disorders, treatment of, 745
APA Factors Promoting Reliance and Positive Outcome, 375–376
Asthma
assessing control in, 647
classification of severity, 638
long-term medications, 641–646
management of, 639
Atomoxetine, 731
Attention-deficit/hyperactivity disorder
comorbid conditions, 730
diagnostic criteria for, 729–730
epidemiology, 730
medications, 730–732
scales, 730
Atypical squamous cells of undetermined significance (ASC-US), 482
Autoimmune thyroiditis (Hashimoto disease, type 1), 454–455
Avoidant personality disorder, 749

B

Bacille Calmette-Guérin vaccine
TB tests after, 613
vaccination during pregnancy, 632
Bacterial vaginosis
diagnostic findings, 591–593
treatment, 594
Barbiturates
intoxication and withdrawal, 775–776
trends in lifetime illicit use, 311
Bardet-Biedl syndrome, 440
Basics of Parenting Adolescents, 375–376
Behavioral change, motivation of, 408
Behavioral therapies, 746
Benzodiazepines, 775
Bidis, use of, 322
Biemond syndrome, 440
Binge-eating disorder, 753
Binging, screening for, 753
Bipolar disorders
depressive, 735
description, 735–738
hypomania, 737
manic, 735, 736
mixed episodes, 737
unipolar depression and, 738
Birth control. *See also* Contraception; Oral contraceptives, combined
use of, 338
web site for teenagers, 564
Birth control pills. *See* Oral contraceptives
Birth rates, women aged 15y-19y, 336
Births to teenagers, 335
Bisexuality, 382
Blood glucose levels
diagnostic ranges, 416
recommended, 418
self-monitoring, 418
Blood pressure charts, 650–653. *See also* Hypertension
Body mass index (BMI). *See also* Obesity
evaluation of obesity, 442
for weight and stature, 362
Body mass index-for-age charts, 360–361
Body piercing, 693
Body surface area, calculation of, 384
Bone age, determination of, 435
Bone, neoplasms of, 795
Borderline personality disorder, 748
Boys. *See also* Gender
ages at sexual maturity, 369
BMI-for-age, 361
BP levels by age/height, 650
height by age chart, 357
prediction of adult height, 384

prepubertal development, 363
stature-for-age charts, 355
testicular volume, 366
weight-for-age charts, 359
Breast cancer, COCs and, 553
Breast development
absent with uterus present, 474–475
ages at stage1/2 transition, 372
present with uterus abnormal, 475
present with uterus present, 475
Breastfeeding, vaccinations during, 634
Bright Futures Strengths During Adolescence, 375–376
Bulimia nervosa, 752, 757
Bupropion, 731

C

C-reactive protein, 799
Calcium requirements
during puberty, 351
food sources of, 789
supplements, 790
Cancers, contraceptives and, 553–554
Candida albicans, 591–593
Candidiasis
diagnostic findings, 591–593
treatment, 594
Cardiology consultations, 823
Cardiorespiratory, **637–663**
Cervical cancer
combined oral contraceptives and, 553
screening guidelines, 480–483
Chlamydia infections
age- and sex-specific rates of, 343–345
age-, race and sex-related rates, 344–345
diagnostic tests, 588
treatment guidelines, 566–568
Cholesterol levels, 655
abnormal, 657
by gender and age, 656
Chronic fatigue syndrome, 811–813
Chronic pain syndromes, 794, 809–814
Cigarettes
30 day prevalence of use, 329, 330
smoking behaviors and, 332
survey on use of, 334
trends in lifetime use, 313
Circle of Courage, 375–376
Clonidine, 732
Clotting factors, impact of COCs, 552
Cocaine
30 day prevalence of use, 326
annual prevalence of use, 319
intoxication and withdrawal, 767–769
trends in lifetime use, 310
Coccidioidomycosis, prophylaxis, 599
COCs. *See* Oral contraceptives, combined
Cognitive behavioral therapy, 746
Concussion
return to sports after, 712, 713
sports-related, 713
Condoms, 338, 555–557
Conduct disorders, 750
Connective tissue disease, tests for, 798–800
Contraception, **484–565.** *See also* Birth control; Oral contraceptives
access by minors to, 389–392
condoms, 555–557
FDA approved, 484
hormone-related complications, 536–537
injectable, 505–517, 558–561
intrauterine devices, 538–551
levonorgestrel-releasing intrauterine system, 563–564
medical eligibility for CICs, 505–517
medical eligibility for COCs, 493–503
medical eligibility for patches, 505–517
medical eligibility for rings, 505–517
patches, 505–517, 561–562
rate of unexpected pregnancies, 485
rings, 505–517
single etonogestrel implant, 564
vaginal rings, 563
web site for teenagers, 564
WHO eligibility criteria, 486–503
Corticosteroids, potency ratings, 689–691
Cough/cold medicines
annual prevalence of illicit use, 321
Crack cocaine
30 day prevalence of use, 326

annual prevalence of use, 319
trends in lifetime use, 310
CRAFFT questions, 406
Criteria for the Assessment and Rating of Behavioral Adjustment, 375–376
Crystal meth (ice)
30 day prevalence of use, 327
annual prevalence of use, 321
trends in lifetime use, 311

D

Dating violence, 272
Death rates, 293–305
Dehydroepiandrosterone (DHEA), 350
Dependent personalities, 749–750
Depomedroxyprogesterone acetate, 558–561
Depressants, intoxication and withdrawal, 774
Depression
description of, 735
screening for, 407
symptoms in adolescents, 415
Dermatology, **677–694**
Dermatomyositis, 804–806
Developmental assets, 385
Dexmethylphenidate, 731
Diabetes mellitus
ADA diagnostic criteria, 416
causes of, 416–417
insulin therapy, 428, 429
management approaches, 432
medications for control of, 419–429
monitoring of, 418
obesity and, 449
prevention of, 418
testing in children and adolescents, 417–418
types of, 416–417
Diabetic ketoacidosis protocol, 432–434
Dialectical behavioral therapy, 746
Diet aids, 291, 754
Dieting
nutrition/exercise and, 290
trends in, 289
Dimethyltryptamine (DMT), 779
Diphtheria vaccines, 613
Driving, alcohol use and, 271
Drug interactions, with COCs, 554–555
Drug use, illicit
stages of, 783–784
stages of change, 785, 786–787
trends in 30 day prevalence of use, 324–331
trends in annual prevalence, 306, 317–323
trends in lifetime prevalence, 308–316
Drugs of abuse, clinical effects, 758–759
Dysfunctional uterine bleeding (DUB), 458
definition of, 463–464
differential diagnoses, 462–463, 464
treatment of, 465
Dysmenorrhea, 476, 477
Dysthymic disorder
diagnostic criteria, 732
treatment in primary care, 745

E

Eating disorders, 751–757
medical complications, 756
physical examination in, 755
screening for, 754
Ecstasy (MDMA)
30 day prevalence of use, 325
annual prevalence of use, 318
trends in lifetime use, 309
Endocrine/metabolic system, 350, **416–456**
Endometrial cancer, COCs and, 553
Enteritis, treatment guidelines, 586–587
Enteropathic arthritis, 803
Epididymal cysts, 672
Epididymitis
characteristics, 674, 676
treatment guidelines, 585
Epstein-Barr virus, patterns of viral antibodies, 610
Erythema multiforme, 687
Erythema nodosum, 687, 808
Erythrocyte sedimentation rate (ESR), 798–799
Estrogens, in COCs, 518
Etonogestrel implant, 564
Euthyroid disease, tests for, 453
Exercise, excessive, 290, 754
Eyes, protection during sports, 710–711

F

Familial short stature, 437–438
Families, psychosocial history and, 400–401
Fasting
for more than 24 hours, 291

medical complications, 756
screening for, 753
Femur, muscles around, 720
Fibromyalgia, 809–812
Follicle-stimulating hormone (FSH), 350
Follicular hyperkeratosis, 692
Food labels, 793
Foot
bony anatomy of, 725
range of motion, 718
Forearm, motion of, 717
Formulary, **823–859**
FRAMES mnemonic, 408–409
Functional hypothalamic amenorrhea, 464
Fungal infections
dermatologic, 683–686
topical therapies, 684

G

Gay identity, stages of development, 383
Gender. *See also* Boys; Girls
alcohol use before 13yrs, 334
BMI cut-offs, 442
Chlamydia infection rates, 344
contraceptive use and, 338
deaths and death rates by, 293–305
dieting and, 288
experience of sexual violence and, 272
fasting and diet aid use, 291
feelings of sadness/hopelessness and, 273
first marijuana use, 333
gonorrhea infection rates and, 346–347
HIV/AIDS diagnosis and, 341
induced vomiting and laxative use, 292
lipid levels and, 656
number of outpatient visits and, 388
nutrition/exercise and, 290
obese and overweight students and, 288
overweight in high school and, 288
peak expiratory flow rates, 640
predicted adult heights and, 384, 435
prepubertal stages of development, 363, 364, 365
projected U.S. population, 264
receipt of HIV/AIDS education, 339
sexual behavior and, 337
sexual maturation and, 352
sexually-transmitted diseases and, 341–349
smoking behaviors and, 332, 334
stature-for-age charts, 354–355
suicidal ideation and, 274
suicide attempts and, 275
syphilis infection rates and, 348–349
weight gain velocity and, 351
Gender identity, 382
stages of identity development, 383
transgender, 384
Generalized anxiety disorder, 740
Genital HSV infection, 575–577
Genital warts, 568–575
Genitourinary system, **664–676**
GHB, prevalence of use, 322
Girls. *See also* Gender
ages at sexual maturity, 367, 368
body mass index-for-age, 360
BP levels by age/height, 650
height-by-age charts, 356
prediction of adult height, 384
stages of prepubertal development, 363
stature-for-age charts, 354
weight-for-age charts, 358
Glucocorticoid excess, height and, 438
Glucose, blood levels, 416
Glycemic control guidelines, 419
Gondotropin releasing hormone (GnRH), 350, 351
Gonococcal infections, 568–571
Gonorrhea. *See also Neisseria gonorrhoea*
age- and sex-specific rates of, 343
age-, race- and sex-related rates, 346–347
treatment guidelines, 568–571
Growth and development
biological and psychosocial, **350–385**
BMI-for-age charts, 360–361
constitutional delay of, 436
developmental assets, 385
height-by-age charts, 356, 357
prepubertal stages of, 363, 365
syndromes-associated abnormalities, 439–440
weight-for-age charts, 358–359

Growth hormone deficiency, 438
Growth hormone, in puberty, 351
Growth velocity, 434
Gynecology, **457–483**

H

Hair loss, acquired, 692
Hallucinogens
  30 day prevalence of use, 325
  annual prevalence of use, 318
  effects, 779
  trends in lifetime use, 309
Hand, bony anatomy of, 720
Hashimoto disease, type 1 (autoimmune thyroiditis), 454–455
Headaches, 814–819
HEADS FIRST mnemonic, 402–403
HEADS/HEADSS mnemonic, 401–402
Health indicators
  adolescents, 269–270
  young adults and adolescents, 266–268
Health statistics, adolescents, **261–349**
Healthy People 2010 health indicators, 266–268
Height
  adult, prediction of, 384
  BP levels by age, 650, 651
  by age for girls, 356, 357
  by gender, 435
  changes during puberty, 351–352
  evaluation of curves, 437
  genetic short stature, 437–438
  peak expiratory flow rates, 640
Hematuria, microscopic, 668, 669
Hemoglobin A1c, 418
Henoch-Schonlein vasculitis, 807–808
Hepatitis A virus, 601, 628
Hepatitis B virus, 608, 628, 634
Hernia
  characteristics, 673, 675
  hydrocele and, 671
Heroin
  30 day prevalence of use, 326
  annual prevalence of use, 319
  intoxication and withdrawal, 764–766
  trends in lifetime use, 310
Herpes simplex virus, treatment, 575–577
Heterosexuality, 382
High-density lipoprotein (HDL) levels, 656
High-grade squamous intraepithelial lesions (HSILs), 482
Hip, range of motion, 718
Hirsuitism
  causes of, 469
  evaluation of, 468, 470–471, 474
Hisptoplasma capsulatum
  prophylaxis, 599
Histrionic personality disorder, 748
HIV/AIDS
  defining conditions for AIDS, 595
  diagnosis of, 340, 341, 342
  education in schools about, 339
  lab evaluation after exposure, 606
  occupational exposures, 604
  prophylaxis, 565, 605
  prophylaxis of opportunistic diseases in, 597–603
  surveillance case definition, 595
Homosexuality, 382. *See also* Gay identity, stages of development
  HIV/AIDS diagnosis and, 342
  stages of identity development, 383
Human papillomavirus (HPV)
  prophylaxis, 599, 601
  treatment guidelines, 568–575
  vaccination during pregnancy, 628
Hydrocele, 671, 672
Hyperactivity, 728
Hyperlipidemia, 450, 661
Hypermenorrhea, 458
Hypersensitivity syndromes, 691
Hypertension. *See also* Blood pressure charts
  causes of, 652
  classification of, 649
  clinical evaluation of, 653–654
  management in adolescents, 655
  obesity and, 449
  recommendations, 649
Hypomenorrhea, 458
Hypothalamic-pituitary-gonadal (HPG) axis, 350–351
Hypothyroidism, 438, 453, 454

I

Identity. *See also* Gender identity
components of, 382
transgender, 384
Immunizations, 613–635
catch-up schedules, 624–625
contraindications, 613–616
during breastfeeding, 634
during pregnancy, 627–633
for travelers, 616–617
prenatal serologic screening, 634
reporting adverse events, 615
schedules for, 613–616, 622
vaccines, doses and intervals, 623
web site information, 617
Implanon, 564
Impulse control issues, 728
Inattentiveness issues, 728
Infections, causes of, 794
Infectious diseases, **566–636**
Infectious mononucleosis, 714
Influenza virus
prophylaxis, 599
vaccination during pregnancy, 628–629
vaccination recommendations, 613
Inhalants
30 day prevalence of use, 324
annual prevalence of illicit use, 317
intoxication and withdrawal, 777–778
trends in lifetime use, 308
Injectable contraceptives, 505–517
Insulin therapy, 428
conventional regimens, 431–432
dosage hints, 429
intensive regimens, 429
meal coverage, 431
storage of insulin, 430
types of insulin, 428
Insulin-like growth factors (IGFs), 351
Interpersonal therapy, 746
Intrauterine devices (IUDs), 538–551
Iron requirements, 351, 791–792

J

Japanese encephalitis, 632
Jimsonweed, 779
Juvenile ankylosing spondylitis, 802–803
Juvenile idiopathic arthritis
classification, 800
differential diagnoses, 800–801
types of, 801–802

K

Kallman syndrome, 440
Kawasaki disease, 808
Keratosis pilaris, 692
Ketamine
annual prevalence of use, 322
intoxication and withdrawal, 774
Knee
musculature of, 721
pain diagram, 727
range of motion, 718
Kreteks, prevalence of use, 322

L

Laurence-Moon syndrome, 440
Laxatives, 292, 754
Lesbian identity, 383
Levonorgestrel-releasing intrauterine system (IUS), 563–564
Levothyroxine, requirements for, 456
Lipid distributions, 656, 657–659
Lipid screening, 655–663
Lipoprotein distributions, 656
Low-density lipoprotein (LDL)
levels, 656
by gender and age, 656
management goals, 663
management of elevated levels, 662
pharmacologic treatment and, 660
Lower extremities
compartments of, 722
pain diagram, 727
range of motion, 718
LSD
30 day prevalence of use, 325
annual prevalence of use, 318
intoxication and withdrawal, 771–772
trends in lifetime use, 309
Luteinizing hormone (LH), 350

M

Major depressive disorder
recommendations, 734
treatment in primary care, 745
US Preventive Services Task Force, 734
Major depressive episodes, 731

Malaria, prophylaxis, 602
Mania
  criteria, 736
  description of, 735
Marijuana/hashish
  30 day prevalence of use, 324, 329
  annual prevalence of use, 317
  intoxication and withdrawal, 762–764
  survey on first use of, 333
  trends in lifetime use, 308
Measles vaccination, 629
Medications used by adolescent medicine clinicians, **823–859**
Melanomas, 693
Menarche, timing of, 352
Meningococcal disease
  chemoprophylaxis regimens, 607
  disease risk after contact with, 607
  vaccination during pregnancy, 629, 632
Menorrhagia, 458, 462–463
Menstrual cycles
  evaluation of disorders, 458–462
  irregularities in, 457–458
  normal, 457
Mental health
  common diagnoses, 728–746
  core symptoms, 728
  psychotherapeutic modalities, 746
  psychotropic medications, and substance abuse, **728–787**
  screening/diagnostic questions, 742–744
  treatment in primary care, 745
Mescaline, effects, 779
Metabolic syndrome, 443–446
Methadone, intoxication and withdrawal, 766–767
Methamphetamines
  30 day prevalence of use, 327
  annual prevalence of use, 320
  trends in lifetime use, 311
Methaqualone
  30 day prevalence of use, 327
  annual prevalence of use, 321
  trends in lifetime use, 311
Methylphenidate, 730–731
Metrorrhagia, 458
Microscopic hematuria, 668, 669
Middle childhood checklist, 413
Migraine headaches, 814
  diagnostic criteria, 816
  history checklist, 817
  indications for additional tests, 817–818
  treatment of, 819–820
Mirena, 563–564
Mnemonics, 401–405
Molluscum contagiosum, 692
Morning glory seeds, 779
Mortality rates. *See* Death rates
Mosteller's formula for BSA, 384
Mullerian agenesis, 475
Mullerian fusion abnormalities, 475
Mumps vaccination, 629
Muscle diseases, causes of, 795
Musculoskeletal and sports medicine, **695–727**
Mushrooms, psychedelic, 779
Mycobacterium avium prophylaxis, 598
Mycobacterium tuberculosis prophylaxis, 598

N

Narcissistic personality, 749
Narcotics
  30 day prevalence of illicit use, 326–327
  annual prevalence of illicit use, 319–320
  trends in lifetime use, 310–311
Nausea, treatment of, 535–536
Neisseria gonorrhoea
  diagnostic tests, 588
  treatment guidelines, 568–571
Neoplasms of bone, 795
NFALD, obesity and, 449
Nitrites
  30 day prevalence of use, 325
  annual prevalence of use, 318
  effects, 780
  trends in lifetime use, 309
Nitrous oxide, 780
Nutmeg, 779
Nutrition, **788–793**
  during puberty, 351
  reading label information, 793
NuvaRing, 563

O

Obesity
  cardiometabolic conditions related to, 449–450
  causes of, 447–448
  ICD-9 codes related to, 451
  in high school, 288
  measurement of, 441–443
  physical examination in, 448
  review of systems, 447

Obsessive compulsive disorder, 738, 745
Obsessive-compulsive personality disorder, 750
Office visits, **386–415**
Oligomenorrhea, 457, 464
Oppositional defiant disorders, 750–751
Oral contraceptives, combined, 338. *See also* Contraception
 alteration in lab tests, 552
 androgenic activity of progestins, 519
 by estrogen dose, 518
 cancer risk and, 553–554
 contraindications, 504
 drug interactions, 554–555
 extended cycling, 557–558
 for DUB, 465
 for EC in the U.S., 520–521
 health benefits of, 552–553
 low-dose combined, 493–503
 missed-pill instructions, 555
 monitoring for complications from, 407
 progestogen-only, 522–535
 starting, 551
 use of, 338
Ortho Evra, 561–562
Orthopedic conditions, causes of, 795
OSAS, obesity and, 449
Ovarian cancer, COCs and, 554
Ovarian hyperandrogenism, 466–468
Overuse syndromes, causes of, 794
Overweight
 in high school, 288
 self-assessment of, 289
OxyContin, 320

P

PACES mnemonic, 405
Palpation landmarks, sport-related injuries, 716
Panic attack, symptoms of, 741
Panniculitis, 808
Paranoid personality disorder, 747
Parent-adolescent relationships, 400–401
Parents, psychosocial history and, 400–401
PCP
 30 day prevalence of use, 325
 annual prevalence of use, 318
 intoxication and withdrawal, 772–774
 trends in lifetime use, 309
Peak expiratory flow rates, 640
Pediatric symptom checklist, 410–412
Pelvic inflammatory disease (PID), 580–585
Peripheral neuropathies, 795
Personality disorders, 747–750
Pertussis
 postexposure prophylaxis, 621
 vaccines, 613, 619–620
Peyote, 779
Photoprotection, 693
Pigmented lesions, 693
Pityriasis (tinea) versicolor, 683
Pityriasis rosea, 694
Pneumococcal disease, vaccination, 629
Pneumocystis pneumonia prophylaxis, 597
Poliovirus vaccination, 629
Polyarteritis, 807–808
Polycystic ovary syndrome (PCOS), 449
Polymenorrhea, 457, 462–463
Polymyositis, 804–806
Posttraumatic stress disorder
 diagnostic criteria, 739
 treatment in primary care, 745
Prader-Willi syndrome, 439
Prediabetes, diagnostic criteria, 416
Predicted heights, by gender, 435
Pregnancy
 contraceptive use and, 485
 immunization during, 627–633
 trends in teenagers, 335
Premenstrual dysphoric syndrome, 476–480
Premenstrual syndrome, 476–480
Prenatal serologic screening, 634
Preventive services
 number of outpatient visits, 388
 recommendations, 387–388
Proctitis treatment guidelines, 586–587
Proctocolitis treatment guidelines, 586–587
Progestins, androgenic activity of, 519
Progestogen-only contraceptives (POCs), 522–535
Proteinuria
 disorders causing, 664–665
 persistent, evaluation of, 667
 testing methods, 666
Psilocin, 779
Psilocybin, 779
Psoriasis, 694
Psychodynamic therapy, 746

Psychosocial history, 400–401
Psychosomatic conditions, 795
Psychotherapeutic modalities, 746
Puberty
causes of delay, 440–441
fast facts, 350–353
onset of menses, 457
Pubic hair, 371, 373

R

Race/ethnicity
ages at sexual maturity, 368, 370
alcohol use before 13yrs, 334
births to women aged 15–19yrs, 336
causes of deaths, 296–305
Chlamydia infection rates, 344–345
contraceptives use and, 338
deaths and death rates by, 293–295
dieting and, 288
experience of sexual violence and, 272
fasting and diet aid use and, 291
feelings of sadness/hopelessness and, 273
first marijuana use, 333
gonorrhea infection rates and, 346–347
HIV/AIDS diagnosis and, 341, 342
induced vomiting and laxative use and, 292
nutrition/exercise and, 290
obese and overweight students and, 288
overweight in high school and, 288
projected U.S. population, 263, 265
receipt of HIV/AIDS education, 339
risk behaviors and, 276–286
sexual behavior and, 337
smoking behavior and, 332, 334
suicidal ideation and, 274
suicide attempts and, 275
syphilis infection rates and, 348–349
U.S. population, 2010, 262
Rape laws, 398–399
Reactive arthritis, 803
READY for Life Checklist, 375–376
Rebound headaches, 814
Reflex sympathetic dystrophy, 813–814
Reiter syndrome, 803
Reproductive health, web sites, 564–565
Retinoids, topical, 681
Rheumatic diseases, causes of, 794
Rheumatology and miscellaneous clinical conditions, **794–822**
Risk behaviors, prevalence of, 276–286
Ritalin, prevalence of illicit use, 319–320
Rohypnol
30 day prevalence of illicit use, 328
annual prevalence of illicit use, 322
trends in lifetime illicit use, 312
Rubella
prenatal serologic screening, 634
vaccination during pregnancy, 630

S

Sadness/hopelessness survey, 273
SAFE TEENS mnemonic, 404
SAFE TIMES mnemonic, 403
Schizoid personality disorder, 747
Schizotypal personality disorder, 747–748
Scleroderma, 806–807
Scrotum
causes of swelling, 670
miscellaneous appendages, 673
normal anatomy of, 671
painful masses, 672–674, 675
painless masses, 672–674, 675
Sedatives
30 day prevalence of illicit use, 327
annual prevalence of illicit use, 321
trends in lifetime illicit use, 311
Sex roles, 382. *See also* Gender identity
Sexual intercourse
before 13yrs, 337
forced, 272
rates in high school students, 337
use of alcohol before, 339
Sexual maturation
ages at entry into, 367, 368–369

ages at stage1/2 transition, 371–372
breast development and, 272
changes during puberty, 352
genitalia development and, 274
pubic hair growth and, 271, 273
testicular volume changes, 366
Sexual orientation, 382. *See also* Gender; Heterosexuality; Homosexuality; Transgender identity
Sexual violence, survey of, 272
Sexually-transmitted diseases
age- and sex-related rates, 343–349
minors' access to services, 393–394
treatment guidelines, 566–587
vaginal discharge, 591–593
vaginal wet preps, 589–590
SHADSSS mnemonic, 404
Shingles vaccination, 633
Short stature, 437–438, 438–439
Shoulder
anatomy of, 719
motion of, 717
pain diagram, 726
SIGECAPS mnemonic, 407, 732–733
Single etonogestrel implant, 564
Skeletal dysplasias, 439
Skeleton, changes during puberty, 351–352
Smallpox vaccination, 632
Smokeless tobacco, 331
Smoking
attempts to stop, 332
cigarettes per day, 332
survey on, 334
SPACE DIGS mnemonic, 407
Spermatocele cysts, 672, 675
Spondyloarthropathies, 802–804
Sporadic arthritis, 804
Sport-related injuries
musculoskeletal problems, 715
palpation landmarks, 716
Sports
categories of eye-injury risk, 709
classification by contact, 696
classification by CV demands, 708
eye protectors, 710
participation in, 697–707
return to play, 712, 713, 714
Statistics, adolescent health, **261–349**
Stature
body mass index for, 362
changes during puberty, 351–352
Stature-for-age charts, 354–355
Statutory rape laws, 398–399
Steroids
30 day prevalence of illicit use, 329
annual prevalence of illicit use, 322
biosynthetic pathways, 473
topical, 688
trends in lifetime illicit use, 313
Strengths checklist
for individual adolescents, 375–376
support in office settings, 377–379
Streptococcus pneumoniae prophylaxis, 598
Stress fractures, sports-related, 715
Substance abuse, 758–787
definitions, 738
sample brief advice, 783
screening for, 406
stages of, 783–784
stages of change, 785, 786–787
Substance dependence, 738
Suicidal ideation, survey of, 274
Suicide attempts, survey of, 275
Sunscreen facts, 693–694
Syncope
cardiology consultation, 823
differential diagnosis, 819, 821–822
Syndrome of vanishing testes, 476
Syphilis
age-, race- and sex-related rates, 348–349
treatment guidelines, 577–580
Systemic diseases, causes of, 795
Systemic lupus erythematosus, 804

T

Tattoos, 693
Tension-type headaches, 814
Testes, vanishing, 476
Testicular feminization, 476
Testicular torsion, 674, 676
Testicular tumors, 672, 675
Tetanus & diphtheria (Td) vaccination, 630
Tetanus, diphtheria & pertussis (TdaP) vaccine
contraindications, 621
special situation

recommendations, 619–620
vaccination, 631
Tetanus vaccines, 613, 618, 619–620
Thyroglobulin test, 453
Thyroid disorders, 452–456
Thyroid nodules, 455
Thyroiditis, autoimmune, 454–455
Thyrotoxicosis, 455
Thyrotropin test, 452–453
Tinea corporis, 685
Tinea cruris, 686
Tinea pedis, 684
Tinea unguium, 685, 686
Tinea versicolor, 683
Toxoplasma gondi encephalitis, 597
Trachomonas, diagnostic findings, 591–593
Tranquilizers
30 day prevalence of illicit use, 328
annual prevalence of illicit use, 321
trends in lifetime illicit use, 312
Transdermal contraceptive patches, 561–562
Transgender identity, 384
Trauma, causes of, 795
Travelers, immunizations for, 616–617, 627
Triceps skinfold thickness, 442
Trichomonas vaginalis, 591–593
Trichomoniasis
diagnostic findings, 591–593
treatment, 594
Triglycerides, by gender and age, 656
Tuberculin tests
in BCG vaccine recipients, 613
positive results, 611
recommendations, 612
Tuberculosis, latent infections, 612
Turner syndrome (45,X), 440
Typhoid vaccination, 632

U

Unipolar depression, bipolar disorders and, 738
Upper extremities, ranges of motion, 717
Upper-/lower body segment measures, 435, 439
Urinalysis
microscopic hematuria, 668–669
presistent proteinuria, 667
testing for proteinuria, 666
Urticaria, 686–687
US Preventive Services Task Force, 734

V

Vaccinations, 613–635. *See also* Immunizations
Vaccinia virus vaccination, 632
Vaginal discharge
diagnostic findings, 591–593
treatment for infections, 594
Vaginal rings, 563
Varicella-zoster virus
prophylaxis, 600
vaccination during pregnancy, 631
Variocele, 674, 675
Vasculitis syndromes, 807–808
Vasculitis, causes of, 794
Venlafaxine, 731
Vicodin, prevalence of illicit use, 320
Virilization, evaluation of, 468
Vitamin D supplements, 790
Vomiting, induced, 292, 754, 756

W

Waist circumferences, 443
Warts, 687
Weight
body mass index for, 362
evaluation of curves, 437
for age charts, 358–359
gain during puberty, 351
gain velocity during puberty, 351
Weight loss
medications related to, 452
surgical approaches for, 452
Weight-control measures, 753
Weight-for-height ratios, 434, 438, 439
World Health Organization (WHO)
acute rheumatic fever criteria, 797
on contraceptive use, 486–517
Wrist
bony anatomy of, 720
motion of, 717

Y

Yellow fever vaccination, 633
Youth Risk Behavior Survey
on alcohol use, 334
on alcohol use and driving, 271

on fasting and supplements to lose weight, 291
on feelings of sadness/hopelessness, 273
on marijuana use, 333
on nutrition and exercise, 290
on obese and overweight students, 288
on receipt of HIV/AIDS education, 339
on risk behavior prevalence, 276–286
on sexual violence, 272
on smoking behaviors, 332
on suicidal ideation, 274
on suicide attempts, 275
on use of contraceptives, 338
on use of induced vomiting and laxatives, 292

Z

Zoster vaccination, 633

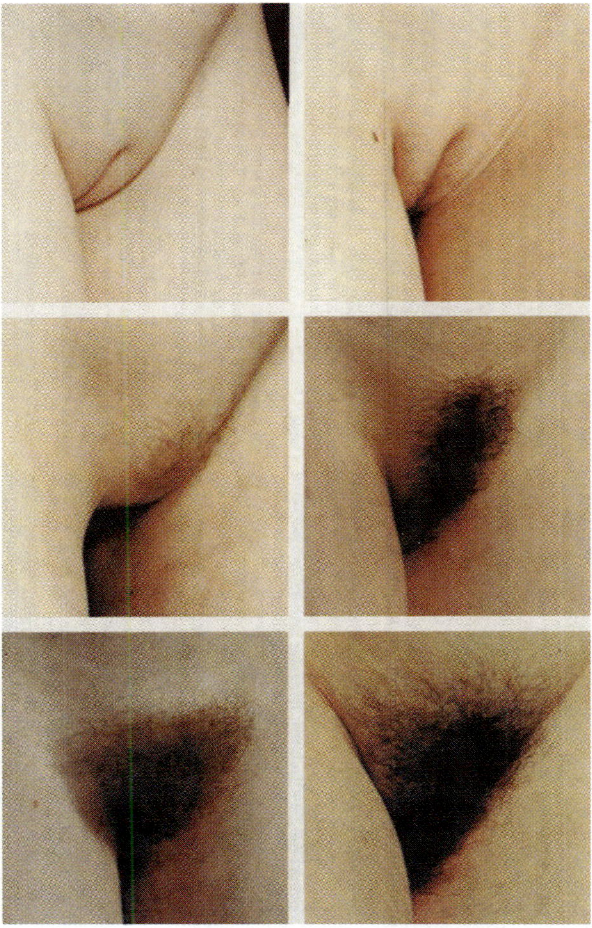

Fig 2.9. Stages of pubertal pubic hair development in girls. (Reproduced with permission from Roede MJ, van Wieringen JC. Growth diagrams 1980: Netherlands third nation-wide survey. *Tijdschr Soc Gezondheidsz*. 1985;63[suppl]:6–7).

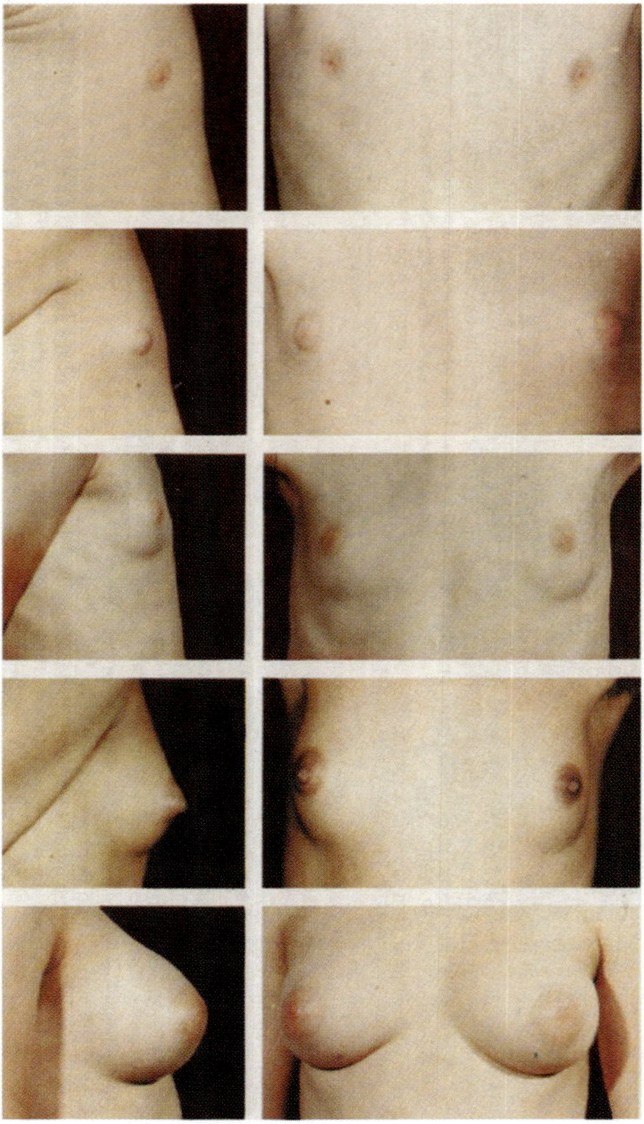

Fig 2.10. Stages of pubertal breast development in girls. (Reproduced with permission from Roede MJ, van Wieringen JC. Growth diagrams 1980: Netherlands third nation-wide survey. *Tijdschr Soc Gezondheidsz*. 1985;63[suppl]:6–7).

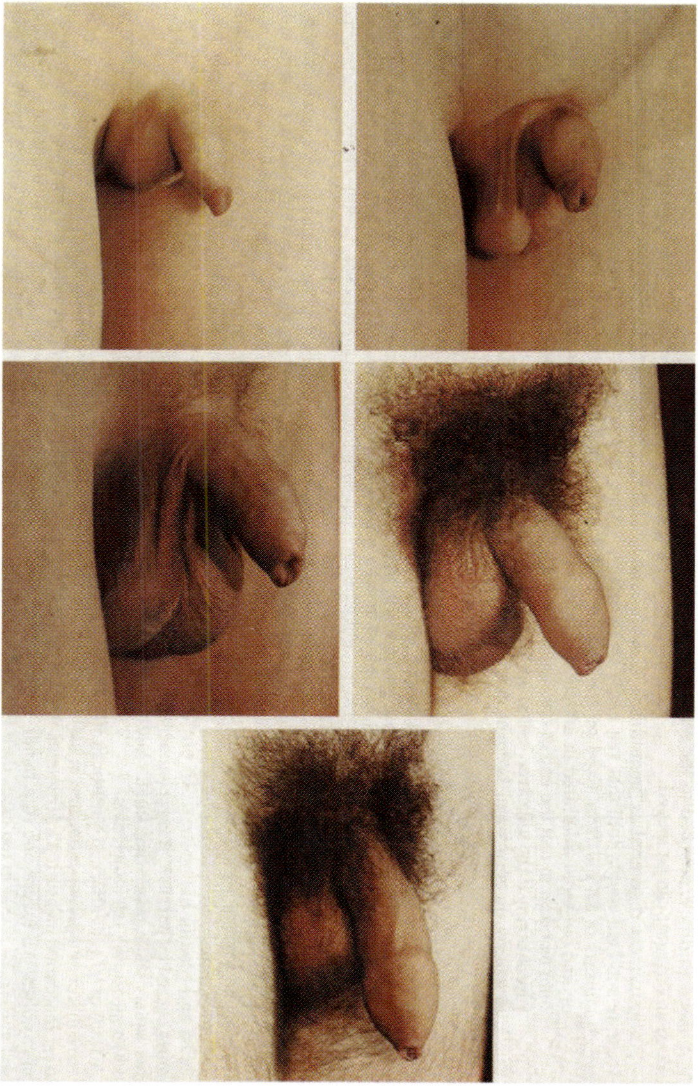

Fig 2.11. Stages of pubertal genital development in boys. (Reproduced with permission from Roede MJ, van Wieringen JC. Growth diagrams 1980: Netherlands third nation-wide survey. *Tijdschr Soc Gezondheidsz.* 1985;63[suppl]:6–7).

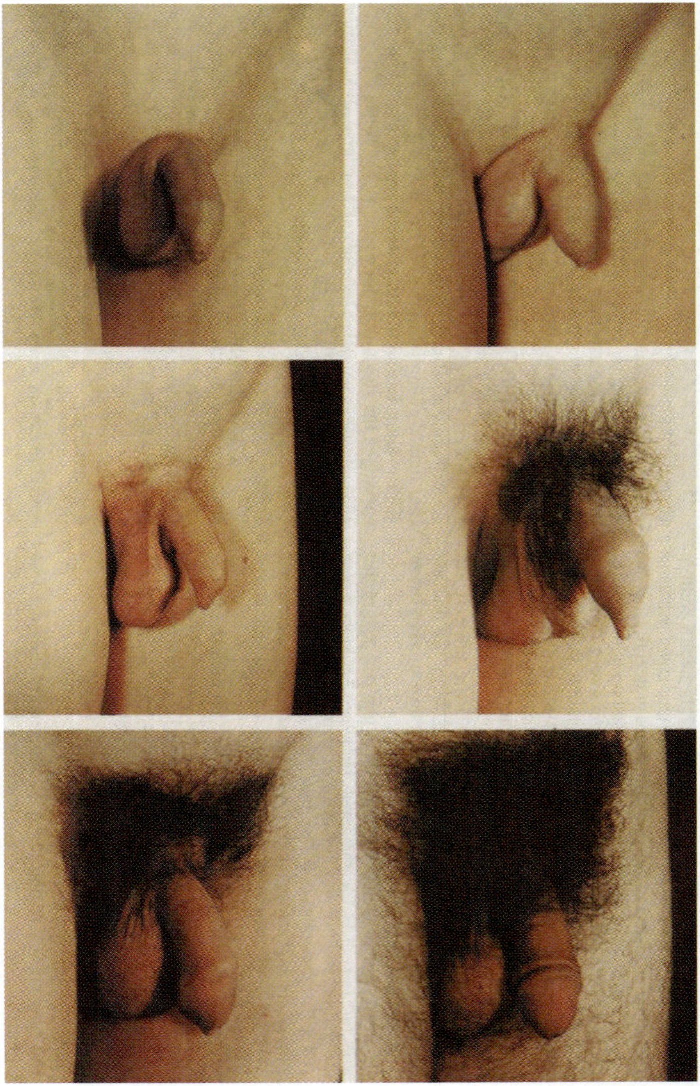

Fig 2.12. Stages of pubertal pubic hair development in boys. (Reproduced with permission from Roede MJ, van Wieringen JC. Growth diagrams 1980: Netherlands third nation-wide survey. *Tijdschr Soc Gezondheidsz*. 1985;63[suppl]:6–7).

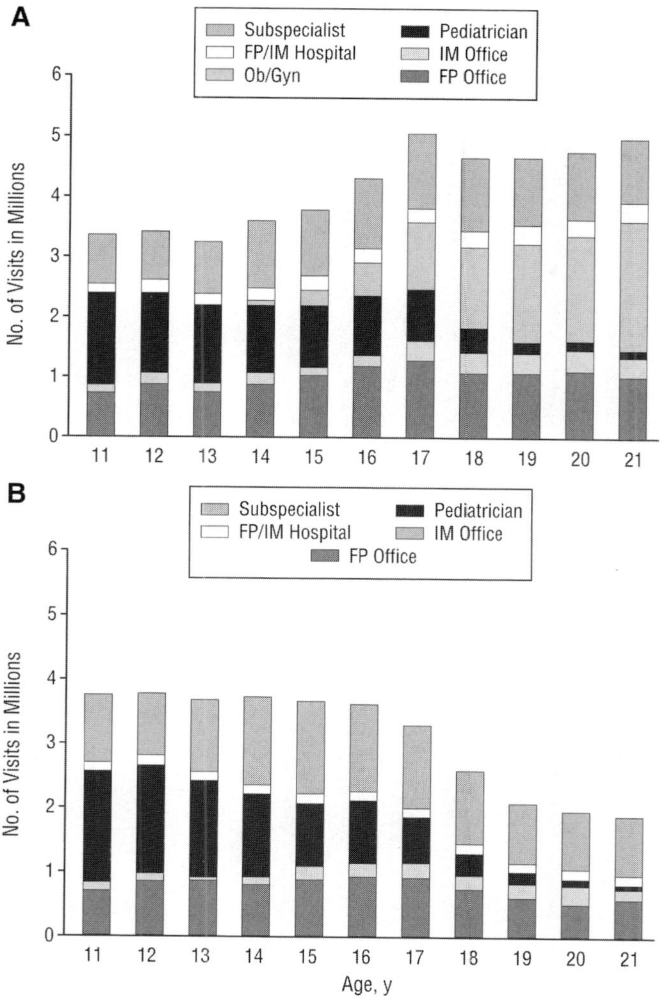

'ig 3.1. Mean number of annual adolescent outpatient visits according to gender, ge, and physician type, 1994–2003, National Ambulatory Medical Care Survey NAMCS) and National Hospital Ambulatory Medical Care Survey (NHAMCS). A, 'isits by females; B, visits by males. FP/IM hospital indicates family practice or nternal medicine hospital-based sample from the NHAMCS (with FP/IM combined);)b/Gyn, obstetrician-gynecologist; IM office, internal medicine office; FP office, amily practice office-based sample from the NAMCS. (Reproduced with ermission from Rand CM, Shone LP, Albertin C. National health care visit atterns for adolescents. *Arch Pediatr Adolesc Med.* 2007;161[3]:252–259).

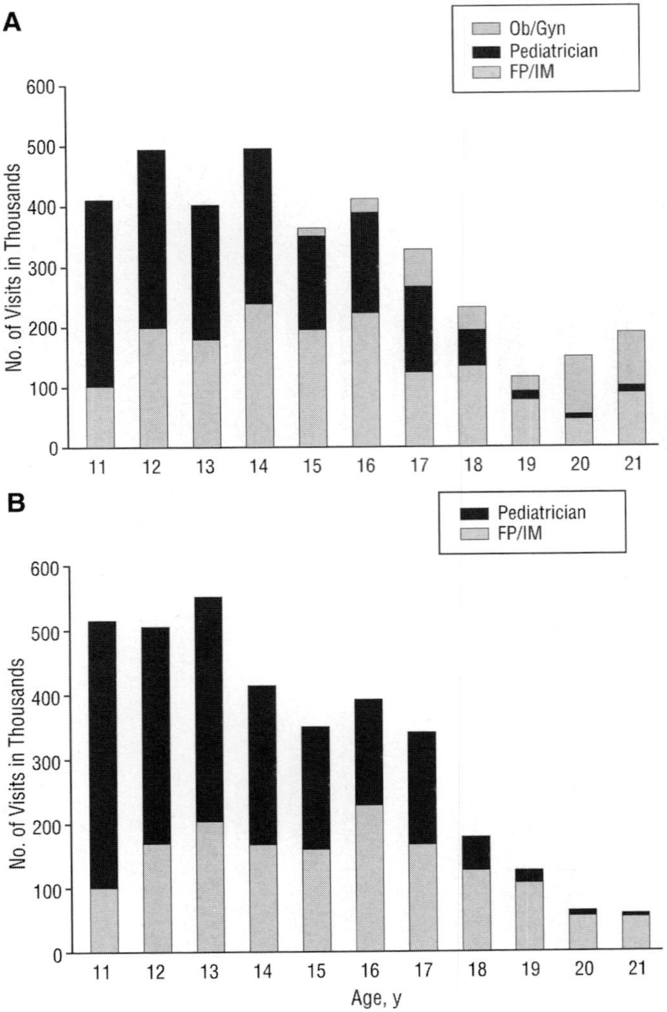

Fig 3.2. Mean number of annual adolescent preventive outpatient visits according to gender, age, and physician type, 1994–2003, National Ambulatory Medical Care Survey and National Hospital Ambulatory Medical Care Survey. A, Visits by females; B, visits by males. FP/IM indicates family practice and internal medicine practice combined; Ob/Gyn, obstetrician-gynecologist. (Reproduced with permission from Rand CM, Shone LP, Albertin C. National health care visit patterns for adolescents. *Arch Pediatr Adolesc Med.* 2007;161[3]:252–259).

	Pen Device and Insulin(s) Available	Recommended Storage	Specific Guidelines for Pen Device Use	
SoloStar® by Sanofi Aventis	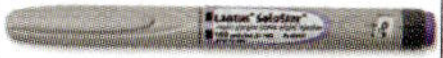 ***Apidra®** (Prefilled Pen) May deliver up to 80 units/dose in 1-unit increments. This is a **disposable** pen device. *Pending release to market	**If not in use:** Refrigerate pen at 36-46°F. Good until expiration date **If in use:** Store pen at 59-86°F. **Apidra®** - good for 28 days **Lantus®** - good for 28 days	**To prime the pen device:** **1)** Turn the dosing knob clockwise to two units [2]. **2)** Holding the pen with the needle facing upwards, tap the side of the pen to help force air bubbles upward. **3)** Press in on the dosing knob and hold for at least five seconds. **4)** If insulin exits the needle, you are ready to dial and inject your dose. **5)** If insulin does not exit the needle, repeat priming up to three times. **6)** If still no insulin appears, replace the pen needle with a new pen needle. **7)** Repeat priming process. If unsuccessful after several attempts, do not use the pen and call customer service.	**Customer Service:** 1-800-633-1610
OptiClik® by Sanofi Aventis	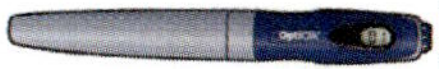 **Apidra®** (3-mL Cartridges) **Lantus®** (3-mL Cartridges) May deliver up to 80 units/dose in 1-unit increments. This is a **reusable** pen device.	**If not in use:** Refrigerate cartridges at 36-46°F. Good until expiration date Do not refrigerate pen. **If in use:** Store pen and cartridges at 59-86°F. **Apidra®** - good for 28 days **Lantus®** - good for 28 days	**To load cartridges:** **1)** Turn clockwise and push in on the pen cartridge to attach to pen body. The pen cartridge should click into place once it is fully attached. **2)** To remove a cartridge, press the release button next to where the pen cartridge and body meet. **To prime the pen device:** **1)** Press the dial release button on the back of the pen device, behind the unit display. **2)** Turn the dosing knob clockwise to two units [2]. **3)** Holding the pen with the needle facing upwards, tap the side of the pen to help force air bubbles upward. **4)** Press in on the dosing knob and hold for at least five seconds. **5)** If insulin exits the needle, you are ready to dial and inject your dose. **6)** If insulin does not exit the needle, repeat priming up to three times. **7)** If still no insulin appears, replace the pen needle with a new pen needle. **8)** Repeat priming process. If unsuccessful after several attempts, do not use the pen and call customer service.	
	Pen Device and Incretin(s) Available	**Recommended Storage**	**Specific Guidelines for Pen Device Use**	
Byetta® Pen by Amylin Pharmaceuticals	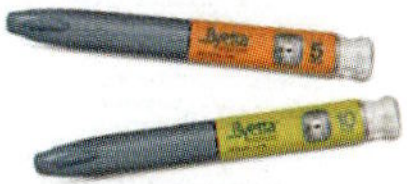 **Byetta® 5 mcg** (Prefilled Pen) **Byetta® 10 mcg** (Prefilled Pen) May deliver fixed doses of 5 or 10 mcg. Device capacity of 60 fixed doses This is a **disposable** pen device.	**If not in use:** Refrigerate pen at 36-46°F. Good until expiration date **If in use:** Store pen at 59-86°F. **Byetta®** - good for 30 days	**To prime the pen device:** **1)** Turn the dosing knob clockwise until a right arrow [→] appears in the center of the dosing window. **2)** Pull the dosing knob outward until an upward arrow [↑] appears in the center of the dosing window. **3)** Dial clockwise to a 5-mcg [5] or 10-mcg dose [10], depending on the pen device. **4)** Holding the pen with the needle facing upwards, tap the side of the pen to help force air bubbles upward. **5)** Press in on the dosing knob and hold for at least five seconds. **6)** Incretin should appear at the end of the needle tip, and a triangle [▲] should appear in the dosing window to indicate that the pen is working properly. **7)** If incretin exits the needle, you are ready to dial and inject your dose. **8)** If incretin does not exit the needle, replace the pen needle with a new pen needle. **9)** Repeat priming process. If unsuccessful, do not waste additional doses. Call customer service for additional instructions.	**Customer Service:** 1-800-868-1190
SymlinPen® by Amylin Pharmaceuticals	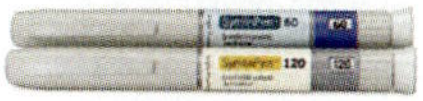 **SymlinPen® 60** (Prefilled Pen) May deliver fixed doses of 15, 30, 45, and 60 mcg. **SymlinPen® 120** (Prefilled Pen) May deliver fixed doses of 60 and 120 mcg. This is a **disposable** pen device.	**If not in use:** Refrigerate pen at 36-46°F. Good until expiration date **If in use:** Store pen at 59-86°F. **Symlin®** - good for 30 days	**To prime the pen device:** **1)** Turn the ribbed dosing knob clockwise to the lowest available dose on each pen, [15] mcg on the **SymlinPen® 60** or [60] mcg on the **SymlinPen® 120**. **2)** Pull the smooth dosing knob outward until it clicks, then turn the dosing knob clockwise until a | < 15 or a | < 60 on the dosing knob lines up with the [15] or [60] mcg dose in the dosing window of each pen device. **3)** Holding the pen with the needle facing upwards, tap the side of the pen to help force air bubbles upward. **4)** Press in on the smooth dosing knob and hold for at least 10 seconds. **5)** If incretin exits the needle as a stream, you are ready to dial and inject your dose. **6)** If incretin does not exit the needle as a stream, you may repeat priming up to six times. Try switching the pen needle for a new pen needle during these additional primes. **7)** If still unsuccessful, do not waste additional doses. Call customer service for additional instructions.	**Customer Service:** 1-800-349-8919

Reproduced with permission Christopher M. Antoszek, University of Connecticut 2008 Pharm.D. Candidate, March 2008.

Fig 4.1. Types of insulin pens and cartridges.

	Pen Device and Insulin(s) Available	Recommended Storage	Specific Guidelines for Pen Device Use	
FlexPen® by Novo Nordisk	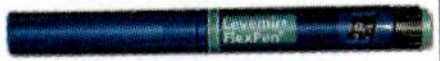 **Levemir®** (Prefilled Pen) **Novolog®** (Prefilled Pen) **Novolog® Mix70/30** (Prefilled Pen) May deliver up to 60 units/dose in 1-unit increments. This is a **disposable** pen device.	**If not in use:** Refrigerate pen at 36-46°F. Good until expiration date **If in use:** Store pen at 59-86°F. **Levemir®** - good for 42 days **Novolog®** - good for 28 days **Novolog® Mix70/30** - good for 14 days	**To load cartridges in the NovoPen® 3 and NovoPen® Junior:** 1) Unscrew cartridge holder from pen body. 2) Insert smaller end of insulin cartridge into cartridge holder. 3) Use cartridge plunger to push back screw, if extended. 4) Screw cartridge holder back onto pen body by turning on clockwise. **To prime all four devices:** 1) Turn the dosing knob clockwise to two units [2]. 2) Holding the device with the needle facing upwards, tap the side of the device to help force air bubbles upward. 3) Press in on the dosing knob and hold for at least five seconds, six seconds with the **Innolet®**. 4) If insulin exits the needle, you are ready to dial and inject your dose. 5) If insulin does not exit the needle, repeat priming up to three times. 6) If still no insulin appears, replace the pen needle with a new pen needle. 7) Repeat priming process. If unsuccessful after several attempts, do not use the device and call customer service.	**Customer Service:** 1-800-727-6500
NovoPen® 3 by Novo Nordisk	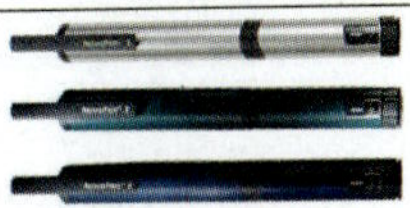 **Novolin® 70/30** (3-mL Cartridges) **Novolin® N** (3-mL Cartridges) **Novolin® R** (3-mL Cartridges) **Novolog®** (3-mL Cartridges) May deliver up to 70 units/dose in 1-unit increments. This is a **reusable** pen device.	**If not in use:** Refrigerate cartridges at 36-46°F. Good until expiration date **If in use:** Store pen and cartridges at 59-86°F. **Novolin® 70/30** - good for 10 days **Novolin® N** - good for 14 days **Novolin® R** - good for 28 days **Novolog®** - good for 28 days		
NovoPen® Junior by Novo Nordisk	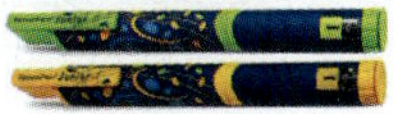 **Novolin® 70/30** (3-mL Cartridges) **Novolin® N** (3-mL Cartridges) **Novolin® R** (3-mL Cartridges) **Novolog®** (3-mL Cartridges) May deliver up to 35 units/dose in ½-unit increments. This is a **reusable** pen device.	**If not in use:** Refrigerate cartridges at 36-46°F. Good until expiration date **If in use:** Store pen and cartridges at 59-86°F. **Novolin® 70/30** - good for 10 days **Novolin® N** - good for 14 days **Novolin® R** - good for 28 days **Novolog®** - good for 28 days		
Innolet® by Novo Nordisk	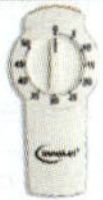 **Novolin® 70/30** (Prefilled Device) **Novolin® N** (Prefilled Device) May deliver up to 50 units/dose in 1-unit increments. Do not use with 12 or less units left in the device. This is a **disposable** device.	**If not in use:** Refrigerate device at 36-46°F. Good until expiration date **If in use:** Store device at 59-86°F. **Novolin® 70/30** - good for 10 days **Novolin® N** - good for 14 days		

Fig 4.1. (*Continued*).

General Guidelines for Pen Device Use			
1) Always wash your hands before handling pen devices. **2)** Check the expiration date on pen devices and cartridges before use. **3)** Always examine the contents of pen devices and cartridges before use: • The following incretins and insulins should appear clear, colorless, and free of particles throughout use: **Apidra®, Byetta®, Humalog®, Lantus®, Levemir®, Novolin® R, Novolog®, and Symlin®** • The following insulins should appear uniformly cloudy or milky after mixing: **Humalog® Mix50/50™, Humalog® Mix75/25™, Humulin® 70/30, Humulin® N, Novolin® 70/30, Novolin® N, and Novolog® Mix70/30** **4)** If using cloudy insulin, gently roll the pen device between the palms of your hands 10 times. In addition, invert the device 10 times to ensure the proper mixing of insulin. **5)** All pen devices and cartridges are compatible with the following pen needles: **BD Ultra-Fine™ III Mini Pen Needles** [5 mm (3/16 in) X 31G], **BD Ultra-Fine™ III Short Pen Needles** [8 mm (5/16 in) X 31G], **BD Ultra-Fine™ Original Pen Needles** [12.7 mm (1/2 in) X 29G], **NovoFine® 31 Pen Needles** [6 mm X 31G], and **NovoFine® 30 Pen Needles** [8 mm X 30G] **6)** Prior to attaching a new pen needle, use an alcohol swab to clean the rubber seal on the end of the insulin cartridge or pen device. Save the outer shield of the pen needle for recapping after use. **7)** Priming should be performed before administering each dose, with exception to the incretin pens that are only primed before the first time of use. **8)** Dial your prescribed dose as directed. If you have dialed pass your dose on any pen device, with exception to the **OptiClik®**, you can easily dial backwards without releasing any medication. **9)** Inject your dose as directed. For injections, press in and hold on the dosing knob for at least five seconds to ensure full delivery of the incretin or insulin before removing the needle from the skin; exceptions include six seconds for the **Innolet®** and 10 seconds for the **SymlinPen®**. **10)** Following an injection, discard the used pen needle in a biohazard container. Use a new pen needle each time you inject to prevent air bubbles from collecting inside of the pen device or cartridges.			
	Pen Device and Insulin(s) Available	**Recommended Storage**	**Specific Guidelines for Pen Device Use**
Original Pen by Eli Lilly & Company	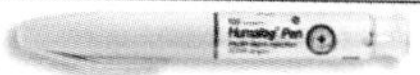 **Humalog®** (Prefilled Pen) **Humalog® Mix75/25™** (Prefilled Pen) **Humalog® Mix50/50™** (Prefilled Pen) **Humulin® N** (Prefilled Pen) **Humulin® 70/30** (Prefilled Pen) May deliver up to 60 units/dose in 1-unit increments. This is a **disposable** pen device.	**If not in use:** Refrigerate pen at 36-46°F. Good until expiration date **If in use:** Store pen at 59-86°F. **Humalog®** - good for 28 days **Humalog® Mix75/25™** - good for 10 days **Humalog® Mix50/50™** - good for 10 days **Humulin® N** - good for 14 days **Humulin® 70/30** - good for 10 days	**To prime the pen device:** **1)** Turn the dosing knob clockwise until an arrow [→] appears in the center of the dosing window. **2)** Pull the dosing knob outward until a zero [0] appears in the center of the dosing window. **3)** Dial clockwise to two units [2]. **4)** Holding the pen with the needle facing upwards, tap the side of the pen to help force air bubbles upward. **5)** Press in on the dosing knob and hold for at least five seconds. **6)** Insulin should appear at the end of the needle tip, and a diamond [♦] should appear in the dosing window to indicate that the pen is working properly. **7)** If insulin exits the needle, you are ready to dial and inject your dose. **8)** If insulin does not exit the needle, repeat priming up to three times. **9)** If still no insulin appears, replace the pen needle with a new pen needle. **10)** Repeat priming process. If unsuccessful after several attempts, do not use the pen and call customer service.
KwikPen® by Eli Lilly & Company	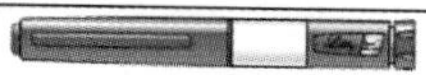 **Humalog®** (Prefilled Pen) **Humalog® Mix75/25™** (Prefilled Pen) **Humalog® Mix50/50™** (Prefilled Pen) May deliver up to 60 units/dose in 1-unit increments. This is a **disposable** pen device.	**If not in use:** Refrigerate pen at 36-46°F. Good until expiration date **If in use:** Store pen at 59-86°F. **Humalog®** - good for 28 days **Humalog® Mix75/25™** - good for 10 days **Humalog® Mix50/50™** - good for 10 days	**To set the date and time on the HumaPen® Memoir™:** Refer to the directions provided in the package insert. **To load cartridges in the HumaPen® Memoir™ and Luxura™ HD:** **1)** Unscrew cartridge holder from pen body. **2)** Insert smaller end of insulin cartridge into cartridge holder. **3)** Use cartridge plunger to push back screw, if extended. **4)** Screw cartridge holder back onto pen body by turning on clockwise. **To prime all three pen devices:** **1)** Turn the dosing knob clockwise to two units [2]. **2)** Holding the pen with the needle facing upwards, tap the side of the pen to help force air bubbles upward. **3)** Press in on the dosing knob and hold for at least five seconds. **4)** If insulin exits the needle, you are ready to dial and inject your dose. **5)** If insulin does not exit the needle, repeat priming up to three times. **6)** If still no insulin appears, replace the pen needle with a new pen needle. **7)** Repeat priming process. If unsuccessful after several attempts, do not use the pen and call customer service.
HumaPen® Memoir™ by Eli Lilly & Company	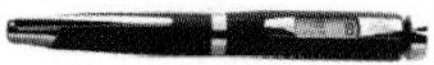 **Humalog®** (3-mL Cartridges) May deliver up to 60 units/dose in 1-unit increments. This is a **reusable** pen device.	**If not in use:** Refrigerate cartridges at 36-46°F. Good until expiration date Do not refrigerate pen. **If in use:** Store cartridges in pen at 59-86°F. **Humalog®** - good for 28 days	
HumaPen® Luxura™ HD by Eli Lilly & Company	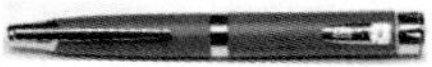 **Humalog®** (3-mL Cartridges) May deliver up to 30 units/dose in ½-unit increments. This is a **reusable** pen device.	**If not in use:** Refrigerate cartridges at 36-46°F. Good until expiration date Do not refrigerate pen. **If in use:** Store cartridges in pen at 59-86°F. **Humalog®** - good for 28 days	

Customer Service: 1-800-545-5979

Reproduced with permission Christopher M. Antoszek, University of Connecticut 2008 Pharm.D. Candidate, March 2008.

Fig 4.1. (*Continued*).

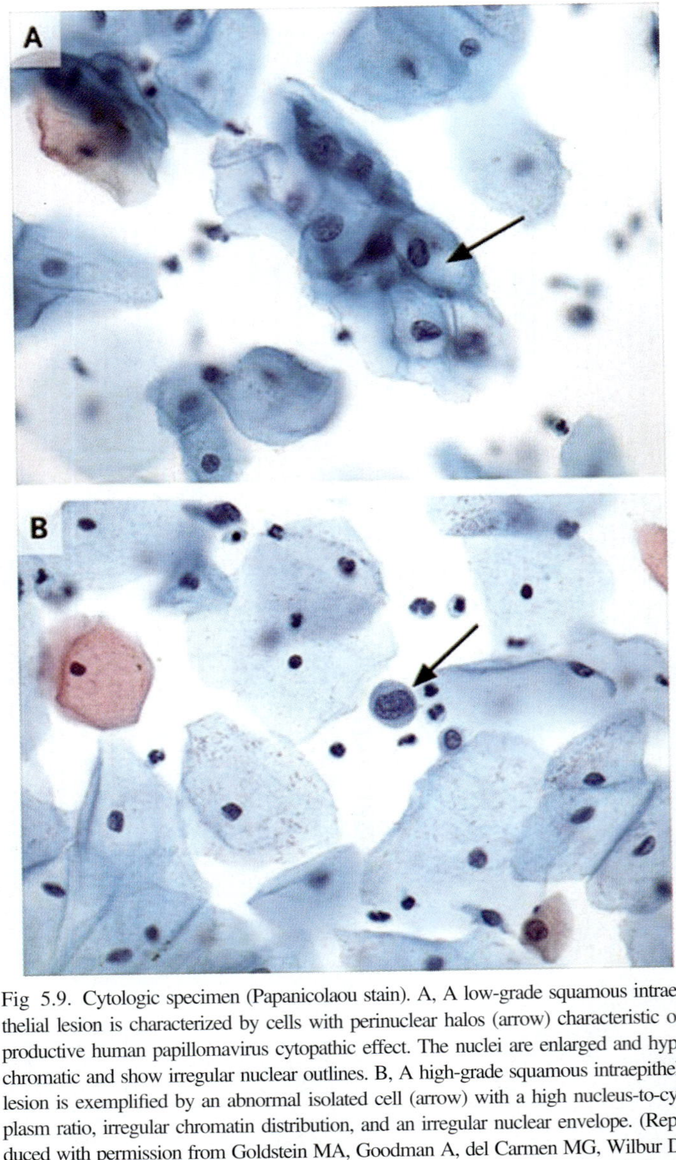

Fig 5.9. Cytologic specimen (Papanicolaou stain). A, A low-grade squamous intraepithelial lesion is characterized by cells with perinuclear halos (arrow) characteristic of a productive human papillomavirus cytopathic effect. The nuclei are enlarged and hyperchromatic and show irregular nuclear outlines. B, A high-grade squamous intraepithelial lesion is exemplified by an abnormal isolated cell (arrow) with a high nucleus-to-cytoplasm ratio, irregular chromatin distribution, and an irregular nuclear envelope. (Reproduced with permission from Goldstein MA, Goodman A, del Carmen MG, Wilbur DC. Case records of the Massachusetts General Hospital: case 10–2009—a 23-year-old woman with an abnormal Papanicolaou smear. *N Engl J Med*. 2009;360[13]:1339).

My Asthma Plan ENGLISH

Patient Name: ____________

Medical Record #: ____________

Provider's Name: ____________ DOB: ____________

Provider's Phone #: ____________ Completed by: ____________ Date: ____________

Controller Medicines	How Much to Take	How Often	Other Instructions
		____ times per day **EVERY DAY!**	❑ Gargle or rinse mouth after use
		____ times per day **EVERY DAY!**	
		____ times per day **EVERY DAY!**	
		____ times per day **EVERY DAY!**	

Quick-Relief Medicines	How Much to Take	How Often	Other Instructions
❑ Albuterol (ProAir, Ventolin, Proventil) ❑ Levalbuterol (Xopenex)	❑ 2 puffs ❑ 4 puffs ❑ 1 nebulizer treatment	Take ONLY as needed (see below — starting in Yellow Zone or before excercise)	NOTE: If you need this medicine more than two days a week, call physician to consider increasing controller medications and discuss your treatment plan.

Special instructions when I am *doing well*, *getting worse*, *having a medical alert.*

GREEN ZONE

Doing *well.*

- No cough, wheeze, chest tightness, or shortness of breath during the day or night.
- Can do usual activities.

Peak Flow (for ages 5 and up):
is ______ or more. (80% or more of personal best)

Personal Best Peak Flow (for ages 5 and up): ______

PREVENT asthma symptoms every day:

☐ Take my controller medicines (above) every day.

☐ Before exercise, take ______ puff(s) of ______________

☐ Avoid things that make my asthma worse. (See back of form.)

YELLOW ZONE

Getting *worse.*

- Cough, wheeze, chest tightness, shortness of breath, or
- Waking at night due to asthma symptoms, or
- Can do some, but not all, usual activities.

Peak Flow (for ages 5 and up):
______ to ______ (50 to 79% of personal best)

CAUTION. Continue taking every day controller medicines, AND:

☐ Take ____ puffs or ____ one nebulizer treatment of quick relief medicine. If I am not back in the *Green Zone* within 20-30 minutes take ____ more puffs or nebulizer treatments. If I am not back in the *Green Zone* within one hour, then I should:

☐ Increase ______________

☐ Add ______________

☐ Call ______________

☐ Continue using quick relief medicine every 4 hours as needed. Call provider if not improving in ______ days.

RED ZONE

Medical Alert

- Very short of breath, or
- Quick-relief medicines have not helped, or
- Cannot do usual activities, or
- Symptoms are same or get worse after 24 hours in Yellow Zone.

Peak Flow (for ages 5 and up):
less than ________ (50% of personal best)

MEDICAL ALERT! Get help!

☐ Take quick relief medicine: ______ puffs every ______ minutes and get help immediately.

☐ Take ______________

☐ Call ______________

Danger! Get help immediately! Call 911 if trouble walking or talking due to shortness of breath or if lips or fingernails are gray or blue. For child, call 911 if skin is sucked in around neck and ribs during breaths or child doesn't respond normally.

Health Care Provider: My signature provides authorization for the above written orders. I understand that all procedures will be implemented in accordance with state laws and regulations. Student may self carry asthma medications: ❑ Yes ❑ No self administer asthma medications: ❑ Yes ❑ No (This authorization is for a maximum of one year from signature date.)

Healthcare Provider Signature ____________ Date ____________

ORIGINAL (Patient) / CANARY (School/Child Care/Work/Other Support Systems) / PINK (Chart)

Fig 8.4. Sample asthma action plan (English). (Reproduced with permission from Regional Asthma Management and Prevention (RAMP), a program of the Public Health Institute. The RAMP Asthma Action Plan was supported by Cooperative Agreement Number 1U58DP001016-01 from the Centers for Disease Control and Prevention. The contents of the RAMP Asthma Action Plan are solely the responsibility of the authors and do not necessarily represent the official views of the Centers for Disease Control and Prevention. For more information, go to www.rampasthma.org).

Plan de tratamiento contra el asma

SPANISH

Patient Name: ____________

Medical Record #: ____________

Nombre del proveedor: ____________

DOB: ____________

N.º de teléfono del proveedor: ____________ Completado por: ____________ Fecha: ____________

Medicamentos de control	Cantidad que se debe tomar	Con qué frecuencia se deben tomar	Otras instrucciones
		______ veces por día TODOS LOS DÍAS	❑ Hacerse gárgaras o enjuagarse la boca después de tomar el medicamento
		______ veces por día TODOS LOS DÍAS	
		______ veces por día TODOS LOS DÍAS	
		______ veces por día TODOS LOS DÍAS	

Medicamentos de alivio rápido	Cantidad que se debe tomar	Con qué frecuencia se deben tomar	Otras instrucciones
❑ Albuterol (ProAir, Ventolin, Proventil) ❑ Levalbuterol (Xopenex)	❑ 2 inhalaciones ❑ 4 inhalaciones ❑ 1 tratamiento con nebulizador	Deben tomarse SÓLO en caso de ser necesario (ver debajo; comenzar en la Zona amarilla o antes de hacer ejercicio)	NOTA: Si necesita tomar este medicamento más de dos días a la semana, llame a su médico para consultar sobre la necesidad de un aumento de dosis para los medicamentos de control, y para conversar sobre su plan de tratamiento.

Instrucciones especiales en caso de que *Se sienta bien*, *empeore o*, *tenga una emergencia médica.*

ZONA VERDE

Se siente ***bien.***

- No tiene tos, resuellos, opresión en el pecho ni dificultad para respirar durante el día o la noche.
- Puede realizar las actividades habituales.

Capacidad pulmonar máxima (para personas de 5 años en adelante): es ______ o más. (80% o más de su mejor nivel de capacidad pulmonar máxima)
Su mejor nivel de capacidad pulmonar máxima (para las personas de 5 años en adelante): ______

Debe ***PREVENIR*** los síntomas del asma todos los días:

- ☐ Tome los medicamentos de control (mencionados arriba) todos los días.
- ☐ Antes de hacer ejercicio, adminístrese ______ dosis de ______
- ☐ Evite aquello que pueda empeorar el asma. (Ver el reverso del formulario)

ZONA AMARILLA

Su estado ***empeora.***

- Tiene tos, resuellos, opresión en el pecho, dificultad para respirar o
- Se despierta por las noches debido a los síntomas del asma, o
- Puede realizar algunas de sus actividades habituales, pero no todas.

Capacidad pulmonar máxima (para personas de 5 años en adelante): ______ a ______ (50% al 79% de su mejor nivel de capacidad pulmonar máxima)

PRECAUCIÓN. Continúe tomando los medicamentos de control todos los días, Y:

- ☐ Reciba ___ inhalaciones o ___ el medicamento de alivio rápido por medio de nebulizador. Si no vuelve a la *Zona verde* en el plazo de 20 o 30 minutos, debe tomar ___ inhalaciones o tratamientos con nebulizador más. Si no vuelve a la *Zona verde* en una hora, entonces debe:
- ☐ Aumentar ______ ______
- ☐ Agregar ______
- ☐ Llamar ______
- ☐ Continúe usando los medicamentos de alivio rápido cada 4 horas según sea necesario. Llame al proveedor si no mejora en ______ días.

ZONA ROJA

Emergencia médica

- Mucha dificultad para respirar, o
- Los medicamentos de alivio rápido no le han ayudado, o
- No puede realizar las actividades habituales, o
- Los síntomas son los mismos o empeoran después de 24 horas.

Capacidad pulmonar máxima (para personas de 5 años en adelante): menos de ______ (50% de su mejor nivel de capacidad pulmonar máxima)

ALERTA MÉDICA ¡Pida ayuda!

- ☐ Tome medicamentos de alivio rápido: ______ inhalaciones cada ______ minuto y pida ayuda de inmediato.
- ☐ Tome ______
- ☐ Llame ______

Peligro. ¡Pida ayuda de inmediato! Llame al 911 si tiene problemas para caminar o hablar debido a la dificultad para respirar , o si tiene los labios o las uñas grises o morados. Si se trata de un niño, llame al 911 en caso de que se le hunda la piel de alrededor del cuello y las costillas durante la respiración, o si el niño no responde normalmente.

Health Care Provider: My signature provides authorization for the above written orders. I understand that all procedures will be implemented in accordance with state laws and regulations. Student may self carry asthma medications: ❑ Yes ❑ No self administer asthma medications: ❑ Yes ❑ No (This authorization is for a maximum of one year from signature date.)

______________________ ______________________

Healthcare Provider Signature Date

ORIGINAL (Patient) / CANARY (School/Child Care/Work/Other Support Systems) / PINK (Chart)

Fig 8.5. Sample asthma action plan (Spanish). (Reproduced with permission from Regional Asthma Management and Prevention (RAMP), a program of the Public Health Institute. The RAMP Asthma Action Plan was supported by Cooperative Agreement Number 1U58DP001016-01 from the Centers for Disease Control and Prevention. The contents of the RAMP Asthma Action Plan are solely the responsibility of the authors and do not necessarily represent the official views of the Centers for Disease Control and Prevention. For more information, go to www.rampasthma.org).

National Cholesterol Education Program

ATP III Guidelines At-A-Glance Quick Desk Reference

Step 1 **Determine lipoprotein levels–obtain complete lipoprotein profile after 9- to 12-hour fast.**

ATP III Classification of LDL, Total, and HDL Cholesterol (mg/dL)

LDL Cholesterol – Primary Target of Therapy	
<100	Optimal
100-129	Near optimal/above optimal
130-159	Borderline high
160-189	High
≥190	Very high
Total Cholesterol	
<200	Desirable
200-239	Borderline high
≥240	High
HDL Cholesterol	
<40	Low
≥60	High

Step 2 **Identify presence of clinical atherosclerotic disease that confers high risk for coronary heart disease (CHD) events (CHD risk equivalent):**

- Clinical CHD
- Symptomatic carotid artery disease
- Peripheral arterial disease
- Abdominal aortic aneurysm.

Step 3 **Determine presence of major risk factors (other than LDL):**

Major Risk Factors (Exclusive of LDL Cholesterol) That Modify LDL Goals
Cigarette smoking
Hypertension (BP ≥140/90 mmHg or on antihypertensive medication)
Low HDL cholesterol (<40 mg/dL)*
Family history of premature CHD (CHD in male first degree relative <55 years; CHD in female first degree relative <65 years)
Age (men ≥45 years; women ≥55 years)

** HDL cholesterol ≥60 mg/dL counts as a "negative" risk factor; its presence removes one risk factor from the total count.*

- Note: in ATP III, diabetes is regarded as a CHD risk equivalent.

NATIONAL INSTITUTES OF HEALTH
NATIONAL HEART, LUNG, AND BLOOD INSTITUTE

Fig 8.8. Adult Treatment Panel III guidelines at-a-glance quick desk reference. (Reproduced from National Heart Lung and Blood Institute. Third Report of the Expert Panel on Detection, Evaluation, and Treatment of High Blood Cholesterol in Adults (Adult Treatment Panel III). Available at: www.nhlbi.nih.gov/guidelines/cholesterol/index.htm. Accessed July 17, 2009).

Step 4

If 2+ risk factors (other than LDL) are present without CHD or CHD risk equivalent, assess 10-year (short-term) CHD risk (see Framingham tables).
Three levels of 10-year risk:

- >20% — CHD risk equivalent
- 10-20%
- <10%

Step 5

Determine risk category:

- Establish LDL goal of therapy
- Determine need for therapeutic lifestyle changes (TLC)
- Determine level for drug consideration

LDL Cholesterol Goals and Cutpoints for Therapeutic Lifestyle Changes (TLC) and Drug Therapy in Different Risk Categories.

Risk Category	LDL Goal	LDL Level at Which to Initiate Therapeutic Lifestyle Changes (TLC)	LDL Level at Which to Consider Drug Therapy
CHD or CHD Risk Equivalents (10-year risk >20%)	<100 mg/dL	≥100 mg/dL	≥130 mg/dL (100-129 mg/dL: drug optional)*
2+ Risk Factors (10-year risk ≤20%)	<130 mg/dL	≥130 mg/dL	10-year risk 10-20%: ≥130 mg/dL 10-year risk <10%: ≥160 mg/dL
0-1 Risk Factor†	<160 mg/dL	≥160 mg/dL	≥190 mg/dL (160-189 mg/dL: LDL-lowering drug optional)

* *Some authorities recommend use of LDL-lowering drugs in this category if an LDL cholesterol <100 mg/dL cannot be achieved by therapeutic lifestyle changes. Others prefer use of drugs that primarily modify triglycerides and HDL, e.g., nicotinic acid or fibrate. Clinical judgment also may call for deferring drug therapy in this subcategory.*

† *Almost all people with 0-1 risk factor have a 10-year risk <10%, thus 10-year risk assessment in people with 0-1 risk factor is not necessary.*

Step 6

Initiate therapeutic lifestyle changes (TLC) if LDL is above goal.

TLC Features

- TLC Diet:
  - Saturated fat <7% of calories, cholesterol <200 mg/day
  - Consider increased viscous (soluble) fiber (10-25 g/day) and plant stanols/sterols (2g/day) as therapeutic options to enhance LDL lowering
- Weight management
- Increased physical activity.

Fig 8.8. (*Continued*).

Step 7

Consider adding drug therapy if LDL exceeds levels shown in Step 5 table:

- Consider drug simultaneously with TLC for CHD and CHD equivalents
- Consider adding drug to TLC after 3 months for other risk categories.

Drugs Affecting Lipoprotein Metabolism

Drug Class	Agents and Daily Doses	Lipid/Lipoprotein Effects	Side Effects	Contraindications
HMG CoA reductase inhibitors (statins)	Lovastatin (20-80 mg) Pravastatin (20-40 mg) Simvastatin (20-80 mg) Fluvastatin (20-80 mg) Atorvastatin (10-80 mg) Cerivastatin (0.4-0.8 mg)	LDL ↓18-55% HDL ↑5-15% TG ↓7-30%	Myopathy Increased liver enzymes	Absolute: • Active or chronic liver disease Relative: • Concomitant use of certain drugs*
Bile acid sequestrants	Cholestyramine (4-16 g) Colestipol (5-20 g) Colesevelam (2.6-3.8 g)	LDL ↓15-30% HDL ↑3-5% TG No change or increase	Gastrointestinal distress Constipation Decreased absorption of other drugs	Absolute: • dysbeta-lipoproteinemia • TG >400 mg/dL Relative: • TG >200 mg/dL
Nicotinic acid	Immediate release (crystalline) nicotinic acid (1.5-3 gm), extended release nicotinic acid (Niaspan®) (1-2 g), sustained release nicotinic acid (1-2 g)	LDL ↓5-25% HDL ↑15-35% TG ↓20-50%	Flushing Hyperglycemia Hyperuricemia (or gout) Upper GI distress Hepatotoxicity	Absolute: • Chronic liver disease • Severe gout Relative: • Diabetes • Hyperuricemia • Peptic ulcer disease
Fibric acids	Gemfibrozil (600 mg BID) Fenofibrate (200 mg) Clofibrate (1000 mg BID)	LDL ↓5-20% *(may be increased in patients with high TG)* HDL ↑10-20% TG ↓20-50%	Dyspepsia Gallstones Myopathy	Absolute: • Severe renal disease • Severe hepatic disease

* *Cyclosporine, macrolide antibiotics, various anti-fungal agents, and cytochrome P-450 inhibitors (fibrates and niacin should be used with appropriate caution).*

Fig 8.8. (*Continued*).

Step 8

Identify metabolic syndrome and treat, if present, after 3 months of TLC.

Clinical Identification of the Metabolic Syndrome – Any 3 of the Following:

Risk Factor	Defining Level
Abdominal obesity*	Waist circumference†
Men	>102 cm (>40 in)
Women	>88 cm (>35 in)
Triglycerides	≥150 mg/dL
HDL cholesterol	
Men	<40 mg/dL
Women	<50 mg/dL
Blood pressure	≥130/≥85 mmHg
Fasting glucose	≥110 mg/dL

* *Overweight and obesity are associated with insulin resistance and the metabolic syndrome. However, the presence of abdominal obesity is more highly correlated with the metabolic risk factors than is an elevated body mass index (BMI). Therefore, the simple measure of waist circumference is recommended to identify the body weight component of the metabolic syndrome.*

† *Some male patients can develop multiple metabolic risk factors when the waist circumference is only marginally increased, e.g., 94-102 cm (37-39 in). Such patients may have a strong genetic contribution to insulin resistance. They should benefit from changes in life habits, similarly to men with categorical increases in waist circumference.*

Treatment of the metabolic syndrome

- Treat underlying causes (overweight/obesity and physical inactivity):
  - Intensify weight management
  - Increase physical activity.
- Treat lipid and non-lipid risk factors if they persist despite these lifestyle therapies:
  - Treat hypertension
  - Use aspirin for CHD patients to reduce prothrombotic state
  - Treat elevated triglycerides and/or low HDL (as shown in Step 9).

Fig 8.8. (*Continued*).

Step 9

Treat elevated triglycerides.

ATP III Classification of Serum Triglycerides (mg/dL)

<150	Normal
150-199	Borderline high
200-499	High
≥500	Very high

Treatment of elevated triglycerides (≥150 mg/dL)

- Primary aim of therapy is to reach LDL goal
- Intensify weight management
- Increase physical activity
- If triglycerides are ≥200 mg/dL after LDL goal is reached, set secondary goal for non-HDL cholesterol (total – HDL) 30 mg/dL higher than LDL goal.

Comparison of LDL Cholesterol and Non-HDL Cholesterol Goals for Three Risk Categories

Risk Category	LDL Goal (mg/dL)	Non-HDL Goal (mg/dL)
CHD and CHD Risk Equivalent (10-year risk for CHD >20%)	<100	<130
Multiple (2+) Risk Factors and 10-year risk ≤20%	<130	<160
0-1 Risk Factor	<160	<190

If triglycerides 200-499 mg/dL after LDL goal is reached, consider adding drug if needed to reach non-HDL goal:

- intensify therapy with LDL-lowering drug, or
- add nicotinic acid or fibrate to further lower VLDL.

If triglycerides ≥500 mg/dL, first lower triglycerides to prevent pancreatitis:

- very low-fat diet (≤15% of calories from fat)
- weight management and physical activity
- fibrate or nicotinic acid
- when triglycerides <500 mg/dL, turn to LDL-lowering therapy.

Treatment of low HDL cholesterol (<40 mg/dL)

- First reach LDL goal, then:
- Intensify weight management and increase physical activity
- If triglycerides 200-499 mg/dL, achieve non-HDL goal
- If triglycerides <200 mg/dL (isolated low HDL) in CHD or CHD equivalent consider nicotinic acid or fibrate.

Fig 8.8. (*Continued*).

Men

Estimate of 10-Year Risk for Men

(Framingham Point Scores)

Age	Points
20-34	-9
35-39	-4
40-44	0
45-49	3
50-54	6
55-59	8
60-64	10
65-69	11
70-74	12
75-79	13

Total Cholesterol	Points				
	Age 20-39	Age 40-49	Age 50-59	Age 60-69	Age 70-79
<160	0	0	0	0	0
160-199	4	3	2	1	0
200-239	7	5	3	1	0
240-279	9	6	4	2	1
≥280	11	8	5	3	1

	Points				
	Age 20-39	Age 40-49	Age 50-59	Age 60-69	Age 70-79
Nonsmoker	0	0	0	0	0
Smoker	8	5	3	1	1

HDL (mg/dL)	Points
≥60	-1
50-59	0
40-49	1
<40	2

Systolic BP (mmHg)	If Untreated	If Treated
<120	0	0
120-129	0	1
130-139	1	2
140-159	1	2
≥160	2	3

Point Total	10-Year Risk %
<0	< 1
0	1
1	1
2	1
3	1
4	1
5	2
6	2
7	3
8	4
9	5
10	6
11	8
12	10
13	12
14	16
15	20
16	25
≥17	≥ 30

10-Year risk _____%

Women

Estimate of 10-Year Risk for Women

(Framingham Point Scores)

Age	Points
20-34	-7
35-39	-3
40-44	0
45-49	3
50-54	6
55-59	8
60-64	10
65-69	12
70-74	14
75-79	16

Total Cholesterol	Points				
	Age 20-39	Age 40-49	Age 50-59	Age 60-69	Age 70-79
<160	0	0	0	0	0
160-199	4	3	2	1	1
200-239	8	6	4	2	1
240-279	11	8	5	3	2
≥280	13	10	7	4	2

	Points				
	Age 20-39	Age 40-49	Age 50-59	Age 60-69	Age 70-79
Nonsmoker	0	0	0	0	0
Smoker	9	7	4	2	1

HDL (mg/dL)	Points
≥60	-1
50-59	0
40-49	1
<40	2

Systolic BP (mmHg)	If Untreated	If Treated
<120	0	0
120-129	1	3
130-139	2	4
140-159	3	5
≥160	4	6

Point Total	10-Year Risk %
< 9	< 1
9	1
10	1
11	1
12	1
13	2
14	2
15	3
16	4
17	5
18	6
19	8
20	11
21	14
22	17
23	22
24	27
≥25	≥ 30

10-Year risk _____%

U.S. DEPARTMENT OF HEALTH AND HUMAN SERVICES
Public Health Service
National Institutes of Health
National Heart, Lung, and Blood Institute

NIH Publication No. 01-3305
May 2001

Fig 8.8. (*Continued*).

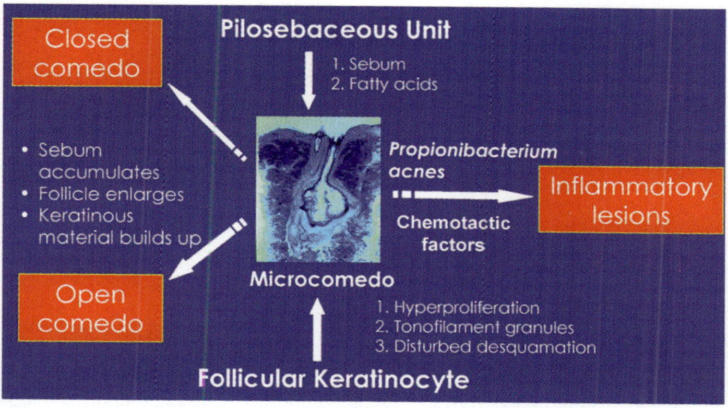

Fig 10.1. Pathogenesis of acne (From Gollnick H, Cunliffe W, et al. Management of acne: a report from a global alliance to improve outcomes in acne. *J Am Acad Dermatol.* 2003;49:S1–S38, with permission from Elsevier.)

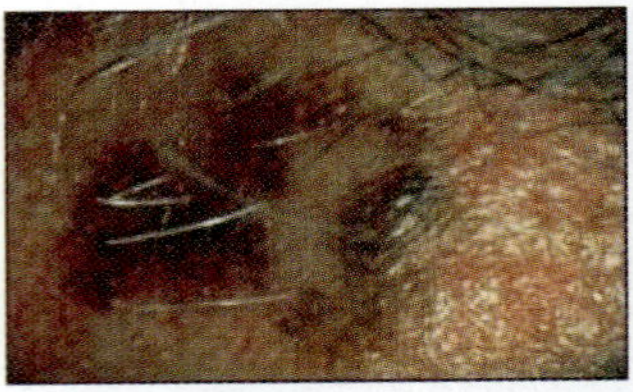

Fig 10.2. **Asymmetry**—The shape of one half does not match the other. (US National Institutes of Health, National Cancer Institute. What you need to know about melanoma. Available at: www.cancer.gov/cancertopics/wyntk/melanoma/page8. Accessed August 5, 2009.)

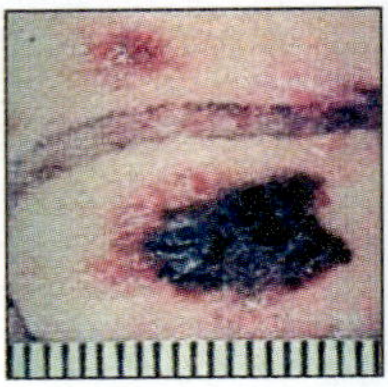

Fig 10.3. **Border**—The edges are often ragged, notched, blurred, or irregular in outline; the pigment may spread into the surrounding skin. (US National Institutes of Health, National Cancer Institute. What you need to know about melanoma. Available at: www.cancer.gov/cancertopics/wyntk/melanoma/page8. Accessed August 5, 2009.)

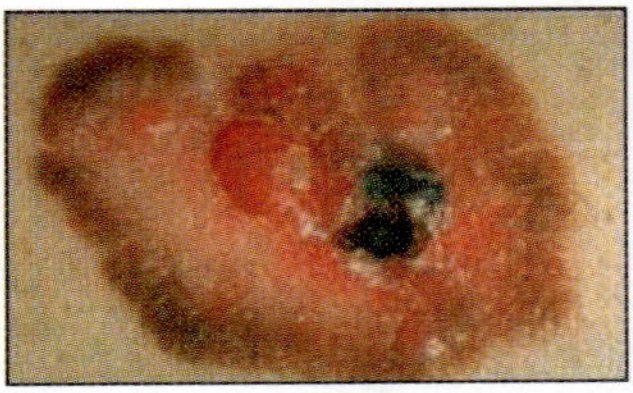

Fig 10.4. **Color**—The color is uneven. Shades of black, brown, and tan may be present. Areas of white, grey, red, pink, or blue also may be seen. (US National Institutes of Health, National Cancer Institute. What you need to know about melanoma. Available at: www.cancer.gov/cancertopics/wyntk/melanoma/page8. Accessed August 5, 2009.)

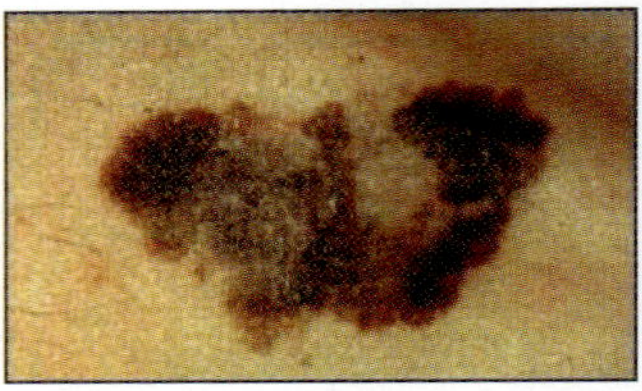

Fig 10.5. **Diameter**—There is a change in size, usually an increase. Melanomas are usually larger than the eraser of a pencil (1/4 inch or 5 millimeters). (US National Institutes of Health, National Cancer Institute. What you need to know about melanoma. Available at: www.cancer.gov/cancertopics/wyntk/melanoma/page8. Accessed August 5, 2009.)

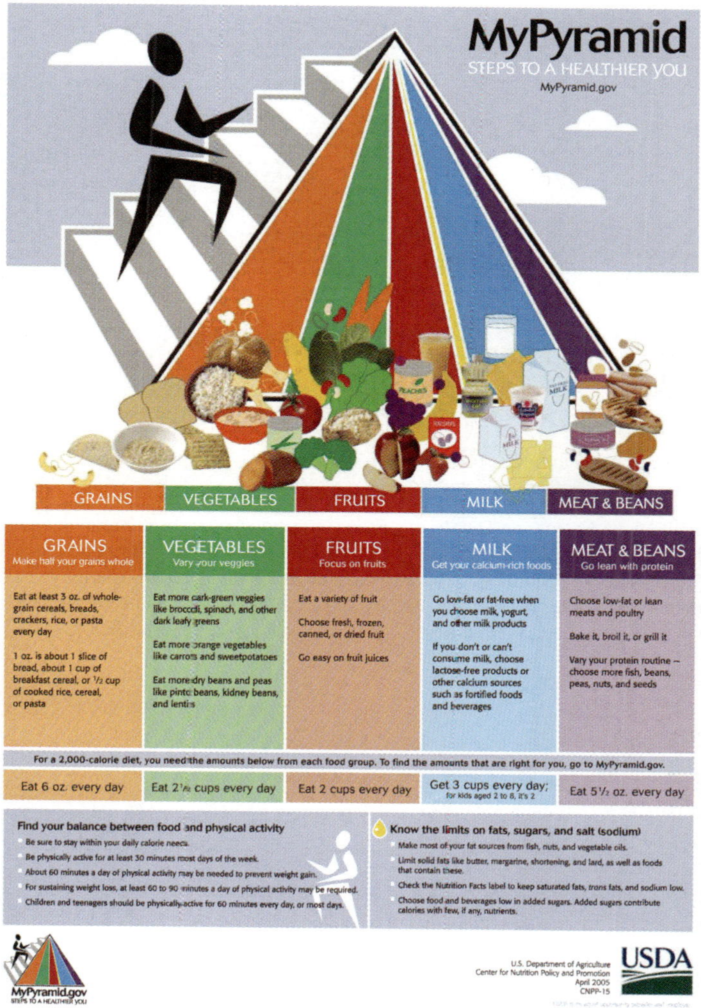

Fig 13.1. A pyramid approach to sound nutrition and a healthy lifestyle. Available at: www.mypyramid.gov/downloads/MiniPoster.pdf. Accessed July 30, 2009.

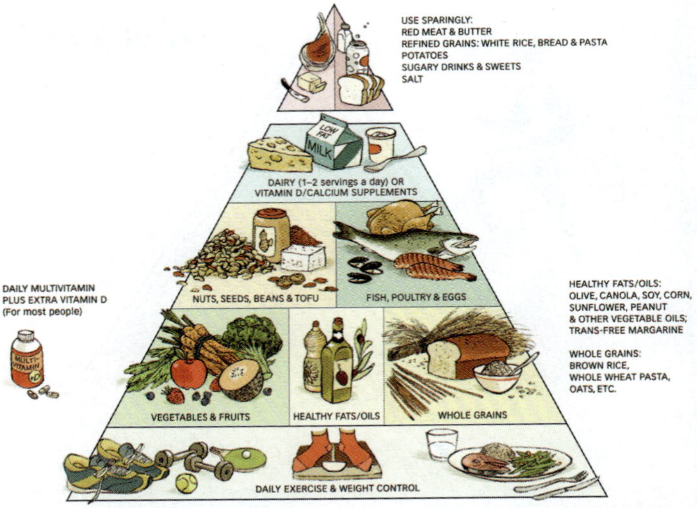

Fig 13.2. Adapted from The Healthy Eating Pyramid. (Copyright © 2008. For more information about The Healthy Eating Pyramid, please see The Nutrition Source, Department of Nutrition, Harvard School of Public Health, http://www.thenutritionsource.org, and Eat, Drink, and Be Heathly, by Walter C. Willett, M.D. and Patrick J. Skerrett (2005), Free Press/Simon & Schuster Inc.)